Handbook of
Biologics & Biosimilars in Dermatology

Handbook of Biologics & Biosimilars in Dermatology

SECOND EDITION

Editor-in-Chief

Shekhar Neema MD EBDVD
Professor
Department of Dermatology
Base Hospital
Lucknow, Uttar Pradesh, India

Brig (Dr) Manas Chatterjee MD DNB(DVL)
Consultant Dermatologist
Base Hospital Delhi Cantt
Brigadier Armed Forces Medical Services
New Delhi, India

Assistant Editors

Ankan Gupta MD DNB
Associate Professor
Department of Dermatology
Christian Medical College
Vellore, Tamil Nadu, India

Siddharth Mani MD(DVL)
Assistant Professor
Department of Dermatology
Indian Naval Hospital Ship (INHS) Sanjivani
Kochi, Kerala, India

Foreword

Murlidhar Rajagopalan

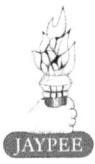

JAYPEE BROTHERS MEDICAL PUBLISHERS
The Health Sciences Publisher
New Delhi | London

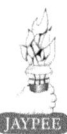 **Jaypee Brothers Medical Publishers (P) Ltd**

Headquarters
EMCA House
23/23-B, Ansari Road, Daryaganj
New Delhi 110 002, India
Landline: +91-11-23272143
+91-11-23272703, +91-11-23282021
+91-11-23245672
E-mail: jaypee@jaypeebrothers.com

Corporate Office
Jaypee Brothers Medical Publishers (P) Ltd.
4838/24, Ansari Road, Daryaganj
New Delhi 110 002, India
Phone: +91-11-43574357
Fax: +91-11-43574314
E-mail: jaypee@jaypeebrothers.com

Overseas Office
JP Medical Ltd.
83, Victoria Street, London
SW1H 0HW (UK)
Phone: +44-20 3170 8910
E-mail: info@jpmedpub.com

EU GPSR Authorised Representative
Logos Europe, 9 rue Nicolas Poussin
17000, La Rochelle, France
Phone: +33 (0) 6 67 93 73 78
E-mail: Contact@logoseurope.eu

Website: www.jaypeebrothers.com
Website: www.jaypeedigital.com

© 2024, Jaypee Brothers Medical Publishers

The views and opinions expressed in this book are solely those of the original contributor(s)/author(s) and do not necessarily represent those of editor(s) or publisher of the book.

All rights reserved. No part of this publication may be reproduced, stored or transmitted in any form or by any means, electronic, mechanical, photocopying, recording or otherwise, without the prior permission in writing of the publishers.

All brand names and product names used in this book are trade names, service marks, trademarks or registered trademarks of their respective owners. The publisher is not associated with any product or vendor mentioned in this book.

Medical knowledge and practice change constantly. This book is designed to provide accurate, authoritative information about the subject matter in question. However, readers are advised to check the most current information available on procedures included and check information from the manufacturer of each product to be administered, to verify the recommended dose, formula, method and duration of administration, adverse effects and contraindications. It is the responsibility of the practitioner to take all appropriate safety precautions. Neither the publisher nor the author(s)/editor(s) assume any liability for any injury and/or damage to persons or property arising from or related to use of material in this book.

This book is sold on the understanding that the publisher is not engaged in providing professional medical services. If such advice or services are required, the services of a competent medical professional should be sought.

Every effort has been made where necessary to contact holders of copyright to obtain permission to reproduce copyright material. If any have been inadvertently overlooked, the publisher will be pleased to make the necessary arrangements at the first opportunity.

Inquiries for bulk sales may be solicited at: jaypee@jaypeebrothers.com

Handbook of Biologics & Biosimilars in Dermatology / Shekhar Neema, Manas Chatterjee

First Edition: 2018

Second Edition: **2024**

ISBN: 978-93-5696-903-2

DEDICATED TO

My family
and
My teacher, Col BAK Prasad, who introduced me to scientific reasoning
"You will live in our hearts forever"

—**Shekhar Neema**

Our families who tolerate our periods of absence from their immediate surrounds with equanimity and understanding

—**Manas Chatterjee**

Contributors

Aarti Zope DNB(General Medicine)
Fellowship in Rheumatology
Consultant Rheumatologist
Bliss Rheumat-Dermat Clinic
Thane, Maharashtra, India

Abhishek De MD FAGE
Associate Professor
Department of Dermatology
Calcutta National Medical College
Kolkata, West Bengal, India

Abir Saraswat MD DNB
Consultant Dermatologist
Indushree Skin Clinic
Lucknow, Uttar Pradesh, India

Ankan Gupta MD DNB
Associate Professor
Department of Dermatology
Christian Medical College
Vellore, Tamil Nadu, India

Anupama Molpariya
MD(Dermatology and STD)
Specialist Dermatologist
AdLife Hospital, Muscat
Muscat, Oman

Anupam Das MBBS MD
Dermatology(Gold Medalist)
Assistant Professor
Department of Dermatology
KPC Medical College and Hospital
Kolkata, West Bengal, India

Aradhana Rout MD
Assistant Professor
Department of Dermatology
Military Hospital, Jammu
Jammu and Kashmir, India

Sqn Ldr (Dr) Aseem Sharma MD
DNB MBA FAGE IFAAD
Chief Dermatologist
Skin Saga Centre for Dermatology
Mumbai, Maharashtra, India
Ex-Assistant Professor of
Dermatology
LTMMC and GH

Bhavni Oberoi MD DNB MNAMS
MRCP(SCE)
Assistant Professor and Head
Department of Dermatology
INHS Kalyani
Visakhapatnam, Andhra Pradesh,
India

Bhojani Amee MD
Resident
Department of Dermatology
DY Patil Hospital
Navi Mumbai, Maharashtra, India

Bhushan Madke MD
Professor and Head
Department of Dermatology
Jawaharlal Nehru Medical College
and Acharya Vinoba Bhave Rural
Hospital
Wardha, Maharashtra, India

Contributors

Biju Vasudevan MD
Professor and Head
Department of Dermatology
Armed Forces Medical College
Pune, Maharashtra, India

Brijesh Nair MD
Head
Department of Dermatology
Command Hospital
Kolkata, West Bengal, India

Debatraya Paul MD DNB
MNAMS(Dermatology, Venereology and Leprosy)
Assistant Professor
Department of Dermatology and STDs
Military Hospital
Jaipur, Rajasthan, India

Dipali Rathod MD
Assistant Professor
Department of Dermatology
Seth GS Medical College and KEM Hospital
Mumbai, Maharashtra, India

Dipankar De MD
Professor
Department of Dermatology, Venereology and Leprology
Postgraduate Institute of Medical Education and Research (PGIMER)
Chandigarh, India

Disha Chakraborty MD
Senior Resident
Department of Dermatology
National Medical College
Kolkata, West Bengal, India

D Joshika Bhandary MD
Consultant Dermatologist
Tvaksh Advanced Skin and Hair Clinic
Mumbai, Maharashtra, India

Himadri MD
Consultant Dermatologist
Department of Dermatology
St Stephen Hospital
New Delhi, India

Hitaishi Mehta MD DNB MRCP(SCE)
Senior Resident
Department of Dermatology, Venereology and Leprology
Postgraduate Institute of Medical Education and Research (PGIMER)
Chandigarh, India

Indrashish Podder MD DNB
Assistant Professor
Department of Dermatology
College of Medicine and Sagore Dutta Hospital
Kolkata, West Bengal, India

Jaya Krishna MBBS MD
Senior Resident
Christian Medical College
Vellore, Tamil Nadu, India

Khushboo Minni MD
Honorary Consultant
Department of Pediatric Dermatology
BJ Wadia Hospital for Children and Nowrosjee Wadia Maternity Hospital
Parel, Mumbai, Maharashtra, India

Kingshuk Chatterjee MBBS
DNB MNAMS FAGE FRCP(Edinburgh) FRCP(Glasgow) FRCP(London)
Associate Professor
Department of Dermatology
Nil Ratan Sircar Medical College
Kolkata, West Bengal, India

Kiran Godse MD PhD FRCP(Glasgow)
Professor in Dermatology
Department of Dermatology
Dr DY Patil Medical College and Hospital
Navi Mumbai, Maharashtra, India

Krupashankar DS MD DVD FAGE
Senior Consultant and Dermatologist
Dr Krupa Shankar Skin Diagnostic Center
Bengaluru, Karnataka, India

Brig (Dr) Manas Chatterjee MD DNB
Consultant Dermatologist
Base Hospital Delhi Cantt
Brigadier Armed Forces Medical Services
New Delhi, India

Manish Khandare MBBS MD
Assistant Professor
Department of Dermatology
All India Institute of Medical Sciences (AIIMS)
Bhopal, Madhya Pradesh, India

Manish Manrai MBBS MD DM
Professor
Department of Gastroenterology
Command Hospital
Lucknow, Uttar Pradesh, India

Muhammed Razmi T MBBS MD(PGIMER) DNB MNAMS EBDVD
Consultant Dermatologist and Clinical Head
IQRAA Aesthetics, IQRAA International Hospital and Research Center
Dr Afra'z ZIVA Skin and Hair Clinic
Kannur, Kerala, India

Murlidhar Rajagopalan MD
Senior Consultant Dermatologist
Department of Dermatology
Apollo Hospital
Chennai, Tamil Nadu, India

Narayanan B MD
Senior Resident
Department of Dermatology, Venereology and Leprology
Postgraduate Institute of Medical Education and Research (PGIMER)
Chandigarh, India

Surg Cdr (Dr) Padmapriya Srinivasan MD DNB
Assistant Professor
Department of Dermatology
INHS Asvini
Mumbai, Maharashtra

Prathyusha Manikuppam MD DM
(Clinical Immunology and Rheumatology)
Assistant Professor
Department of Immunology and Rheumatology
Kasturba Medical College
Mangaluru, Karnataka, India

Rajat Kandhari MBBS MD MSc(UK)
Consultant Dermatologist
Dr Kandhari's Skin and Dental Clinic
New Delhi, India

Rajesh Verma MD
Professor, Department of Dermatology, Venereology and Leprosy, Command Hospital
Panchkula, Haryana, India

Ravina Surve MBBS MD(DVL) DNB(DVL)
Senior Resident
Kanachur Institute of Medical Sciences
Mangaluru, Karnataka, India

Resham Vasani MD DNB FCPC DDV
Consultant Dermatologist
Bhojani Clinic
Mumbai, Maharashtra, India

Contributors

Riti Bhatia MD
Associate Professor
Department of Dermatology,
Venereology and Leprosy
All India Institute of Medical Sciences
Rishikesh, Uttarakhand, India

Rohit Kothari MD MRCP(SCE)
(Dermatology)
Assistant Professor
Department of Dermatology
Command Hospital Air Force
Bengaluru, Karnataka, India

Ruchi Hemdani MBBS MD(DVL)
Assistant Professor
Himalayan Institute of Medical
Sciences
Dehradun, Uttarakhand, India

Sandipan Dhar MBBS MD DNB
FRCP(Edinburgh)
Professor and Head
Department of Pediatric
Dermatology
Institute of Child Health
Kolkata, West Bengal, India

Santanu Banerjee MD DNB
Senior Advisor
Department of Dermatology
Military Hospital
Jaipur, Rajasthan, India

SG Parasramani MD DDV FAAD
Dermatologist
Lilavati Hospital and Research Centre
Mumbai, Maharashtra, India

Sharmila Patil MBBS DDVL MD(Skin and VD)
Dermatologist, Cosmetologist, Trichologist
Bliss - Dermocosmetic Laser Center
Hair and Skin Clinic
Thane, Maharashtra, India

Shekhar Neema MD EBDVD
Professor
Department of Dermatology
Base Hospital
Lucknow, Uttar Pradesh, India

Shivraj Padiyar MD DM(Clinical Immunology and Rheumatology)
Associate Professor
Department of Immunology and Rheumatology
Kasturba Medical College
Mangaluru, Karnataka, India

Shreya Poddar MD DNB
Consultant Dermatologist
Asansol District Hospital
Asansol, West Bengal, India

Siddharth Mani MD(DVL)
Assistant Professor
Department of Dermatology
Indian Naval Hospital Ship (INHS)
Sanjivani
Kochi, Kerala, India

Snigdha Saxena MBBS
MD(Dermatology and STD) MRCP(SCE)
Consultant Dermatologist
Nav Imperial Hospital and
Research Centre
Jaipur, Rajasthan, India

Sunil Dogra MD DNB FRCP
Professor
Department of Dermatology,
Venereology and Leprology
Postgraduate Institute of Medical
Education and Research (PGIMER)
Chandigarh, India

Surbhi Rajput MD(Dermatology)
Senior Resident
Military Hospital
Meerut, Uttar Pradesh, India

Swaroop HS MD
Senior Medical Advisor
Novo Nordisk India
Bengaluru, Karnataka, India

Swetalina Pradhan MD
Associate Professor and Head
Department of Dermatology
All India Institute of Medical Sciences
Patna, Bihar, India

Vikas Pathania MD
Professor and Head
Department of Dermatology
Base Hospital
Lucknow, Uttar Pradesh, India

Vinay Singh MBBS MD
Senior Consultant
Vibrance Wellness Vista
New Delhi, India

Vishal Gupta MD
Associate Professor
Department of Dermatology and Venereology
All India Institute of Medical Sciences
New Delhi, India

Foreword

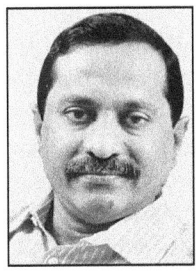

Murlidhar Rajagopalan MD
Senior Consultant Dermatologist
Department of Dermatology
Apollo Hospital
Chennai, Tamil Nadu, India

I am happy to write a foreword for the second edition of *"Handbook of Biologics & Biosimilars in Dermatology"*. The first edition was highly successful and useful for dermatologists across India, and it was but natural to come out with a second edition of the book, given the rapid advances in the field in the last few years. This is meant to be a ready reckoner for both the novice and expert in immunodermatology in India. One has to remember that small molecules are also making a headway into dermatology in India, and it is but natural that the book should touch on these also as a natural corollary to guiding us on biologic usage. All drugs currently available for dermatological indications in India have been covered along with guidance on the optimum utilization of these drugs for conditions in which they are indicated in terms of choice of agent in view of best practice principles as on date.

Conditions such as psoriasis are saddled with multiple options in terms of biological therapy and it is frequently difficult to decide which of these drugs would be best fit in a given clinical scenario. Also, some of the drugs have multiple indications, and it is only in certain conditions that they are best suited. This brings in the use of biologics in off-label indications in dermatology. A clear understanding of the drug and the pathogenesis of the disease is needed for this to happen well, and the results have to be well documented to get an ethical approval. In the last few years, newer biologics have been approved as our understanding of psoriasis pathogenesis has improved. So, decision-making on which drug to use where is important. I hope that understanding the drugs will make this feasible. This book will help in that direction. In such cases, opinions will always differ but charting the well trodden path ensures the best possible outcome for the patients. That path has to be shown by those who have walked it with success and our distinguished galaxy of authors have done just that.

This book highlights what a clinician needs to know and presents it in lucid form for the reader who would have little time to go through detailed nuances that may not be necessary for the practical prescriber. No essential has been missed and at the same time, superfluities have been avoided to ensure a rapid read of contents required at the time of prescription decision-making. That makes this text most handy and a must-have on the table-top of the hands-on clinician for whom this work is primarily meant.

It is ardently hoped and expected that this effort by the authors and editors would bear fruit in terms of the more rational use of these wonderful molecules for the benefit of the patients who should be the final beneficiaries of medical knowledge.

The development of biologics in dermatology will not stop here and new drugs will enter the market. We will also gain a lot from real-world evidence in India. This makes the book vitally important for the Indian dermatologist.

I wish the editors and all the contributors all the best in this venture.

Happy reading!

Preface to the Second Edition

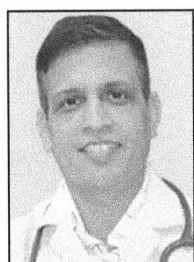

Shekhar Neema

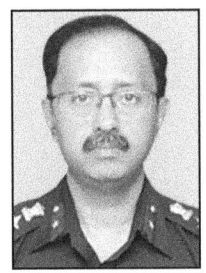

Manas Chatterjee

The first edition of "*Handbook of Biologics & Biosimilars in Dermatology*" was a work borne out of necessity. With progressively more number of patients in India and other developing countries being prescribed biologics and biosimilars as well as the introduction of small molecules since the previous edition, the need was felt to update the handbook with newer information so that the specialist treating the patient has the current information available to him in a small form factor which enables quick referencing when faced with a patient and the confident prescription of these drugs, which were not available when the vast majority of dermatologists and other specialties dealing with these drugs trained to become specialists. The addition of small molecules into our armamentarium has enabled the usage of drugs which have a narrow spectrum of immunosuppressive effect leading to reduced adverse effects. This has broadened the use of these agents due to their more affordable price range and excellent therapeutic benefit. Also, with the gradual overall development of the country, there has been an increase in the number of patients who have been inquiring about biologics as well as biosimilars to get quick response of their condition. Progressively, the negative attitude to these drugs has given way to awareness and acceptance. Many more specialists today than when the first edition came out prescribe these agents with regularity. With professions where complete clearance of skin conditions is not only desirable but essential in the minds of patients, the demand and usage of these drugs are increasing rapidly. As knowledge of biologics, biosimilars, and small molecules improves, there is more benefit to patients due to the judicious use of these agents.

We have attempted to address queries that we have been getting from dermatologists in formal and informal gatherings regarding how to best use these drugs in their specific circumstances. We have attempted to address these in this edition and would love to receive comments on whether we have been able to address issues pertaining to the practicing dermatologist. Just like the previous edition, we disclose that we have no conflict of interest in writing this book and the project has been conceptualized and completed without any grants or support.

Just as the previous edition received an overwhelming response, it is hoped that this second edition of "*Handbook of Biologics & Biosimilars in Dermatology*" will find its way to the table-tops and not bookshelves of academic and practicing dermatologists alike and be helpful to them in making more informed choices in biologic use.

Jai Hind!

Shekhar Neema
Manas Chatterjee

Preface to the First Edition

The *Handbook of Biologics and Biosimilars in Dermatology* is a work borne out of necessity. The usage of biologics and biosimilars in India as well as other countries in the developing world is steadily increasing. Unlike in the West where expenditure on prescription of biologics is reimbursable, the cost of the same is usually borne by the patient in our situation. More prudence, therefore, becomes imperative in decision-making. A clear understanding which stems out of accurate knowledge of these molecules and their exact mode and mechanism of action becomes necessary.

In addition, this knowledge and understanding must be dovetailed to the comorbidities and financial constraints, which are different in our patient population. This entails a different perspective to biologic and biosimilar usage in our country. This spurred us to attempt to write this handbook which is meant to be a concise guide for dermatology practitioners, who are stepping into the era of biologics, biosimilars and similar targeted therapies.

An attempt has been sincerely made to ensure that concerns that we come across in our day-to-day clinical interactions with our patients are addressed. Things, such as cost-effectiveness have been dealt with to provide perspective to the specialist, as well as provide material to better counsel patients when these medications are prescribed. It was our endeavor to provide up-to-date information to readers. However, the field of biologic is expanding at a rapid pace and it is possible that some newer developments have been missed despite our best efforts. We also disclose that we have no conflict of interest in writing this book and the project has been conceptualized and completed without any grants or support.

It is hoped and expected that this handbook will find its way to the table-tops and not bookshelves of academic and practicing dermatologists alike and be helpful to them in making more informed choices in biologic use.

Jai Hind!

Shekhar Neema MD(Dermatology)
Manas Chatterjee MD DNB(DVL)

Acknowledgments

We are grateful to Dr Ankan Gupta and Dr Siddharth Mani, assistant editors who have worked tirelessly on this project for the last one year.

I am grateful to Dr Sweta Mukherjee for taking her time out for language editing and proofreading some portions of this book.

Last but not the least, I would also like to extend my special gratitude to Shri Jitendar P Vij (Group Chairman), Mr Ankit Vij (Managing Director), MS Mani (Group President), Ms Chetna Malhotra (Senior Director—Professional Publishing, Marketing and Business Development), Ms Pooja Bhandari [Director–Production (Books and Journals)] and Ms Himani Pandey (Development Editor), for their help and assistance in completing the project within the time frame.

We are thankful to Mr Sabyasachi Hazra [Associate Director, Publishing and Digital Sales, Jaypee Brothers Medical Publishers (P) Ltd].

Shekhar Neema
Manas Chatterjee

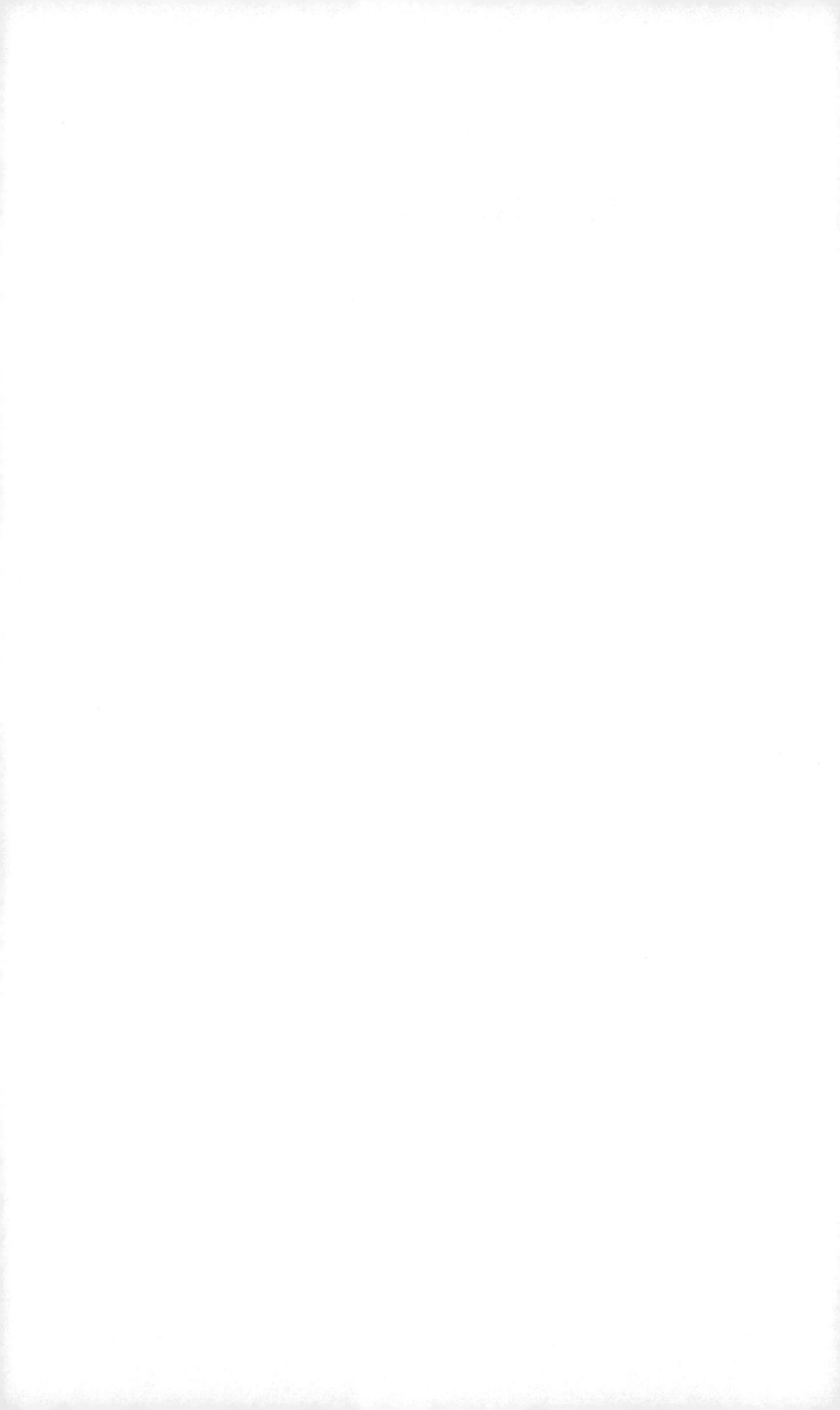

Contents

Section 1: Basics of Biologics

1. **History and Development of Biologics** — 3
   Biju Vasudevan, Ankan Gupta

2. **Classification of Biologics** — 9
   Aradhana Rout

3. **Concept and Development of Biosimilars** — 17
   Brijesh Nair

Section 2: Biologics in Psoriasis

4. **Pathogenesis of Psoriasis** — 33
   Rajat Kandhari, Snigdha Saxena, Anupama Molpariya

5. **Etanercept** — 51
   Santanu Banerjee, Debatraya Paul

6. **Infliximab** — 65
   Biju Vasudevan, Shekhar Neema

7. **Adalimumab** — 75
   Vinay Singh

8. **IL-17 Blockers: Secukinumab** — 84
   SG Parasramani, D Joshika Bhandary

9. **Ixekizumab** — 96
   Aseem Sharma, Ravina Surve

10. **Anti-CD6 Monoclonal Antibody: Itolizumab** — 106
    Krupashankar DS, Swaroop HS

11. **Interleukin-36 Receptor Antagonist: Spesolimab** — 114
    Ruchi Hemdani

12. **Newer Biologics in Psoriasis** — 122
    Siddharth Mani, Abir Saraswat

Section 3: Biologics in Immunobullous Disorders

13. **Biologics in the Management of Pemphigus—Anti-CD20 Monoclonal Antibody: Rituximab** — 145
    Dipankar De, Hitaishi Mehta, Muhammed Razmi T

14. **Newer Biologics in the Management of Immunobullous Disorders** — 167
    Surbhi Rajput

Section 4: Biologics in Urticaria

15. **Anti-IgE Monoclonal Antibody: Omalizumab** — 179
    Kiran Godse, Bhojani Amee

16. **Newer Biologics in Urticaria** — 186
    Shreya Poddar, Indrashish Podder

Section 5: Biologics in Atopic Dermatitis

17. **Interleukin-4 Inhibitor: Dupilumab** — 199
    Sandipan Dhar, Disha Chakraborty, Abhishek De

18. **Newer Biologics in the Management of Atopic Dermatitis** — 212
    Disha Chakraborty, Abhishek De

Section 6: Biologic Approach to Management of Various Diseases

19. **Psoriasis** — 231
    Murlidhar Rajagopalan, Shekhar Neema, Ankan Gupta, Manish Khandare, Manas Chatterjee

20. **Immunobullous Disorders** — 252
    Himadri, Ankan Gupta

21. **Hidradenitis Suppurativa** — 262
    Sharmila Patil, Aarti Zope

22. **Use of Biologics in Dermatological Aspects of Autoimmune Rheumatic Diseases** — 275
    Shivraj Padiyar, Prathyusha Manikuppam

Section 7: Biologics and Chronic Infections

23. **Management of Latent Tuberculosis Infection** — 287
    Bhushan Madke, Swetalina Pradhan

24. **Biologics in Presence of Hepatitis B and C Infection** — 300
    Shekhar Neema, Manish Manrai

Section 8: Biologics in Special Situation

25. **Biologics in Children: Which, When, Why?** 313
    Khushboo Minni, Resham Vasani

26. **Biologics in Pregnancy, Lactation, and Other Situations** 341
    Shekhar Neema, Vikas Pathania

Section 9: Miscellaneous Issues with Biologics

27. **Miscellaneous Uses of Biologics** 357
    Manas Chatterjee, Dipali Rathod

28. **Adverse Effects of Biologics: Feared or Real?** 369
    Sunil Dogra, Narayanan B

29. **Adult Immunization Prior to Initiation of Biologic Therapy** 397
    Ankan Gupta, Himadri

30. **Cost Effectiveness and Quality of Life with Biologic Therapy** 409
    Ankan Gupta, Jaya Krishna, Shekhar Neema

Section 10: Small Molecules and IVIG

31. **Janus Kinase Inhibitors** 437

    Part A: Classification of Janus Kinase Inhibitors 437
    Siddharth Mani, Manish Khandare

    Part B: Tofacitinib 442
    Siddharth Mani, Manish Khandare

    Part C: Other JAK Inhibitors: Baricitinib, Abrocitinib, and Upadacitinib 454
    Ruchi Hemdani

    Part D: Newer Janus Kinase Inhibitors 467
    Padmapriya Srinivasan

32. **Phosphodiesterase-4 Inhibitors** 482
    Anupam Das, Kingshuk Chatterjee

33. **Mammalian Target of Rapamycin Inhibitors: Sirolimus** 489
    Riti Bhatia, Vishal Gupta

34. **Newer Small Molecules in Pipeline** 501
    Bhavni Oberoi

35. **Intravenous Immunoglobulins** 512
    Rohit Kothari, Rajesh Verma

36. **Ready Reckoner for Biologics and Small Molecules** 525
    Bhavni Oberoi, Shekhar Neema

Index 531

SECTION 1

Basics of Biologics

CHAPTER 1

History and Development of Biologics

Biju Vasudevan, Ankan Gupta

INTRODUCTION

Biologics are proteins and/or their derivatives that regulate the immune system or support tumor-specific defense. They are also known as "biological" or "recombinant therapeutics" and there are multiple definitions to it, being a constant source of controversy among the semantic purists. Biologics do not represent one homogeneous drug group, rather includes unrelated molecules such as monoclonal antibodies, growth factors, fusion proteins, interferons, and expression vectors generating proteins in situ.[1]

The first documented use of the term "biologics" was in 1912 when the pharmacological editor of the California State Journal of Medicine, Fred Lackenbach, used it in connection with national healthcare legislation and the control of vaccine production in the United States (US).[2] For a long time, there was no equivalent expression in Europe, and terms such as Naturstojfe, Wirkstoffe (biologische Arzneimittel), or medicaments biologiques were used; all of them had different meanings and connotations, but sharing a common reference to "natural products." Over the past century, biologics are so ubiquitous that our bodies have increasingly become exposed to them without us realizing the same, for example, the use of vitamins, vaccines, insulin, etc. In present context, however, the "natural products" of yesteryears cease to be recognized as biologics with new definitions excluding them. The aim of this chapter is not intended to go into the controversial semantics, but to introduce the reader to the history of this therapeutic revolution.

HISTORY OF BIOLOGICS

Under an Act of Congress in 1902, all viruses, sera, and toxins used in the United States were required to conform to established standards. It was officially designated as "An Act to Regulate the Sale of Viruses, Serums, Toxins and Analogous Products in the District of Columbia, to Regulate Interstate Traffic in Said Articles, and for Other Purposes."[3] This law marked the beginning of a regimen for licensing of drugs that ultimately evolved into the Food and Drug Administration (FDA), which today is responsible for the control of biologics in the US.[4] When the FDA celebrated the 75th anniversary of the Food and Drugs Act of 1920 in 1995, it also celebrated the "Biologics Control Act" of 1902. Though in the original law of July 1, 1902, there was no mention of "biologics," "biological," or "biological products," which implicitly suggested the continuity in the regulation of biological products. It was with this new legislative framework in place, subsequent years witnessed the emergence of various labels to describe these products.

In 1917, the Biological Department of Eli Lilly (a pharmaceutical bigwig of his times) and Company published a small treatise on "Elements of Biologics" designed to provide the company's representatives with standard knowledge about biological or natural products like antitoxins and vaccines.[5] By 1921, 41 establishments were licensed to sell >102 different sera, toxins, and analogous products. Of these establishments, 32 were located in the US, one in Canada, one in England, three in France, one in Italy, two in Switzerland, and one in Germany, posing a challenge to federal regulators. In 1923, Public Health Reports compiled a list of national agencies and organizations associated with the regulation of "biologics."[6]

The isolation of the first-ever biologic was of the hormone insulin, which was achieved by Frederick Banting and Charles Best in Toronto in 1921.[7] The second biologic was erythropoietin, the existence of which was first proposed in 1906 by Paul Carnot based on his transfusion experiments in rabbits.[8] From 1921 to 1934, other biological substances such as vitamin D (1927), estrone (1929), androsterone (1931), ascorbic acid (1932), and progesterone (1934) were isolated and synthesized, but it was in 1934, when the National Institutes of Health (NIH) issued the first licenses to manufacturers for the production of a human blood product, which was a preparation of protein from human placental extract that was designed to immunize against measles.[9,10] In 1937, work on biologics control was granted its own division within the NIH, the Division of Biologics Control. Institutionalizing the control of biologics involved expanding existing regulations on vaccines, sera, and antitoxins to include arsenical drugs, blood, and blood products. Meanwhile, in Europe, the physician and entrepreneur Gerhard Maclaus (1890–1942) published a famous three-volume textbook of biological remedies (Lehrbuch der biologischen Heilmittel); and in 1939, a research institute for biological remedies was founded at the Paracelsus.[11]

The decades after the Second World War, especially from the 1950s to the 1980s, there were dynamic years for biologics, as the quantity and quality of biologics and the challenges for regulators continued to grow. After the spectacular introduction of penicillin in the 1940s, the biotechnological exploitation of fungal metabolisms invigorated the search for magic bullets.[12] Similarly, the invention of cortisone raised expectations and drove pharmaceutical industries in their search for "natural products" from exotic plants. Another advance in postwar research that significantly influenced the development of biologics was made in 1949 at Boston Children's Hospital, where scientists successfully grew a human virus, the Lansing type 2 poliovirus, in a human tissue cell culture.[13] In the mid-1960s, pioneering work resulted in the first experimental live virus vaccine against German measles (rubella).

In July 1972, both the authority to administer the drug provisions of the Federal Food, Drug, and Cosmetic Act (FDCA) for all biological products and the responsibility for implementing the Biologics Act was delegated to the FDA. The Division of Biologics Standards was then transferred from the NIH to the FDA and renamed the Bureau of Biologics (BoB). Insulin was inarguably the first protein that embodied the aspirations of the new biology. A team at the University of California, San Francisco, associated with Herbert Boyer, who in April 1976 founded the small company GeneTech (Genetic Engineering Technology), used the bacterium *Escherichia coli* to produce insulin and claimed success in September 1978. The FDA finally approved the drug in 1982. By 1988, live proteins such as insulin, human growth hormone, hepatitis B vaccine, alpha-interferon, and tissue plasminogen activator had been approved as drugs by the FDA.

The discovery that revolutionized the antibody therapy came after decoding of the human genome, which revealed that there are 30,000 different genes encoding possibly 50,000 different proteins and that disease may result when one of these proteins is defective or present in abnormally high or low concentration. This ability to identify the cause of disease has presented a number of targets for possible therapies. The first monoclonal antibodies (mAbs), Ortho Biotech's muromonab-CD3 (Orthoclone), was approved by the FDA in 1986.[14] The original concept of antibodies as molecules that bind to specific targets emerged through the pioneering work of Paul Ehrlich, Emil von Behring, Shibasaburo Kitasato, and Karl Landsteiner.[15] Further, recombinant deoxyribonucleic acid technology has allowed a new generation of protein-based medicines and in Cambridge, the United Kingdom, scientists developed a relatively simple method for custom-producing antibodies in the laboratory.[16] More recent advances led to the development of part-mouse, part-human mAbs called chimeras [e.g., rituximab (Rituxan) and cetuximab (Erbitux)], as well as humanized antibodies [e.g., trastuzumab (Herceptin) and bevacizumab (Avastin)] that contain a bare minimum of nonhuman amino acid sequences. In 2002, the first completely human therapeutic mAb, Abbott's adalimumab (Humira), received market approval. Today, there are over a dozen mAbs, with collective oncology market sales in 2006 of over US $7.8 billion and sharp growth predicted over the next decade.[17]

In 1988, the FDA had again split biologics from the more general drug review process. Since then, the FDA has been busy distributing and redistributing the responsibility for an ever-growing number of biological products. The FDA Center for Biologics Evaluation and Research (CBER) became responsible for some therapeutic proteins, such as monoclonal antibodies, but control of these was later transferred to the Center for Drug Evaluation and Research (CDER).[18]

DEVELOPMENT OF BIOSIMILARS

The realm of biologics has evolved throughout the 20th century. With the advent of biosimilars, there is a big competition to challenge the parent molecules.[19] Biologics and their biosimilars are large complex molecules and require a different regulatory framework to produce constant quality. Most regulations in the 21st century have addressed this by recognizing an intermediate ground of testing for biosimilars that require more testing than for small-molecule generics, but less testing than for registering completely new therapeutics.[20] In 2003, the European Medicines Agency introduced an approval pathway for biosimilars, termed similar biological medicinal products, that is based on a thorough demonstration of "comparability" of the "similar" product to an existing approved product.[21] Within the United States, the Patient Protection and Affordable Care Act of 2010 is developed for biosimilars for comparison with the FDA-licensed reference biological product.[22]

PRESENT DAY BIOLOGICS

Necessity is the mother of invention and new clinical situations where the conventional treatment options fail and/or are contraindicated, newer drugs are being developed and the already existing ones are being tried as a hope rather an expectation. Results are giving rise to research, eventually handing the clinicians a new set of arsenal. Diseases such as psoriasis, where target-specific drugs are now universally being used with a more favorable side effect profile, thus providing an effective and safe alternative choice for treatment. Alefacept (Amevive) was the first biologic approved by the FDA in 2003 for the treatment of moderate-to-severe chronic plaque psoriasis. However, in November 2011, Astellas Pharma US, manufacturer of alefacept, announced its decision to cease sales of the drug. There are currently 11 biologics approved for the treatment of psoriasis (etanercept, adalimumab, infliximab, secukinumab, ixekizumab, brodalumab, ustekinumab, risankizumab, tildrakizumab, guselkumab, and bimekizumab) and the list is growing rapidly. If there is one biologic in dermatology that is closest to challenging the conventional immunosuppressants as the first choice drug, it would be the use of rituximab in pemphigus. Treatment of hidradenitis suppurativa, pyoderma gangrenosum, skin cancers, collagen vascular dermatoses, severe cutaneous adverse reactions, alopecia areata, and chronic urticaria and atopic dermatitis have been a challenge over the years and this "therapeutic revolution" with biologics and biosimilars is expected to make life easier for patients as well as clinicians.

CONCLUSION

With the increase in our understanding of dermatological diseases; biologics are making rapid inroads in to the treatment of common as well as complex dermatological diseases. The use of biologics is going to increase rapidly as they become more accessible to population living in developing countries.

REFERENCES

1. Boehncke WH, Radeke HH. Introduction: definition and classification of biologics. In: Boehncke WH, Radeke HH (Eds). Biologics in General Medicine. Berlin, Heidelberg: Springer; 2007. pp. 1-2.
2. Korwek EL. What are biologics? A comparative legislative, regulatory and scientific analysis. Food Drug Law J. 2007;62(2):257-304.
3. Carpenter DP. Reputation and gatekeeping authority: the Federal Food, Drug and Cosmetic Act of 1938 and its aftermath. In: Carpenter DP (Ed). Reputation and Power: Organizational Image and Pharmaceutical Regulation at the FDA. Princeton, NJ: Princeton University Press; 2010. p. 137.
4. Kondratas RA. Biologics Control Act of 1902. In: Young JH (Ed). The Early Years of Federal Food and Drug Control. Madison, WI: American Institute of the History of Pharmacy; 1982. pp. 8-27.
5. Heiser VG. The health work of the League of Nations. Proceedings of the American Philosophical Society. 1926;65 (Supplement):1-9.
6. Sneader W. (2001). History of insulin. Encyclopedia of Life Sciences. [online] Available from http://mrw.interscience.wiley.com/emrw/9780470015902/els/article/a0003623/current/abstract?hd=All,w&hd=All,sneader [Last accessed January, 2024].
7. Jelkmann W. Erythropoietin after a century of research: younger than ever. Eur J Haematol. 2007;78(3):183-205.
8. Miyake T, Kung CK, Goldwasser E. Purification of human erythropoietin. J Biol Chem. 1977;252(15):5558-64.
9. Meng H. Das ärztliche Volksbuc. Gemeinverständliche Darstellung der Gesundheitspflege und Heilkunde. Stuttgart: Hippokrates; 1924.
10. Timmermann C. Rationalizing 'folk medicine' in interwar Germany: faith, business, and science at "Dr. Madaus & Co." Soc Hist Med. 2001;14(3):459-82.
11. Bud R. Penicillin: Triumph and Tragedy. Oxford: Oxford University Press; 2007.
12. Gradmann C. Magic bullets and moving targets: antibiotic resistance and experimental chemotherapy 1900-1940. Dynamis. 2011;31(2):305-21.
13. Commissioner O of the. Science and the Regulation of Biological Products. FDA [Internet]. 2018 Dec 1 [cited 2024 Jan 27]; Available from: https://www.fda.gov/about-fda/histories-product-regulation/science-and-regulation-biological-products.
14. Smith S. Ten years of Orthoclone OKT3 (muromonab CD3): a review. J Transpl Coord. 1996;6(3):109-19.
15. Kaufmann SH. Immunology's foundation: the 100-year anniversary of the Nobel Prize to Paul Ehrlich and Elie Metchnikoff. Nat Immunol. 2008;9(7):705-12.
16. Köhler G, Milstein C. Continuous cultures of fused cells secreting antibody of predefined specificity. Nature. 1975;256(5517):495-7.
17. Gricks C, Cann CI, Merrin A. Antibody Therapies in Oncology. Waltham (MA): Decision Resources, Inc.; 2008.
18. Biopharma. Transfer of Biopharmaceuticals (Biologics) within FDA from CBER to CDER. [online] Available from www.biopharma.com/CBERtoCDER.html [Last accessed January, 2024].

19. Calo-Fernández B, Martínez-Hurtado JL. Biosimilars: company strategies to capture value from the biologics market. Pharmaceuticals. 2012;5(12):1393-408.
20. The US Biosimilars Act: Challenges Facing Regulatory Approval. Pharm Med. 2012;26(3):145-52.
21. European Medicines Agency. (2012). Questions and answers on biosimilar medicines (similar biological medicinal products). [online] Available from https://www.medicinesforeurope.com/wp-content/uploads/2016/03/WC500020062.pdf [Last accessed January, 2024].
22. United States Food and Drug Administration. Approval Pathway for Biosimilar and Interchangeable Biological Products. Maryland: USFDA; 2010.

CHAPTER 2

Classification of Biologics

Aradhana Rout

INTRODUCTION

Biologics/biological response modifiers are components of living organisms, which target specific points of inflammation cascade by imitating or inhibiting naturally occurring proteins. Biologics include a wide range of substances such as serum, vaccine, toxin, antitoxin, blood and blood components, allergenic products, somatic cells, gene therapy, tissues, and recombinant therapeutic proteins.

Properties of biologics are as follows:
- *Target specificity*: Biologics are more specific in their site of action as compared to other systemic therapies, thereby reducing drug interaction.
- *Immunogenicity*: This puts biologics at an increased susceptibility to infections and malignancies (exacerbation/de novo).

CLASSIFICATION

Biologics are divided into groups as shown in **Flowchart 1**.[1]

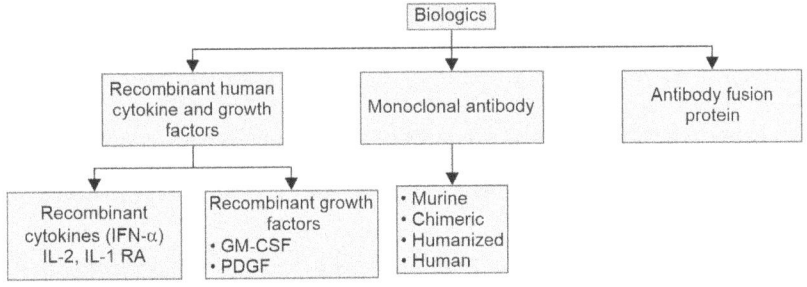

FLOWCHART 1: Classification of biologics.
(GM-CSF: granulocyte-macrophage colony-stimulating factor; IL: interleukin; IFN-α: interferon alpha; PDGF: platelet-derived growth factor; RA: receptor antagonist)

Monoclonal Antibodies

Monoclonal antibodies are produced by a single clone of cells. They work by targeting specific cell-surface receptors. In early days of biologics, purely murine monoclonal antibodies were used resulting in rapid removal from blood through immune response due to development of antimurine antibodies. The monoclonal antibodies used now have genes that have different amounts of murine sequences in the variable region and may be categorized into the following four classes:
1. *Murine antibodies*: Composed of solely murine component
2. *Chimeric antibodies*: 30% murine part fused with human antibodies
3. *Humanized antibodies*: 10% murine part fused with human antibodies
4. *Human antibodies*: Solely composed of human antibodies

Nomenclature of Monoclonal Antibody

It includes following components:
- *Stem:* All monoclonal antibody names end with the stem—*mab*.
- *Substem:* Monoclonal antibody nomenclature uses different parts of the preceding word depending on structure and function. These are officially called as substems.
- *Source substem:* Prefix mentioned below preceding the "-mab" denotes origin of the antibodies.
- *Target substem*: It precedes the source of the antibodies and denotes the medicine's target **(Table 1)**.
- *Prefix*: The prefix carries no special meaning. It should be unique for each medicine and contributes to a well-sounding name. Antibodies with the same source and target substems are only distinguished by their prefix.
- *Additional word*: A second word following the name of the antibody indicates that another substance is attached.
- An antibody can be PEGylated (attached to molecules of polyethylene glycol) to slow down its degradation by enzymes and to decrease its immunogenicity; this is shown by the word pegol, for example, certolizumab pegol.

The principal monoclonal antibodies with therapeutic relevance in dermatology are summarized in **Table 2**.

TABLE 1: Nomenclature of monoclonal antibody.			
Type	Source substem	Example	Target substem
Murine	-o-	Muromonab	
Chimeric	-xi-	Infliximab	Immune (-l-)
Humanized	-zu-	Efalizumab	Immune (-l-)
Human	-u-	Ustekinumab	Interleukin(-k-)

TABLE 2: The principal monoclonal antibodies in dermatology.[2]

Receptor	Name of biologic	Type of monoclonal antibody	Uses
Anti-tumor necrosis factor-alpha (TNF-α)	Infliximab	Human–mouse monoclonal antibody	Psoriasis, psoriatic arthritis, recalcitrant subcorneal pustular dermatosis, atopic dermatitis, hidradenitis suppurativa (HS), pemphigus vulgaris, pyoderma gangrenosum, sarcoidosis, Behçet's disease
	Adalimumab	Human immunoglobulin G (IgG)-1 monoclonal antibody	Psoriasis, psoriatic arthritis, HS, neutrophilic dermatosis, sarcoidosis, Behçet's disease
	Certolizumab pegol	PEGylated antigen binding fragment of humanized monoclonal antibody	Psoriasis, psoriatic arthritis, sarcoidosis, Behçet's disease
	Golimumab	Fully human monoclonal antibody	Psoriasis arthritis (under phase III trial)
Anti-lymphocyte function-associated antigen-1(LFA-1) (CD11a)	Efalizumab	Humanized IgG1 monoclonal antibody	Psoriasis, lichen planus, discoid lupus erythematosus, dermatomyositis
Anti CD20	Rituximab	Humanized monoclonal antibody	Lymphoma, systemic lupus erythematosus (SLE), autoimmune bullous diseases
	Ofatumumab	Human monoclonal	Pemphigus vulgaris
	Obinutuzumab	Humanized monoclonal	Pemphigus vulgaris, paraneoplastic pemphigus
BAFF (B-cell activating factor) inhibitor	Belimumab	Human monoclonal	SLE
PD-1 receptor inhibitor	Pembrolizumab	Humanized monoclonal	• Cutaneous squamous cell carcinoma (SCC) • Melanoma • Merkel cell carcinoma
	Nivolumab		• Melanoma
	Cemiplimab	Human monoclonal	• Cutaneous SCC • Basal cell carcinoma

Continued

SECTION 1: Basics of Biologics

Continued

Receptor	Name of biologic	Type of monoclonal antibody	Uses
PD-1 receptor antagonist plus LAG-3 (lymphocyte activation gene) inhibitor	Avelumab	Human monoclonal	Merkel cell carcinoma
	Nivolumab-relatlimab		Melanoma
CTLA-4 inhibitor (cytotoxic T lymphocyte-associated antigen 4)	Ipilimumab	Human monoclonal	Melanoma
CD 52	Alemtuzumab	Recombinant humanized immunoglobulin	CTCL
Anti-interleukin (IL)-12 and anti-IL-23	Ustekinumab	Human monoclonal antibody that binds with high specificity and affinity to the P40 subunit of both interleukin 12 (IL-12) and IL-23	Psoriasis
	Guselkumab	Human IgG1 lambda monoclonal antibody that blocks the p19 subunit of IL-23	Psoriasis
	Tildrakizumab	Humanized IgG1, monoclonal antibody designed to selectively block IL-23 by binding to the p19 subunit	Psoriasis
	Risankizumab	Humanized IgG1 monoclonal antibody that selectively inhibits IL-23 by binding to the p19 subunit	Psoriasis
Anti-IL-17	Secukinumab	Human IgG1 monoclonal antibody that binds IL-17A	Psoriasis, HS, pityriasis rubra pilaris (PRP), Behçet disease, alopecia areata, and allergic contact dermatitis
	Ixekizumab	Humanized IgG4 monoclonal antibody that neutralizes IL-17A	Psoriasis (under phase III trial), HS, PRP, Behçet disease, alopecia areata, and allergic contact dermatitis
	Brodalumab	Human monoclonal antibody that binds to IL-17 A receptor and blocks the biologic activities of IL-17A, IL-17F, IL-17A/F, and IL-17E (also known as IL-25)	Psoriasis (under phase III trial), HS, PRP, Behçet disease, alopecia areata, and allergic contact dermatitis

Continued

Continued

Receptor	Name of biologic	Type of monoclonal antibody	Uses
IL-36 inhibitor	Spesolimab	Human monoclonal	Generalized pustular psoriasis
Anti-CD2	Siplizumab	Humanized IgG1 monoclonal antibody	Psoriasis, graft-versus-host disease
Anti-CD4	Muromonab	Humanized antihuman IgG4 monoclonal antibody	Psoriasis
Anti-CD6	Itolizumab	Humanized recombinant IgG1 monoclonal antibody	Psoriasis
Anti-CD25	Basiliximab	Chimeric mouse-human monoclonal antibody	Plaque psoriasis, palmoplantar pustular psoriasis
	Daclizumab	Humanized monoclonal antibody	Psoriasis
Anti-CD80r	Galiximab	Primatized monoclonal antibody with a human IgG1 constant region	Psoriasis
Anti-immunoglobulin E	Omalizumab	Recombinant, humanized, monoclonal antibody	• Atopic dermatitis • Chronic urticaria
Anti IL-4/13	Dupilumab	Recombinant, human, monoclonal antibody	Atopic dermatitis, moderate to severe eczema
Anti-IL-13	Tralokinumab	Recombinant, human, monoclonal antibody	Atopic dermatitis
	Lebrikizumab	Recombinant, humanized, monoclonal antibody	Atopic dermatitis
Anti-IL-31	Nemolizumab	Recombinant, humanized, monoclonal antibody	Atopic dermatitis
	Etokimab	Recombinant, human, monoclonal antibody	Atopic dermatitis
Anti-IL-22	Fezakinumab	Recombinant, human, monoclonal antibody	Atopic dermatitis

Fusion Antibody Proteins

Fusion proteins, also known as chimeric proteins, are proteins that are created by the fusion of two or more genes that originally code for separate protein. For example, the fusion of receptor domain of a human protein with the constant region of human immunoglobulin G (IgG) results in formation of fusion antibody protein.[3] It binds specifically to a ligand or a coreceptor. Recombinant fusion proteins have also been produced by combining human proteins with bacterial toxins. The name of fusion protein in which human antibodies are bound to human receptors end with "cept", for example, etanercept. The fusion proteins most commonly used in dermatology are summarized in **Table 3**.

Recombinant Human Cytokines and Growth Factors

Cytokines are small nonimmunoglobulin proteins and glycoproteins produced by a broad range of cells in the human body. In response to any immune stimulus, cytokines are released transiently into the tissue microenvironment and act through receptors to modulate balance between humoral and cell-mediated immune system. Recombinant cytokines or cytokine antagonists produced by recombinant deoxyribonucleic acid

TABLE 3: The principal fusion proteins in dermatology.

Components	Name of biologic	Type of fusion protein	Uses
Two identical tumor necrosis factor-alpha (TNF-α) type II (p75) receptor peptides and fragment crystallizable (Fc) portion of the human immunoglobulin G (IgG)-1	Etanercept	Fully human dimeric fusion protein	Moderate and severe plaque psoriasis in patients >4 years, psoriatic arthritis, single dose in Stevens–Johnson syndrome, Behçet's disease, sarcoidosis
First extracellular domain of lymphocyte function-associated antigen 3 (LFA-3) with hinge Ch1 and Ch2 sequences of human IgG1p	Alefacept	Recombinant fusion protein	Psoriasis; graft-versus-host disease; lichen planus; alopecia areata; atopic dermatitis; Hailey–Hailey disease
Extracellular domain of CTLA4 and the Fc region of IgG4	Abatacept	Recombinant fusion protein	Rheumatoid arthritis, acute graft-versus-host disease
Human interleukin (IL)-2 gene and the enzymatically active ADP-ribosyl transferase domain of the diphtheria toxin	Denileukin diftitox	Recombinant fusion toxin	Cutaneous T-cell lymphoma

TABLE 4: The principal recombinant cytokines and growth factors used in dermatology.

Cytokines/ Growth factors/ Enzyme inhibitors	Type of biologic	Uses
Interferons	Interferon-α	Verruca vulgaris, cutaneous T cell lymphoma, Kaposi sarcoma, basal cell carcinoma, melanoma, systemic mastocytosis, hypereosinophilic syndrome, discoid lupus erythematosus, atopic dermatitis
	Interferon-γ	Chronic granulomatous disease
Interleukins	Interleukin-1 receptor antagonist (IL1-RA), anakinra	Rheumatoid arthritis, cryopyrin-associated periodic syndromes, interleukin-1 receptor antagonist deficiency
	Interleukin 2 (IL-2), daclizumab, basiliximab	Cutaneous T-cell lymphoma, metastatic melanoma
Granulocyte macrophage colony-stimulating factor (GM-CSF)	Recombinant human GM-CSF	Wound (leg ulcer), melanoma, Sézary syndrome
Platelet-derived growth factor (PDGF)	Recombinant PDGF-BB	Diabetic foot ulcer

technology have been used as immunomodulators for malignant and inflammatory dermatoses.[4] The principal recombinant cytokines and growth factors used in dermatology are summarized in **Table 4**.

Intravenous Immunoglobulins

Intravenous immunoglobulin (IVIG) is a fractionated blood product consisting of IgG antibodies that was first used in antibody-deficiency disorders. It is a protein derivative consisting of high concentrations of IgG (>95%) and trace amounts of IgA and IgM made from large pools of human plasma antibodies.[5] IVIG is currently Food and Drug Administration (FDA) approved in dermatology for graft-versus-host disease Kawasaki disease and dermatomyositis. Other uses include connective tissue disorders, autoimmune bullous disorders, atopic dermatitis, toxic epidermal necrolysis, and pyoderma gangrenosum.[6]

CONCLUSION

The availability of biologic drugs is increasing rapidly. Understanding basics of biologics is key to safe use of these new and exciting molecules.

REFERENCES

1. Stern DK, Tripp JM, Ho VC, Lebwohi M. The use of systemic immune moderators in dermatology. In: Maclean DI, Maddin WS (Eds). Dermatologic Clinics, Volume 23. US: Elsevier; 2005. p. 275.
2. Sehgal VN, Pandhi D, Khurana A. Biologics in dermatology: An integrated review. Indian J Dermatol. 2014;59(5):425-41.
3. Coondoo A. Biologics in dermatologic therapy – an update. Indian J Dermatol. 2009;54(3): 211-20.
4. Trefzer U, Hofmann M, Sterry W, Asadullah K. Cytokine and anticytokine therapy in dermatology. Expert Opin Biol Ther. 2003;3(5):733-43.
5. Smith DI, Swamy PM, Heffernan MP. Off-label uses of biologics in dermatology: Interferon and intravenous immunoglobulin (part 1 of 2). J Am Acad Dermatol. 2007;56(1):e55-79.
6. Dhar S. Intravenous immunoglobulin in dermatology. Indian J Dermatol. 2009;54(1):77-9.

CHAPTER 3

Concept and Development of Biosimilars

Brijesh Nair

INTRODUCTION

Biosimilars are biopharmaceuticals that have been assessed by regulatory agencies to have efficacy and safety similar to their reference products and are expected to be marketed at substantially lower prices. They are not 100% identical, but essentially the same biological substance, though there may be minor differences due to their complex nature and production methods. They have come into the limelight because of patent expiry of originator biological molecules. The new wave of biosimilars will largely consist of monoclonal antibodies, which are mainly used in the oncology and immunology setting. Biologicals have revolutionized the field of medicine and dermatology in particular, with significant impact in the management of psoriasis, psoriatic arthritis (PsA), and urticarial and immunobullous disorders. The expected benefits of biosimilars are reductions in costs and consequently better access to biotherapeutics. However, uptake of biosimilars in the market has been slower than expected, which may, at least partly, be attributed to a lack of trust in the efficacy and safety of biosimilars as well as their interchangeability with the originator product by both patients and clinicians, which needs to be addressed meticulously. The difference in philosophy of biosimilar development is the focus on detection of potential differences in efficacy rather than the demonstration of efficacy, per se. "The demonstration of comparability does not necessarily mean that the quality attributes of the pre-change and post-change product are identical, but that they are highly similar and that the existing knowledge is sufficiently predictive to ensure that any differences in quality attributes have no adverse impact upon safety or efficacy of the drug product."

As such, a biosimilar development is therefore not so much "abridged" but rather "tailored" toward a distinct scientific objective—that is, to establish biosimilarity, not to re-establish benefit for the patient. The current concept of development of biosimilar monoclonal antibodies/soluble receptor fusion proteins (mAbs/cepts) follows the principle that extensive state-of-the-art physicochemical, analytical, and functional comparison of the molecules is complemented by comparative nonclinical and clinical data that establishes equivalent efficacy and safety in a clinical "model" indication that is most sensitive to detect any minor differences (if these exist) between biosimilar and its reference mAb also at the clinical level.[1,2]

DEFINITION: BIOSIMILARS

The European Medicines Agency (EMA) defines biosimilars as "biological medicinal products that contain a version of the active substance of an already authorized, original biological medicinal product (reference medicinal product). A biosimilar agent is similar to the reference medicinal product in terms of quality characteristics, biological activity, safety and efficacy based on a comprehensive comparability exercise."

The intention of the biosimilar development is to show similarity with the reference product, not to independently demonstrate patient benefit. The scientific principles for establishing biosimilarity are the same as those for demonstrating comparability after a change in the manufacturing process of an already licensed biological originator molecule. According to US legislation, biosimilars must utilize the same mechanism or mechanisms of action for the condition or conditions of use prescribed, recommended, or suggested in the proposed labeling and are prescribed for conditions that have been previously approved for the reference product. Furthermore, the route of administration, the dosage form, and the strength of the biosimilar should be the same as those of the reference product.[3-5]

Why is Biosimilar Development Complex?
Biologicals are derived from living cells or organisms and consist of relatively large and often highly complex molecular entities that may be difficult to fully characterize. Because of inherent variability of the biologic system and the manufacturing process, any resulting biological will display a certain degree of variability (microheterogeneity), even between different batches of the same product. Because of unavoidable differences in the manufacturing processes, a biosimilar and the respective originator product, the reference product, will not be entirely identical. However, the amino acid sequence is expected to be the same, and only small differences in the microheterogeneity pattern of the molecule may be acceptable. A very thorough comparison of the structural and functional characteristics and the product and process-related impurities of the biosimilar and the reference product is essential. Any differences found will need to be explained and justified with regard to the potential impact on the clinical performance of the biosimilar. Hence, the data requirements for demonstration of biosimilarity will usually be more extensive than for demonstration of comparability of a given biological before and after manufacturing changes by the same manufacturer. Data requirements for the development and

licensing of biosimilars are considerably greater than for small chemically synthesized generic molecules. For a generic, physicochemical identification and demonstration of a similar pharmacokinetic profile (bioequivalence) to the originator product are usually sufficient to conclude on therapeutic equivalence. In contrast, a biosimilar needs to be developed based on a more extensive head-to-head comparison with the reference product, to ensure close resemblance in physicochemical and biologic characteristics, safety, and efficacy. The focus of biosimilar development is not to establish patient's benefit per se—this has already been done for the originator product—but to convincingly demonstrate high similarity to the reference product as basis for relying, in part, on its efficacy and safety experience.

Clinicians need to be aware that clinical data are not the only cornerstone of a biosimilar development to be relied on. Extensive characterization and comparison of the physicochemical properties and biologic activity of the biosimilar and the originator product play a fundamental role in this, and close similarity in these aspects is a prerequisite for any reduction in the amount of nonclinical and clinical data requirements. Clinical data provide complementary information. The biosimilar development program is scientifically tailored using up-to-date analytical tools and sensitive test models to best detect even small potential product-related differences between the biosimilar and the reference product.[6-11]

PRECLINICAL ANALYTICAL ASSESSMENT

Preclinical analytical assessments are used to determine similarity to an originator biologic and are critical for regulatory approval of biosimilars. Approximately 40 different analytical methods are utilized to assess 100 different drug attributes. The International Psoriasis Council suggested guidelines for standardization of preclinical assessments of emerging biosimilars through the development of a biosimilar index. Companies in the business of making biosimilars are not in possession of the original cell line utilized for the originator compound, and thus their biologic, derived from a new cell line, is not identical to the original product. Instead of relying on any one key piece of data, the weight of all the analytical assessments is considered when determining whether the biosimilar is "similar" to the originator compound, the choice of the cell line, the culture media, the culture temperature, and the purification processes can all be altered, with each change potentially affecting the quality of the end product. The primary amino acid composition of a biosimilar medication is precisely bioengineered, but other features of biologics such as three-dimensional protein folding, glycosylation, charge, and presence of impurities are more variable during the manufacturing process. These particular features of a biologically produced product may affect both the antigen binding and immunogenicity of a given drug, and thus may affect both drug efficacy and safety in clinical use. Evaluating post-translational modifications via mass spectrometry, including testing for glycosylation, acetylation, sulfation, phosphorylation, glycation, and charge, is essential in the characterization of biologics and biosimilars. Testing for drug product stability (e.g., shelf life and alterations with temperature) and product devices (e.g., autoinjectors, prefilled syringes) are also needed in order to determine similarity between the biosimilar product and originator biological product.[12-14]

Biosimilar index is an algorithm where each comparison is weighted with regard to its criticality, and where variability for each assay/test, (e.g., <10% or 1 SD) is standardized. Using this index, biosimilars would be rated and scored regarding their preclinical analytical similarity to the originator biologic.[15]

SOME TERMINOLOGIES DEFINED

- *Biomimics*: These are versions of mAbs or fusion proteins available in countries where regulation is less strict. Biomimics are also known as "biocopies," "intended copies," or "nonregulated biologics." Kikuzubam was a rituximab biomimic that demonstrated adverse events different from originator molecule of rituximab, and hence regulatory authorities had to revoke the approval, thus demonstrating the complexity of the biomimic explosion. It also needs to be stated that different adverse effect profile of a biomimic raises questions on its biosimilarity.
- *Reference product (alternative terms—"originator" or "innovator" product)*: The initial biopharmaceutical that has been approved by regulatory agencies for specific indications; preclinical and clinical data regarding the reference product provides the basis for comparison of a biosimilar agent in the approval process.
- *Biosimilar (alternative terms—"similar biotherapeutic product," "subsequent entry biologic," "follow-on biologic," and "biocomparables")*: A mAb or fusion protein that has undergone a complete development process based on comparability to preclinical and clinical data of the reference product, with sufficient bioequivalence to meet regulatory approval.
- *Interchangeability*:[16-19] Interchangeability is the concept that a biosimilar drug and its parent biologic compound are so similar that a patient could be switched from one originator drug to another biosimilar drug and back during chronic therapeutic use, perhaps an indefinite number of times, without any untoward clinical side effects occurring due to this interchange of products. This designation allows a biosimilar agent to be substituted for its reference product by the pharmacist without prescriber input. Unlike small-molecule drugs, a biopharmaceutical that is repeatedly interchanged with a similar biological agent might elicit immunogenicity that could compromise the efficacy and safety of both the medications. Thus, the prevalent American College of Rheumatology (ACR) and European League Against Rheumatism (EULAR) consensus

is that frequent switching between the original protein product and the biosimilar agent should be avoided, as even subtle differences, such as impurities introduced during manufacturing, can trigger an immune response to biosimilar agents.
- *Switch*: Therapeutic transition from a reference product to a biosimilar agent or vice versa based on prescriber decision. A "switch" study demonstrating no loss of efficacy or no increase in risk would support the transition from biological to other.
- *Substitution*: Interchange of a biosimilar agent with its reference product by someone other than the prescribing health professional. If a biosimilar agent is determined to be "interchangeable" with its reference product, a pharmacist would be allowed to substitute a prescribed biological therapy for a biosimilar agent without involving the prescribing physician.[20,21]

METHODOLOGY OF PROVING BIOSIMILARITY

For approval, a comprehensive dossier of analytical, preclinical, pharmacokinetic, pharmacodynamics, and clinical data that demonstrates comparable efficacy and safety of the biosimilar and its off-patent reference biopharmaceutical is required. The EMA has prescribed certain steps that are mandatory for approval of a biosimilar. This process is depicted in **Table 1**.

TABLE 1: Steps for approval of biosimilar.

Stages	Steps
Preclinical stage	
In vitro studies	• Assessing binding to targets • Assess signal transduction and functional activity/viability
Determine if in vivo studies are needed	Necessary only if factors of concern are identified, for example, new post-translational modification structures
In vivo studies	Focus of study depends on the need for additional information.
Phase 1	
Pharmacokinetic/ Pharmacodynamics studies	• Single dose crossover or parallel group designs preferred • Pharmacodynamic markers selected on the basis of their clinical relevance • Affinity is a key determinant of the PK and PD profile of mAbs and soluble receptors • Close reproduction of conformational structure for biosimilar mAbs and cepts is needed to ensure comparable biological effect
Phase 3	
Safety and efficacy studies	• No clinically significant difference in efficacy to reference product • Compare severity and frequency of adverse events, in particular for immunogenicity/safety

(cepts: soluble receptor constructs; mAbs: monoclonal antibodies; PD: pharmacodynamics; PK: pharmacokinetics)

IMMUNOGENICITY

It is important to understand the complexity of production of both biological reference product and biosimilar, which precludes exact replication. Earlier batches of reference product have also changed due to the process changes and hence the current version of a biological reference product is not identical to the earlier batches of the same product. This underlines the need for rigorous pharmacological equivalence and biocomparability studies (for clinical comparison) in the approval process of a biological/biosimilar.

Immunogenicity may be influenced by patient-, disease-, or product-related factors. Patient- and disease-related factors are already known from the experience gained with the originator product and therefore do not need to be reinvestigated for the biosimilar. The focus of the evaluation is thus on potential product-related factors, such as structural or impurities/contaminants, most of which are readily detected by state-of-the-art analytical methods. Differences in immunogenicity can also be due to extraneous factors such as impurities in the manufacturing process of the prefilled syringes. This demonstrates the complexity of biosimilarity confirmation process.

In order to gain full insight into the long-term outcomes, particularly the immunogenicity profile of biosimilars, it is recommended that comparative clinical data should be collected for >1 year especially for antitumor necrosis factor (anti-TNF) therapies. Immunogenicity data beyond 1 year lacks scientific rationale and would raise the bar for biosimilars above that expected for innovator drugs, with obvious negative consequences for the affordability of these products.[22-26]

PHARMACOVIGILANCE

Pharmacovigilance, embedded in postmarketing surveillance, is of critical importance for biosimilars. As the abbreviated clinical development program of biosimilar agents is less able to identify small safety risks (compared with the development of reference products), appropriate pharmacovigilance measures need to be implemented after approval is granted. The means of pharmacovigilance are company-initiated risk management plans, postmarketing research, and surveillance of existing databases (registries) created to monitor patients receiving biologic agents.

The pharmacoequivalence and bioequivalence of the biosimilar to reference product intuitively suggests similarity in safety profile from product-related and patient-population-related perspectives. However, variability in immunogenicity due to batch-to-batch variability is a cause for concern. Thus, the safety of biosimilars needs to be actively and comprehensively followed up on an ongoing basis. Adverse event reports, if any, should include, in addition to the International Nonproprietary Name (INN), other indicators, such as brand name, manufacturer's name, lot number, and country of origin of the batch used.[27,28]

Nomenclature

To avoid confusion between biosimilar agents and their reference products during pharmacovigilance, specific nomenclature is necessary to distinguish each biosimilar from its reference drug and from each other. It has been suggested that a Greek letter or a combination of several letters could be appended to the end of the INN of each biopharmaceutical. Alternatively, a "biologic qualifier" (BQ) [a four-digit code proposed by the World Health Organization (WHO)] could be used to distinguish reference products and biosimilars from one another. Overall, the general agreement is that use of the INN alone is insufficient to differentiate biosimilars, and that traceability of each biosimilar needs to be secured. However, even though an internationally standardized system of nomenclature for biosimilars is urgently needed, this system has not yet been established, making postmarketing surveillance, risk evaluation, and management strategies for biosimilars more difficult.[29-31]

Extrapolation

Extrapolation is defined as the ability to utilize clinical study data for one disease to gain agency approval for another disease not explicitly studied in clinical trials. Extrapolation is the foundation of the biosimilar regulatory framework and is here defined as granting regulatory approval for indications of the reference medicine that are not specifically studied during the clinical development of the biosimilar medicine. The United States Food and Drug Administration (US FDA) issued guidance stating that data from a clinical trial of a biosimilar agent conducted in one disease could be used to support approval for additional indications for which the reference product has already been licensed. To obtain approval for any additional indication, the licensed biosimilar must follow the traditional regulatory pathway for biopharmaceuticals. The FDA mandates two randomized, placebo-controlled clinical trials (conducted in patients with the disease for which the indication is being sought) that demonstrate both efficacy and safety of the biological agent in that disease state. Thus, if a biosimilar agent was not approved initially for all indications for which the reference biopharmaceutical is licensed, the biosimilar manufacturer must conduct clinical trials in each additional individual disease state to support a biological license application for each separate indication. Similarly, if the reference biopharmaceutical is approved for an additional indication after its biosimilar has already been licensed, extrapolation of indications no longer applies; the manufacturer of the licensed biosimilar must conduct new clinical trials in this new indication to get approval. Thus, extrapolation of indication requires convincing scientific justification, which should address the mechanism of action, toxicities, and immunogenicity in each indication of use.[32-38]

For mAb, extrapolation is more complex as their mechanism of action may depend on multiple sites of the molecule. Often, no direct pharmacodynamic marker exists for their activity, which means that clinical studies are designed around (insensitive) clinical end points, which makes it particularly challenging to study these products. How the different structure–activity relationships of antibodies contribute to efficacy and safety in the different indications is often not fully understood.[39,40]

Regulatory Issues

CT-P13 (an infliximab biosimilar) was the first mAb biosimilar to be approved, but not all national regulatory agencies granted extrapolation to all infliximab indications. Infliximab biosimilar (Remsima) had been approved in a total of 47 countries as of May 2014, and marketing applications were pending in an additional 23 countries. Thus, as of May 2015, CT-P13 has been approved for use in approximately 70 countries worldwide. Agencies allowed extrapolation of indications for CT-P13 to six additional diseases for which the reference infliximab is approved but in which CT-P13 was not studied, namely PsA, psoriasis, adult and juvenile Crohn disease, and adult and juvenile ulcerative colitis. This decision established a regulatory precedent for the extrapolation of indications for a therapeutic monoclonal antibody based on results of one successful phase III trial in a sensitive population [in rheumatoid arthritis (RA)] and on additional pharmacokinetic, efficacy, safety, and immunogenicity data acquired in a phase I trial of patients with a different disease [ankylosing spondylitis (AS)]. Extrapolation of indications for biosimilars is possible, but concerns have been raised regarding the potential efficacy and safety of a biosimilar in diseases for which it has not been studied. It is opined that the outcome of a biosimilarity exercise should be binary: you either are, or you are not biosimilar to a given reference product. Selective approval for extrapolation to indications is at odds with this concept. Allowing products on the market that do not have the same authorized indications will create considerable confusion about the concept of biosimilarity. The success of biosimilars will depend on how they will be able to be interchanged with the reference product and other biosimilars in clinical practice. If multiple biosimilars are allowed in the market with different approved uses, this will create a complex situation that will add hurdles for the successful practitioner uptake of biosimilars.[41-44]

INDIAN SCENARIO FOR BIOSIMILARS

There has been burgeoning interest in biosimilars in Indian dermatology scenario. Biosimilars of infliximab, etanercept, rituximab, and adalimumab have been launched. The permissive nature of regulation in India has resulted in proliferation of intended copies without published biocomparability research supporting their use. The possibility of revoking an approval on recognition of inefficacy or adverse events is a definite possibility in the current scenario. Indian guidelines allow a biosimilar product to be

TABLE 2: Biosimilars currently approved for use in India.

Product	Brand name/manufacturer	Biosimilarity status
Adalimumab	Exemptia (Zydus)	Biosimilarity proven
	Adalirel (Reliance), Adfrar P (Torrent)	Intended copies/biomimics
Etanercept	Etacept (Cipla), Intacept (Intas)	Intended copies/biomimics
Rituximab	Reditux (Dr Reddy's), Rituxirel (Reliance), Mabtas RA (Intas)	Intended copies/biomimics
Infliximab	Infimab (Sun/Epirus/Reliance)	Biocomparability studies with switching carried out in rheumatoid arthritis. Similar study in psoriasis planned
Omalizumab	Omalirel, Emzumab	Intended copies

authorized if the reference product is licensed and widely marketed for at least 4 years in a country with a well-established regulatory framework, although not marketed in India (e.g., Humira).[45] The biosimilars currently approved for use in India are depicted in **Table 2**.

ZRC-3197, developed and marketed by Zydus Cadila (India) in India as exemptia to treat RA, juvenile inflammatory arthritis, PsA, and AS, is described as a "fingerprint match" of the reference adalimumab (Humira, Abbvie Inc, USA) "in terms of safety, purity and potency." The primary and secondary structures of ZRC-3197 and reference adalimumab are identical, and no differences were detected in aggregation or in the profile of low-molecular-weight fragments between these two biopharmaceuticals. Based on this, ZRC-3197 was approved for RA, juvenile idiopathic arthritis, AS, PsA, hidradenitis suppurativa, ulcerative colitis, and Crohn disease, but interestingly not for the treatment of psoriasis. The reason for not authorizing the product for psoriasis is not clear.[46-48]

BIOSIMILARS IN PSORIASIS

There is a paucity of biosimilar trials pertaining to psoriasis. In dermatology, direct data on psoriasis patients is missing. Most approvals are based on extrapolation. The question has been raised whether results obtained from such diverse patient populations treated with the same biologic may be compared at all. In general, psoriasis patients have been exposed to previous treatment protocols [e.g., ultraviolet (UV) therapy]. They also tend to exhibit different patient characteristics that may make them more susceptible to adverse drug reactions than other patient groups (e.g., alcohol abuse, liver toxicity). The fact that, for instance, inflammatory bowel diseases respond to infliximab and adalimumab but not to etanercept, whereas etanercept, on the other hand, is effective in psoriasis and RA also clearly underlines the differences between the mechanistic of various autoimmune diseases. The underpowered biosimilarity studies are ill-equipped to detect safety signals. Although not all ongoing biosimilar trials may have been registered, the present situation in terms of registered trials is unsatisfactory and will leave clinicians with a high degree of uncertainty with respect to their treatment decisions. It is now up to the clinical community to start collecting data on efficacy and particularly safety with independent trials and patient registries.

Biosimilars ideally must be studied in the preferred ("most sensitive") indication to assess comparable safety and efficacy. In case of TNF inhibitors, it is psoriasis with a reliable, easily assessable clinical endpoint [Psoriasis Area and Severity Index (PASI)]. Future of biosimilar development might focus more on this "sensitivity" aspect of psoriasis.[49-51]

BIOSIMILARS FOR PSORIASIS: CLINICAL STUDIES TO DETERMINE SIMILARITY

The International Psoriasis Consortium (IPC) has defined biosimilarity in psoriasis biosimilars on a clinical level recently. The amount and the type of clinical data generated in clinical studies involving biosimilars will inherently be less than the clinical data obtained for originator biologics. Owing to the regulatory emphasis on extrapolation eventuating in cost reduction, utilizing biosimilars in practice for diseases where little or no clinical data exist is a reality that clinicians must learn to accept. The IPC has suggested psoriasis as a future model for TNF blocker testing owing to (1) high effect sizes in clinical trials, (2) lack of cointervention, (3) commonality of the disease, (4) ease of conduct of trials with an easily reproducible outcome endpoint (PASI score). IPC also suggested that a biosimilar trial should also be at least as long as the primary endpoint in the reference product's pivotal trials and be based on the same safety measures collected during these original trials. For example, TNF blocker biosimilar trials should include safety outcomes such as deaths, malignancies, opportunistic infections, reactivation of tuberculosis and hepatitis B virus, major adverse cardiac events, and injection site reactions. In many cases, to demonstrate clinical equivalence on efficacy and safety of the biosimilar and the reference biologic adequately powered, randomized, parallel group, preferably double-blinded, comparative clinical trials are needed.[52-54]

CONCLUSION

The principles of establishing biosimilarity are to demonstrate structural and functional similarity to a reference product using the most discriminatory analytical methods. These data are supported where necessary by focused clinical evaluation using conditions that are adequately sensitive to evaluate real risks that cannot be addressed solely by analytical data. Unanswered questions remain, particularly regarding extrapolation of indications,

> **BOX 1** **Problem areas in biosimilar products.**
> - Consistent demonstration of pharmaceutical quality and quality assurance of the manufacturing process by biosimilar firm
> - Ensuring batch to batch product consistency
> - Lack of data on substitution, switching, interchangeability and subsequent adverse events/immunogenicity
> - Extrapolation of data from index disease to other indications
> - *Intense postmarketing surveillance for safety issues*: Pharma company, the primary stakeholder as opposed to practitioner driven registries
> - Problems with inconsistent nomenclature
> - Trial design complexity in demonstration of equivalence and interchangeability
> - Inter-regulator variations in licensing for extrapolation based on in vitro assays
> - Practitioner and patient apprehension regarding efficacy and safety of biosimilars
> - Grant of license by regulator subject to a post-authorization safety surveillance commitment

switching and interchangeability, naming and traceability, and long-term safety of biosimilars. Even after licensing, biosimilars (owing to the batch to batch variability inherent to biopharmaceuticals) must be subjected to intense postmarketing surveillance and pharmacovigilance. Further studies, including postmarketing surveillance using data acquired from registries, are needed to give healthcare providers confidence to accept these biosimilar agents into their armamentarium. The tighter regulation of intended copies and biomimics must be ensured to avoid safety issues that might blight the development of genuine biosimilar agents. The appropriately regulated and rationally extrapolated biosimilar development milieu will go a long way in reducing healthcare costs in the therapy of inflammatory diseases and can augment health policy decision-making. Despite the increasing number of countries that have adopted biosimilar guidelines, there are clear differences in local requirements in terms of weight of evidence and data interpretation, labeling, and naming of biosimilars. Such divergent regulatory decisions on the biosimilarity exercise do not assist in solving the trepidation that exists at the level of healthcare professionals and patients about biosimilars. There is a need for a global harmonization exercise for deciding upon the determinants of the concept of biosimilarity and for standardizing the regulatory requirements of biosimilars **(Box 1)**.

REFERENCES

1. Simoens S. Biosimilar medicines and cost-effectiveness. Clinicoecon Outcomes Res. 2011;3:29-36.
2. Schneider CK, Kalinke U. Toward biosimilar monoclonal antibodies. Nat Biotechnol. 2008;26(9):908-85.
3. European Medicines Agency. (2014). Guidelines on similar biological medicinal products. [online] Available from www.ema.europa.eu/docs/en_GB/document_library/Scientific_guideline/2014/10/WC500176768.pdf [Last accessed January, 2024].

4. US Senate. Biologics Price Competition and Innovation Act of 2009. 2009;703:3590-686.
5. United States Food and Drug Administration. (2012). Guidance for Industry on Biosimilars: Q & As Regarding Implementation of the BPCI Act of 2009: Questions and Answers Part I. [online] Available from http://www.fda.gov/Drugs/GuidanceComplianceRegulatoryInformation/Guidances/ucm259809 [Last accessed January, 2024].
6. United States Food and Drug Administration. Draft guidance on biosimilar product development. [online] Available from http://www.fda.gov/Drugs/DevelopmentApprovalProcess/HowDrugsareDevelopedandApproved/ApprovalApplications/TherapeuticBiologicApplications/Biosimilars/default.htm [Last accessed January, 2024].
7. European Medicines Agency. (2005). Committee for Medicinal Products for Human Use. Guideline on similar biological medicinal products containing biotechnology-derived proteins as active substance: quality issues. [online] Available from http://www.ema.europaeu/pdfs/human/biosimilar/4934805en.pdf [Last accessed January, 2024].
8. International Conference on Harmonisation. (2004). Comparability of Biotechnological/Biological Products Subject to Changes in their Manufacturing Process Q5E. [online] Available from https://database.ich.org/sites/default/files/Q5E%20Guideline.pdf [Last accessed January, 2024].
9. Schellekens H. Biosimilar therapeutics: what do we need to consider? NDT Plus. 2009;2(1):i27-i36.
10. Wadhwa M, Thorpe R. The challenges of immunogenicity in developing biosimilar products. IDrugs. 2009;12(7):440-4.
11. European Medicines Agency. (2015). European public assessment reports. [online] Available from http://www.ema.europa.eu/ema/index.jsp?curl=pages/medicines/landing/epar_search.jsp&mid=WC0b01ac058001d124 [Last accessed January, 2024].
12. O'Connor A, Rogge M. Nonclinical development of a biosimilar: the current landscape. Bioanalysis. 2013;5(5):537-44.
13. Schiestl M, Stangler T, Torella C, et al. Acceptable changes in quality attributes of glycosylated biopharmaceuticals. Nat Biotechnol. 2011;29(4):310-2.
14. Calvo B, Zuniga L. Therapeutic monoclonal antibodies: strategies and challenges for biosimilars development. Curr Med Chem. 2012;19(26):4445-50.
15. Blauvelt A, Cohen AD, Puig L, et al. Biosimilars for psoriasis: preclinical analytical assessment to determine similarity. Br J Dermatol. 2016;174(2):282-6.
16. US Department of Health and Human Services. The Affordable Care Act. [online] Available from https://www.hhs.gov/healthcare/about-the-aca/index.html [Last accessed January, 2024].
17. American College of Rheumatology. (2015). ACR Position Statement—Biosimilars. [online] Available from http://www.rheumatology.org/Practice/Clinical/Position/Biosimilars_02_2015/.pdf [Last accessed January, 2024].
18. Tóthfalusi L, Endrényi L, Chow SC. Statistical and regulatory considerations in assessments of interchangeability of biological drug products. Eur J Health Econ. 2014;15(1):S5-11.
19. Anderson S, Hauck WW. Consideration of individual bioequivalence. J Pharmacokinet Biopharm. 1990;18(3):259-73.
20. Castañeda-Hernandez G, Szekanecz Z, Mysler E, Azevedo VF, Guzman R, Gutierrez M, et al. Biopharmaceuticals for rheumatic diseases in Latin America, Europe, Russia, and India: innovators, biosimilars, and intended copies. Joint Bone Spine. 2014;81(6):471-7.
21. Barile-Fabris LA, Irazoque-Palazuelos F, Vasquez RH, Vazquez SC, and Gúzman R, et al. Incidence of adverse events in patients treated with intended copies of biologic therapeutic agents in Colombia and Mexico. Arthritis Rheumatol. 2014;66,S662.

22. Braun J, Baraliakos X, Kudrin A, Kim H, and Lee SJ, et al. Striking discrepancy in the development of anti-drug antibodies (ADA) in patients with rheumatoid arthritis (RA) and ankylosing spondylitis (AS) in response to infliximab (INF) and its biosimilar CTP13. Arthritis Rheumatol. 2014;66:3538-9.
23. Udata C, Yin D, Cai C, Salts S, Hua SY, Rehman MI, et al. Immunogenicity assessment of PF06438179, a potential biosimilar to infliximab, in healthy volunteers. Ann Rheum. 2015;74(2):702.
24. Mok CC, Van der Kleij D, Wolbink GJ. Drug levels, anti-drug antibodies, and clinical efficacy of the anti-TNF a biologics in rheumatic diseases. Clin. Rheumatol. 2013;32(10):1429-35.
25. European Medicines Agency. Committee for Medicinal Products for Human Use. (2017). Guideline on immunogenicity assessment of biotechnology derived therapeutic proteins. [online] Available from https://www.ema.europa.eu/en/documents/scientific-guideline/guideline-immunogenicity-assessment-therapeutic-proteins-revision-1_en.pdf [Last accessed January, 2024].
26. Ben-Horin S, Yavzori M, Benhar I, Fudim E, Picard O, Ungar B, et al. Cross-immunogenicity: antibodies to infliximab in Remicade-treated patients with IBD similarly recognise the biosimilar Remsima. Gut. 2015;65(7):1132-8.
27. Minghetti P, Rocco P, Cilurzo F, Vecchio LD, Locatelli F. The regulatory framework of biosimilars in the European Union. Drug Dis Today. 2012;17(1-2):63-70.
28. European Medicines Agency. Good pharmacovigilance practices. [online] Available from https://www.ema.europa.eu/en/human-regulatory-overview/post-authorisation/pharmacovigilance-post-authorisation/good-pharmacovigilance-practices [Last accessed January, 2024].
29. World Health Organization. (2012). 55th Consultation on International Nonproprietary Names for Pharmaceutical Substances, Geneva. [online] Available from https://www.who.int/docs/default-source/international-nonproprietary-names-%28inn%29/55th-executive-summary.pdf [Last accessed January, 2024].
30. Pineda C, Caballero-Uribe CV, de Oliveira MG, Lipszyc PS, Lopez JJ, Mataos Moreira MM, et al. Recommendations on how to ensure the safety and effectiveness of biosimilars in Latin America: a point of view. Clin Rheumatol. 2015;34(4):635-40.
31. European Biopharmaceutical Enterprises. Tell me the whole story: the role of product labelling in building user confidence in biosimilars in Europe. Gen Biosimil Initiative J. 2014;3:188-92.
32. Weise M, Kurki P, Wolff-Holz E, Bielsky MC, Schneider CK. Biosimilars: the science of extrapolation. Blood. 2014;124(22):3191-6.
33. European Medicines Agency. Committee for Medicinal Products for Human Use. (2014). Guideline on similar biological medicinal products containing biotechnology-derived proteins as active substance: nonclinical and clinical issues. [online] Available from https://www.ema.europa.eu/en/documents/scientific-guideline/guideline-similar-biological-medicinal-products-containing-biotechnology-derived-proteins-active-substance-quality-issues-revision-1_en.pdf [Last accessed January, 2024].
34. US Department of Health and Human Services. (2015). Biosimilars: questions and answers regarding implementation of the Biologics Price Competition and Innovation Act of 2009. [online] Available from https://www.federalregister.gov/documents/2015/04/30/2015-10064/biosimilars-questions-and-answers-regarding-implementation-of-the-biologics-price-competition-and [Last accessed January, 2024].
35. Danese S, Gomollon F. ECCO position statement: The use of biosimilar medicines in the treatment of inflammatory bowel disease (IBD). J. Crohns Colitis. 2013;7(7):586-9.
36. Fiorino G, Danese S. The biosimilar road in inflammatory bowel disease: the right way? Best Pract Res Clin Gastroenterol. 2014;28(3):465-71.

37. Strober BE, Armour K, Romiti R, Smith C, Tebbey PW, Menter A, et al. Biopharmaceuticals and biosimilars in psoriasis: what the dermatologist needs to know. J Am Acad Dermatol. 2012;66(2):317-22.
38. American College of Rheumatology. (2011). Position statement. Biosimilars. Available from http://www.rheumatology.org/Practice/Clinical/Position/Position_Statements [Last accessed January, 2024].
39. Minghetti P, Rocco P, Del Veccio L, Locatelli F. Biosimilars and regulatory authorities. Nephron Clin Pract. 2011;117(1):c1-c7.
40. World Health Organization. (2009) Guidelines on evaluation of similar biotherapeutic products (SBPs). 2009. [online] Available from http://www.who.int/biologicals/areas/biological_therapeutics/BIOTHERAPEUTICS_FOR_WEB_22APRIL2010.pdf [Last accessed January, 2024].
41. Dörner T, Kay J. Biosimilars in rheumatology: current perspectives and lessons learnt. Nat Rev Rheumatol. 2015;11(12):713-24.
42. Health Canada. Inflectra. (2015). Drugs and Health Products. Available from http://www.hc-sc.gc.ca/dhp-mps/prodpharma/sbd-smd/drugmed/sbd_smd_2014_inflectra_159493-eng.php [Accessed in May, 2017].
43. Scott BJ, Klein AV, Wang J. Biosimilar monoclonal antibodies: A canadian regulatory perspective on the assessment of clinically relevant differences and indication extrapolation. J Clin Pharmacol. 2014;55(3):S123-32.
44. Hazlewood GS, Rezaie A, Borman M, Panaccione R, Ghosh S, Seow CH, et al. Comparative effectiveness of immunosuppressants and biologics for inducing and maintaining remission in Crohn's disease: a network meta-analysis. Gastroenterology. 2015;148(2):344-54.e5; quiz e14-5.
45. Government of India. (2012). Guidelines on similar biologics: regulatory requirements for Marketing Authorization in India. [online] Available from http://geacindia.gov.in/resource-documents/biosafety-regulations/guidelines-and-protocols/CDSCO-DBTSimilarBiologicsfinal.pdf [Last accessed January, 2024].
46. Bandyopadhyay S, Mahajan M, Mehta T, Singh AK, Parikh A, Gupta AK, et al. Physicochemical and functional characterization of a biosimilar adalimumab ZRC3197. Biosimilars. 2015;5:1-18.
47. Zydus Cadila. (2014). Zydus launches world's first biosimilar of Adalimumab. [online] Available from http://zyduscadila.com/wp-content/uploads/2015/05/PressNote09-12-14.pdf [Last accessed January, 2024].
48. Jani RH, Gupta R, Bhatia G, Rathi G, Ashok Kumar P, Sharma R, et al. A prospective, randomized, double-blind, multicentre, parallel-group, active controlled study to compare efficacy and safety of biosimilar adalimumab (Exemptia; ZRC-3197) and adalimumab (Humira) in patients with rheumatoid arthritis. Int J Rheumat Dis. 2015;19(11):1157-68.
49. ClinicalTrials.gov. (2017). Study to demonstrate equivalent efficacy and to compare safety of biosimilar adalimumab (GP2017) and Humira (ADACCESS). [online] Available from http://ClinicalTrials.gov/show/NCT02016105 [Last accessed January, 2024].
50. ClinicalTrials.gov. (2013). Study to demonstrate equivalent efficacy and to compare safety of biosimilar etanercept (GP2015) and Enbrel (EGALITY). [online] Available from https://classic.clinicaltrials.gov/ct2/show/NCT01891864
51. Radtke MA, Augustin M. Biosimilars in psoriasis: what can we expect? J Dtsch Dermatol Ges. 2014;12:306-12.
52. Casadevall N, Thorpe R, Schellekens H. Biosimilars need comparative clinical data. Kidney Int. 2011;80(5):553.
53. Ebbers HC, Muenzberg M, Schellekens H. The safety of switching between therapeutic proteins. Expert Opin Biol Ther. 2012;12(11):1473-85.
54. Ebbers HC, Crow SA, Vulto AG, Schellekens H. Interchangeability, immunogenicity and biosimilars. Nat Biotechnol. 2012;30(12):1186-90.

SECTION 2

Biologics in Psoriasis

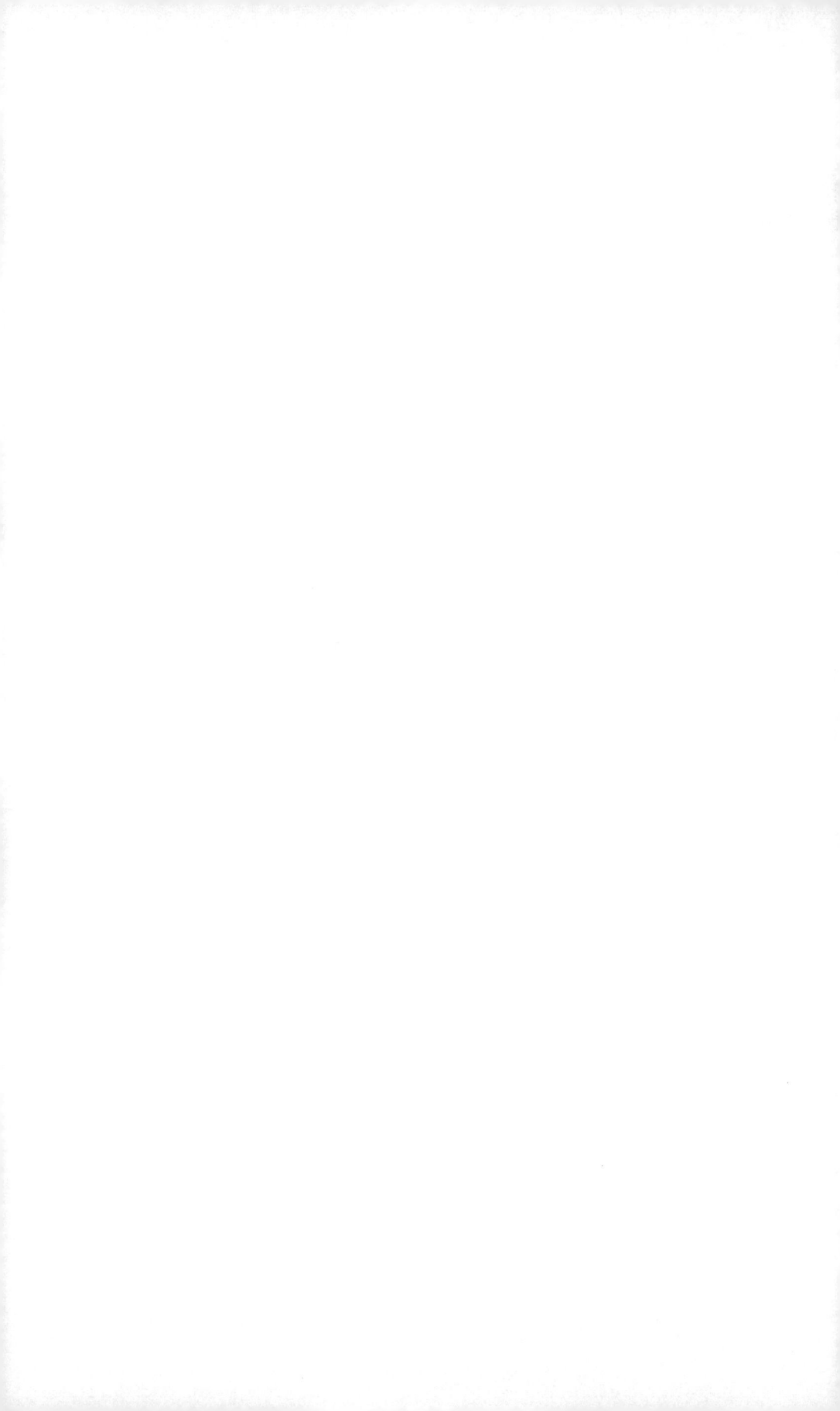

CHAPTER 4

Pathogenesis of Psoriasis

Rajat Kandhari, Snigdha Saxena, Anupama Molpariya

INTRODUCTION

Psoriasis is a common, chronic, inflammatory, and proliferative disorder of the skin, associated with systemic manifestations. In simplified terms, the psoriatic phenotype presents itself as a result of a complex interplay of genetic and environmental triggers (such as trauma, stress, infections, and drugs), followed by a cytokine cascade, resulting in various morphological variants of psoriasis **(Fig. 1)**.[1,2] Our understanding of psoriasis pathogenesis has come a long way, from psoriasis being a disease associated with abnormal proliferation and disturbed terminal differentiation, with the keratinocyte at the forefront and treatments such as coal tar, anthralin, and methotrexate forming the mainstay of therapy; to an era where the T lymphocytes were considered the main culprit and were tackled by drugs such as cyclosporine, alefacept, and efalizumab; this was subsequently followed by type 1 T helper (Th1) cytokines [tumor necrosis factor-alpha (TNF-α)] dominating the pathogenesis of psoriasis and molecules, such as etanercept and infliximab got introduced to tackle the disorder. Today the concept of psoriasis being solely a Th1-driven disease is considered inconsistent, and there is enough

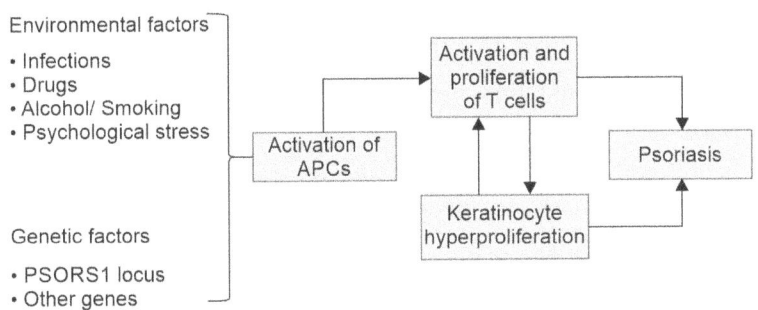

FIG. 1: A simplified illustration of the psoriatic pathogenesis.
(APCs: antigen-presenting cells; PSORS1: psoriasis susceptibility 1)

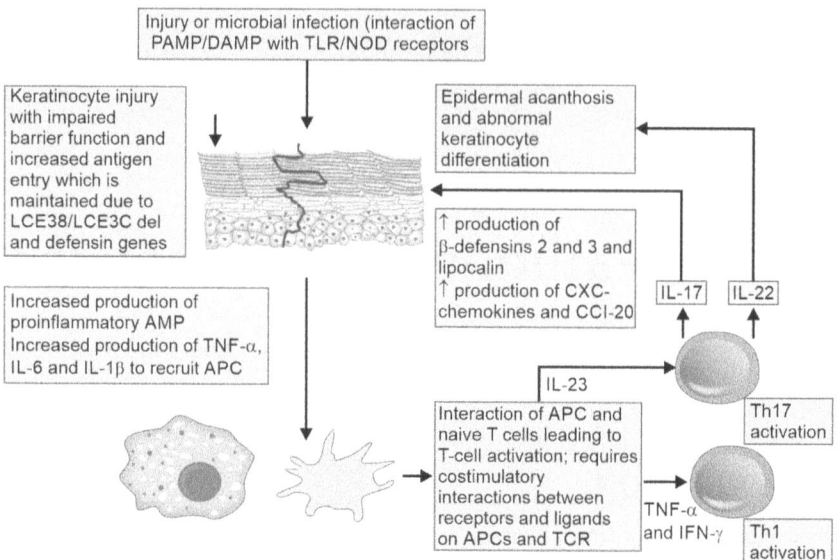

FIG. 2: Pathogenesis of psoriasis.[24]
[APC: antigen-presenting cell; CCl20: chemokine (C-C motif) ligand 20; DAMP: damage-associated molecular pattern; IFN-γ: interferon-gamma; IL: interleukin; LCE: late cornified envelope; NOD: nucleotide-binding oligomerization domain; PAMP: pathogen-associated molecular patterns; TCR: T-cell receptor; TNF-α: tumor necrosis factor-alpha; TLR: toll-like receptors; Th1: type 1 T helper]

evidence to support the key role of the interleukin (IL)-12, IL-23, and IL-17 in the psoriasis pathogenesis. Moreover, this understanding has led to the treatment of psoriasis becoming "targeted" to certain cytokines and certain pathways, leading to improved outcomes and safety.

It is considered that various antigens activate effector T cells in the skin, leading to release of inflammatory cytokines that promote further recruitment of immune cells, keratinocyte proliferation, and sustained chronic inflammation **(Fig. 2)**.

ETIOLOGY OF PSORIASIS

Environmental Factors

Infections

It has been proposed that certain variants of psoriasis, particularly guttate and chronic plaque psoriasis, are fueled by persistent intracellular streptococcal infection.[3]

Both initiation and acute exacerbations of psoriasis have been associated with β-hemolytic streptococcal throat infection. Bacterial superantigens are able to stimulate T-cell proliferation without prior intracellular processing by an antigen-presenting cell (APC), and this seems to be the underlying mechanism for triggering psoriasis.

T cells that infiltrate and exacerbate psoriatic skin disease may originate in the tonsils. Streptococcal infection can induce a skin-homing phenotype in these T cells, in which both streptococcal and skin-specific epitopes interact through a process called molecular mimicry.[4] This infection is not eliminated by standard antibiotic therapy; however, tonsillectomy may be effective in some patients.[5] Psoriasis may occur not only following throat infection, as was originally described, but also as a result of perianal streptococcal infection and streptococcal vulvovaginitis.[6] Further, human immunodeficiency virus (HIV) infection is associated with paradoxical aggravation or worsening of psoriasis, as it causes a reduction in the Th cells. Suggested explanations for this occurrence include HIV-induced reduction in regulatory T cells, an increased number of memory CD8+ T cells, effects of HIV on dendritic cell populations, HIV proteins acting as superantigens or shared genetic variants between psoriasis and HIV responder status.[7]

Other infections which may contribute as triggers of psoriasis include bacterial infections such as *Staphylococcus aureus, Helicobacter pylori,* and fungal infections such as *Malassezia* and *Candida.*[8]

Drugs

Certain drugs may trigger or exacerbate psoriasis. The latency period between starting the medication and onset of psoriasis is highly variable between different drugs; hence, it may sometimes be difficult to establish a drug-related cause. Psoriatic lesions may persist even after discontinuation of the implicated drug. Psoriasis triggered by drugs may present as chronic plaque psoriasis, palmoplantar psoriasis, nail psoriasis, scalp psoriasis, pustular psoriasis, and erythrodermic psoriasis.[9]

Drugs like antimalarials, lithium salts, interferon-alpha (INF-)α, TNF-α inhibitors, and tetracyclines may induce or exacerbate psoriasis. Beta-blockers, nonsteroidal anti-inflammatory drugs (NSAIDs), and angiotensin-converting enzyme (ACE) inhibitors, digoxin, clonidine, carbamazepine, valproic acid, calcium-channel blockers, granulocyte colony-stimulating factor (G-CSF), potassium iodide, ampicillin, penicillin, progesterone, morphine, and acetazolamide have also been implicated in smaller studies.[10]

Lithium acts directly by blocking cell differentiation and this results in dysregulation of inflammatory cytokines and reduced cyclic adenosine monophosphate (cAMP) levels. Beta blockers, both cardioselective and noncardioselective, initiate a delayed type hypersensitivity reaction and a reduction in cAMP levels with consequent increase in epidermal cell turnover. Antimalarials inhibit the enzyme transglutaminase, thereby triggering psoriasis. NSAIDs exacerbate psoriasis by inhibiting cyclo-oxygenase pathway, leading to accumulation of leukotrienes.[11]

Alcohol

Alcohol consumption is associated with moderate-to-severe psoriasis.[12] In alcoholics, psoriasis tends to be more severe and is associated with depression and cardiovascular diseases.[13]

Smoking

It has been demonstrated that smoking increases the chances of a person developing psoriasis, psoriatic arthritis, and palmoplantar pustulosis. Moreover, the disease tends to be more severe in smokers.[14,15]

Other Factors

Psychological Stress

There is a role of psychological stress as a trigger for psoriasis in genetically predisposed individuals through immunological and inflammatory mechanisms.[16] Psoriasis has been associated with depression, anxiety, and suicidal tendency and psychological stress may cause disease flares.[17,18]

Meditation, weight loss, and yoga lead to decreased Psoriasis Area Severity Index (PASI) scores.[19] This may be explained by the numerous neurocutaneous connections forming the brain-skin axis.[20,21]

The immune modulatory neurotransmitters may be involved in the pathogenesis of psoriasis as psoriatic lesions may resolve after a sensory loss or nerve damage in the same area.[22,23]

Further, stress may also impact the efficacy of the various treatments given for psoriasis. A slow response to psoralen with ultraviolet A (PUVA) therapy due to stress has been noted.[24]

Thus, there is a need to recognize stress early and initiate specific treatment for it in appropriate cases, and this may considerably improve management of psoriasis.[25]

Sunlight

Sun exposure generally causes improvement in psoriatic lesions but 5–20% patients may show worsening.[10] Some patients may develop psoriatic lesions over the lesions of polymorphous light eruption due to Koebner's phenomenon.[26]

Physical Trauma

Koebner's phenomenon is seen in up to 25% psoriatic patients,[27] more commonly seen in human leukocyte antigen (HLA)-C:06:02 positive patients.[28] It is hypothesized that mechanical trauma activates innate immunity with subsequent adaptive immune activation, keratinocyte hyperproliferation, and angiogenesis, leading to new psoriatic lesions at the sites of trauma.[10]

Genetic Factors

Multiple inherited alleles as well as environmental risk factors play a synergistic role in the causality of psoriasis. A strong genetic component has been implicated in the etiology of psoriasis, with reported >60% heritability.[29]

The involvement of genetic factors contributing to the disease has been demonstrated by a higher rate of disease prevalence in cases with a positive family history[30,31] and increase in lifetime risk of psoriasis if both parents of an individual are affected.[32] Higher concordance rate of 72% among monozygotic twins, compared to 22% among dizygotic twins, has also been seen.[33] The development and severity of psoriasis have also been linked to the sex of the contributing parent, wherein men are more likely than women to transmit psoriasis to the offspring. An earlier age of onset was seen when the disease was inherited from the father, consistent with "genetic anticipation".[34]

Psoriasis demonstrates a genetic spectrum, wherein one end of the spectrum is represented by rare families in which changes in a single gene may be sufficient to cause the disease (monogenic), whereas at the other end exists the more common form in which an obvious family history may be lacking, and it is likely that changes in multiple genes interacting both with each other and the environment are required for disease expression (polygenic).[35]

At least nine genomic regions or loci [psoriasis susceptibility (PSORS) 1-9), which co-segregated with psoriasis have been identified. Out of these, the most well studied is PSORS-1, which maps to the class I major histocompatibility complex (MHC) and codes for genes involved in antigen presentation. PSORS-1 is responsible for 35–50% of disease heritability.[29,36]

Three genes, namely *HLA-Cw6*, *CCHCR1* (coiled-coil alpha-helical rod protein 1) and *CDSN* (corneodesmosin), are present within this region. *HLA-Cw6* encodes a class I MHC protein involved in antigen presentation, *CCHCR1* encodes coiled-coil alpha-helical rod protein 1, which is highly expressed in psoriatic epidermis and regulates keratinocyte proliferation, and *CDSN* encodes corneodesmosin, a late differentiation epidermal glycoprotein overexpressed in the granular and cornified layers of the epidermis involved in keratinocyte adhesion.[1,2]

Human leukocyte antigen-C*06:02 is understood to be the most significant causal susceptibility allele, among all the PSORS genes. HLA-C plays a role in immune responses by presenting antigens to CD8+ T cells, which are the main inflammatory T cells that migrate into the epidermis and also by interacting with natural killer (NK) cell receptors.[37]

Human leukocyte antigen-Cw6 has been associated with early-onset psoriasis (type-1 psoriasis), guttate psoriasis, psoriatic arthritis, and Koebner phenomenon, and these patients are more likely to show improvement during pregnancy. Psoriatic arthritis patients with HLA-Cw6 positivity, besides early-onset disease, have been shown to present with development of cutaneous features before arthritis.

A higher response to methotrexate, anti-IL-12/23, and anti IL-17 drugs and a lower response to anti-TNF-α agents have been reported with HLA-Cw6 positivity.[38,39]

Various non-*MHC* genes have also found to be involved in the pathogenesis of psoriasis, albeit with a lesser role. These include genes related to skin barrier and innate/adaptive immunity.[40]

Pustular psoriasis has been associated with three disease genes, namely *IL36RN*, *AP1S3*, and *CARD14*, using next-generation sequencing techniques. The *IL36RN* gene encodes for the IL-36 receptor antagonist, which plays a role in modulating the activity of IL-1 cytokines. Mutations in *IL36RN* gene have been linked to pustular psoriasis in many populations.[41]

Thus, the advances in genetics have opened the door for the development of innovative and transformative treatment options for psoriasis.[29]

PATHOGENETIC PATHWAY

There are multiple molecular processes occurring simultaneously to produce the basic pathological and phenotypic features of psoriatic lesions. No single cause has been identified, and it is accepted that genetic and environmental factors act together to produce immune dysregulation in the presence of a defective skin barrier.[11]

Role of Damage-associated Molecular Patterns/Pathogen-associated Molecular Patterns and Maturation of Antigen-presenting Cells

Whenever there is microbial or mechanical insult, damage-associated molecular patterns (DAMPs) and pathogen-associated molecular patterns (PAMPs) interact with their receptors, such as toll-like receptors (TLRs) and nucleotide-binding oligomerization domain (NOD)-like receptors (NLRs), causing activation of keratinocytes and the epidermal innate immune system, and thus increased secretion of antimicrobial proteins/peptides (AMPs).[11] This interaction also leads to the liberation of potent chemoattractants and inflammatory cytokines, such as TNF-α, IL-8, and IL-1β.

In a genetically predisposed individual:
- Exposure to PAMPs leads to a heightened inflammatory response and defective skin barrier repair with increased expression of keratins 6 and 17 and the late cornified envelope 3 (LCE3) family proteins. This aberrant skin repair allows a sustained exposure to PAMPs, which are engulfed by APCs like Langerhans and dendritic cells.
- Subsequent to the environmental triggers, there is release of heat-shock proteins and under the influence of aforementioned cytokines, the APCs undergo a process of maturation involving upregulation of C-C chemokine receptor type 7 (CCR7), B7 molecules, and intercellular adhesion molecule 1 (ICAM-1).

These mature APCs are then ready to interact with the naïve T cells in the neighboring lymph nodes, resulting in T-cell activation.

Migration of Antigen-presenting Cells to the Local Lymph Nodes and the "Immunological Synapse"

Once the APCs attain maturity, they find their way via the afferent lymphatics to the nearby draining lymph nodes to interact with the naïve T cells.

This process requires interaction between the MHC antigens on APCs with the T-cell receptors (TCRs). In addition, costimulatory interactions between receptors and ligands on APCs and TCRs are important. These include interaction of lymphocyte function antigen (LFA)-3 and cluster of differentiation 2 (CD2), between ICAM-1 and LFA-1, and between B7 and CD28 **(Table 1)**.[42]

The interaction between the APCs and naïve T cells results in activation of naïve T cells to pathogenic T cells. This is facilitated by the presence of polymorphisms in *IL-23* genes and HLA-Cw6. Once the T cells are activated, both CD4+ (Th1 cells and Th17 cells) and CD8+ T cells infiltrate the skin and secrete Th1 and Th17 cytokines, which activate the keratinocytes **(Fig. 3)**.

Maturation of T-cells and Migration into the Inflamed Skin

The IL-12 released by the mature Langerhans cells binds to IL-12R cell surface receptors on the activated T cells leading to differentiation of T cells into type 1 effector T helper cells. The maturation of the T cells results in expression of new surface proteins, namely the cutaneous lymphocyte-associated antigen (CLA), which enables the T cells to exit the blood vessels and migrate to the skin. This is mediated by the interaction between the CLA on the T cell and E-selectin on the endothelial cells. Interferon gamma (IFN-γ) and TNF-α (released from antigen-activated T cells) induce chemokine expression from endothelial cells and keratinocytes, and this chemokine gradient enhances trafficking of the T cells to the epidermis. The entry of T cells into the epidermis is mediated by the ICAM-1 on the keratinocytes and LFA-1 on the T cells. Further α3β7 integrin (on Tc1 cells) binds to E-cadherin on keratinocytes,

TABLE 1: The immunological synapse.	
Signal	Interaction
Primary	• T-cell receptor (TCR) and MHC I/II interaction • ICAM-1 and LFA-1 interaction—maintains adhesion between the T cell and the APC
Secondary/Costimulatory	• B7-CD28 interactions leads to positive activation signals to T cells • LFA-3/CD2 • CD40/CD40L • Upregulates transcription of cytokines involved in T-cell activation, IL-2, TNF-α, IFN-γ, and GM-CSF
Third set of signals	• IL-2 (made by activated T cells) binds to IL-2R surface receptors and regulates mitotic activation of T cells • IL-12 (made by mature Langerhans cells) binds to IL-12R surface receptors on activated T cell, leading to differentiation of T cells into type 1 effectors

(APC: antigen-presenting cell; CD2: cluster of differentiation 2; CD40L: cluster of differentiation 40 ligand; GM-CSF: granulocyte-macrophage colony-stimulating factor; ICAM-1: intercellular adhesion molecule 1; IFN-γ: interferon gamma; IL-2: interleukin 2; IL-2R: interleukin 2 receptor; LFA-1: lymphocyte function antigen 1; MHC: major histocompatibility complex; TNF-α: tumor necrosis factor-alpha; TCR: T-cell receptor)

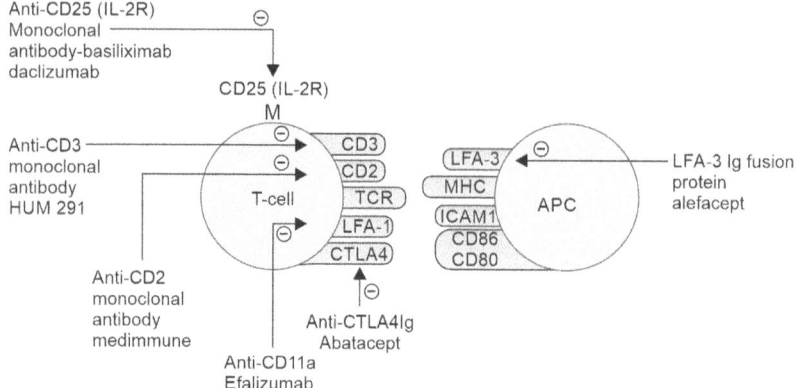

FIG. 3: Inhibition of T-cell activation and costimulation.
(APC: antigen-presenting cell; CD2: cluster of differentiation 2; CTLA4Ig: cytotoxic T-lymphocyte antigen 4-immunoglobulin; ICAM-1: intercellular adhesion molecule 1; IL-2R: interleukin 2 receptor; LFA-1: lymphocyte function antigen 1; MHC: major histocompatibility complex; TCR: T-cell receptor)

which is increased in the psoriatic epidermis, facilitating transport of T cells into the epidermis and resulting in an injury response program and release of various cytokines, which serve as signals for chronic epidermal hyperplasia.

Role of Keratinocytes

While the T cells have been at the forefront of the complex psoriasis pathogenesis, the keratinocyte plays an important and supportive role as well.[43]

Role in T-cell Trafficking

The keratinocytes under the influence of IFN-γ express ICAM-1, which interacts with the LFA-1 on the T cells, allowing the entry of the T cells into the epidermis.

Further, keratinocytes release cytokines and result in the production of a chemokine gradient, which is responsible for adhesion of leukocytes to endothelial cells and their trafficking into the epidermis.

Role in Neutrophil Accumulation

Keratinocytes release IL-8, a cytokine which is responsible for the attraction and accumulation of neutrophils in the epidermis, forming the characteristic "Munro's microabscess" associated with the psoriatic pathology.

Role in Angiogenesis

There is considerable evidence to demonstrate the role of vascular endothelial growth factor (VEGF) driving the angiogenesis associated with psoriasis.[44] The psoriatic epidermis has greater angiogenic activity compared with the skin of normal subjects, uninvolved skin, and treated psoriatic skin.[45,46]

Keratinocytes in the lesional skin are a major source of proangiogenic cytokines in psoriasis, including:
- VEGF
- Endothelial cell-stimulating angiogenesis factor (ESAF)
- Thymidine phosphorylase (PDECGE/TP)
- TNF-α
- Transforming growth factor alpha (TGF-α)
- Platelet-derived growth factor (PDGF)

Vascular endothelial growth factor has been demonstrated to be overexpressed in basal keratinocytes and result in chronic skin inflammation and tortuous capillaries. Moreover, serum VEGF levels have been correlated with the disease severity.[47]

Further, VEGF increases the expression of VEGF receptor (VEGFR) in keratinocytes, and the keratinocytes in turn regulates VEGF expression, giving support to the claim that VEGF has a role in keratinocyte proliferation.[48]

Cross-talk between Keratinocytes and T Cells

The role of keratinocytes in the initiation as well as maintenance phases of psoriasis is well recognized.

Initiation Phase

External trigger factors stimulate the keratinocytes to release LL-37 (the only cathelicidin-derived antimicrobial peptide in humans) and self-DNA. When LL-37 is conjugated with self-DNA, it triggers the activation of TLR9 in plasmacytoid dendritic cells (pDCs). This, in turn, leads to the production of IFN-α, which activates myeloid dendritic cells (mDCs) to generate IL-12 and IL-23. These cytokines play a role in activating Th1 and Th17 immune responses, respectively.

Maintenance Phase

On activation, Th1 cells produce IFN-γ and TNF-α, while Th17 cells release Th17 cytokines (IL-17A, IL-17F, IL-22, and IL-26) that act on keratinocytes. This, in turn, triggers keratinocytes to produce chemokines, cytokines, and antimicrobial peptides that recruit neutrophils, macrophages, or additional Th1 and Th17 cells to the site of inflammation. Further, these cytokines may directly act on keratinocytes to modulate keratinocyte proliferation and differentiation.[49]

Thus, there is a cross-talk between keratinocytes and IL-17-producing Th17 cells, which fuels cutaneous inflammation and epidermal hyperplasia by facilitating both immune and nonimmune functions.

Role of Th17 Cells and Interleukin-23

Following evidence points toward the involvement of Th17 cells and IL-23 in the pathogenesis of psoriasis:

- Elevated levels of IL-23 and Th17-related cytokines were observed in cutaneous lesions and serum of psoriatic patients.
- Association of IL-23 receptor (*IL23R*) gene variants with psoriasis
- Evidence of a functional role of Th17 cells in autoimmunity and its significance with the comorbidities have been observed.

The development and maintenance of Th17 cells have been linked to IL-23.[50,51] The surface marker for Th17 cells is CD 161.[52,53] The cytokine IL-23, a heterodimer composed of p19 and p40 subunits, shares the p40 subunit with IL-12 and has been implicated in pathophysiology of various autoimmune diseases in both mice and humans.[54] On exposure to TGF-β, Th17 cells develop from a committed CD4+ T cell population and IL-23 plays a major role at this step.[55,56]

Interleukin-23 is produced by dendritic cells, macrophages, and keratinocytes. IL-23, when it binds to IL23R, results in JAK2-mediated phosphorylation of tyrosine residues located in intracellular domain of IL23R subunit. The phosphorylated tyrosine residues serve as a docking site for signal transducer and activator of transcription (STAT)-3 molecules, which in turn get translocated to nucleus of Th17 cells, resulting in transcription, and thus production of various cytokines (IL-17A, IL-17F, IL-22, and IL-26). These cytokines in turn increase the expression of proinflammatory cytokines, cerebrospinal fluids (CSFs), and chemokines and are also responsible for neutrophil activation.[57]

Interestingly, it has been seen that IL-17A is elevated in the skin but not in the sera of psoriasis patients, and this observation is consistent with the finding that drugs such as cyclosporin and anti-TNF-α agents decrease proinflammatory cytokines in lesional skin and not in the periphery.[58]

Cytokines released by Th17 cells along with those secreted by Th1 cells act on keratinocytes, thereby leading to changes characteristic of psoriasis such as epidermal hyperproliferation, acanthosis, and hyperparakeratosis.[54]

The activated keratinocytes further produce IL-23, which mediates a cross talk with Th17 lymphocytes. Moreover, Th17 cells induce keratinocytes to produce IL-8 for recruitment of neutrophils, cathelicidin for activation of pDCs, and VEGF with resulting angiogenesis.[54]

In view of the aforementioned changes, one may speculate that the concept of psoriasis as a Th1-driven disease is inconsistent with evidence obtained since the discovery of Th17 cells, which appear to play a key role in the maintenance of psoriasis **(Fig. 2)**.

Role of Regulatory T cells (Treg Cells) in Psoriasis

Regulatory T cells or Treg cells are helper T cells, which are characterized by a high expression of CD25 (alpha chain of IL-2 receptor). The development of Treg cells is controlled by FoxP3, a transcription factor of the fork head/winged-helix family. Cytokines released by Treg cells include IL-10 and TGF-β, which suppress the activities of other effector immune cells and thereby aid in peripheral tolerance. Severe autoimmunity may develop in the absence of FoxP3 expressing Treg cells.

During various inflammatory stimuli, Treg cells retain their lineage stability and suppressive function; however, they may gain effector phenotypes and lose FoxP3 expression. On exposure to IL-6, a proinflammatory cytokine highly expressed in psoriatic skin, there is Treg plasticity to a Th17-like phenotype.[59]

Role of Janus Kinase-signal Transducer and Activator of Transcription Pathway

The Janus kinase-signal transducer and activator of transcription (JAK-STAT) pathway is an intracellular signaling system that interacts with extracellular factors to regulate gene expression in various immune-mediated inflammatory diseases, by downstream signaling of receptors for type I and type II cytokines, including IL-6, IL-10, IL-12, IL-22, IL-23, and IFN. Many of these cytokines have a role to play in the pathogenesis of certain inflammatory and autoimmune diseases including psoriasis.[60]

The IL-23/Th17 axis plays an important role in the pathogenesis of psoriasis. IL-23 promotes the differentiation of Th17 cells, which in turn produce IL-17 and IL-22. These cytokines induce proliferation of keratinocytes and other typical features of psoriasis. The role of JAKs in the pathogenesis of psoriasis and the therapeutic potential of JAK inhibitors is highlighted by the fact that the IL-23 receptor depends on a JAK2 and TYK2 heterodimer for signal transduction.[60]

Further, tyrosine kinase 2 (TYK2) plays a crucial role in mediating signaling and downstream responses of the IL-12, IL-23, and type I IFN receptors. Inflammation in psoriasis is initiated and maintained by IL-12 and IL-23 signaling pathways. An association between TYK2 mutations that impair function, and protection from psoriasis has been shown by genetic linkage studies.[61]

Role of the Skin Barrier

Psoriasis is characterized by a compromised barrier function, which leads to alteration of the innate and adaptive immunity. As discussed earlier, psoriasis is linked with genes specifically present on epidermal cells, namely *CDSN* genes, β-defensin cluster genes, and *LCE3B* and *3C* genes.[62]

Abnormal Keratinization

Abnormal keratinization presents with an increased expression of early differentiation markers (such as CDSN and small proline-rich proteins, cystatin A, and transglutaminase 1) and decreased expression of late differentiation markers (such as loricrin and filaggrin). This abnormal barrier leads to increased transepidermal water loss (TEWL), which is directly proportional to the clinical severity.[11]

Antimicrobial Proteins

The two major groups of AMPs, defensins, and cathelicidins provide a chemical barrier to infection or injury. Psoriatic lesions are characterized by increased levels of human β-defensin-2.[63] High defensin levels may be responsible for lower risk of skin infections in psoriatic plaque, but they also possess potent proinflammatory activity. Similarly, cathelicidin LL-37 is overexpressed in psoriatic skin.[64] It binds to extracellular self-DNA released from dying cells and thereby converts self DNA into a potent stimulus for pDCs. An autoinflammatory cascade is thus triggered by the release of type I interferons by these pDCs.[11]

Abnormal Barrier Repair

The *LCE* gene cluster, composed of six groups (LCE1-6, with a total of 18 members) is a part of the epidermal differentiation complex, and its deletion has been linked with psoriasis.[65] Increased expression of *LCE3* gene and reduced expression of other *LCE* genes is seen in psoriatic plaques.[66] This may lead to incomplete barrier repair after minor trauma, which in turn causes penetration of various antigens and induces an inflammatory response.

Role of Adaptive and Innate Immunity

The psoriasis pathogenesis depicts a balance between the innate and acquired immune systems. The imbalance in the adaptive immune system is characterized by a skewed Th1 response.[67-69]

Further, cytokines/chemokines produced by keratinocytes in the epidermis act on both the innate and acquired immune systems, stimulating dendritic cells, neutrophils, and other innate mediators, as well as T cells.[43]

The roles of the adaptive and innate immune systems and their cells have been highlighted in **Table 2**.[70-82]

TABLE 2: Immune systems, cytokines, and their probable roles in the psoriatic pathogenesis.

Role of adaptive immunity		
Cell types	Cytokine production	Probable role
CD 4+ T cells		
Th1 cells	IFN-γ	Keratinocyte hyperproliferation, concomitant inflammation, and dermal proliferation of small vessels[70,71]
Th17 cells	IL-17, IL-21, IL-22, and IL-6	Responsible for increased AMP levels, keratinocyte hyperproliferation, neutrophil chemotaxis, and angiogenesis
Th22 cells	IL-22	Mediates keratinocyte proliferation and epidermal hyperplasia

Continued

Continued

Regulatory T cells (FoxP3+ Treg)	IL-17	Role in keratinocyte hyperproliferation, skin inflammation, and immune response amplification
CD 8+ T cells	IL-17, IL-22, IFN-γ, and TNF-α	CD8+ T cells with assistance from the CD4+ T cells play a role in induction and maintenance of the disease. The cytokines released result in keratinocyte hyperproliferation and skin inflammation, with TNF-α playing a role in dendritic cell maturation[71]
γδ T cells	IL-17, IL-22, and TNF-α	γδ T cells may act in an amplification loop for IL-17 synthesis and provide a possible mechanism mediating autoimmune inflammation. Further the cytokines play a role in keratinocyte hyperproliferation
Role of innate immunity		
Cell types	**Cytokines**	**Probable role**
mDCs	TNF-α, IL-23, and IL-20	Psoriatic skin contains a highly increased number of CD11c+ mDCs in the dermis.[79] They contribute to autoantigen presentation and activation of T cells in situ[80]
pDCs	Type 1 IFNs	Play a role in initiating the psoriatic pathogenesis[64]
LCs		They act as APCs, which stimulate naïve T cells[11,76]
Keratinocytes	IL-6, IL-8, TGF-α, TGF-β, and IL-1	Act as APCs and play a crucial role in the entry of T cells into the epidermis, upregulation of adhesion molecules, keratinocyte hyperproliferation, and skin inflammation
NK cells	IFN-γ, TNF-α, and IL-17	Coexpress TCR and NK lineage markers and represent a component of innate immunity. Play a role in immune-regulatory functions and an intermediary role between innate and acquired immune system, resulting in keratinocyte hyperproliferation and skin inflammation[82]
Macrophages	TNF-α	They serve as APCs, regulate epidermal proliferation and differentiation, and influence T-cell proliferation[73]
Neutrophils	IL-8	These are the effector cells of innate immunity, which produce IL-8, S100 proteins and proteases, which act on keratinocytes to induce inflammatory genes or increase their proliferation[43]
Mast cells	Proteases, histamine, prostaglandins, leukotrienes, chemokines, MHC class II molecules	Believed to play an immune regulatory role in psoriasis[74] as they are able to promote as well as suppress inflammation • Act as APCs • Recruit cells of immune system • Suppress inflammation and keratinocyte growth

(APCs: antigen-presenting cells; CD: cluster of differentiation; IFN-γ: interferon gamma; mDCs: myeloid dendritic cells; MHC: major histocompatibility complex; LCs: Langerhans cells; NK cells: natural killer cells; pDCs: plasmacytoid dendritic cells; TCR: T-cell receptor; TNF-α: tumor necrosis factor-alpha; TGF-β: transforming growth factor beta; Th1: type 1 T helper)

Psoriasis and the Gut Microbiota

Many studies have shown an alteration of the gut microbiota in psoriasis patients. These alterations have been shown to be similar to those in inflammatory bowel disease, obesity, and some cardiovascular disorders. The triggering factor for the onset of disease seems to be the "leaky gut syndrome" and bacterial translocation, as they are promoters of chronic systemic inflammation. Significant findings concerning altered gut physiology in psoriatic patients include microbiota dysbiosis, decline in production of short-chain fatty acids (SCFAs), increased amount of trimethylamine-N-oxide (TMAO), and dysregulation of pathways affecting the balance between lymphocyte populations. In a randomized placebo controlled trial, wherein 90 psoriatic patients were administered a mixture of three probiotic strains—*Bifidobacterium longum*, *Bifidobacterium lactis*, and *Lactobacillus rhamnosus*, a significant reduction of PASI and a lower risk of relapse were observed in patients who received the probiotic strains as compared to controls.[83]

CONCLUSION

While our understanding of psoriasis has grown by leaps and bounds, there remains a lot more to be understood. Due to its multifactorial nature, a cure of psoriasis still eludes us. It is important as clinicians to understand the varying pathways mentioned earlier to provide our patients with a sustainable and holistic treatment plan to achieve optimal treatment outcomes.

REFERENCES

1. Griffiths CE, Barker JN. Pathogenesis and clinical features of psoriasis. Lancet (London, England). 2007;370(9583):263-71.
2. Monteleone G, Pallone F, MacDonald TT, Chimenti S, Costanzo A. Psoriasis: from pathogenesis to novel therapeutic approaches. Clin Sci (Lond). 2011;120(1):1-11.
3. Sigurdardottir SL, Thorleifsdottir RH, Valdimarsson H, Johnston A. The role of the palatine tonsils in the pathogenesis and treatment of psoriasis. Br J Dermatol. 2013;168(2):237-42.
4. Rademaker M, Agnew K, Anagnostou N, Andrews M, Armour K, Baker C, et al. Psoriasis and infection. A clinical practice narrative. Australas J Dermatol. 2019;60(2):91-8.
5. Thorleifsdottir RH, Sigurdardottir SL, Sigurgeirsson B, Olafsson JH, Sigurdsson MI, Petersen H, et al. Improvement of psoriasis after tonsillectomy is associated with a decrease in the frequency of circulating T cells that recognize streptococcal determinants and homologous skin determinants. J Immunol. 2012;188(10):5160-5.
6. Lee EB, Wu KK, Lee MP, Bhutani T, Wu JJ. Psoriasis risk factors and triggers. Cutis. 2018;102(5S):18-20.
7. Chen H, Hayashi G, Lai OY, Dilthey A, Kuebler PJ, Wong TV, et al. Psoriasis patients are enriched for genetic variants that protect against HIV-1 disease. PLoS Genet. 2012;8(2):e1002514.
8. Fry L, Baker BS. Triggering psoriasis: the role of infections and medications. Clin Dermatol. 2007;25(6):606-15.

9. Kamiya K, Kishimoto M, Sugai J, Komine M, Ohtsuki M. Risk Factors for the Development of Psoriasis. Int J Mol Sci. 2019;20(18).
10. Burden A, Kirby B. Psoriasis and Related Disorders. In: Griffiths CEM, Barker J, Bleiker T, Chalmers R, Creamer D (Eds). Rook's Textbook of Dermatology, 9th edition. London: Blackwell Science Ltd.; 2004. pp. 35.1-35.48.
11. Mahajan R, Handa S. Pathophysiology of psoriasis. Indian J Dermatol Venereol Leprol. 2013;79 Suppl 7:S1-9.
12. Naldi L, Parazzini F, Brevi A, Peserico A, Veller Fornasa C, Grosso G, et al. Family history, smoking habits, alcohol consumption and risk of psoriasis. Br J Dermatol. 1992;127(3):212-7.
13. Tobin AM, Kirby B. Psoriasis: an opportunity to identify cardiovascular risk. Br J Dermatol. 2009;161(3):719.
14. Tobin A-M, Veale DJ, Fitzgerald O, Rogers S, Collins P, O'Shea D, et al. Cardiovascular disease and risk factors in patients with psoriasis and psoriatic arthritis. J Rheumatol. 2010;37(7):1386-94.
15. Higgins E. Alcohol, smoking and psoriasis. Clin Exp Dermatol. 2000;25(2):107-10.
16. Rousset L, Halioua B. Stress and psoriasis. Int J Dermatol. 2018;57(10):1165-72.
17. Fortune DG, Richards HL, Griffiths CEM. Psychologic factors in psoriasis: consequences, mechanisms, and interventions. Dermatol Clin. 2005;23(4):681-94.
18. Meyer N, Paul C, Feneron D, Bardoulat I, Thiriet C, Camara C, et al. Psoriasis: an epidemiological evaluation of disease burden in 590 patients. J Eur Acad Dermatol Venereol. 2010;24(9):1075-82.
19. Bostoen J, Bracke S, De Keyser S, Lambert J. An educational programme for patients with psoriasis and atopic dermatitis: a prospective randomized controlled trial. Br J Dermatol. 2012;167(5):1025-31.
20. Roosterman D, Goerge T, Schneider SW, Bunnett NW, Steinhoff M. Neuronal control of skin function: the skin as a neuroimmunoendocrine organ. Physiol Rev. 2006;86(4):1309-79.
21. Jiang WY, Raychaudhuri SP, Farber EM. Double-labeled immunofluorescence study of cutaneous nerves in psoriasis. Int J Dermatol. 1998;37(8):572-4.
22. Raychaudhuri SP, Raychaudhuri SK. Role of NGF and neurogenic inflammation in the pathogenesis of psoriasis. Prog Brain Res. 2004;146:433-7.
23. Joseph T, Kurian J, Warwick DJ, Friedmann PS. Unilateral remission of psoriasis following traumatic nerve palsy. Br J Dermatol. 2005;152(1):185-6.
24. Fortune DG, Richards HL, Kirby B, McElhone K, Markham T, Rogers S, et al. Psychological distress impairs clearance of psoriasis in patients treated with photochemotherapy. Arch Dermatol. 2003;139(6):752-6.
25. Eskin M, Savk E, Uslu M, Küçükaydoğan N. Social problem-solving, perceived stress, negative life events, depression and life satisfaction in psoriasis. J Eur Acad Dermatol Venereol. 2014;28(11):1553-9.
26. Ros AM, Eklund G. Photosensitive psoriasis. An epidemiologic study. J Am Acad Dermatol. 1987;17(5 Pt 1):752-8.
27. Weiss G, Shemer A, Trau H. The Koebner phenomenon: review of the literature. J Eur Acad Dermatol Venereol. 2002;16(3):241-8.
28. Gudjónsson JE, Kárason A, Antonsdóttir AA, Rúnarsdóttir EH, Gulcher JR, Stefánsson K, et al. HLA-Cw6-positive and HLA-Cw6-negative patients with Psoriasis vulgaris have distinct clinical features. J Invest Dermatol. 2002;118(2):362-5.
29. Dand N, Mahil SK, Capon F, Smith CH, Simpson MA, Barker JN. Psoriasis and Genetics. Acta Derm Venereol. 2020;100(3):adv00030.
30. Nanda A, Kaur S, Kaur I, Kumar B. Childhood psoriasis: an epidemiologic survey of 112 patients. Pediatr Dermatol. 1990;7(1):19-21.
31. al-Fouzan AS, Nanda A. A survey of childhood psoriasis in Kuwait. Pediatr Dermatol. 1994;11(2):116-9.

32. Swanbeck G, Inerot A, Martinsson T, Wahlström J. A population genetic study of psoriasis. Br J Dermatol. 1994;131(1):32-9.
33. Brandrup F, Hauge M, Henningsen K, Eriksen B. Psoriasis in an unselected series of twins. Arch Dermatol. 1978;114(6):874-8.
34. Burden AD, Javed S, Bailey M, Hodgins M, Connor M, Tillman D. Genetics of psoriasis: paternal inheritance and a locus on chromosome 6p. J Invest Dermatol. 1998;110(6):958-60.
35. Barker JN. Genetic aspects of psoriasis. Clin Exp Dermatol. 2001;26(4):321-5.
36. Trembath RC, Clough RL, Rosbotham JL, Jones AB, Camp RD, Frodsham A, et al. Identification of a major susceptibility locus on chromosome 6p and evidence for further disease loci revealed by a two stage genome-wide search in psoriasis. Hum Mol Genet. 1997;6(5):813-820.
37. Huang Y-W, Tsai T-F. HLA-Cw1 and Psoriasis. Am J Clin Dermatol. 2021;22(3):339-47.
38. van Vugt LJ, van den Reek JMPA, Hannink G, Coenen MJH, de Jong EMGJ. Association of HLA-C*06:02 Status With Differential Response to Ustekinumab in Patients With Psoriasis: A Systematic Review and Meta-analysis. JAMA Dermatol. 2019;155(6):708-15.
39. Burlando M, Russo R, Clapasson A, Carmisciano L, Stecca A, Cozzani E, et al. The HLA-Cw6 Dilemma: Is It Really an Outcome Predictor in Psoriasis Patients under Biologic Therapy? A Monocentric Retrospective Analysis. J Clin Med. 2020;9(10):3140.
40. Babaie F, Omraninava M, Gorabi AM, Khosrojerdi A, Aslani S, Yazdchi A, et al. Etiopathogenesis of Psoriasis from Genetic Perspective: An updated Review. Curr Genomics. 2022;23(3):163-74.
41. Twelves S, Mostafa A, Dand N, Burri E, Farkas K, Wilson R, et al. Clinical and genetic differences between pustular psoriasis subtypes. J Allergy Clin Immunol. 2019;143(3):1021-6.
42. Lebwohl M. Psoriasis. Lancet (London, England). 2003;361(9364):1197-204.
43. Lowes MA, Bowcock AM, Krueger JG. Pathogenesis and therapy of psoriasis. Nature. 2007;445(7130):866-73.
44. Heidenreich R, Röcken M, Ghoreschi K. Angiogenesis drives psoriasis pathogenesis. Int J Exp Pathol. 2009;90(3):232-48.
45. Canavese M, Altruda F, Ruzicka T, Schauber J. Vascular endothelial growth factor (VEGF) in the pathogenesis of psoriasis--a possible target for novel therapies? J Dermatol Sci. 2010;58(3):171-6.
46. Marina ME, Roman II, Constantin A-M, Mihu CM, Tătaru AD. VEGF involvement in psoriasis. Clujul Med. 2015;88(3):247-52.
47. Creamer D, Allen MH, Groves RW, Barker JN. Circulating vascular permeability factor/vascular endothelial growth factor in erythroderma. Lancet (London, England). 1996;348(9034):1101.
48. Sabat R, Philipp S, Höflich C, Kreutzer S, Wallace E, Asadullah K, et al. Immunopathogenesis of psoriasis. Exp Dermatol. 2007;16(10):779-98.
49. Ni X, Lai Y. Keratinocyte: A trigger or an executor of psoriasis? J Leukoc Biol. 2020;108(2):485-91.
50. Blauvelt A. T-helper 17 cells in psoriatic plaques and additional genetic links between IL-23 and psoriasis. J Invest Dermatol. 2008;128(5):1064-7.
51. Bettelli E, Carrier Y, Gao W, Korn T, Strom TB, Oukka M, et al. Reciprocal developmental pathways for the generation of pathogenic effector TH17 and regulatory T cells. Nature. 2006;441(7090):235-8.
52. Hugh JM, Weinberg JM. Update on the pathophysiology of psoriasis. Cutis. 2018;102(5S):6-12.
53. Cosmi L, De Palma R, Santarlasci V, Maggi L, Capone M, Frosali F, et al. Human interleukin 17-producing cells originate from a CD161+CD4+ T cell precursor. J Exp Med. 2008;205(8):1903-16.

54. Di Cesare A, Di Meglio P, Nestle FO. The IL-23/Th17 axis in the immunopathogenesis of psoriasis. J Invest Dermatol. 2009;129(6):1339-50.
55. Manel N, Unutmaz D, Littman DR. The differentiation of human T(H)-17 cells requires transforming growth factor-beta and induction of the nuclear receptor RORgammat. Nat Immunol. 2008;9(6):641-9.
56. Yang L, Anderson DE, Baecher-Allan C, Hastings WD, Bettelli E, Oukka M, et al. IL-21 and TGF-beta are required for differentiation of human T(H)17 cells. Nature. 2008;454(7202):350-2.
57. Weaver CT, Hatton RD, Mangan PR, Harrington LE. IL-17 family cytokines and the expanding diversity of effector T cell lineages. Annu Rev Immunol. 2007;25:821-52.
58. Zaba LC, Cardinale I, Gilleaudeau P, Sullivan-Whalen M, Suárez-Fariñas M, Fuentes-Duculan J, et al. Amelioration of epidermal hyperplasia by TNF inhibition is associated with reduced Th17 responses. J Exp Med. 2007;204(13):3183-94.
59. Nussbaum L, Chen YL, Ogg GS. Role of regulatory T cells in psoriasis pathogenesis and treatment. Br J Dermatol. 2021;184(1):14-24.
60. Kvist-Hansen A, Hansen PR, Skov L. Systemic Treatment of Psoriasis with JAK Inhibitors: A Review. Dermatol Ther (Heidelb). 2020;10(1):29-42.
61. Krueger JG, McInnes IB, Blauvelt A. Tyrosine kinase 2 and Janus kinase–signal transducer and activator of transcription signaling and inhibition in plaque psoriasis. J Am Acad Dermatol. 2022;86(1):148-57.
62. Sano S. Psoriasis as a barrier disease. Dermatologica Sin. 2015;33(2):64-9.
63. Jansen PAM, Rodijk-Olthuis D, Hollox EJ, Kamsteeg M, Tjabringa GS, de Jongh GJ, et al. Beta-defensin-2 protein is a serum biomarker for disease activity in psoriasis and reaches biologically relevant concentrations in lesional skin. PLoS One. 2009;4(3):e4725.
64. Lee E, Trepicchio WL, Oestreicher JL, Pittman D, Wang F, Chamian F, et al. Increased expression of interleukin 23 p19 and p40 in lesional skin of patients with psoriasis vulgaris. J Exp Med. 2004;199(1):125-30.
65. Bergboer JGM, Tjabringa GS, Kamsteeg M, van Vlijmen-Willems IM, Rodijk-Olthuis D, Jansen PA, et al. Psoriasis risk genes of the late cornified envelope-3 group are distinctly expressed compared with genes of other LCE groups. Am J Pathol. 2011;178(4):1470-7.
66. Nair RP, Duffin KC, Helms C, Ding J, Stuart PE, Goldgar D, et al. Genome-wide scan reveals association of psoriasis with IL-23 and NF-kappaB pathways. Nat Genet. 2009;41(2):199-204.
67. Uyemura K, Yamamura M, Fivenson DF, Modlin RL, Nickoloff BJ. The cytokine network in lesional and lesion-free psoriatic skin is characterized by a T-helper type 1 cell-mediated response. J Invest Dermatol. 1993;101(5):701-5.
68. Schlaak JF, Buslau M, Jochum W, Hermann E, Girndt M, Gallati H, et al. T cells involved in psoriasis vulgaris belong to the Th1 subset. J Invest Dermatol. 1994;102(2):145-9.
69. Vanaki E, Ataei M, Sanati MH, Mansouri P, Mahmoudi M, Zarei F, et al. Expression patterns of Th1/Th2 transcription factors in patients with guttate psoriasis. Acta Microbiol Immunol Hung. 2013;60(2):163-74.
70. Ghoreschi K, Mrowietz U, Röcken M. A molecule solves psoriasis? Systemic therapies for psoriasis inducing interleukin 4 and Th2 responses. J Mol Med (Berl). 2003;81(8):471-80.
71. Jadali Z, Eslami MB. T cell immune responses in psoriasis. Iran J Allergy Asthma Immunol. 2014;13(4):220-30.
72. Clark RA, Kupper TS. Misbehaving macrophages in the pathogenesis of psoriasis. J Clin Invest. 2006;116(8):2084-7.
73. Harvima IT, Nilsson G, Suttle M-M, Naukkarinen A. Is there a role for mast cells in psoriasis? Arch Dermatol Res. 2008;300(9):461-78.
74. Cai Y, Fleming C, Yan J. New insights of T cells in the pathogenesis of psoriasis. Cell Mol Immunol. 2012;9(4):302-9.

75. Ghoreschi K, Laurence A, Yang X-P, Hirahara K, O'Shea JJ. T helper 17 cell heterogeneity and pathogenicity in autoimmune disease. Trends Immunol. 2011;32(9):395-401.
76. Fujita H, Nograles KE, Kikuchi T, Gonzalez J, Carucci JA, Krueger JG. Human Langerhans cells induce distinct IL-22-producing CD4+ T cells lacking IL-17 production. Proc Natl Acad Sci U S A. 2009;106(51):21795-800.
77. Sugiyama H, Gyulai R, Toichi E, Garaczi E, Shimada S, Stevens SR, et al. Dysfunctional blood and target tissue CD4+CD25high regulatory T cells in psoriasis: mechanism underlying unrestrained pathogenic effector T cell proliferation. J Immunol. 2005;174(1):164-73.
78. Cai Y, Shen X, Ding C, Qi C, Li K, Li X, et al. Pivotal role of dermal IL-17-producing γδ T cells in skin inflammation. Immunity. 2011;35(4):596-610.
79. Lowes MA, Chamian F, Abello MV, Fuentes-Duculan J, Lin SL, Nussbaum R, et al. Increase in TNF-alpha and inducible nitric oxide synthase-expressing dendritic cells in psoriasis and reduction with efalizumab (anti-CD11a). Proc Natl Acad Sci U S A. 2005;102(52):19057-62.
80. Nestle FO, Turka LA, Nickoloff BJ. Characterization of dermal dendritic cells in psoriasis. Autostimulation of T lymphocytes and induction of Th1 type cytokines. J Clin Invest. 1994;94(1):202-9.
81. Wollenberg A, Wagner M, Günther S, Towarowski A, Tuma E, Moderer M, et al. Plasmacytoid dendritic cells: a new cutaneous dendritic cell subset with distinct role in inflammatory skin diseases. J Invest Dermatol. 2002;119(5):1096-102.
82. Peternel S, Kastelan M. Immunopathogenesis of psoriasis: focus on natural killer T cells. J Eur Acad Dermatol Venereol. 2009;23(10):1123-7.
83. Polak K, Bergler-Czop B, Szczepanek M, Wojciechowska K, Frątczak A, Kiss N. Psoriasis and Gut Microbiome-Current State of Art. Int J Mol Sci. 2021;22(9).

CHAPTER 5

Etanercept

Santanu Banerjee, Debatraya Paul

INTRODUCTION

Etanercept is a human tumor necrosis factor-alpha (TNF-α) receptor p75 Fc fusion protein produced by recombinant deoxyribonucleic acid (DNA) technology in a Chinese hamster ovary (CHO) mammalian expression system.

MOLECULAR STRUCTURE

It is a dimer of a chimeric protein genetically engineered by fusing the extracellular ligand binding domain of human tumor necrosis factor receptor-2 (TNFR2/75) to the Fc domain of human immunoglobulin G1 (IgG1). This Fc component contains the hinge, CH2, and CH3 regions, but not the CH1 region of IgG1. It contains 934 amino acids and molecular weight is 150 kDa.

HISTORY

Etanercept was developed at Immunex and in late 1998 released it for commercial use, soon after the release of infliximab. It was first approved by the Food and Drug Administration (FDA) in 1998 for rheumatoid arthritis. It later got approval for psoriatic arthritis (PsA) in 2002, moderate-to-severe plaque psoriasis in 2004, and pediatric psoriasis in 2016.[1]

PHARMACOLOGY

Etanercept binds and neutralizes both TNF-α and TNF-β, binding to both soluble and receptor bound TNF-α. Since, it is dimeric in nature the affinity of etanercept to TNF-α is 100 times greater than the natural monomeric cellular receptor whereas the Fc region of IgG1 gives it a stability.

PHARMACOKINETICS

The drug attains peak plasma level at 2 days. It has a half-life of 4.8 days and absolute bioavailability after subcutaneous etanercept is 58%. The etanercept–TNF-α complex undergoes proteolysis in blood and is excreted in urine and bile.

MECHANISM OF ACTION

Tumor necrosis factor-α is a naturally occurring cytokine which binds to two different receptors and initiates a cascade of cellular signals which results in production and release of inflammatory cytokines and recruitment of a host of inflammatory cells. Elevated TNF-α levels are found both in affected skin and serum of patients with psoriasis. The disease severity and remission are directly proportional to the serum levels of TNF-α.[2]

Two distinct TNF receptors (TNFRs) exist naturally as monomeric molecules on cell surfaces and in soluble forms, a 55 kDa protein (p55) and a 75 kDa protein (p75). Biological activity of TNF is dependent upon binding to either cell surface TNFR or the soluble form. Etanercept is a dimeric soluble form of the p75 TNFR that can bind competitively to TNF molecules with an affinity of 50–100 times more than its natural receptors. Etanercept inhibits binding of TNF-α and TNF-β to cell surface TNFRs, thus rendering TNF biologically inactive. TNF inhibition causes decrease in proinflammatory cytokines, adhesion molecules, decreased release of vascular endothelial growth factor, and prevents activation of dendritic cells and their production of interleukin-23 (IL-23). It results in apoptosis of dendritic cells in psoriatic plaques and reduced expression of nuclear factor-kappa B (NF-κB).[3]

USES

- *FDA-approved indications*:
  - Chronic plaque psoriasis (4 years or older)
  - Psoriatic arthritis[4]
  - Rheumatoid arthritis
  - Juvenile idiopathic arthritis (JIA) (2 years or older)
  - Ankylosing spondylitis
- *Off-label indications*:
  - Neutrophilic dermatoses:
    - Aphthous stomatitis
    - Behçet's disease
    - Pyoderma gangrenosum
  - Bullous dermatoses:
    - Bullous pemphigoid
    - Pemphigus vulgaris
    - Cicatricial pemphigoid

- *Granulomatous dermatoses*:
  - Granuloma annulare (generalized)
  - Sarcoidosis
- Connective tissue diseases:
  - Dermatomyositis
  - Relapsing polychondritis
  - Scleroderma
- Miscellaneous conditions:
  - Stevens–Johnson syndrome and toxic epidermal necrolysis (TEN)
  - Graft-versus-host disease
  - Hidradenitis suppurativa
  - Multicentric reticulohistiocytosis
  - Synovitis, acne, pustulosis, hyperostosis, and osteitis (SAPHO) syndrome
  - Pityriasis rubra pilaris
  - Kawasaki disease
  - Erythema nodosum leprosum

PSORIASIS

Etanercept was first approved by the FDA in 2004 for the treatment of chronic plaque psoriasis. It has been used in different dosing schedule in different studies, most common being 50 mg subcutaneously twice a week for 12 weeks followed by 50 mg weekly. This has been explained in **Table 1**.

Monotherapy

Etanercept shown good response when used as monotherapy as demonstrated in many clinical trials. There was improvement from baseline psoriasis

TABLE 1: Efficacy of etanercept in psoriasis.

Dose	PASI 50	PASI 75	Reference
• 50 mg twice a week • 25 mg twice a week • 25 mg once a week	• 64.2% • 52.6% • 40.9%	• 49% (after 12 weeks) • 34% • 14%	Leonardi et al. (2003)[1]
25 mg twice weekly	–	26% (12 weeks)	Mease P (2000)[4]
50 mg twice a week	–	49% (12 weeks)	Papp et al. (2005)[5]
50 mg once a week	90%	60%	
	After 12 weeks, dose was reduced to 25 mg twice a week. At the end of 24 weeks, there was no reduction in the efficacy of etanercept.		

Note: Long-term safety of etanercept was mentioned by Kivelevitch D et al. in their study showcasing use of etanercept for 72 weeks, 96 weeks and up to 156 weeks.[6]

(PASI 50: psoriasis area and severity index 50; PASI-75: psoriasis area and severity index 75).

area and severity index 75 (PASI 75) or more in 34% of the etanercept group receiving 25 mg twice weekly and 49% of the etanercept group receiving 50 mg twice weekly, as compared with 4% of the patients in the placebo group at 12 weeks.[1,5,7]

Combination Therapy

To augment the effect of biologics and reduce the cost associated with its usage, it can be used in combination therapy with conventional systemic therapy.

Etanercept and Methotrexate

To improve efficacy etanercept can be combined with methotrexate. On combining methotrexate (7.5–15 mg weekly) to etanercept 50 mg twice a week, 70.2% patients achieved PASI 75 after 12 weeks as compared to 54.3% patients on monotherapy with etanercept. PASI 50 and PASI 90 were achieved in 92.4% and 34% respectively in patient on combination therapy as compared to 83.8% and 23.1% in patients on monotherapy. Nonserious adverse events were slightly higher in combination group as compared to monotherapy.[8]

Etanercept and Acitretin

The combination therapy has a potential benefit of giving protection against skin cancer by acitretin and also helps in reducing the dose of etanercept to once weekly when combined with acitretin in the dose of 0.4 mg/kg.[9] Etanercept has been used in lower dosage of 25 mg with acitretin and produced good results.[10]

Etanercept and Narrowband Ultraviolet B

Etanercept 50 mg once a week on combining with narrowband ultraviolet B (NB-UVB) three times a week, results in PASI 75, 90, and 100 in 81.8%, 57.6%, and 24.6% patients respectively after 12 weeks.[11] Etanercept 25 mg twice a week has been combined with NB-UVB and was found to be very effective. Due to theoretical risk of increasing risk of malignancy with this combination, this combination should be limited to shortest period of time.[12] As the implication of malignancy in treatment with TNF-α blockers alone or in combination with NB-UVB complex with levels of TNF-α having varied effects on tumoral growth, it is recommended to restrict this highly effective combination for short duration up to 24 weeks, to obtain a quicker response and to avoid long-term complications. The European Academy of Dermatology and Venereology (EADV) guidelines on management of psoriasis mention that TNF-α blockers and NB-UVB may or may not be combined and it is not as strict a contraindication as cyclosporine with NB-UVB.[13,14]

Continuous versus Intermittent Therapy

Etanercept should be used continuously for sustained clinical benefit; however, patient may need to discontinue therapy for some reason. In a study conducted by Gordon et al., psoriasis returns gradually after 3 months of stopping etanercept and retreatment with etanercept is as effective as initial treatment. An open-label trial by Moore et al. using etanercept continuously or intermittently concluded that continuous therapy is more effective.[15,16] In a study conducted by Wolfram Sterry et al. it was found that initial treatment of psoriasis with etanercept 50 mg twice weekly showed more rapid clearance of skin lesions as compared to 50 mg once weekly. However, 50 mg once weekly regimen showed better response in joint and tendon rheumatic symptoms.[17]

Adherence

Adherence is important for biologics treatment. A retrospective analysis conducted by Esposito et al. on survival rate of anti-TNF-α treatment revealed that global adherence was 72.9% after 28.9 months of therapy. Etanercept showed longest survival (mean 51.4 months), as compared to infliximab (36.8 months) and adalimumab (34.7 months). Main reason for discontinuation were inefficacy or adverse events.[18] In a study conducted by Fiorenzo Santoleri et al., adherence levels were found to be 0.83 for adalimumab versus 0.84 for etanercept in PsA patients.[19]

PSORIATIC ARTHRITIS

It was approved by the FDA for management of PsA in 2002. Etanercept in dose of 25 mg twice a week, resulted in ACR20 (20% improvement) in 59% patients at the end of 12 weeks. Results were sustained till 48 weeks and it also inhibited radiographic progression.[4] Dose of 50 mg twice a week and once a week were compared in a randomized controlled trial (RCT) by Sterry et al. There was no significant difference in patient with PsA treated with once a week or twice a week dose. However, psoriatic lesions showed much more improvement with twice weekly regimen for 12 weeks. In patient with PsA without or minimal psoriasis, 50 mg once a week is an adequate treatment.[16]

Combination therapy with etanercept and methotrexate showed greater efficacy in patients with PsA as far as the American College of Rheumatology (ACR) and minimal disease activity (MDA) response rates and extent of radiographic progression are concerned.[20]

ERYTHRODERMIC PSORIASIS

Good response was seen in 14 patients of erythrodermic psoriasis treated with etanercept,[21] Romero-Mate et al. reported a patient with PASI 100 over 34 months.[22]

NAIL PSORIASIS

Good response was noted in two patients at 48 weeks of treatment with etanercept in case of nail psoriasis with Nail Psoriasis Severity Index (NAPSI) improvement of 92.9% and 56.6% as noted by Coelho et al.[23]

Mease et al., examined the efficacy of methotrexate monotherapy relative to that of etanercept monotherapy and their combination in 588 patients. There was no significant difference in modified NAPSI (mNAPSI) changes between the two monotherapies at week 24, while combining therapy showed a greater decrease in mNAPSI compared with methotrexate monotherapy (-1.7 vs. -1.1, $p = 0.02$).[20]

PSORIASIS WITH COMORBIDITIES

- *Psoriatic arthritis*: Mease et al., explored efficacy and safety of etanercept and reported improvement in ACR and PASI.[20]
- *Inflammatory bowel disease (IBD)*: Etanercept is not as effective. Adalimumab and infliximab are preferred TNF inhibitor for IBD
- *Malignancy*: TNF-α inhibitor may increase the risk of nonmelanoma skin cancer (NMSC).[24] It should be used when malignancy in remission for 5 years.
- *Cardiac diseases*: Wu and Poon reported less hazard ratio of myocardial infarction for patients with psoriasis who were treated with TNF-α inhibitor compared to those who were not.[25] TNF-α inhibitors are contraindicated in class 3 or 4 New York Heart Association (NYHA) congestive heart failure (CHF) patients.[26]
- *Multiple sclerosis*: TNF-α inhibitors are contraindicated in patients with MS.[27] Even though a causal relationship between TNF-α inhibitors and demyelinating diseases has not been established, there are many case reports (>50) and a case series of 15 patients having demyelinating disorder as optic neuritis, Guillain–Barré syndrome, multiple sclerosis, and others with this group of biologic.[28]
- *Systemic lupus erythematosus*: Drug-induced lupus is associated with etanercept.[29] Drug-induced lupus has been described in the literature with infliximab, etanercept, and adalimumab. Many patients on TNF-α inhibitors might show antinuclear antibody (ANA) positivity; however, in absence of clinical signs and symptoms it does not preclude the use of these drugs.[30]

OFF-LABEL DERMATOLOGIC USES

Off-label dermatologic uses of etanercept are presented in **Table 2**.

TABLE 2: Off-label dermatologic uses.	
Neutrophilic dermatoses	
Behçet's disease	Remission of oral ulcers treated with 25 mg twice weekly documented complete remission 3–5 weeks after starting treatment[31]
• Pyoderma gangrenosum (PG) • Granuloma annulare	• Etanercept was found to be as not effective as other tumor necrosis factor (TNF) antagonists in PG[31] • Generalized granuloma annulare—etanercept 50 mg biweekly for 12 weeks[32]
Necrobiosis lipoidica diabeticorum	Etanercept used 25 mg twice weekly after 6 days of surgical debridement along with prednisolone. Etanercept was continued for 16 months[33]
Sweet's syndrome	Complete clearance with subcutaneous etanercept 50 mg twice weekly and 25 mg twice weekly, both doses[34]
Graft-versus-host disease (GVHD)	
Acute GVHD	Complete remission of steroid-refractory acute GVHD with etanercept[35] and in case of acute GVHD after liver transplant with etanercept 25 mg subcutaneously for 8 weeks[36]
Chronic GVHD	Steroid dependent chronic GVHD treated with etanercept showed >50% of symptoms with etanercept 25 mg twice weekly for 4 weeks and then once weekly for subsequent 4 weeks[37,38]
Severe drug reactions	
Stevens–Johnson syndrome/toxic epidermal necrolysis (SJS/TEN)	• Single dose etanercept 50 mg was used by Nicola et al.[39] with good response • Etanercept was also found superior to corticosteroids[40] and along with systemic steroids, showed improved outcome[41] in SJS/TEN • Cui Cui Tain et al. showed in their study that conjunction with etanercept reduced the duration of hospitalization, exposure time of high dose steroids and overall amount of systemic steroid in patients with SJS/TEN[42] • Etanercept 50 mg subcutaneously along with single dose methylprednisolone 125 mg were used successfully to treat TEN and concurrent hyperinflammatory syndrome by Rachel et al[43]
Miscellaneous	
Vasculitis	Refractory giant cell arthritis,[44] deficiency of adenosine deaminase 2 diseases,[45] polyarteritis nodosa,[46] Takayasu's arteritis[47]
Hidradenitis suppurativa (HS)	Severe treatment refractory HS were treated with etanercept 25 mg twice weekly.[48] Adalimumab and infliximab are preferred
Pityriasis rubra pilaris	Etanercept was used in case of refractory pityriasis rubra pilaris[49]
Pulmonary sarcoidosis	Small phase II trial of etanercept[50] 25 mg subcutaneously twice weekly
Lupus pernio with arthropathy	Etanercept 25 mg twice weekly[51]

Continued

Continued

Mucous membrane pemphigoid	Etanercept 25 mg twice weekly, 6 doses along with oral prednisolone.[52] Rituximab is a preferred biologic
Scleroderma	Etanercept 25 mg subcutaneous twice weekly for 6 months showed clinical improvement.[53] Rituximab is a preferred biologic
Dermatomyositis	Alleviation of both skin and muscle symptoms with etanercept[54] with 25 mg weekly for a month, then 50 mg weekly for 6 months and 75 mg subsequently

AVAILABILITY

- *Trade name:* Enbrel
- *Marketed by:* Amgen, Wyeth, and Takeda
- *Biosimilars/Intended copies:* Intacept (Intas pharmaceuticals) and Etacept (Cipla)

BIOSIMILARS OF ETANERCEPT

- LBEC0101 had been developed as a biosimilar product.[55]
- The FDA-approved biosimilar Erelzi (etanercept-szzs). A phase III equivalence trial conducted in 531 adult patients with psoriasis comparing Erelzi to etanercept.[56]

PREPARATION

- Single use prefilled 25 mg (0.5 mL) and 50 mg syringe (1 mL). The pH of the solution is 6.3 ± 0.3.
- Preservative free lyophilized powder containing 25 mg/vial, reconstituted with 1 mL of bacteriostatic water supplied along with the vial.

STORAGE

It should be stored at 2–8°C and should not be frozen. It should be allowed to return to room temperature before injecting, to reduce the discomfort. It should be kept in the carton to protect from light. Shelf life is 36 months.

ADMINISTRATION

Site

- Anterior aspect of middle thigh, abdomen 5 cm away radius from umbilicus, and outer aspect of upper arm. Rotate injection site at least 1 inch from last injection site. Do not inject into a tender, bruised skin.
- The injection should be brought to room temperature before use.
- Injection site should be rotated at least 1 inch away from the last injection site.[57]

PRETREATMENT EVALUATION

Clinical
Rule out infections such as tuberculosis (TB), cardiac failure, and demyelinating disease.

Investigations
- Complete hemogram
- Urine routine and microscopic examination
- *Liver function tests (LFTs):* Including hepatitis B virus (HBV) and hepatitis C virus (HCV) panel
- Renal function test
- Chest X-ray, Mantoux test, and interferon gamma release assay (IGRA) test for TB
- Human immunodeficiency virus (HIV)
- Pregnancy test (urine or blood)

MONITORING DURING ETANERCEPT THERAPY

- Fortnightly for one month, monthly for 3 months and three monthly afterward
- Hemogram and LFT with enzymes
- Chest X-ray and IGRA annually

CONTRAINDICATIONS

- Known hypersensitivity
- Patients with active serious infections warranting systemic antibiotic therapy
- Pregnancy
- Children < 4 years
- *Cardiovascular disease*: CHF (NYHA III or IV)
- *Neurological disorders*: Contraindicated in patients with demyelinating diseases such as multiple sclerosis or with first-degree relative with such disease and seizure disorder
- *Malignancy*: Anti-TNF treatment should be avoided in patients with a current or previous history of malignancy, unless there is a high likelihood of cure or the malignancy was diagnosed and treated >10 years ago.
- Any concurrent administration of IL-1 receptor antagonist
- *TB*: Patient with active TB should not be given etanercept. Those with latent TB should be treated with single drug or two drugs antitubercular treatment before initiating etanercept. Etanercept can be started 2 months after starting treatment.

DRUG INTERACTIONS

Etanercept is metabolized by proteolysis. Hence it does not interfere with metabolism or excretion of most of the drugs. Trials with anakinra along with etanercept showed increased risk of serious infections.[58]

SPECIAL SITUATIONS

Pregnancy and Lactation

It is a category B drug. Etanercept concentration in umbilical cord serum was 3–32% of the maternal serum when mother was exposed during pregnancy, suggesting low transplacental transmission.[59] Breast milk concentration is very low and it is undetectable in child's serum.[60] Registry data published by Hyrich et al. included 32 patients who were exposed to anti-TNF-α therapy during pregnancy. 91% patients elected to continue pregnancy and out of these 76% delivered healthy child and 24% had first-trimester abortions. There is no evidence of maternal harm or major congenital malformations. Although they are likely to be safe in pregnancy but it is to be used with caution.[61]

Pediatric Population

In November 2016, the FDA approved etanercept for management of psoriasis in pediatric population (4–17 years), making it first biologic to be approved for management of pediatric psoriasis. It is the FDA approved for management of JIA in children older than 2 years. Dose to be used is 0.8 mg/kg/week, maximum being 50 mg/week. Etanercept is safe, effective, and has sustained benefit up to 5 years in management of psoriasis.[62,63]

Level of evidence 1b and strength of recommendation A of etanercept in case of pediatric patients (adapted from Oxford Centre for Evidence-Based Medicine, 2011) **(Table 3)**.

Geriatric Population

To be used cautiously in elderly population in general.

Use in Diabetic Patients

Reports of hypoglycemia following initiation of treatment.

TABLE 3: Etanercept in pediatric patient.		
Recommendation	Level of evidence	References
Etanercept for pediatric patients (>6 years age)	I–III	Paller et al. (2016)[63]
Etanercept dose • 0.8 mg/kg/week • 0.4 mg/kg 2×/week • *Maximum dose*: 50 mg/week	I and III	Hawrot et al. (2006)[64]

Hepatitis B and C Infection

Etanercept can cause reactivation of hepatitis B and C infection. All patients should be screened for hepatitis B before administering etanercept and in chronic hepatitis B carrier, it should be given along with antiviral therapy. Transaminases should be monitored during entire therapy.

Anti-TNF-α therapy is safe in patients with chronic HCV infection; however, close monitoring of transaminases and viral load are indicated in these patients.[65]

Immunization

Live vaccines should not be given concurrently with etanercept.

Human Immunodeficiency Virus Infection

There is limited experience for use of etanercept in HIV positive patients. Existing literature suggests that etanercept can be safely used in HIV seropositive patients, even without concomitant antiretroviral therapy. A phase I study in 16 patients with HIV-associated TB were treated with 25 mg twice weekly for 24 weeks etanercept along with anti-TB treatment.[66] However, CD4 count and viral load should be closely monitored in this scenario and antiretroviral therapy should be used concomitantly.[67]

CONCLUSION

Etanercept is one of the most widely used biologic and has excellent safety records. It can be used in special population. It can be used intermittently or continuously without loss of efficacy and can be combined with conventional therapy. Biosimilars of etanercept are emerging on the market.

REFERENCES

1. Leonardi CL, Powers JL, Matheson RT, Goffe BS, Zitnik R, Wang A, et al. Etanercept as monotherapy in patients with psoriasis. N Engl J Med. 2003;349(21):2014-22.
2. Krueger JG. The immunologic basis for the treatment of psoriasis with new biologic agents. J Am Acad Dermatol. 2002;46(1):1-23.
3. Keystone EC. Safety of biologic therapies--an update. J Rheumatol Suppl. 2005;74:8-12.
4. Mease P. Psoriatic arthritis: the role of TNF inhibition and the effect of its inhibition with etanercept. Clin Exp Rheumatol. 2002;20(6 Suppl 28):S116-121.
5. Papp KA, Tyring S, Lahfa M, Prinz J, Griffiths CEM, Nakanishi AM, et al. A global phase III randomized controlled trial of etanercept in psoriasis: safety, efficacy, and effect of dose reduction. Br J Dermatol. 2005;152(6):1304-12.
6. Kivelevitch D, Mansouri B, Menter A. Long term efficacy and safety of etanercept in the treatment of psoriasis and psoriatic arthritis. Biologics. 2014;8:169-82.
7. Feldman SR, Kimball AB, Krueger GG, Woolley JM, Lalla D, Jahreis A. Etanercept improves the health-related quality of life of patients with psoriasis: results of a phase III randomized clinical trial. J Am Acad Dermatol. 2005;53(5):887-9.
8. Gottlieb AB, Langley RG, Strober BE, Papp KA, Klekotka P, Creamer K, et al. A randomized, double-blind, placebo-controlled study to evaluate the addition of methotrexate

to etanercept in patients with moderate to severe plaque psoriasis. Br J Dermatol. 2012;167(3):649-57.
9. Smith ECA, Riddle C, Menter MA, Lebwohl M. Combining systemic retinoids with biologic agents for moderate to severe psoriasis. Int J Dermatol. 2008;47(5):514-8.
10. Lee JH, Youn JI, Kim TY, Choi JH, Park CJ, Choe YB, et al. A multicenter, randomized, open-label pilot trial assessing the efficacy and safety of etanercept 50 mg twice weekly followed by etanercept 25 mg twice weekly, the combination of etanercept 25 mg twice weekly and acitretin, and acitretin alone in patients with moderate to severe psoriasis. BMC Dermatol. 2016;16:11.
11. De Simone C, D'Agostino M, Capizzi R, Capponi A, Venier A, Caldarola G. Combined treatment with etanercept 50 mg once weekly and narrow-band ultraviolet B phototherapy in chronic plaque psoriasis. Eur J Dermatol. 2011;21(4):568-72.
12. Gambichler T, Tigges C, Scola N, Weber J, Skrygan M, Bechara FG, et al. Etanercept plus narrowband ultraviolet B phototherapy of psoriasis is more effective than etanercept monotherapy at 6 weeks. Br J Dermatol. 2011;164(6):1383-6.
13. Montfort A, Colacios C, Levade T, Andrieu-Abadie N, Meyer N, Ségui B. The TNF paradox in cancer progression and immunotherapy. Front Immunol. 2019;10:1818.
14. Patel RV, Clark LN, Lebwohl M, Weinberg JM. Treatments for psoriasis and the risk of malignancy. J Am Acad Dermatol. 2009;60(6):1001-17.
15. Moore A, Gordon KB, Kang S, Gottlieb A, Freundlich B, Xia HA, et al. A randomized, open-label trial of continuous versus interrupted etanercept therapy in the treatment of psoriasis. J Am Acad Dermatol. 2007;56(4):598-603.
16. Gordon KB, Gottlieb AB, Leonardi CL, Elewski BE, Wang A, Jahreis A, et al. Clinical response in psoriasis patients discontinued from and then reinitiated on etanercept therapy. J Dermatol Treat. 2006;17(1):9-17.
17. Sterry W, Ortonne JP, Kirkham B, Brocq O, Robertson D, Pedersen RD, et al. Comparison of two etanercept regimens for treatment of psoriasis and psoriatic arthritis: PRESTA randomised double blind multicentre trial. BMJ. 2010;340:c147.
18. Esposito M, Gisondi P, Cassano N, Ferrucci G, Del Giglio M, Loconsole F, et al. Survival rate of antitumour necrosis factor-α treatments for psoriasis in routine dermatological practice: a multicentre observational study. Br J Dermatol. 2013;169(3):666-72.
19. Santoleri F, Romagnoli A, Costantini A. Adalimumab and etanercept adherence, persistence and switch in the treatment of psoriatic arthritis: 10-year real-life analysis. Expert Opin Drug Saf. 2020;19(1):93-7.
20. Mease PJ, Gladman DD, Collier DH, Ritchlin CT, Helliwell PS, Liu L, et al. Etanercept and Methotrexate as Monotherapy or in Combination for Psoriatic Arthritis: Primary Results From a Randomized, Controlled Phase III Trial. Arthritis Rheumatol. 2019;71(7):1112-24.
21. Talat H, Wahid Z, Feroz F, Sajid M. Erythrodermic Psoriasis and Hepatitis C Infection Treated with Pegylated Interferon and Anti-TNFα α(Etanercept) Therapy. J Coll Physicians Surg Pak. 2017;27(9):S77-9.
22. Romero-Maté A, García-Donoso C, Martinez-Morán C, Hernández-Núñez A, Borbujo J. Long-term management of erythrodermic psoriasis with anti-TNF agents. Dermatol Online J. 2010;16(6):15.
23. Coelho JD, Diamantino F, Lestre S, Ferreira AM. Treatment of severe nail psoriasis with etanercept. Indian J Dermatol Venereol Leprol. 2011;77:72.
24. Asgari MM, Ray GT, Geier JL, Quesenberry CP. Malignancy rates in a large cohort of patients with systemically treated psoriasis in a managed care population. J Am Acad Dermatol. 2017;76(4):632-8.
25. Wu JJ, Poon KYT, Channual JC, Shen AYJ. Association between tumor necrosis factor inhibitor therapy and myocardial infarction risk in patients with psoriasis. Arch Dermatol. 2012;148(11):1244-50.
26. Desai SB, Furst DE. Problems encountered during anti-tumour necrosis factor therapy. Best Pract Res Clin Rheumatol. 2006;20(4):757-90.

27. Tristano AG. Neurological adverse events associated with anti-tumor necrosis factor α treatment. J Neurol. 2010;257(9):1421-31.
28. Bechtel M, Sanders C, Bechtel A. Neurological complications of biologic therapy in psoriasis: a review. J Clin Aesthet Dermatol. 2009;2(11):27-32.
29. Shakoor N, Michalska M, Harris CA, Block JA. Drug-induced systemic lupus erythematosus associated with etanercept therapy. Lancet Lond Engl. 2002;359(9306):579-80.
30. Costa MF, Said NR, Zimmermann B. Drug-induced lupus due to anti-tumor necrosis factor α agents. Semin Arthritis Rheum. 2008;37(6):381-7.
31. Scheinberg MA. Treatment of recurrent oral aphthous ulcers with etanercept. Clin Exp Rheumatol. 2002;20(5):733-4.
32. Hubbard VG, Friedmann AC, Goldsmith P. Systemic pyoderma gangrenosum responding to infliximab and adalimumab. Br J Dermatol. 2005;152(5):1059-61.
33. Shupack J, Siu K. Resolving Granuloma Annulare with Etanercept. Arch Dermatol. 2006;142(3):393-403.
34. Cummins DL, Hiatt KM, Mimouni D, Vander Kolk CA, Cohen BA, Nousari CH. Generalized necrobiosis lipoidica treated with a combination of split-thickness autografting and immunomodulatory therapy. Int J Dermatol. 2004;43(11):852-4.
35. Yamauchi PS, Turner L, Lowe NJ, Gindi V, Jackson JM. Treatment of recurrent Sweet's syndrome with coexisting rheumatoid arthritis with the tumor necrosis factor antagonist etanercept. J Am Acad Dermatol. 2006;54(3 Suppl 2):S122-126.
36. Andolina M, Rabusin M, Maximova N, Di Leo G. Etanercept in graft-versus-host disease. Bone Marrow Transplant. 2000;26(8):929.
37. Thin L, Macquillan G, Adams L, Garas G, Seow C, Cannell P, et al. Acute graft-versus-host disease after liver transplant: novel use of etanercept and the role of tumor necrosis factor alpha inhibitors. Liver Transpl. 2009;15(4):421-6.
38. Chiang KY, Abhyankar S, Bridges K, Godder K, Henslee-Downey JP. Recombinant human tumor necrosis factor receptor fusion protein as complementary treatment for chronic graft-versus-host disease. Transplantation. 2002;73(4):665-7.
39. Natsis N, Ikediobi O, Dorschner R. 31783 Etanercept in toxic epidermal necrolysis: In support of standard of care. J Am Acad Dermatol. 2022;87(3):AB56.
40. Cw W, Ly Y, Cb C, Hc H, Si H, Ch Y, et al. Randomized, controlled trial of TNF-α antagonist in CTL-mediated severe cutaneous adverse reactions. J Clin Invest. 2018;128(3):985-96.
41. Ao S, Gao X, Zhan J, Ai L, Li M, Su H, et al. Inhibition of tumor necrosis factor improves conventional steroid therapy for Stevens-Johnson syndrome/toxic epidermal necrolysis in a cohort of patients. J Am Acad Dermatol. 2022;86(6):1236-45.
42. Tian CC, Ai XC, Ma JC, Hu FQ, Liu XT, Luo YJ, et al. Etanercept treatment of Stevens-Johnson syndrome and toxic epidermal necrolysis. Ann Allergy Asthma Immunol. 2022;129(3):360-365.e1.
43. Choi R, Garritano J, Laird M, Johnston M, Tkachenko E, Damsky W, et al. Treatment of toxic epidermal necrolysis and concurrent COVID-19-associated hyperinflammatory syndrome with systemic corticosteroids and etanercept. JAAD Case Rep. 2022;29:139-41.
44. Fujita M, Tabuchi Y, Yagita M. Successful treatment of refractory giant cell arteritis with etanercept. Rheumatol Int. 2016;36(8):1177-9.
45. Pichard DC, Ombrello AK, Hoffmann P, Stone DL, Cowen EW. Early Onset Stroke, Polyarteritis Nodosa, and Livedo Racemosa. J Am Acad Dermatol. 2016;75(2):449-53.
46. Valor L, Monteagudo I, de la Torre I, Fernández CG, Montoro M, Longo JL, et al. Young male patient diagnosed with cutaneous polyarteritis nodosa successfully treated with etanercept. Mod Rheumatol. 2014;24(4):688-9.
47. Comarmond C, Plaisier E, Dahan K, Mirault T, Emmerich J, Amoura Z, et al. Anti TNF-α in refractory Takayasu's arteritis: cases series and review of the literature. Autoimmun Rev. 2012;11(9):678-84.
48. Cusack C, Buckley C. Etanercept: effective in the management of hidradenitis suppurativa. Br J Dermatol. 2006;154(4):726-9.

49. Petrof G, Almaani N, Archer CB, Griffiths WAD, Smith CH. A systematic review of the literature on the treatment of pityriasis rubra pilaris type 1 with TNF-antagonists. J Eur Acad Dermatol Venereol. 2013;27(1):e131-5.
50. Utz JP, Limper AH, Kalra S, Specks U, Scott JP, Vuk-Pavlovic Z, et al. Etanercept for the treatment of stage II and III progressive pulmonary sarcoidosis. Chest. 2003;124(1):177-85.
51. Khanna D, Liebling MR, Louie JS. Etanercept ameliorates sarcoidosis arthritis and skin disease. J Rheumatol. 2003;30(8):1864-7.
52. Canizares MJ, Smith DI, Conners MS, Maverick KJ, Heffernan MP. Successful Treatment of Mucous Membrane Pemphigoid with Etanercept in 3 Patients. Arch Dermatol. 2006;142(11):1457-61.
53. Sapadin AN, Fleischmajer R. Treatment of Scleroderma. Arch Dermatol. 2002;138(1):99-105.
54. Norman R, Greenberg RG, Jackson JM. Case reports of etanercept in inflammatory dermatoses. J Am Acad Dermatol. 2006;54(3 Suppl 2):S139-142.
55. Song YW, Park YB, Kim J. LBEC0101, an etanercept biosimilar for the treatment of rheumatoid arthritis. Expert Opin Biol Ther. 2021;21(1):1-8.
56. Hung A, Vu Q, Mostovoy L. A Systematic Review of U.S. Biosimilar Approvals: What Evidence Does the FDA Require and How Are Manufacturers Responding? J Manag Care Spec Pharm. 2017;23(12):10.
57. Yamauchi PS, Gindi V, Lowe NJ. The treatment of psoriasis and psoriatic arthritis with etanercept: practical considerations on monotherapy, combination therapy, and safety. Dermatol Clin. 2004;22(4):449-59.
58. Burls A, Jobanputra P. The trials of anakinra. Lancet. 2004;364(9437):827-8.
59. Nishide M, Yagita M, Kumanogoh A. Continuous Use of Etanercept During Pregnancy Does Not Affect TNF-Alpha Levels in Umbilical Cord Blood. Biol Targets Ther. 2022;16:17-9.
60. Berthelsen BG, Fjeldsøe-Nielsen H, Nielsen CT, Hellmuth E. Etanercept concentrations in maternal serum, umbilical cord serum, breast milk and child serum during breastfeeding. Rheumatol Oxf Engl. 2010;49(11):2225-7.
61. Hyrich KL, Symmons DPM, Watson KD, Silman AJ; British Society, for Rheumatology Biologics Register. Pregnancy outcome in women who were exposed to anti-tumor necrosis factor agents: results from a national population register. Arthritis Rheum. 2006;54(8):2701-2.
62. Bellodi Schmidt F, Shah KN. Biologic response modifiers and pediatric psoriasis. Pediatr Dermatol. 2015;32(3):303-20.
63. Paller AS, Siegfried EC, Pariser DM, Rice KC, Trivedi M, Iles J, et al. Long-term safety and efficacy of etanercept in children and adolescents with plaque psoriasis. J Am Acad Dermatol. 2016;74(2):280-7.e1-3.
64. Hawrot AC, Metry DW, Theos AJ, Levy ML. Etanercept for psoriasis in the pediatric population: experience in nine patients. Pediatr Dermatol. 2006;23(1):67-71.
65. Salvi M, Macaluso L, Luci C, Mattozzi C, Paolino G, Aprea Y, et al. Safety and efficacy of anti-tumor necrosis factors α in patients with psoriasis and chronic hepatitis C. World J Clin Cases. 2016;4(2):49-55.
66. Wallis RS, Kyambadde P, Johnson JL, Horter L, Kittle R, Pohle M, et al. A study of the safety, immunology, virology, and microbiology of adjunctive etanercept in HIV-1-associated tuberculosis. AIDS Lond Engl. 2004;18(2):257-64.
67. Clinicalinfo.HIV.gov. (2022). Plasma HIV-1 RNA (Viral Load) and CD4 Count Monitoring. [online] Available from https://clinicalinfo.hiv.gov/en/guidelines/hiv-clinical-guidelines-adult-and-adolescent-arv/plasma-hiv-1-rna-cd4-monitoring. [Last accessed January, 2024].

CHAPTER 6

Infliximab

Biju Vasudevan, Shekhar Neema

INTRODUCTION

Infliximab is chimeric (25% mouse and 75% human) monoclonal antibody against tumor necrosis factor alpha (TNF-α). It was approved for treatment of Crohn's disease in 1998 and was subsequently approved for ulcerative colitis, ankylosing spondylitis, rheumatoid arthritis, psoriatic arthritis (PsA), and chronic plaque psoriasis.

PHARMACOLOGY

Infliximab is an immunoglobulin G (IgG)-1 monoclonal antibody which neutralizes both soluble and receptor bound TNF-α, it does not neutralize TNF-β. It being a protein, it is not metabolized by cytochrome P450 enzymes. Because of this advantage, the development of different toxic or inactive metabolites following genetic polymorphisms of P450 isoenzymes and the consequent variability in metabolism are reduced. In comparison to the small molecules, the likelihood of complex drug interactions is less.

CHARACTERISTICS

- *Molecular weight:* 150 kDa
- *Half-life:* 7 days in 5 mg/kg group, 9 days in 10 mg/kg group
- Distribution in vascular compartment and metabolized by proteolysis.

USES

- *Food and Drug Administration (FDA)-approved indications*:
  - Chronic plaque psoriasis
  - Psoriatic arthritis

- *Off-label indications*:
  - Erythrodermic psoriasis and generalized pustular psoriasis (approved in Japan)
  - Nail psoriasis
  - Hidradenitis suppurativa
  - Synovitis, acne, pustulosis, hyperostosis, and osteitis (SAPHO) syndrome
  - Neutrophilic dermatoses: Pyoderma gangrenosum and Behçet's disease
  - Systemic vasculitis
  - Granulomatous dermatoses: Sarcoidosis and granuloma annulare
  - Connective tissue diseases: Dermatomyositis, scleroderma, and systemic lupus erythematosus (SLE)
  - Graft-versus-host disease (GVHD), toxic epidermal necrolysis (TEN), Reiter's disease, and pityriasis rubra pilaris (PRP).

Psoriasis

Infliximab was approved for management of chronic plaque psoriasis by the FDA in September 2006. It is administered in dose of 3–5 mg/kg on 0, 2, and 6 weeks and thereafter every 8 weeks. Improvement is assessed by psoriasis area and severity index (PASI) and 75% improvement in PASI from baseline (PASI 75) is a standard measure of efficacy of the drug used for treatment of psoriasis **(Table 1)**.

- *Continuous therapy or intermittent therapy:* Intermittent therapy or as and when infusion is more practical in our scenario where economic constraints prevail over best possible options. Menter et al. published data in 2004 on continuous and intermittent therapy of infliximab in 3 mg/kg and 5 mg/kg group. PASI 75 response was better maintained in continuous therapy group (5 mg/kg—89.6%, 3 mg/kg—80.6%) as compared to intermittent group (5 mg/kg—76.4%, 3 mg/kg—72.4%). Development of antidrug antibody (ADA) is associated with infusion reaction and loss of response. ADAs were detected in 35.8% and 41.5% patients in 5 mg/kg in continuous and intermittent group and 51.5% and 46.2% in 3 mg/kg in

TABLE 1: Efficacy of infliximab in chronic plaque psoriasis.

Dose	PASI 75	PASI 90	Reference
5 mg/kg	80% (after 10 weeks)	57% (after 10 weeks)	EXPRESS (2005)[1]
	• PASI 75 and 90 was sustained till week 50 • In this study, patient also showed significant improvement in nail psoriasis. Improvement in nail psoriasis and severity index in 42% patients		
3 mg/kg	72% (after 10 weeks)		Gottlieb AB (2004)[2]
	Improvement was observed as early as 2 weeks		

(PASI: psoriasis area and severity index)

continuous and intermittent group.[3] Another study, conducted by Reich et al. (RESTORE2) in which patients were randomized to receive 5 mg/kg infliximab as continuous or intermittent therapy. Study was terminated because of high incidence of infusion reaction in intermittent group.[4]

- *Adherence and drug survival:* Adherence is very important for treatment success. Apart from economic considerations, there are various other factors such as safety and efficacy which result in treatment discontinuation in real world. Etanercept showed longest survival (1,565 days), followed by infliximab (1,120 days) and adalimumab (1,056 days) in a retrospective study. Most common cause for drug discontinuation was lack of efficacy. Discontinuation due to adverse effect was highest with infliximab followed by adalimumab and etanercept.[5] Higher severity at the disease onset (PASI >12), high level of initial psoriasis clearance (PASI 90) and combination of methotrexate are independent predictor of long-term survival of infliximab in real life.[6]
- *Dose escalation*: Loss of efficacy is a common problem with infliximab due to development of antidrug antibodies. Many patients with loss of efficacy have low serum trough levels. Dose escalation of infliximab to 10 mg/kg is an important treatment strategy in these patients. A Japanese study conducted by Torii et al. found that higher dosage leads to meaningful response in patients who fail to respond to standard dosage regimen.[7]
- *Combination treatment*: Infliximab can be combined with low dose methotrexate, acitretin, and narrow band ultraviolet B therapy in management of psoriasis. Methotrexate reduced development of antidrug antibodies and increases drug survival. Acitretin is treatment of choice in generalized pustular psoriasis and can be combined with infliximab when rapid control of the disease is desired.[8,9]

Psoriatic Arthritis

Psoriatic arthritis develops in almost 30% patients with psoriasis. Infliximab was approved by the FDA for treatment of PsA in 2005. PsA treatment is assessed by the American College of Rheumatology (ACR) criteria. ACR 20, ACR 50, and ACR 70 signifies >20%, 50%, and 70% improvement, respectively. Treatment with infliximab at 5 mg/kg resulted in ACR 20, ACR 50, and ACR 70 in 65%, 46% and 29% at the end of 16 weeks. This improvement was sustained till week 50 [infliximab multinational psoriatic arthritis controlled trial (IMPACT) study].[10] Another study which was conducted with larger sample size (IMPACT II) had similar effect in improvement of PsA. It also showed improvement in enthesopathy, quality of life, and delayed radiographic progression of PsA.[11]

Off-label Indications

- *Erythrodermic psoriasis and generalized pustular psoriasis*: Infliximab is considered biologic of choice in the management of these severe forms of psoriasis. It is approved in Japan for the management of both erythrodermic and generalized pustular psoriasis. It leads to rapid and sustained response in erythrodermic as well as generalized pustular psoriasis.[12]

- *Nail psoriasis*: An open-label study of infliximab in psoriasis patients with recalcitrant nail involvement showed improvement in most cases after 22 weeks of treatment, however, complete clearance was seen in only 10% patients.[13] A network meta-analysis comparing all biologics for the treatment of nail psoriasis found ixekizumab to be most effective and infliximab to be least effective biologic in the management of nail psoriasis.[14]
- *Hidradenitis suppurativa*:
  - Infliximab has been used successfully for management of hidradenitis suppurativa not responding to topical and systemic antibiotics.
  - Dose: 5 mg/kg on 0, 2, and 6 weeks results in almost 50% improvement after 8 weeks of initial infusion in 26% patients. There is moderate to marked improvement in induration, sinus discharge and pain in 3–7 days after every infusion.[15]
  - Adalimumab is the FDA approved for the treatment of hidradenitis suppurativa. Dose used is 160 mg subcutaneous on day 0, 80 mg on day 15 followed by 40 mg weekly starting on day 29.[16]
- *Neutrophilic dermatoses*: It can be used for management of pyoderma gangrenosum not responding to prednisolone and other immunosuppressive agents. It has also been used for management of sight threatening uveitis in Behçet's disease.[17,18]
- *Systemic vasculitis*: It can be used as salvage therapy in management of refractory systemic vasculitides such as Wegener's granulomatosis and microscopic polyangiitis.[19]
- *Granulomatous dermatoses*: Refractory sarcoidosis has been treated with infliximab. However, tuberculosis needs to be ruled out objectively before administering infliximab as it increases the risk of reactivation of latent tuberculosis. Infliximab has also been used for management of recalcitrant granuloma annulare, which does not respond to first-line therapy.[20,21]
- *Connective tissue diseases*:
  - Dermatomyositis: It can be used for management of dermatomyositis refractory to treatment such as corticosteroids, methotrexate, cyclosporine, intravenous immunoglobulin, azathioprine, and cyclophosphamide.[22,23]
- *Miscellaneous*:
  - GVHD: Infliximab has been used for management of acute GVHD not responding to steroids. However, phase III study showed no benefit from addition of infliximab to steroids in management of early acute GVHD.[24]

- TEN: Single dose infliximab 5 mg/kg early in disease has resulted in rapid improvement in TEN in many case reports. However, the risk of infection remains high with use of this modality for the treatment of TEN.[25]
- Reiter's syndrome: Infliximab can be used for management of cutaneous and joint manifestation of Reiter's syndrome, not responding to steroids and methotrexate.[26]
- PRP: It has been used successfully for management of type 1 adult PRP not responding to acitretin, methotrexate and cyclosporine or as first-line therapy for management of PRP.[27]

ADMINISTRATION

- Available as 100 mg lyophilized powder in 20 mL vial.
- Lyophilized powder is stored in refrigerator and reconstituted with 10 mL sterile water.
- Administered as intravenous infusion at the dose of 3–5 mg/kg at 0, 2, 6 weeks and 8 weekly thereafter.
- Total dose required after reconstitution is mixed in 250 mL normal saline and infused over not <2 hours and ideally over 4 hours.
- Infusion should be started within 3 hours of reconstitution.
- Premedication with hydrocortisone, pheniramine and paracetamol should be done to reduce the risk and severity of infusion reactions.

Tests to be done Prior to Administration

- Complete blood count (CBC)
- Liver function test (LFT)
- Blood urea and serum creatinine
- Hepatitis B surface antigen and anti-hepatitis C virus immunoglobulin M
- *Rule out active and latent tuberculosis:*
  - History of past tuberculosis, history of contact with active case of tuberculosis
  - History of fever, weight loss, and night sweats
  - Chest X-ray posteroanterior (PA) view
  - Purified protein derivative (PPD) or interferon-gamma release assays (IGRAs)

MONITORING DURING INFLIXIMAB THERAPY

Patients who are on infliximab should be closely monitored for infusion-related reactions and development of any infection, especially tuberculosis. Patients have high-risk of development of extrapulmonary or disseminated tuberculosis and should be asked for history of weight loss, fever and night sweats during each visit.

- CBC and LFT—before every infusion
- Chest X-ray PA view and IGRA—annually

ADVERSE EFFECTS

- *Infusion reaction*:
    - Defined as reaction occurring during infusion or within 1 hour after infusion. It is the most common adverse reaction seen in approximately 20% patients.
    - Fever and chills are most common symptoms of infusion reaction, other rare symptoms being cardiopulmonary symptoms (chest pain, hypotension, and dyspnea), pruritus, and urticaria.
    - Serious infusion reactions are seen in <1% of patients and includes anaphylaxis, convulsions, and hypotension.
    - Patient who develops antidrug antibodies have higher risk of infusion reaction. Concomitant immunosuppressive medication reduces the severity of infusion reaction.
    - Patient who are on long-term maintenance therapy have less risk of development of infusion reaction as compared to patients who are on intermittent therapy.
- *Antidrug antibodies*:
    - Anti-infliximab antibodies develop in almost 40% patients within 1 year of therapy.
    - Development of antidrug antibodies is associated with loss of efficacy. Concomitant use of immunosuppressive therapy such as methotrexate, cyclosporine, and azathioprine can reduce the formation of antidrug antibodies and addition of an immunomodulator can restore clinical response with anti-TNF-α blockers.[28,29]
- *Infections*:
    - Tuberculosis: Increased risk of reactivation of latent tuberculosis by almost 20 times and also of extrapulmonary and disseminated tuberculosis.[30]
    - Invasive fungal infections: Increased risk of development of disseminated candidiasis, histoplasmosis, and invasive aspergillosis.[31]
    - Hepatitis B infection: Patient with chronic carrier state due to hepatitis B, when administered infliximab can lead to reactivation of hepatitis B and liver failure.[32]
- *Malignancy*: There has been concern that anti-TNF-α drugs can lead to increase in risk of development of malignancies. However, meta-analyses and literature evaluation does not either refute or verify the risk of development of malignancies resulting from use of anti-TNF-α blockers.[33]
- *Congestive heart failure*: It can cause worsening of heart failure. Contraindicated in patients with the New York Heart Association (NYHA) class III or IV failure.[34]

- *Demyelinating diseases*: There are various reports of diseases such as multiple sclerosis (MS), optic neuritis, and Guillain–Barré syndrome developing in patients who were administered infliximab. Use of TNF-α blockers can lead to worsening of MS. It can also lead to unmasking of MS in patient with family history of demyelinating disorders.[35]
- *Hepatotoxicity*: Anti-TNF-α drugs are an uncommon cause of drug-induced liver injury (DILI). It can result in both hepatocellular as well as cholestatic type of DILI; however, hepatocellular injury is more common. Infliximab is more common cause of DILI out of etanercept, adalimumab, and infliximab. Majority of cases of DILI are autoimmune type with positive antinuclear antibody (ANA) and anti-smooth muscle antibody.[36]
- *Autoimmunity*: ANA and anti-double-stranded deoxyribonucleic acid (DNA) positivity can be seen in almost 60% and 10% patients on infliximab, respectively. However, development of clinical SLE is very rare.
- *Serum sickness type reaction*: Since infliximab is a chimeric protein, it can result in serum sickness type of reaction, especially when it is used intermittently. Patient presents with fever, severe joint pains, and myalgia 3–10 days after infliximab infusion and these symptoms cannot be explained by an alternative diagnosis.[37]
- *Induction of psoriasis by infliximab*: Use of anti-TNF-α drugs can lead to paradoxical induction of psoriasis in patients with inflammatory bowel disease.[38]

CONTRAINDICATIONS

- *Absolute*: Hypersensitivity to murine proteins and active infections
- *Relative*: Congestive heart failure and family history of demyelinating disease

SPECIAL SITUATIONS

- *Pregnancy and lactation*: It is pregnancy category B drug and has been safely used even intentionally during pregnancy without fetal harm. However, infliximab passes through placenta and live vaccines should be avoided in neonates for 6 months whose mother have been given infliximab during pregnancy.[39] Infliximab should be stopped at 16 weeks of pregnancy to reduce risk of neonatal immunosuppression.
- *Children*: Approved for use in children >6 years old in Crohn's disease and ulcerative colitis. Can also be used in psoriasis in children if clinically indicated.
- *Latent tuberculosis*: Infliximab should not be used in patient with latent tuberculosis (PPD or IGRA positive), because of high-risk of reactivation of tuberculosis. Patient should be treated with isoniazid monotherapy for 6–9 months or isoniazid-rifampicin for 3–4 months. Infliximab therapy can be initiated once treatment for latent tuberculosis infection has been completed for at least 2 months.

- *Hepatitis B and hepatitis C infection*: Infliximab can lead to flare of hepatitis in patients with chronic hepatitis B carrier state. It should be used cautiously in patient with chronic carrier state, in consultation with hepatologist. Regular monitoring of aminotransferases and prophylactic antiviral therapy should be used if indicated.

    Patients with chronic hepatitis C generally do not develop acute flare due to use of infliximab; however, caution during use of infliximab in patient with chronic hepatitis C carrier is important.[40]
- *Human immunodeficiency infection*: Infliximab should not be used in patients who are human immunodeficiency virus (HIV) positive. However, in patient in whom it is clinically indicated it can be used along with antiretroviral therapy.[41]
- *Immunization*: Live vaccines should be avoided while patient is on infliximab therapy. Patient should be immunized against hepatitis B, pneumococcus, and influenza prior to initiation of therapy.

CONCLUSION

Infliximab is an effective drug when rapid control of the psoriasis is required. It is also very effective in the management of severe forms of psoriasis such as generalized pustular psoriasis and erythrodermic psoriasis. Use of infliximab requires screening for infections particularly latent tuberculosis infection and monitoring during infusion. While contemplating infliximab use, patient should be primed for continuous therapy rather than as when required.

REFERENCES

1. Reich K, Nestle FO, Papp K, Ortonne JP, Evans R, Guzzo C, et al; EXPRESS study investigators. Infliximab induction and maintenance therapy for moderate-to-severe psoriasis: a phase III, multicentre, double-blind trial. Lancet. 2005;366(9494):1367-74.
2. Gottlieb AB, Evans R, Li S, Dooley LT, Guzzo CA, Baker D, et al. Infliximab induction therapy for patients with severe plaque-type psoriasis: a randomized, double-blind, placebo-controlled trial. J Am Acad Dermatol. 2004;51(4):534-42.
3. Menter A, Feldman SR, Weinstein GD, Papp K, Evans R, Guzzo C, et al. A randomized comparison of continuous vs. intermittent infliximab maintenance regimens over 1 year in the treatment of moderate-to-severe plaque psoriasis. J Am Acad Dermatol. 2007;56(1):31-e1.
4. Reich K, Wozel G, Zheng H, van Hoogstraten HJF, Flint L, Barker J. Efficacy and safety of infliximab as continuous or intermittent therapy in patients with moderate-to-severe plaque psoriasis: results of a randomized, long-term extension trial (RESTORE2). Br J Dermatol. 2013;168(6):1325-34.
5. Esposito M, Gisondi P, Cassano N, Ferrucci G, Del Giglio M, Loconsole F, et al. Survival rate of antitumour necrosis factor-α treatments for psoriasis in routine dermatological practice: a multicentre observational study. Br J Dermatol. 2013;169(3):666-72.
6. Reich K, Conrad C, Kristensen LE, Smith SD, Puig L, Rich P, et al. Network meta-analysis comparing the efficacy of biologic treatments for achieving complete resolution of nail psoriasis. J Dermatolog Treat. 2022;33(3):1652-60.

7. Torii H, Nakano M, Yano T, Kondo K, Nakagawa H; SPREAD Study Group. Efficacy and safety of dose escalation of infliximab therapy in Japanese patients with psoriasis: Results of the SPREAD study. J Dermatol. 2017;44(5):552-9.
8. Kołt-Kamińska M, Żychowska M, Reich A. Infliximab in Combination with Low-Dose Acitretin in Generalized Pustular Psoriasis: A Report of Two Cases and Review of the Literature. Biologics. 2021;15:317-27.
9. Skrabl-Baumgartner A, Weger W, Salmhofer W, Jahnel J. Childhood generalized pustular psoriasis: longtime remission with combined infliximab and methotrexate treatment. Pediatr Dermatol. 2015;32(1):e13-4.
10. Antoni CE, Kavanaugh A, Kirkham B, Tutuncu Z, Burmester GR, Schneider U, et al. Sustained benefits of infliximab therapy for dermatologic and articular manifestations of psoriatic arthritis: results from the infliximab multinational psoriatic arthritis controlled trial (IMPACT). Arthritis Rheum. 2005;52(4):1227-36.
11. Antoni C, Krueger GG, de Vlam K, Birbara C, Beutler A, Guzzo X, et al. Infliximab improves signs and symptoms of psoriatic arthritis: results of the IMPACT 2 trial. Ann Rheum Dis. 2005;64(8):1150-7.
12. Torii H, Nakagawa H; Japanese Infliximab Study Investigators. Long-term study of infliximab in Japanese patients with plaque psoriasis, psoriatic arthritis, pustular psoriasis and psoriatic erythroderma. J Dermatol. 2011;38(4):321-34.
13. Fabroni C, Gori A, Troiano M, Prignano F, Lotti T. Infliximab efficacy in nail psoriasis. A retrospective study in 48 patients. J Eur Acad Dermatol Venereol. 2011;25(5):549-53.
14. Reich K, Conrad C, Kristensen LE, Smith SD, Puig L, Rich P, et al. Network meta-analysis comparing the efficacy of biologic treatments for achieving complete resolution of nail psoriasis. J Dermatolog Treat. 2022;33(3):1652-60.
15. Grant A, Gonzalez T, Montgomery MO, Cardenas V, Kerdel FA. Infliximab therapy for patients with moderate to severe hidradenitis suppurativa: a randomized, double-blind, placebo-controlled crossover trial. J Am Acad Dermatol. 2010;62(2):205-17.
16. van Rappard DC, Leenarts MF, Meijerink-van 't Oost L, Mekkes JR. Comparing treatment outcome of infliximab and adalimumab in patients with severe hidradenitis suppurativa. J Dermatolog Treat. 2012;23(4):284-9.
17. Hubbard VG, Friedmann AC, Goldsmith P. Systemic pyoderma gangrenosum responding to infliximab and adalimumab. Br J Dermatol. 2005;152(5):1059-61.
18. Sfikakis PP, Theodossiadis PG, Katsiari CG, Kaklamanis P, Markomichelakis NN. Effect of infliximab on sight-threatening panuveitis in Behcet's disease. Lancet. 2001;358(9278):295-6.
19. Josselin L, Mahr A, Cohen P, Pagnoux C, Guaydier-Souquières G, Hayem G, et al. Infliximab efficacy and safety against refractory systemic necrotising vasculitides: long-term follow-up of 15 patients. Ann Rheum Dis. 2008;67(9):1343-6.
20. Doty JD, Mazur JE, Judson MA. Treatment of sarcoidosis with infliximab. Chest. 2005;127(3):1064-71.
21. Amy de la Breteque M, Saussine A, Rybojad M, Kramkimel N, Pennamen MDV, Bagot M, et al. Infliximab in recalcitrant granuloma annulare. Int J Dermatol. 2016;55(2):220-2.
22. Riley P, McCann LJ, Maillard SM, Woo P, Murray KJ, Pilkington CA, et al. Effectiveness of infliximab in the treatment of refractory juvenile dermatomyositis with calcinosis. Rheumatology. 2008;47(6):877-80.
23. Dold S, Justiniano ME, Marquez J, Espinoza LR. Treatment of early and refractory dermatomyositis with infliximab: a report of two cases. Clin Rheumatol. 2007;26(7):1186-8.
24. Couriel DR, Saliba R, de Lima M, Giralt S, Andersson B, Khouri I, et al. A phase III study of infliximab and corticosteroids for the initial treatment of acute graft-versus-host disease. Biol Blood Marrow Transplant. 2009;15(12):1555-62.

25. Hunger RE, Hunziker T, Buettiker U, Braathen LR, Yawalkar N. Rapid resolution of toxic epidermal necrolysis with anti-TNF-Alpha treatment. J Allergy Clin Immunol. 2005;116(4):923-4.
26. Gill H, Majithia V. Successful use of infliximab in the treatment of Reiter's syndrome: a case report and discussion. Clin Rheumatol. 2008;27(1):121-3.
27. Petrof G, Almaani N, Archer CB, Griffiths WAD, Smith CH. A systematic review of the literature on the treatment of pityriasis rubra pilaris type 1 with TNF-antagonists. J Eur Acad Dermatol Venereol. 2013;27(1):e131-5.
28. Wolbink GJ, Vis M, Lems W, de Groot E, Nurmohamed MT, Stapel S, et al. Development of antiinfliximab antibodies and relationship to clinical response in patients with rheumatoid arthritis. Arthritis Rheumatol. 2006;54(3):711-5.
29. Ben–Horin S, Waterman M, Kopylov U, Yavzori M, Picard O, Fudim E, et al. Addition of an immunomodulator to infliximab therapy eliminates antidrug antibodies in serum and restores clinical response of patients with inflammatory bowel disease. Clin Gastroenterol Hepatol. 2013;11(4):444-7.
30. Carmona L, Gómez-Reino JJ, Rodríguez-Valverde V, Montero D, Pascual-Gómez E, Mola EM, et al. Effectiveness of recommendations to prevent reactivation of latent tuberculosis infection in patients treated with tumor necrosis factor antagonists. Arthritis Rheum. 2005;52(6):1766-72.
31. Filler SG, Yeaman MR, Sheppard DC. Tumor necrosis factor inhibition and invasive fungal infections. Clin Infect Dis. 2005;41(Supplement 3):S208-12.
32. Esteve M, Saro C, Gonzalez-Huix F, Forné M, Viver JM. Chronic hepatitis B reactivation following infliximab therapy in Crohn's disease patients: need for primary prophylaxis. Gut. 2004;53(9):1363-5.
33. Askling J, Fahrbach K, Nordstrom B. Cancer risk with tumor necrosis factor alpha (TNF) inhibitors: meta-analysis of randomized controlled trials of adalimumab, etanercept, and infliximab using patient level data. Pharmacoepidemiol Drug Saf. 2011;20(2):119-30.
34. Heslinga SC, Sijl AM, De Boer K, Van Halm VP, Nurmohamed MT. Tumor necrosis factor blocking therapy and congestive heart failure in patients with inflammatory rheumatic disorders: a systematic review. Curr Med Chem. 2015;22(16):1892-902.
35. Bradshaw MJ, Mobley BC, Zwerner JP, Sriram S. Autopsy-proven demyelination associated with infliximab treatment. Neurol Neuroimmunol Neuroinflamm. 2016;3(2):e205.
36. French JB, Bonacini M, Ghabril M, Foureau D. Hepatotoxicity associated with the use of anti-TNF-a agents. Drug Saf. 2016;39(3):199-208.
37. Lichtenstein L, Ron Y, Kivity S, Ben-Horin S, Israeli E, Fraser GM, et al. Infliximab-related infusion reactions: systematic review. J Crohns Colitis. 2015;9(9):806-15.
38. Barthel C, Biedermann L, Frei P. Induction or exacerbation of psoriasis in patients with Crohn's disease under treatment with anti-TNF antibodies. Digestion. 2014;89(3):209-15.
39. Mahadevan U, Kane S, Sandborn WJ, Cohen RD, Hanson K, Terdiman JP, et al. Intentional infliximab use during pregnancy for induction or maintenance of remission in Crohn's disease. Aliment Pharmacol Ther. 2005;21(6):733-8.
40. Nathan DM, Angus PW, Gibson PR. Hepatitis B and C virus infections and anti-tumor necrosis factor-α therapy: Guidelines for clinical approach. J Gastroenterol Hepatol. 2006;21(9):1366-71.
41. Gaylis N. Infliximab in the treatment of an HIV positive patient with Reiter's syndrome. J Rheumatol. 2003;30(2):407-11.

CHAPTER 7

Adalimumab

Vinay Singh

INTRODUCTION

Adalimumab is a recombinant, fully human monoclonal immunoglobulin G1 (IgG1) antibody against tumor necrosis factor alpha (TNF-α). It is produced by recombinant technology from Chinese hamster ovary (CHO) cells specific for human TNF. It functions by specifically binding to TNF-α and obstructs its interaction with the p55 and p75 cell surface TNF receptors.

MECHANISM OF ACTION

Intracellular signaling mediated by TNF occurs through interactions with cell-bound TNF receptors. These receptors are present on almost all the cells. The two distinct but structurally similar TNF receptors are designated p55 and p75. These receptors form dimer on the cell surface, where they bind a trimeric TNF molecule, thus initiating signal transduction. Adalimumab binds specifically to TNF-α and blocks its interaction with the p55 and p75 cell surface TNF receptors.

PHARMACOLOGY

- After subcutaneous administration, serum concentration reaches its peak after 5 days
- Average bioavailability—64%
- Mean terminal phase half-life is approximately 2 weeks with a single dose of adalimumab.

THERAPEUTIC INDICATIONS

Approved by Food and Drug Administration
- Rheumatoid arthritis
- Juvenile idiopathic arthritis

- Crohn's disease and ulcerative colitis
- Ankylosing spondylitis
- Psoriatic arthritis
- Chronic plaque psoriasis
- Hidradenitis suppurativa (HS)
- Uveitis

Off-label Indications

- Nail psoriasis
- *Neutrophilic dermatoses:* Behçet's disease, pyoderma gangrenosum
- PAPA syndrome (pyogenic arthritis, pyoderma gangrenosum and acne) and PASH syndrome (pyoderma gangrenosum, acne, and hidradenitis suppurativa)
- Cutaneous vasculitis
- Granulomatous dermatoses

CHRONIC PLAQUE PSORIASIS

Adalimumab was approved by Food and Drug Administration (FDA) for the management of chronic plaque psoriasis in 2008. Efficacy of adalimumab for management of chronic plaque psoriasis is explained in **Table 1**.

TABLE 1: Efficacy of adalimumab for management of chronic plaque psoriasis.

Dose	Schedule	Outcome	Reference
• 80 mg–day 0 • 40 mg week 1 and every other week	• 52-week randomized, placebo controlled trial • 16 weeks: Blinded, 17 weeks onward—open-label extension	• Week 16: 71% patients achieved PASI-75, 45% PASI-90 and 20% PASI-100 • Week 33–52: Patients who achieved PASI-75 at week 33, lost PASI response by week 52 on stopping adalimumab	Menter et al.[1]
80 mg–day 0, 40 mg EOW	Randomized controlled comparative study of adalimumab with methotrexate	• Week 16: 79.6% patients with adalimumab and 35.5% patients in methotrexate group achieved PASI-75 • PASI-100: 16.7% and 7.3% in adalimumab and MTX group, respectively	Saurat et al.[2]
	Dose of methotrexate used was not fixed. It was given in 7.5 mg/week on week 0, 10 mg on week 2 and 15 mg at week 4. Patients who did not achieve PASI-50 by week 8 and week 12, dose was increased to 20 and 25 mg/week, respectively		
40 mg every week or every other week	• Randomized double-blind placebo controlled study • Follow-up: 60 weeks	• 12 weeks: PASI-75 in 53% patients taking adalimumab EOW • 80% in weekly adalimumab group • Response sustained till 60 weeks	Gordon et al.[3]

(EOW: end of the week; MTX: methotrexate; PASI: Psoriasis Area and Severity Index)

Retreatment

Majority of the patients who discontinue therapy relapse, median time to relapse is 141 days. Retreatment results in satisfactory response in majority of the patients. Patients who respond early and have higher Psoriasis Area and Severity Index (PASI) reduction, maintain remission for longer period of time off therapy.[4]

PALMOPLANTAR PSORIASIS

Adalimumab has been used for the management of psoriasis involving hands and feet. Randomized placebo-controlled trial conducted by Leonardi et al. included 75 patients with plaque psoriasis involving hands and feet and 25 placebo. Dose of adalimumab used was 40 mg subcutaneously at week 0, followed by 40 mg every other week starting at week 1. Results revealed that 31% of patients treated with adalimumab were clear or almost clear from disease at the end of 16 weeks compared with 4% of placebo. The outcome for palmoplantar involvement was measured by Erythema, Scaling, Induration, Fissuring (ESIF) score. ESIF 75 was achieved in 29% patients as compared to 4% in placebo.[5]

NAIL PSORIASIS

In March 2017, FDA approved addition of moderate-to-severe fingernail psoriasis data to adalimumab prescribing information, making it first biologic to have fingernail psoriasis data in prescribing information for chronic plaque psoriasis. 26 weeks, multicentric, phase 3 placebo-controlled trial for adalimumab in nail psoriasis was conducted by Elewski et al. in 2016. Adalimumab was administered in a dose of 40 mg every other week. Severity of nail psoriasis was measured by modified Nail Psoriasis Severity Index (m-NAPSI) and Physician Global Assessment (PGA). At 26 weeks, 46.6% in adalimumab group achieved m-NAPSI 75 compared to 3.4% in placebo group. 48.9% patients achieved PGA 0/1 compared to 6.9% in placebo group.[6]

PSORIATIC ARTHRITIS

Adalimumab was approved by FDA for the management of psoriatic arthritis in 2005. The outcome measures used in psoriatic arthritis are ACR 20 (American College of Rheumatology 20% improvement criteria) and modified total sharp score of structural damage of joints. Efficacy of adalimumab in management of psoriatic arthritis is discussed in **Table 2**.

HIDRADENITIS SUPPURATIVA

Adalimumab was approved by FDA for the management of HS in September, 2015. Efficacy of adalimumab in management of HS is discussed in **Table 3**.

TABLE 2: Efficacy of adalimumab in management of psoriatic arthritis.

Dose	Schedule	Outcome	Reference
40 mg every other week	• 24 weeks randomized, double-blind, placebo-controlled trial • Efficacy endpoints was ACR 20 at week 12 and change in sharp score at week 24	• Week 12 and 24—ACR 20 response rate of 58% in adalimumab group versus 14% in placebo group • ACR 50 and ACR 70 response seen in 36% and 17% patients, respectively • Week 24—significant improvement in sharp score	Mease et al.[7] (ADEPT trial)
	• ACR 20, ACR 50 and ACR 70 responses were same in patients receiving adalimumab alone and adalimumab in combination with methotrexate • Open-label extension till 48 weeks—ACR 20, ACR 50 and ACR 70 responses seen in 56%, 44% and 30% patients, respectively. It was safe and well-tolerated till 48 weeks. A 2-year follow-up of this trial was also published demonstrating safety and efficacy of long-term adalimumab		
40 mg every other week	12 weeks, adalimumab for psoriatic arthritis in patients who have failed disease-modifying antirheumatic drug therapy	12 weeks—ACR 20 in 39% of treated patient	Van den Bosch et al.[8]

(ACR: American College of Rheumatology improvement criteria).

TABLE 3: Efficacy of adalimumab in management of hidradenitis suppurativa (HS).

Dose	Schedule	Outcome	Reference
80 mg baseline followed by 40 mg subcutaneously every other week	• Placebo-controlled trial ($n = 21$), 15 adalimumab and 6 placebo • Treatment for 12 weeks and follow-up for 12 weeks	• Significant reduction in Sartorius score at end of 6 weeks and 24 weeks • No significant change after 12 weeks during follow-up period	Miller et al.[9]
• Week 0—160 mg • Week 2—80 mg • Week 4 onward—40 mg weekly	• Placebo-controlled trial • Period 1—till week 12 • Period 2—rerandomization and continue for 24 weeks • Assessment based on HiSCR	• Week 12—PIONEER I—41.8% versus 26% (placebo) • PIONEER II—58.9% versus 27.6% (placebo)	Kimball et al.[10]

(HiSCR: hidradenitis suppurative clinical response)

DOSES AND METHODS OF ADMINISTRATION

- *Psoriatic arthritis*: 40 mg administered every other week
- *Plaque psoriasis*: 80 mg on day 1 followed by 40 mg every other week, starting week 1.

- *HS*:
  - 160 mg on day 1, 80 mg on day 15.
  - 40 mg on day 29 then every week or 80 mg fortnightly

CONTRAINDICATIONS

Adalimumab, sterile solution for injection is contraindicated in the following conditions:
- Hypersensitivity to the active substance or to any of the excipients
- Moderate-to-severe heart failure New York Heart Association (NYHA) class III and above
- Active tuberculosis or other severe infections such as sepsis and opportunistic infections
- Along with live vaccines
- Recent (past 5 years) history of any malignancy or relapse of carcinoma

SPECIAL WARNING AND PRECAUTIONS FOR USE

Infection
- Patients should be treated with adalimumab after active infection including chronic or localized infections are controlled.
- Complete diagnostic evaluation when patients develop a new infection while being treated with adalimumab
- Serious infection like sepsis, pyelonephritis, pneumonia, and opportunistic fungal infections like histoplasmosis may develop.
- In a COVID-19 (coronavirus disease 2019) like situation, one should continue with the biologic as the virus replication stops at day 9. The dose intervals can be adjusted accordingly.

Tuberculosis
- Active or latent tuberculosis infection should be ruled out by history, clinical examination, chest X-ray, purified protein derivative (PPD) or interferon-gamma release assay (IGRA) tests.
- Adalimumab should not be used in patients with active tuberculosis and treatment for latent tuberculosis infection should be started before adalimumab therapy is started.

Hepatitis B Reactivation
Reactivation of hepatitis B can occur in chronic carriers. Hepatologist should be consulted in patients who are hepatitis B surface antigen-positive, before initiating adalimumab.

Neurological Event
Adalimumab is associated with exacerbation or new onset of central or peripheral nervous system demyelinating disorders such as multiple sclerosis and Guillain–Barré syndrome.

Allergic Reactions

Anaphylaxis and allergic reactions are rare. It should be discontinued if serious allergic reactions, such as anaphylaxis, allergic rash, fixed drug reaction, unspecified drug reaction or urticaria, are observed in patients.

Malignancy

There has been concern regarding increase in risk of development of malignancies in patients taking TNF-α blocker. However, meta-analysis does not support or refute this concern.

Hematologic Reactions

Pancytopenia, bicytopenia, or thrombocytopenia has rarely been reported.

Vaccinations

Live vaccines are contraindicated in patients on adalimumab.

Congestive Heart Failure

Increased mortality and worsening congestive heart disease have been reported in patients treated with TNF antagonists including adalimumab. It is contraindicated in NYHA class III or IV congestive heart failure (CHF).

Autoimmunity

- Antidrug antibodies (ADA) develop in almost 30% of patients after 3 years of treatment. Patients with ADA have lower adalimumab level and lower chances of clinical remission.[11]
- Concomitant methotrexate use reduces the immunogenicity of adalimumab.
- Antinuclear antibody (ANA) positivity and lupus-like syndrome can also develop rarely.

Concurrent Administration with Anakinra

Serious infections have been reported with concurrent use of anakinra with etanercept (another TNF blocker). Therefore, adalimumab is not recommended to be used with anakinra.

SPECIAL SITUATIONS

Pediatric Population

Adalimumab has been approved by European Medical Agency for the management of moderate-to-severe psoriasis in children older than 4 years in 2015. While etanercept is approved by USFDA for the management of pediatric psoriasis, adalimumab is not yet.

A phase III randomized double-blind study was conducted by Papp et al. in 114 children with severe psoriasis. Adalimumab was used in the dose of 0.8 mg/kg (maximum 40 mg), 0.4 mg/kg (maximum 20 mg) every other week, and methotrexate in the dose of 0.1–0.4 mg/kg/week. 58% of patients in adalimumab 0.8 mg/kg group achieved PASI-75.[12]

Elderly Population

Adalimumab has been used in patients older than 65 years and found to be safe and effective. Risk of infection is higher in this population and one should be careful about infections and particular emphasis should be placed on immunization.[13]

Surgery

Rheumatoid arthritis patients on biologics undergo orthopedic procedure because of the disease itself. Similar situation can arise in patients with psoriatic arthritis or psoriasis patients requiring elective surgical procedure for unrelated illness. The risk of infections and complications appear to be higher in patients on adalimumab and it should be stopped prior to the surgery. However, data regarding complications are conflicting and there are studies which showed no significant difference in complications in patients on TNF-α blockers. The long half-life of adalimumab should be considered prior to planning a surgery and the patients should be monitored for infections.[14]

Pregnancy

Adalimumab is pregnancy category B drug. TNF-α blockers are not teratogenic drugs and have been used safely in many patients with successful pregnancy outcome. These drugs cross placenta and cord blood levels are higher than maternal serum. These drugs should ideally be stopped prior to conception in view of absence of robust safety data in pregnancy and tendency to cross placenta. In case one needs to continue these drugs in pregnancy to control the disease, immunosuppression in neonate is a major concern and one needs to stop these drugs prior to delivery. Adalimumab should be discontinued at 26–28 weeks of pregnancy.[15]

Lactation

Concentration of TNF-α blockers in breast milk of women taking these drugs were either undetectable or significantly lower than maternal serum. These drugs appear to be safe in lactation, however due to unavailability of large studies; it is not advisable to be used during lactation.[16]

TESTS TO BE DONE PRIOR TO ADMINISTRATION

- Complete blood count
- Liver function test

- Blood urea, serum creatinine
- Hepatitis B surface antigen, anti-hepatitis C virus (HCV)–IgM, human immunodeficiency virus (HIV) 1 and 2
- *Rule out active and latent tuberculosis:*
    - History of past tuberculosis, history of contact with active case of tuberculosis
    - History of fever, weight loss, and night sweats
    - Chest X-ray posteroanterior (PA) view
    - PPD or IGRA

MONITORING DURING ADALIMUMAB THERAPY

Patients who are on adalimumab should be closely monitored for development of any infection especially tuberculosis. Three monthly complete blood count and liver function test and yearly chest X-ray are advisable.

CONCLUSION

Adalimumab, a TNF inhibitor is a fully human monoclonal antibody used in the management of psoriasis. It is approved for the treatment of hidradenitis suppurativa, chronic plaque psoriasis and psoriatic arthritis in dermatology. It has a good safety profile and is effective in the management of these conditions. Reactivation of tuberculosis is a major concern in endemic countries and patient should be monitored carefully when they are on adalimumab.

REFERENCES

1. Menter A, Tyring SK, Gordon K, Kimball AB, Leonardi CL, Langley RG, et al. Adalimumab therapy for moderate to severe psoriasis: a randomized, controlled phase III trial. J Am Acad Dermatol. 2008;58(1):106-15.
2. Saurat JH, Stingl G, Dubertret L, Papp K, Langley RG, Ortonne JP, et al. Efficacy and safety results from the randomized controlled comparative study of adalimumab vs. methotrexate vs. placebo in patients with psoriasis (CHAMPION). Br J Dermatol. 2008;158(3):558-66.
3. Gordon KB, Langley RG, Leonardi C, Toth D, Menter MA, Kang S, et al. Clinical response to adalimumab treatment in patients with moderate to severe psoriasis: double-blind, randomized controlled trial and open-label extension study. J Am Acad Dermatol. 2006;55(4):598-606.
4. Papp K, Crowley J, Ortonne JP, Leu J, Okun M, Gupta SR, et al. Adalimumab for moderate to severe chronic plaque psoriasis: efficacy and safety of retreatment and disease recurrence following withdrawal from therapy. Br J Dermatol. 2011;164(2):434-41.
5. Leonardi C, Langley RG, Papp K, Tyring SK, Wasel N, Vender R, et al. Adalimumab for treatment of moderate to severe chronic plaque psoriasis of the hands and feet efficacy and safety results from reach, a randomized, placebo-controlled, double-blind trial. Arch Dermatol. 2011;147(4):429-36.
6. Elewski BE, Okun MM, Papp K, Baker CS, Crowley JJ, Guillet G, et al. Adalimumab for nail psoriasis: Efficacy and safety from the first 26 weeks of a phase-3, randomized, placebo-controlled trial. J Am Acad Dermatol. 2018;78(1):90-99.e1.

7. Mease PJ, Gladman DD, Ritchlin CT, Ruderman EM, Steinfeld SD, Choy EH, et al.; Adalimumab Effectiveness in Psoriatic Arthritis Trial Study Group. Adalimumab for the treatment of patients with moderately to severely active psoriatic arthritis: results of a double-blind, randomized, placebo-controlled trial. Arthritis Rheum. 2005;52(10): 3279-89.
8. Van den Bosch F, Manger B, Goupille P, McHugh N, Rødevand E, Holck P, et al. Effectiveness of adalimumab in treating patients with active psoriatic arthritis and predictors of good clinical responses for arthritis, skin and nail lesions. Ann Rheum Dis. 2010;69(2):394-9.
9. Miller I, Lynggaard CD, Lophaven S, Zachariae C, Dufour DN, Jemec GB. A double-blind placebo-controlled randomized trial of adalimumab in the treatment of hidradenitis suppurativa. Br J Derm. 2011;165(2):391-8.
10. Kimball AB, Okun MM, Williams DA, Gottlieb AB, Papp KA, Zouboulis CC, et al. Two phase 3 trials of adalimumab for hidradenitis suppurativa. N Engl J Med. 2016;375(5):422-34.
11. Bartelds GM, Krieckaert CL, Nurmohamed MT, van Schouwenburg PA, Lems WF, Twisk JW, et al. Development of antidrug antibodies against adalimumab and association with disease activity and treatment failure during long-term follow-up. JAMA. 2011;305(14):1460-8.
12. Papp K, Thaçi D, Marcoux D, Weibel L, Philipp S, Ghislain PD, et al. Efficacy and safety of adalimumab every other week versus methotrexate once weekly in children and adolescents with severe chronic plaque psoriasis: a randomised, double-blind, phase 3 trial. Lancet. 2017;390(89):40-9.
13. Esposito M, Giunta A, Mazzotta A, Zangrilli A, Babino G, Bavetta M, et al. Efficacy and safety of subcutaneous anti-tumor necrosis factor-alpha agents, etanercept and adalimumab, in elderly patients affected by psoriasis and psoriatic arthritis: an observational long-term study. Dermatology. 2012;225(4):312-9.
14. Ruyssen-Witrand A, Gossec L, Salliot C, Luc M, Duclos M, Guignard S, et al. Complication rates of 127 surgical procedures performed in rheumatic patients receiving tumor necrosis factor alpha blockers. Clin Exp Rheumatol. 2007;25(3):430-6.
15. Soh MC, MacKillop L. Biologics in pregnancy–for the obstetrician. Obstet Gynaecol. 2016;18(1):25-32.
16. Krause ML, Amin S, Makol A. Use of DMARDs and biologics during pregnancy and lactation in rheumatoid arthritis: what the rheumatologist needs to know. Ther Adv Musculoskelet Dis. 2014;6(5):169-84.

CHAPTER 8

IL-17 Blockers: Secukinumab

SG Parasramani, D Joshika Bhandary

INTRODUCTION

Secukinumab is a monoclonal antibody that specifically targets interleukin 17A (IL-17A), a cytokine involved in the pathogenesis of various autoimmune diseases, including psoriasis, psoriatic arthritis (PsA), and ankylosing spondylitis. In 2010, Hueber et al. carried out proof-of-concept research, which showcased the effectiveness of secukinumab in the treatment of chronic plaque-type psoriasis, rheumatoid arthritis, and chronic noninfectious uveitis.[1]

Approved by the Food and Drug Administration (FDA) in 2015, secukinumab has demonstrated impressive efficacy and safety profiles in several clinical trials and has become a widely used therapeutic option for patients with these conditions.

PHARMACOLOGY

Secukinumab is a fully human monoclonal antibody that selectively binds and neutralizes the pro-inflammatory cytokine IL-17A, and is produced in Chinese hamster ovary (CHO) cells, belonging to the immunoglobulin G1 (IgG1)/κ-class. It inhibits the interaction between IL-17A and its receptor, expressed on various cell types including keratinocytes (**Fig. 1**). With a molecular weight of 150 kDa, a single subcutaneous dose of 150 or 300 mg in plaque psoriasis patients led to peak serum concentrations of 13.7 ± 4.8 µg/mL or 27.3 ± 9.5 µg/mL, respectively, between 5 and 6 days post dose.[2] The average absolute bioavailability of secukinumab is estimated to be 73%, and its mean elimination half-life is 27 days (22–31 days) in plaque psoriasis patients.[2,3]

The maximum concentration (C_{max}) of the drug was 27.6 and 55.2 µg/mL after subcutaneous administration of 150 and 300 mg, respectively. With monthly dosing regimens, steady state is achieved after 20 weeks.[2]

The metabolism of human IgG1 monoclonal antibodies like secukinumab occurs similarly to endogenous IgG via intracellular catabolism.[2]

CHAPTER 8: IL-17 Blockers: Secukinumab

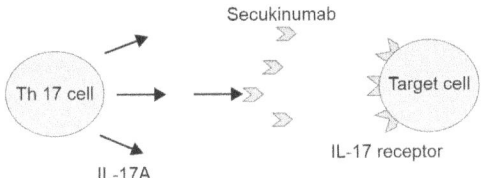

FIG. 1: Mechanism of action of secukinumab.
(IL-17: interleukin 17; Th 17: T helper 17)

Following a single subcutaneous dose of 300 mg secukinumab, the concentrations of the drug in the interstitial fluid of the skin of plaque psoriasis patients were found to be between 28 to 39% of the levels observed in the serum at both 1 and 2 weeks post administration.[2]

MECHANISM OF ACTION

Secukinumab selectively binds to and neutralizes the pro-inflammatory cytokine IL-17A.

USES

Indications Approved by FDA
- Moderate-to-severe plaque psoriasis in patients aged more than 6 years who are candidates for systemic therapy
- Palmoplantar psoriasis
- Nail psoriasis
- Psoriatic arthritis
- Ankylosing spondylitis[4]
- Rheumatoid arthritis

Off-label Indications
- Pustular and erythrodermic psoriasis
- Chronic noninfectious uveitis[5]
- Hidradenitis suppurativa

PSORIASIS

The efficacy of secukinumab in various trials has been tabulated in **Table 1**. At 52 weeks, Psoriasis Area and Severity Index (PASI) 75 was maintained in 80% of patients who received 300 mg of secukinumab and in 60% of patients who received 150 mg of secukinumab; PASI 90 was maintained in 70% in 300 mg of secukinumab and in 50% in 150 mg of secukinumab group.

At 2 years, PASI 75 was maintained in 88.2% of patients in 300 mg and in 75.5% of patients in 150 mg group.

TABLE 1: Efficacy of secukinumab in trials.			
		16 weeks	
Study		PASI 75	PASI 90
ERASURE[6]	300 mg	81.6%	59.2%
	150 mg	71.6%	39.1%
	Placebo	4.5%	1.2%
FIXTURE[6]	300 mg	77.1%	54.2%
	150 mg	67%	41.9%
	Etanercept	44%	20.7%
	Placebo	4.9%	1.5%

(ERASURE: Efficacy of Response and Safety of Two Fixed Secukinumab Regimens in Psoriasis; FIXTURE: Full Year Investigative Examination of Secukinumab versus Etanercept Using Two Dosing Regimens to Determine Efficacy in Psoriasis; PASI: Psoriasis Area and Severity Index)

When secukinumab was withdrawn, relapse occurred within 12 weeks in patients who received 150 mg of the drug and within 18 weeks in those who received 300 mg.[6]

If patients discontinue secukinumab for 3 months, they will require the readministration of complete five induction doses before starting maintenance therapy with the drug. When therapy was restarted with 300 mg of secukinumab, 94.8%, 70.3%, and 38.4% of patients achieved PASI 75, PASI 90, and PASI 100 responses, respectively.[6]

High response rates were sustained over 3 years of continuous secukinumab treatment, with PASI 75/90/100 responses seen in 83%, 63.8%, and 42.6% of patients receiving a 300 mg dose through year 3. Patients receiving a 150 mg dose saw PASI 75/90/100 responses of 62.4%, 36.8%, and 17.9% through year 3.[7]

In the extension study, 168 patients entered at year 1, and 126 patients completed 300 mg (every 4 weeks) treatment by the end of year 5. PASI 75/90/100 responses at year 1 (88.9%, 68.5%, and 43.8%, respectively) were sustained until year 5 (88.5%, 66.4%, and 41%).[8]

Superiority of secukinumab over ustekinumab was demonstrated in both the CLEAR[9] and CLARITY[10] studies, while the FIXTURE (Full Year Investigative Examination of Secukinumab vs. Etanercept Using Two Dosing Regimens to Determine Efficacy in Psoriasis) study[6] showed superiority of secukinumab over etanercept.

In the ECLIPSE trial, guselkumab achieved PASI 90 in 84% of patients at week 48, compared to 70% for secukinumab. Both molecules had similar PASI 75 at weeks 12 and 48, with guselkumab at 85% and secukinumab at 80%.[11]

The IMMerge trial compared risankizumab and secukinumab in moderate-to-severe psoriasis. At 12 weeks, 73.8% of patients in the risankizumab group achieved PASI 90, compared to 65.6% of patients in the secukinumab group. At 52 weeks, PASI 90 was seen in 86.6% of patients who received risankizumab, compared to 57.1% of patients who received secukinumab, demonstrating superior response rates for risankizumab.[12]

PSORIATIC ARTHRITIS

Secukinumab significantly improved joint and skin symptoms in patients with PsA at both 300 and 150 mg doses, resulting in associated improvements in physical function and skin-related quality of life.[13] Furthermore, improvements in signs and symptoms of PsA were demonstrated in both the concomitant methotrexate (MTX) and without MTX subgroups with secukinumab at doses of 300 and 150 mg.[14]

At week 24, the ACR 20 (American College of Rheumatology response criteria) response rates were significantly higher in the group receiving secukinumab at doses of 150 mg (50.0%) and 75 mg (50.5%) than in those receiving placebo (17.3%). Additionally, the secukinumab groups showed significantly better results for secondary endpoints, including ACR 50 response and joint structural damage, compared to the placebo group.[15]

The EXCEED trial[16] pitted secukinumab against adalimumab in individuals with active PsA. Participants were randomly assigned to receive either secukinumab 300 mg subcutaneously at weeks 0, 1, 2, 3, 4, and every 4 weeks thereafter, or adalimumab 40 mg subcutaneously at week 0 and every 2 weeks thereafter. The primary endpoint was the achievement of ACR 20 at week 52, which was met by 67% of patients in the secukinumab group and 62% of patients in the adalimumab group. Furthermore, 31% of secukinumab patients achieved a combined joint and skin response (PASI 100 and ACR 50), while the adalimumab group showed this response in only 19% of patients.

NAIL PSORIASIS

The TRANSFIGURE study[17] showed that both secukinumab 300 mg and secukinumab 150 mg were more effective than placebo in improving Nail Psoriasis Severity Index (NAPSI) percent change at week 16. The NAPSI percent change was −45.4% for secukinumab 300 mg, −38.9% for secukinumab 150 mg, and −11.2% for placebo.

Secondary endpoints such as PASI 75 and modified Investigator Global Assessment (IGA) score of clear or almost clear showed significantly higher responses in both secukinumab 300 mg (PASI 75: 87.1% and IGA 0/1: 74.0%) and secukinumab 150 mg (PASI 75: 77.0% and IGA 0/1: 68.3%), compared to placebo (PASI 75: 5.1% and IGA 0/1: 3.1%). Furthermore, PASI 90 responses were observed in 72.5% of patients receiving secukinumab 300 mg dose, 54.0% of patients receiving secukinumab 150 mg, while in patients on placebo, PASI 90 was seen in only 1.7% of patients.

PALMOPLANTAR PSORIASIS

The GESTURE study[18] showed that at week 16, the percentage of subjects achieving clear or almost clear palms and soles [palmoplantar psoriasis IGA (ppIGA) 0/1] was significantly higher with secukinumab 300 mg (33.3%) and 150 mg (22.1%) compared to placebo (1.5%). In addition, Palmoplantar Psoriasis Area and Severity Index (ppPASI) significantly decreased with secukinumab 300 mg (−54.5%) and 150 mg (−35.3%) compared to placebo (−4.0%). Subjects in the secukinumab groups also had significantly higher Dermatology Life Quality Index (DLQI) 0/1 responses compared to placebo at week 16. Secukinumab markedly improved pain and function of palms and soles as measured by the palmoplantar quality-of-life instrument, and secukinumab 300 mg consistently showed the best outcomes. The safety profile was favorable and similar to previous studies.

SCALP PSORIASIS

In a trial involving 102 patients with moderate-to-severe scalp psoriasis, the Psoriasis Scalp Severity Index (PSSI) 90 response rate was 52.9%, significantly higher than the 2% response rate observed in patients randomized to receive placebo.[19]

PUSTULAR PSORIASIS

In a Japanese study of 12 patients with generalized pustular psoriasis, patients received secukinumab 150 mg weekly from week 0 to 4, followed by once every 4 weeks. Two nonresponsive patients received the 300 mg dose. Improvement was observed as early as week 1, and by week 16, 83.3% of patients achieved "much improved" or "very much improved" as assessed by the Clinical Global Impression. Patients were followed up to week 52, and sustained improvement in generalized pustular psoriasis severity was observed, along with good drug tolerance.[20]

Palmoplantar Pustular Psoriasis

The PRECISE study did not show significant improvement in ppPASI 75 at week 16, but at week 52, the ppPASI 75 response rates for secukinumab 150 and 300 mg doses were 35.0% and 41.8%, respectively.[21]

ADMINISTRATION

The lyophilized powder is a solid white substance that is contained in a 6 mL glass vial. It is stored in a refrigerator in a lyophilized form and can be reconstituted by adding 1 mL of sterile water for injection.

Dosage

To receive the recommended dose, two vials of 150 mg each are administered subcutaneously on the anterolateral aspect of the thigh. Induction phase consists of 300 mg given at weeks 0, 1, 2, 3, and 4 followed by monthly maintenance dosing of 300 mg every 4 weeks.

In the case of PsA, the dose is 150 mg given on week 0, 1, 2, 3, 4, and every 4 weeks thereafter for maintenance dosing.

Tests to be done Prior to Administration

- Complete blood count (CBC)
- Liver function test (LFT)
- Blood urea, serum creatinine
- Hepatitis B surface antigen, anti-hepatitis C virus IgM, human immunodeficiency virus (HIV)
- *Rule out active and latent tuberculosis*:
  - History of past tuberculosis, history of contact with active case of tuberculosis
  - History of fever, weight loss, night sweats
  - Chest X-ray posteroanterior (PA) view
- Purified protein derivative (PPD) or interferon-gamma release assays (IGRA)
- Routine urine and stool examination
- Fasting and post prandial blood sugar
- Electrocardiography (ECG)
- Abdominal sonography
- Urinary pregnancy test (UPT) in females

MONITORING DURING SECUKINUMAB THERAPY

- Patients prescribed with secukinumab require vigilant monitoring for potential candidial infections, particularly if they have diabetes. During every visit, healthcare providers should examine for signs of oral thrush, balanoposthitis, and vulvovaginitis. Additionally, patients should undergo a CBC following the induction phase and then every 12 weeks to screen for neutropenia.
- An annual chest X-ray with a PA view and an IGRA should be conducted to monitor patients' health status.

ADVERSE EFFECTS

- Anti-secukinumab antibodies were detected in four patients after the start of secukinumab treatment in the FIXTURE study (0.4% of the 980 secukinumab-treated patients tested). No patient had neutralizing antibodies. In the ERASURE (Efficacy of Response and Safety of Two Fixed Secukinumab Regimens in Psoriasis) study, anti-secukinumab antibodies that developed during treatment were detected in 2 of 702 (0.3%) secukinumab-treated patients tested.[6]

- *Injection site reactions*: Seven patients (0.7%) in the combined secukinumab groups versus 36 patients (11.1%) in the etanercept group experienced injection site reactions during the entire study.[6]
- *Infections*:[6] No serious infections were reported which warranted stoppage of the therapy.
  - Upper respiratory tract infections:[6] Nasopharyngitis, rhinorrhea, cough
  - Candidiasis:[6] IL-17A plays a key role in host mucocutaneous microbial surveillance.[17] All *Candida* infections in patients treated with secukinumab were mucocutaneous, mild or moderate in severity, responded to standard oral or topical treatment, and did not lead to discontinuation of secukinumab.[22]
  - Oral herpes[23]
- *Gastrointestinal*: Diarrhea[6]
- Headache[6]
- *Others*:[24] Pruritis, hypertension, arthralgia, back pain
- *Neutropenia*: It is an important adverse effect that can occur with IL-17A blockers. IL-17A stimulates granulopoiesis and neutrophil trafficking.[25] Rich et al.[26] found grade 1 or 2 neutropenia in 19 secukinumab patients and 1 placebo patient in the 12-week induction phase and in 30 secukinumab patients in the maintenance phase (weeks 12–32). Dosing was not interrupted or held as no clinically significant adverse events were associated with the development of neutropenia. The incidence of grade 3 neutropenia in patients receiving secukinumab was 0.5% compared with 0.1% in patients receiving placebo. No cases of grade 4 neutropenia were observed with secukinumab.[6] The neutropenia resolved during the course of the study in all cases.[26] [Grade 1 neutropenia: Absolute neutrophil count (ANC) 1,500–2,000 cells/mL; grade 2: 1,000–1,500 cells/mL, grade 3:500–1,000 cells/mL, grade 4: <500 cells/mL]
- Hypersensitivity, urticaria, and angioedema were reported in a very small percentage of patients in the pool of four placebo-controlled phase III trials.[2]

CONTRAINDICATIONS

- Severe hypersensitivity reactions to the active substance or excipients
- If an anaphylactic or other serious allergic reaction occurs, administration of secukinumab should be discontinued immediately and appropriate therapy initiated.
- In clinical studies, urticaria and one case of anaphylactic reaction to secukinumab were observed.

SPECIAL SITUATIONS

Pregnancy and Lactation
Secukinumab falls under pregnancy category B, but there is no available data regarding its use in pregnant women. Animal studies have not shown any direct or indirect harmful effects on pregnancy, embryonic/fetal development, parturition, or postnatal development. However, animal studies may not always predict human response, so the use of secukinumab during pregnancy should only be considered if the benefits outweigh the potential risks.[2] Secukinumab passes through the placenta, and live vaccines should be avoided in neonates whose mothers have been given secukinumab during pregnancy.[2]

Breastfeeding
It is not known whether secukinumab is excreted in human milk. Since immunoglobulins are excreted in human milk, caution should be exercised when administering secukinumab to a woman who is breastfeeding.[2]

Fertility
There is no available data on the effect of secukinumab on human fertility. However, animal studies have not shown any direct or indirect harmful effects on fertility.[2]

Pediatric
Secukinumab can be used in children above 6 years of age.[27]

Vaccinations
Live vaccines should not be administered concurrently with secukinumab.[28] Inactivated or nonlive vaccines may be administered. A study has shown that after meningococcal and inactivated influenza vaccinations, a similar proportion of patients treated with secukinumab and those treated with placebo were able to mount an adequate immune response.[28] Secukinumab does not seem to suppress the humoral immune response to these vaccines.[28] Live or live attenuated vaccines are contraindicated <2 weeks before, during, and for 6 months after discontinuation of biologic therapy. Recommended vaccines are inactivated vaccines, which should be administered 2 weeks before starting therapy to ensure optimal immune responses.

Inflammatory Bowel Disease
Patients with active Crohn's disease and ulcerative colitis should not receive secukinumab, or it should be used with caution since they may experience exacerbation or flare-up of their disease.[29]

Tuberculosis

Secukinumab should not be used in patients with active and latent tuberculosis (PPD- or IGRA-positive). Patients should be asked about their past history of tuberculosis, family history, and recent contact with a tuberculosis patient, or visit to an endemic area where tuberculosis is prevalent. No cases of reactivation of latent tuberculosis were reported in any of the 10 psoriasis studies. Patients with latent tuberculosis were allowed to be randomized, provided that antituberculosis prophylaxis treatment, implemented according to local clinical practice, was ongoing or had been completed before randomization.[30]

Malignant or Unspecified Tumors

The incidence of malignant or unspecified tumors during the first 12 weeks was comparable in the secukinumab 300 mg, 150 mg, and placebo groups. None were reported with etanercept. Over the entire 52 weeks, the exposure-adjusted incidence rate (IR) of malignant or unspecified tumors was comparable in the secukinumab 300 mg, 150 mg, and etanercept groups (0.77, 0.97, and 0.68, respectively). Most tumors were nonmelanoma skin cancers (NMSCs), including basal cell carcinoma (BCC) and squamous cell carcinoma. Most NMSCs were BCC in patients who had undergone previous treatment with phototherapy. No lymphoma was reported.[30]

Adjudicated Major Adverse Cardiovascular Events

In the first 12 weeks of treatment, there were reports of major adverse cardiovascular events (MACEs) in subjects receiving secukinumab 300 mg (0.26%) and placebo (0.10%). However, over the entire 52 weeks, the IR of adjudicated MACEs was similar in subjects receiving secukinumab 300 mg (0.42 per 100 subject-years), 150 mg (0.35), and etanercept (0.34), despite the fact that the secukinumab groups had higher cardiovascular risk factors at the start. It is worth noting that all subjects who experienced MACEs had prior or active cardiovascular disease or risk factors such as hypertension, smoking, obesity, dyslipidemia, or diabetes.[30]

Hepatitis B, Hepatitis C, and HIV Coinfection

There is currently no available data on the use of secukinumab in patients with HIV, hepatitis B, or hepatitis C infection. Clinical studies have not reported any cases of overdose.

TIPS

- Secukinumab should not be used as and when required. If the drug has been discontinued for 3 months, then induction phase of five weekly doses should be repeated to attain the minimum inhibitory concentration

levels. If cost is a factor then instead of 300 mg monthly dose in the maintenance phase, 150 mg of the drug can be used.
- Secukinumab is not combined with MTX as incidence of neutralizing antibodies is very low and also secukinumab alone achieves PASI 90 and PASI 100 response.
- In case of nonresponders to secukinumab 300 mg dose can be given once every 2 weeks (optimize study) or 3 weeks as maintenance dose or even intravenous secukinumab can be given [STATURE (Secukinumab Trial Analyzing the potential of intravenous administration To Upgrade the REsponse in psoriasis) study].[31]

CONCLUSION

Secukinumab is first in class monoclonal antibody against IL-17. It has an impressive efficacy and safety profile in the management of psoriasis. It is approved as a first line treatment for the management of moderate-to-severe psoriasis. It is also being used successfully in difficult to treat psoriasis and hidradenitis suppurativa.

REFERENCES

1. Hueber W, Patel DD, Dryja T, Wright AM, Koroleva I, Bruin G, et al. Effects of AIN457, a fully human antibody to interleukin-17A, on psoriasis, rheumatoid arthritis, and uveitis. Sci Transl Med. 2010;2:52ra72.
2. Novartis Pharmaceuticals Corporation. (2015). Highlights of Prescribing Information. [online] Available from http://www.pharma.us.novartis.com/product/pi/pdf/cosentyx.pdf [Last accessed January, 2024].
3. Wang W, Wang EQ, Balthasar JP. Monoclonal antibody pharmacokinetics and pharmacodynamics. Clin Pharmacol Ther. 2008;84(5):548-58.
4. Baraliakos X, Borah B, Braun J, Baeten D, Laurent D, Sieper J, et al. Long-term effects of secukinumab on MRI findings in relation to clinical efficacy in subjects with active ankylosing spondylitis: an observational study. Ann Rheum Dis. 2016;75(2):408-12.
5. Letko E, Yeh S, Foster CS, Pleyer U, Brigell M, Grosskreutz CL; AIN457A2208 Study Group. Efficacy and safety of intravenous secukinumab in noninfectious uveitis requiring steroid-sparing immunosuppressive therapy. Ophthalmology. 2015;122(5):939-48.
6. Langley RG, Elewski BE, Lebwohl M, Reich K, Griffiths CE, Papp K, et al.; ERASURE Study Group; FIXTURE Study Group. Secukinumab in plaque psoriasis—results of two phase 3 trials. N Engl J Med. 2014;371(4):326-38.
7. Bissonnette R, Luger T, Thaçi D, Toth D, Messina I, Gong Y, et al. (2016). Secukinumab maintains high levels of efficacy through 3 years of treatment: results from an extension to a phase 3 study (SCULPTURE). [online] Available from https://dermcollabstracts.com/abstract/secukinumab-maintains-high-levels-of-efftcacy-through-3-years-of-treatment-results-from-an-extension-to-a-phase-3-study-sculpture/ [Last accessed January, 2024].
8. Bissonnette R, Luger T, Thaçi D, Toth D, Lacombe A, Xia S, et al. Secukinumab demonstrates high sustained efficacy and a favourable safety profile in patients with moderate-to-severe psoriasis through 5 years of treatment (SCULPTURE Extension Study). J Eur Acad Dermatol Venereol. 2018;32(9):1507-14.

9. Thaçi D, Blauvelt A, Reich K, Tsai TF, Vanaclocha F, Kingo K, et al. Secukinumab is superior to ustekinumab in clearing skin of subjects with moderate to severe plaque psoriasis: CLEAR, a randomized controlled trial. J Am Acad Dermatol. 2015;73(3):400-9.
10. Bagel J, Blauvelt A, Nia J, Hashim P, Patekar M, de Vera A, et al. Secukinumab maintains superiority over ustekinumab in clearing skin and improving quality of life in patients with moderate to severe plaque psoriasis: 52-week results from a double-blind phase 3b trial (CLARITY). J Eur Acad Dermatol Venereol. 2021;35(1):135-42.
11. Reich K, Armstrong AW, Langley RG, Flavin S, Randazzo B, Li S, et al. Guselkumab versus secukinumab for the treatment of moderate-to-severe psoriasis (ECLIPSE): results from a phase 3, randomised controlled trial. Lancet. 2019;394(10201):831-39.
12. Warren RB, Blauvelt A, Poulin Y, Beeck S, Kelly M, Wu T, et al. Efficacy and safety of risankizumab vs. secukinumab in patients with moderate-to-severe plaque psoriasis (IMMerge): results from a phase III, randomized, open-label, efficacy–assessor-blinded clinical trial. Br J Dermatol. 2021;184(1):50-9.
13. McInnes IB, Mease PJ, Kirkham B, Kavanaugh A, Ritchlin CT, Rahman P, et al.; FUTURE 2 Study Group. Secukinumab, a human anti-interleukin-17A monoclonal antibody, in patients with psoriatic arthritis (FUTURE 2): a randomised, double-blind, placebo-controlled, phase 3 trial. Lancet. 2015;386:1137-46.
14. Gottlieb AB, McInnes I, Mease P, Mpofu S. Secukinumab improves signs and symptoms of psoriatic arthritis: Results of phase 3 FUTURE 2 study stratified by concomitant methotrexate use. J Am Acad Dermatol. 2016;74(5):AB270.
15. Mease P, McInnes IB, Kirkham B, Kavanaugh A, Rahman P, van der Heijde D, et al.; FUTURE 1 Study Group. Secukinumab inhibition of interleukin-17A in patients with psoriatic arthritis. N Engl J Med. 2015;373(14):1329-39.
16. McInnes IB, Behrens F, Mease PJ, Kavanaugh A, Ritchlin C, Nash P, et al.; EXCEED Study Group. Secukinumab versus adalimumab for treatment of active psoriatic arthritis (EXCEED): a double-blind, parallel-group, randomised, active-controlled, phase 3b trial. Lancet. 2020;395(10235):1496-505.
17. Reich K, Arenberger P, Mrowietz U, Jazayeri S, Augustin M, Parneix A, et al. Secukinumab shows high and sustained efficacy in nail psoriasis: Week 80 results from the TRANSFIGURE study. J Am Acad Dermatol. 2017;76(6):AB232.
18. Gottlieb A, Sullivan J, van Doorn M, Kubanov A, You R, Parneix A, et al. Secukinumab shows significant efficacy in palmoplantar psoriasis: Results from GESTURE, a randomized controlled trial. J Am Acad Dermatol. 2017;76(1):70-80.
19. Bagel J, Duffin KC, Moore A, Ferris LK, Siu K, Steadman J, et al. The effect of secukinumab on moderate-to-severe scalp psoriasis: results of a 24-week, randomized, double-blind, placebo-controlled phase 3b study. J Am Acad Dermatol. 2017;77(4):667-74.
20. Imafuku S, Honma M, Okubo Y, Komine M, Ohtsuki M, Morita A, et al. Efficacy and safety of secukinumab in patients with generalized pustular psoriasis: a 52-week analysis from phase III open-label multicenter Japanese study. J Dermatol. 2016;43(9):1011-7.
21. Mrowietz U, Bachelez H, Burden AD, Rissler M, Sieder C, Orsenigo R, et al. Secukinumab for moderate-to-severe palmoplantar pustular psoriasis: results of the 2PRECISE study. J Am Acad Dermatol. 2019;80(5):1344-52.
22. Huang W, Na L, Fidel PL, Schwarzenberger P. Requirement of interleukin-17A for systemic anti-Candida albicans host defense in mice. J Infect Dis. 2004;190(3):624-31.
23. Blauvelt A. Safety of secukinumab in the treatment of psoriasis. Expert Opin Drug Saf. 2016;15(10):1413-20.
24. International Federation of Psoriasis Associations. 4th World Psoriasis and Psoriatic Arthritis Conference. Stockholm, Sweden: International Federation of Psoriasis Associations; 2015.
25. Ley K, Smith E, Stark MA. IL-17A-producing neutrophil-regulatory Tn lymphocytes. Immunol Res. 2006;34(3):229-42.

26. Rich P, Sigurgeirsson B, Thaci D, Ortonne JP, Paul C, Schopf RE, et al. Secukinumab induction and maintenance therapy in moderate-to-severe plaque psoriasis: a randomized, double-blind, placebo-controlled, phase II regimen-finding study. Br J Dermatol. 2013;168(2):402-11.
27. Bodemer C, Kaszuba A, Kingo K, Tsianakas A, Morita A, Rivas E, et al. Secukinumab demonstrates high efficacy and a favourable safety profile in paediatric patients with severe chronic plaque psoriasis: 52-week results from a Phase 3 double-blind randomized, controlled trial. J Eur Acad Dermatol Venereol. 2021;35(4):938-47.
28. Chioato A, Noseda E, Stevens M, Gaitatzis N, Kleinschmidt A, Picaud H. Treatment with the interleukin-17A-blocking antibody secukinumab does not interfere with the efficacy of influenza and meningococcal vaccinations in healthy subjects: results of an open-label, parallel-group, randomized single-center study. Clin Vaccine Immunol. 2012;19(10):1597-602.
29. Hueber W, Sands BE, Lewitzky S, Vandemeulebroecke M, Reinisch W, Higgins PD, et al.; Secukinumab in Crohn's Disease Study Group. Secukinumab, a human anti-IL-17A monoclonal antibody, for moderate to severe Crohn's disease: unexpected results of a randomised, double-blind placebo-controlled trial. Gut. 2012;61(12):1693-700.
30. van de Kerkhof PC, Griffiths CE, Reich K, Leonardi CL, Blauvelt A, Tsai TF, et al. Secukinumab long-term safety experience: A pooled analysis of 10 phase II and III clinical studies in patients with moderate to severe plaque psoriasis. J Am Acad Dermatol. 2016;75(1):83-98.e4.
31. Thaçi D, Humeniuk J, Frambach Y, Bissonnette R, Goodman JJ, Shevade S, et al.; STATURE study group. Secukinumab in psoriasis: randomized, controlled phase 3 trial results assessing the potential to improve treatment response in partial responders (STATURE). Br J Dermatol. 2015;173(3):777-87.

CHAPTER 9

Ixekizumab

Aseem Sharma, Ravina Surve

INTRODUCTION

Ixekizumab is a humanized immunoglobulin G4 (IgG4) monoclonal antibody that selectively binds and inhibits interleukin-17A (IL-17A), resulting in neutralization of IL-17A homodimers and IL-17A/F heterodimers.[1] IL-17, also known as IL-17A, is a key cytokine that links T-cell activation to neutrophil mobilization and activation.[2] Activated T cells appear to produce cytokines, which lead to hyperproliferation of keratinocytes and endothelial cells. IL-17A is a proinflammatory cytokine produced by T helper (Th) 17 cells, which plays a key role in the pathogenesis of plaque psoriasis. IL-17A pathway is thus a promising therapeutic target in the treatment of plaque psoriasis.[3]

Evaluation of the efficacy of ixekizumab in treatment of moderate-to-severe plaque psoriasis has been done in three pivotal phase III, multicenter, double-blinded, randomized controlled trials (RCTs), UNCOVER-1, UNCOVER-2, and UNCOVER-3, inclusive of 3,866 patients. These trials were of 264 weeks in duration, which included an initial 12 weeks of induction period, 48 weeks of randomized withdrawal period in UNCOVER-1 and UNCOVER-2, and long-term extension period from week 60 to 264 in UNCOVER 1 and UNCOVER-2. In UNCOVER-3, long-term extension was from weeks 12 to 264. In all the three trials, ixekizumab was superior to placebo and etanercept (UNCOVER-2 and UNCOVER-3) in achieving primary and secondary endpoints **(Table 1)**.[4,5]

In total, ixekizumab for adult psoriasis has been studied in 17 trials and 6,892 patients with exposures up to 5 years.[4-6] Ixekizumab has demonstrated superiority in five head-to-head trials in providing patients with complete clearance of psoriasis with clearance of psoriasis in special challenging body areas and resolution of symptoms like skin pain and itch.[4-8]

PHARMACOLOGY

- Ixekizumab is a humanized IgG4 monoclonal antibody that selectively binds to human IL-17A[9] (molecular weight = 146,000 Da).

TABLE 1: 12-week endpoint across all UNCOVER studies.

Trial	UNCOVER-1			UNCOVER-2				UNCOVER-3			
Study group	PBO (n = 431)	IXEQ4W (n = 432)	IXEQ2W (n = 433)	PBO (n = 168)	ETN (n = 358)	IXEQ4W (n = 347)	IXEQ2W (n = 351)	PBO (n = 193)	ETN (n = 382)	IXEQ4W (n = 382)	IXEQ2W (n = 385)
PASI 75	17 (3.9)	357 (82.6)	386 (89.1)	4 (2.4)	149 (41.6)	269 (77.5)	315 (89.7)	14 (7.3)	204 (53.4)	325 (84.2)	336 (87.3)

(ETN: etanercept; IXEQ2W: ixekizumab every 2 weeks after starting dose of 160 mg; IXEQ4W: ixekizumab every 4 weeks after starting dose of 160 mg; PASI: psoriasis area and severity index; PBO: placebo)

- Binding studies confirmed affinity of ixekizumab for human IL-17A and the heteromeric form IL-17A/F. Ixekizumab did not exhibit affinity for other members of the IL-17 family of cytokines (IL-17B, IL-17C, IL-17D, IL-17E, and IL-17F), which share between 20 and 50% homology to IL-17A. Ixekizumab has a bioavailability of 60–81% on subcutaneous administration.[10]
- Following a single subcutaneous dose of 160 mg in subjects with plaque psoriasis, ixekizumab reached peak mean (±SD) serum concentrations (Cmax) of 16.2 ± 6.6 μg/mL by approximately 4 days post dose.[9]
- Steady-state concentrations were achieved by week 8 following the 160 mg starting dose and 80 mg every 2 weeks' dosing regimen; the mean ± SD steady-state trough concentration was 9.3 ± 5.3 μg/mL. Steady-state concentrations were achieved approximately 10 weeks after switching from 80 mg every 2 weeks' dosing regimen to 80 mg every 4 weeks' dosing regimen at week 12. The mean ± SD steady-state trough concentration was 3.5 ± 2.5 μg/mL.[9]
- Ixekizumab shows dose- and time-independent clearance. Like endogenous immunoglobulins, ixekizumab is eliminated via intracellular catabolism.[9]
- Mean elimination half-life is around 13 days.[11]

Indications

Food and Drug Administration-approved Indications[9]
- Patients aged 6 years or older with moderate-to-severe plaque psoriasis who are candidates for systemic therapy or phototherapy
- Active psoriatic arthritis
- Active ankylosing spondylitis
- Active nonradiographic axial spondyloarthritis with objective signs of inflammation

Off-label Indications[12,13]
- Hidradenitis suppurativa
- Pityriasis rubra pilaris
- Erythrodermic psoriasis
- Generalized pustular psoriasis

Dosage and Administration[9]
Administer by subcutaneous injection.

Adult Plaque Psoriasis
The recommended dose is 160 mg (two 80 mg injections) at week 0, followed by 80 mg at weeks 2, 4, 6, 8, 10, and 12, and then 80 mg every 4 weeks.

Pediatric Plaque Psoriasis[9]
- For patients weighing > 50 kg, the recommended dose is 160 mg (two 80 mg injections) at week 0, followed by 80 mg every 4 weeks.

- For patients weighing 25–50 kg, the recommended dose is 80 mg at week 0, followed by 40 mg every 4 weeks.
- For patients weighing < 25 kg, the recommended dose is 40 mg at week 0, followed by 20 mg every 4 weeks.

Psoriatic Arthritis
- Recommended dose is 160 mg by subcutaneous injection (two 80 mg injections) at week 0, followed by 80 mg every 4 weeks.
- For psoriatic arthritis patients with coexistent moderate-to-severe plaque psoriasis, use the dosing regimen for adult plaque psoriasis.

Ixekizumab may be administered alone or in combination with a conventional disease-modifying antirheumatic drug (DMARD) (e.g., methotrexate).

Ankylosing Spondylitis

The recommended dose is 160 mg by subcutaneous injection (two 80 mg injections) at week 0, followed by 80 mg every 4 weeks.

Nonradiographic Axial Spondyloarthritis

The recommended dose is 80 mg by subcutaneous injection every 4 weeks.

ADMINISTRATION

Ixekizumab is a clear and colorless to slightly yellow solution which is available as:
- *Autoinjector injection*: 80 mg/mL solution in a single-dose prefilled autoinjector
- *Prefilled syringe injection*: 80 mg/mL solution in a single-dose prefilled syringe

It is intended for use under the guidance and supervision of a physician. Adult patients may self-inject or caregivers may give injections of ixekizumab 80 mg after training in subcutaneous injection technique using the autoinjector or prefilled syringe.[9]

It should be stored at 2–8°C. Before injection, the autoinjector or prefilled syringe should be removed from the refrigerator and allowed to reach room temperature. Avoid shaking the injection; it should be clear and free of any particulate matter. Injection can be given subcutaneously in the upper arm, thighs, or abdomen on rotation to avoid skin damage. Injection should be avoided in tender, bruised, or on psoriatic plaque.[9,14]

Tests to be done Prior to Administration[15]
- Complete blood count (CBC)
- Liver function test (LFT)
- Blood urea and serum creatinine
- Hepatitis B surface antigen, antihepatitis C virus immunoglobulin M, and human immunodeficiency virus (HIV)

- Rule out active and latent tuberculosis (TB):
  - History of past TB and history of contact with an active case of TB
  - History of fever, weight loss, and night sweats
  - Chest X-ray posteroanterior (PA) view
  - Purified protein derivative (PPD) or interferon-gamma release assays (IGRA), if required
- Fasting and postprandial blood sugar
- Electrocardiography (ECG)
- Urinary pregnancy test (UPT) in females.

ADVERSE EFFECTS

- *Injection site reaction*: Redness and pain at the injection site may be experienced.
- Headache
- *Infections:* Patients may be at an increased risk of infections like candidiasis, upper respiratory tract infections, conjunctivitis, and tinea. These adverse effects were observed in a greater number of patients receiving ixekizumab as opposed to those receiving placebo in the UNCOVER trial. The majority of infections were mild to moderate in severity and did not require discontinuation of treatment.[4,5,10]
- *Hypersensitivity reactions*: Rarely patients may develop serious reactions like anaphylaxis or angioedema, in which case the drug should be stopped.
- *Inflammatory bowel disease (IBD)*: Ixekizumab has been associated with the occurrence and exacerbation of IBDs like Crohn's disease and ulcerative colitis.[16]
- Neutropenia and thrombocytopenia were noted in few patients receiving ixekizumab under the UNCOVER trial. Neutropenia of grades 1 and 2 was more common among the patients who received ixekizumab than the placebo group in UNCOVER trial.
- *Antidrug antibody:* 103 of 1,150 patients (9.0%) in the 2-week dosing group in the three UNCOVER trials during the induction period developed antidrug antibodies against ixekizumab. Lower clinical response was seen in these patients than those who had no or low-to-moderate titers of antidrug antibodies.[4]

CONTRAINDICATIONS FOR IXEKIZUMAB[9]

Serious hypersensitivity reaction to ixekizumab or to any of the excipients is a contraindication.

WARNINGS AND PRECAUTIONS[9]

- *Infections:* Serious infections have occurred. Instruct patients to seek medical advice if signs or symptoms of clinically important chronic

or acute infection occur. If a serious infection develops, discontinue ixekizumab until the infection resolves.
- *TB:* Evaluate for TB prior to initiating treatment.
- *Hypersensitivity:* If a serious allergic reaction occurs, discontinue ixekizumab immediately and initiate appropriate therapy.
- *IBD:* Crohn's disease and ulcerative colitis, including exacerbations, occurred during clinical trials. Monitor closely when prescribing ixekizumab to patients with IBD. Discontinue ixekizumab and initiate appropriate medical management if IBD develops.

SPECIAL SITUATIONS

Pregnancy

Risk Summary[9]

There is no available data on ixekizumab use in pregnant women to inform of any drug-associated risks. Human IgG is known to cross the placental barrier; therefore, ixekizumab may be transmitted from the mother to the developing fetus. Ixekizumab is IgG4 molecule while secukinumab is IgG1 molecule. IgG1 is transmitted preferentially through placenta.

The background risk of major birth defects and miscarriage for the indicated population is unknown. In the US general population, the estimated background risk of major birth defects and miscarriage in clinically recognized pregnancies is 2-4% and 15-20%, respectively.

Animal Data[9]

An embryofetal development study was conducted in cynomolgus monkeys who were administered ixekizumab. No malformations or embryofetal toxicity was observed in fetuses from pregnant monkeys administered ixekizumab weekly by subcutaneous injection during organogenesis to near parturition at doses up to 19 times the maximum recommended human dose (MRHD) (on a mg/kg basis of 50 mg/kg/week). Ixekizumab crossed the placenta in monkeys.

In a pre- and postnatal development toxicity study, pregnant cynomolgus monkeys were administered weekly subcutaneous doses of ixekizumab up to 19 times the MRHD from the beginning of organogenesis to parturition. Neonatal deaths occurred in the offspring of two monkeys administered ixekizumab at 1.9 times the MRHD (on a mg/kg basis of 5 mg/kg/week) and in offspring of two monkeys administered ixekizumab at 19 times the MRHD (on a mg/kg basis of 50 mg/kg/week).

These neonatal deaths were attributed to early delivery, trauma, or congenital defect. The clinical significance of these findings is unknown. No ixekizumab-related effects on functional or immunological development were observed in the infants from birth through 6 months of age.

In a study done by Egeberg et al. to evaluate pregnancy outcomes in patients receiving ixekizumab for psoriasis, psoriatic arthritis, or axial spondyloarthritis, no congenital malformations were noted after maternal exposure to ixekizumab.[17]

An embryofetal development study conducted in pregnant monkeys at doses up to 19 times the MRHD revealed no evidence of harm to the developing fetus. When dosing was continued until parturition, neonatal deaths were observed at 1.9 times the MRHD.

Since human IgG passes through the transplacental route, ixekizumab may be transmitted from mother to fetus; therefore, more studies are required for establishing its safety.

Lactation

Ixekizumab has a molecular weight of 146,000 Da; therefore, its amount in milk is likely to be very low. It is also likely to be destroyed in the infant's gastrointestinal tract partially. However, there is no significant database to prove the safety of ixekizumab in lactating women.[18]

Ixekizumab has not been studied in patients with renal and hepatic impairment. However, elimination of drug is by intracellular catabolism; hence, hepatic or renal impairment may not affect the dosing of ixekizumab.[9]

Pediatric

Randomized double-blinded phase three trial (IXORA-PEDS) showed that ixekizumab was superior to placebo in the treatment of moderate-to-severe pediatric psoriasis, and it has been US Food and Drug Administration (FDA) approved for moderate-to-severe pediatric psoriasis.[13,19,20]

Interactions

In patients taking ixekizumab concurrently with drugs (warfarin and cyclosporine), which are substrates of CYP450 enzyme, dose modification or monitoring serum drug levels may be required. This is especially for drugs with narrow therapeutic indexes. In chronic inflammation, CYP450 enzyme formation may be altered by increased levels of cytokines [ILs, tumor necrosis factor (TNF), interferon (IFN)]; thus, ixekizumab being an IL-17A antagonist may normalize the formation of CYP450 enzyme.[9]

People with autoimmune conditions or those taking immunosuppressive medications may have altered immune responses, which could affect how vaccines work. However, the benefits of vaccination, such as preventing serious illnesses, often outweigh the potential risks. In patients newly diagnosed with immune-mediated diseases, it is recommended that age- and condition-appropriate vaccines be administered prior to initiation of immunosuppressive treatment after assessing immunization status. A study, however, showed that ixekizumab does not suppress the humoral immune response to non-live vaccines, which was assessed by the administration of tetanus and pneumococcal vaccines in healthy subjects.[21] Further studies are required to study its effect on live attenuated vaccines. Live attenuated vaccines can be given after 3–6 months of stopping ixekizumab.

In the United States, ixekizumab is available for moderate-to-severe psoriasis and active psoriatic arthritis since 2016 and 2017, respectively. It is available in India for 8–9 months as well. Many real-world studies have shown efficacy of ixekizumab in various studies across the world **(Table 2)**. Few studies have even found a clinical response to ixekizumab after secukinumab failure in psoriatic patients.

TABLE 2: Few real-world studies of ixekizumab showing its efficacy.

Study by	Number of patients	Type of study	Results
Jorge R Georgakopoulos et al.[22]	n = 60 plaque psoriasis patients	Retrospective study	*At 12 weeks:* • PASI 75: 75%
Andrea Chiricozzi et al.[23]	n = 198 136-Biologic naïve 62-Biologic experienced	Retrospective study	*At 24 months:* • PASI 75: 94.3%, PASI 90: 85.1%, PASI 100: 71.8%
G Deza et al.[24]	n = 100 pts 20-Biologic naïve 80- Biologic experienced	Retrospective study	*At 12–16 weeks:* • PASI 75: 87.5%, PASI 90: 50%, PASI 100: 39.6% *At 24–52 weeks:* • Maintained therapeutic efficacy • PASI 75: 83–88%, PASI 90: 58–59%, PASI 100: 42–47%
Alice B Gottileb et al.[25]	n = 523	Prospective study	*At 12 weeks:* • BSA ≤ 1–54.8% • BSA ≤ 3–75.1% *At 24 weeks:* • Improvement in ≥ 4 points in itch and pain • 63.1% and 64.8% respectively
Gulliver et al.[26]	n = 1,891 1,023-Biologic naïve 573- Biologic experienced	Retrospective study	*Persistence of treatment:* • Biologic naïve, 1 year: 94.6% • Biologic naïve, 2 years: 90.3% • Biologic experienced, 1 year: 87.3% • Biologic experienced, 2 year: 83.5%
Raquel Rivera et al.[27]	301 68.5%-Biologic experienced 31.5%-Biologic naïve	Retrospective	*At 3 months:* • Absolute PASI <2–76.5% • PASI 90: 57.3% *At 12 months:* • Absolute PASI <2–73.4% • PASI 90: 58.7%

(BSA: body surface area; PASI: psoriasis area and severity index)

CONCLUSION

Ixekizumab is a monoclonal antibody. It works by targeting IL-17A which plays a role in inflammatory response associated with certain autoimmune conditions like psoriasis. It is available as autoinjector in form of prefilled syringes making its administration easy. It can be used in recalcitrant cases of psoriasis. Its effects can be seen as early as 4 weeks, however, individual patient response rate may vary. Patients with inflammatory bowel disease may experience exacerbations and should be cautiously used in patients with gastrointestinal symptoms. Overall data regarding ixekizumab usage is encouraging and long-term remission rate needs to be evaluated by further studies.

REFERENCES

1. Dong J, Goldenberg G. New biologics in psoriasis: an update on IL-23 and IL-17 inhibitors. Cutis. 2017;99(2):123-7.
2. Zenobia C, Hajishengallis G. Basic biology and role of interleukin-17 in immunity and inflammation. Periodontol. 2000. 2015;69(1):142-59.
3. Krueger JG, Fretzin S, Suarez-Farinas M, Haslett PA, Phipps KM, Cameron GS, et al. IL-17A is essential for cell activation and inflammatory gene circuits in subjects with psoriasis. J Allergy Clin Immunol. 2012;130(1):145-54.e9.
4. Gordon KB, Blauvelt A, Papp KA, Langley RG, Luger T, Ohtsuki M, et al. Phase 3 trials of ixekizumab in moderate-to-severe plaque psoriasis. N Engl J Med. 2016;375(4):345-56.
5. Griffiths CE, Reich K, Lebwohl M, van de Kerkhof P, Paul C, Menter A, et al; UNCOVER-2 and UNCOVER-3 investigators. Comparison of ixekizumab with etanercept or placebo in moderate-to-severe psoriasis (UNCOVER-2 and UNCOVER-3): Results from two phase 3 randomised trials. Lancet. 2015;386(9993):541-51.
6. Craig S, Warren RB. Ixekizumab for the treatment of psoriasis: up-to-date. Expert Opin Biol Ther. 2020;20(6):549-57.
7. Leonardi C, Reich K, Foley P, Torii H, Gerdes S, Guenther L, et al. Efficacy and safety of ixekizumab through 5 years in moderate-to-severe psoriasis: Long-term results from the UNCOVER-1 and UNCOVER-2 phase-3 randomized controlled trials. Dermatol Ther (Heidelb). 2020;10(3):431-47.
8. Blauvelt A, Lebwohl MG, Mabuchi T, Leung A, Garrelts A, Crane H, et al. Long-term efficacy and safety of ixekizumab: A 5-year analysis of the UNCOVER-3 randomized controlled trial. J Am Acad Dermatol. 2021;85(2):360-8.
9. Eli Lilly and Company. (2016). TALTZ (ixekizumab) injection, for subcutaneous use: US prescribing information. [online] Available from http://www. Ixekizumab.com [Last accessed January, 2024].
10. Syed Y.Y. Ixekizumab: A review in moderate to severe plaque psoriasis. Am J Clin Dermatol. 2017;18(1):147-58.
11. European Medicines Agency. (2015). TALTZ (ixekizumab): Summary of product characteristics. [online] Available from http://www.ema.europa.eu [Last accessed January, 2024].
12. Wu KK, Dao Jr H. Off-label dermatologic uses of IL-17 inhibitors. J Dermatolog Treat. 2022;33(1):41-7.
13. Saeki H, Nakagawa H, Ishii T, Morisaki Y, Aoki T, Berclaz PY, et al. Efficacy and safety of open-label ixekizumab treatment in Japanese patients with moderate-to-severe plaque psoriasis, erythrodermic psoriasis and generalized pustular psoriasis. J Eur Acad Dermatol Venereol. 2015;29(6):1148-55.

14. Preuss CV, Quick J. Ixekizumab. In: StatPearls [Internet]. Treasure Island (FL): StatPearls Publishing; 2023. [online] Available from https://www.ncbi.nlm.nih.gov/books/NBK431088/ [Last accessed January, 2024].
15. Nast A, Smith C, Spuls PI, Avila Valle G, Bata-Csörgö Z, Boonen H, et al. EuroGuiDerm Guideline on the systemic treatment of psoriasis vulgaris–Part 1: Treatment and monitoring recommendations. J Eur Acad Dermatol Venereol. 2020;34(11):2461-98.
16. Deodhar A, Poddubnyy D, Pacheco-Tena C, Salvarani C, Lespessailles E, Rahman P, et al.; COAST-W Study Group. Efficacy and safety of ixekizumab in the treatment of radiographic axial spondyloarthritis: Sixteen-week results from a phase iii randomized, double-blind, placebo-controlled trial in patients with prior inadequate response to or intolerance of tumor necrosis factor inhibitors. Arthritis Rheumatol. 2019;71(4):599-611.
17. Egeberg A, Iversen L, Kimball AB, Kelly S, Grace E, Patel H, et al. Pregnancy outcomes in patients with psoriasis, psoriatic arthritis, or axial spondyloarthritis receiving ixekizumab. J Dermatolog Treat. 2022;33(5):2503-9.
18. U.S. Department of Health and Human Services. Drugs and Lactation Database (LactMed®) [Internet]. Bethesda (MD): National Institute of Child Health and Human Development; 2006. [online] Available from https://www.ncbi.nlm.nih.gov/books/NBK501922/ [Last accessed January, 2024].
19. Paller AS, Seyger MMB, Alejandro Magariños G, Bagel J, Pinter A, Cather J, et al.; IXORA-PEDS study group. Efficacy and safety of ixekizumab in a phase III, randomized, double-blind, placebo-controlled study in paediatric patients with moderate-to-severe plaque psoriasis (IXORA-PEDS). Br J Dermatol. 2020;183(2):231-41.
20. Cather JC, Young CT, Young MS, Cather JC. Ixekizumab for the treatment of pediatric patients with moderate to severe plaque psoriasis. Expert Opin Biol Ther. 2021;21(8):983-90.
21. Gomez EV, Bishop JL, Jackson K, Muram TM, Muram T, Phillips D. response to tetanus and pneumococcal vaccination following administration of ixekizumab in healthy participants. BioDrugs. 2017;31(6):545-54.
22. Briceño Casado M, Gil-Sierra MD, De La Calle Riaguas B, Dominguez-Cantero M. 4CPS-324 Effectiveness and safety of ixekizumab in moderate-to-severe plaque psoriasis. Eur J Hosp Pharm. 2021;28(1):A76-7.
23. Chiricozzi A, Megna M, Giunta A, Carrera CG, Dapavo P, Balato A. Ixekizumab is effective in the long-term management in moderate-to-severe plaque psoriasis: Results from an Italian retrospective cohort study (the LOTIXE study). J Dermatolog Treat. 2023;34(1):2246606.
24. Deza G, Notario J, Lopez-Ferrer A, Vilarrasa E, Ferran M, Del Alcazar E,et al. Initial results of ixekizumab efficacy and safety in real-world plaque psoriasis patients: A multicentre retrospective study. J Eur Acad Dermatol Venereol. 2019;33(3):553-9.
25. Gottlieb AB, Burge R, Malatestinic WN, Zhu B, Zhao Y, McCormack J, et al. Ixekizumab Real-World Effectiveness at 24 Weeks in Patients with Psoriasis: Data from the United States Taltz Customer Support Program. Dermatol Ther (Heidelb). 2023;13(8):1831-46.
26. Gulliver W, Gooderham MJ, Zhu B, Jossart C, Montmayeur S, Burge R, at al. Treatment Persistence of Ixekizumab in Adults with Moderate-to-Severe Plaque Psoriasis Participating in the Canadian Patient Support Program. Dermatol Ther (Heidelb). 2023;13(1):235-44.
27. Rivera R, Velasco M, Vidal D, Carrascosa JM, Daudén E, Vilarrasa E, et al. The effectiveness and safety of ixekizumab in psoriasis patients under clinical practice conditions: A Spanish multicentre retrospective study. Dermatol Ther. 2020;33(6):e14066.

CHAPTER 10

Anti-CD6 Monoclonal Antibody: Itolizumab

Krupashankar DS, Swaroop HS

INTRODUCTION

Itolizumab is a humanized anti-cluster of differentiation 6 (anti-CD6) monoclonal antibody (mAB). It was approved in India by Drug Controller General of India (DCGI) in 2012 for the treatment of moderate-to-severe chronic plaque psoriasis. Till date itolizumab is the only Indian research biologic available in India.

PHARMACOLOGY

Itolizumab is a humanized recombinant anti-CD6 mAB of immunoglobulin G1 (IgG1) isotype which binds to domain of CD6. It contains two heavy chains with 449 amino acids and two light chains with 214 amino acids with a molecular weight of 148 kDa.[1] The initial anti-CD6 mAB was a murine antibody iorT1. It was immunogenic in nature due to its murine origin. With progresses in genetic engineering, the murine content was replaced by human counterparts. The resulting antibody retained the same CD6 affinity of iorT1, with improved side effect profile.[2] Molecular structure of CD6 is shown in **Figure 1**.

MECHANISM OF ACTION

Itolizumab is a humanized monoclonal antibody that recognizes the membrane-distal domain scavenger receptor cysteine-rich 1 (SRCR1) (D1) of CD6, which modulates T lymphocyte activation and proliferation. Itolizumab binds to D1 of CD6, thereby it reduces the interaction of D3 of CD6 to activated leukocyte cell adhesion molecule (ALCAM), which helps in differentiation of T helper cells into T helper 1 cells (Th1) and T helper 17 cells (Th17). Hence, it is an upstream inhibitor. It blocks intracellular mitogen-activated protein kinase (MAPK) and signal transducer and activator of transcription-3 (STAT-3) signaling pathways, thereby it blocks the secretion of proinflammatory cytokines [including tumor necrosis factor alpha

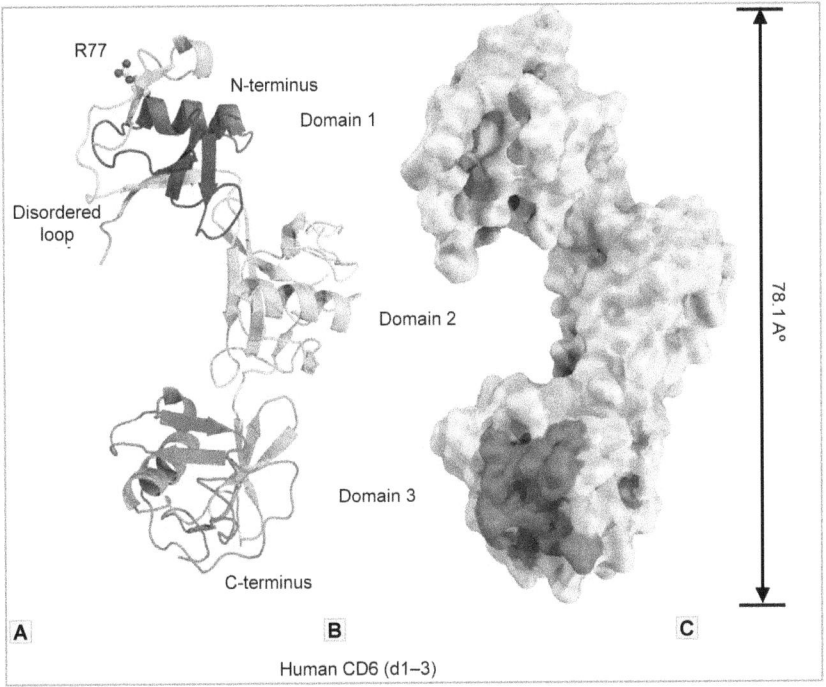

FIGS. 1A TO C: Molecular structure of CD6 (cluster of differentiation 6) with its three domains.[4] (A) Loop structure of CD6; (B) three-dimensional structure of CD6; (C) total length of CD6.

(TNF-α), interferon (IFN-γ), and interleukin-6 (IL-6)] and T cell proliferation. Itolizumab is an immunomodulator; it does not cause T cell depletion and whenever depletion occurs, it is transient in nature.[3] Mechanism of action of itolizumab is illustrated in **Figure 2**.

DOWNREGULATION OF BOTH DOWNSTREAM AND UPSTREAM MEDIATORS IN PSORIASIS

Gupta et al.[5] reported a case report of recalcitrant psoriasis patient successfully treated with cyclosporine for first 15 days followed with itolizumab, where the patient achieved Psoriasis Area and Severity Index (PASI) 90 in 12 weeks and maintained a remission of PASI-90 up to 15 months. The rationale behind this case report is to downregulate both upstream and downstream mediators in psoriasis pathogenesis.

In recalcitrant psoriasis, Th17 skewing of naive T cells leads to the local production of IL-17 ligand; keratinocytes in turn are stimulated by these IL-17 ligands leading to an aberrant differentiation and elevated production of pro-inflammatory factors. These keratinocyte-derived factors in turn stimulate further IL-17-producing cells, which establish a self-sustaining inflammatory feedback loop at keratinocytes. This in turn leads to recalcitrant psoriasis.

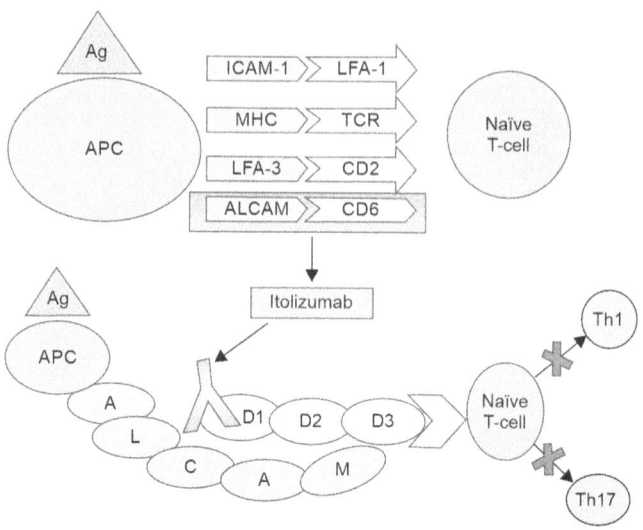

FIG. 2: Mechanism of action of itolizumab.
(Ag: antigen; ALCAM: activated lymphocyte cell adhesion molecule; APC: antigen-presenting cell; CD2: cluster of differentiation 2; CD6: cluster of differentiation 6; ICAM: intercellular adhesion molecule; LFA-1: lymphocyte function-associated antigen 1; LFA-3: lymphocyte function-associated antigen 3; MHC: major histocompatibility complex; TCR: T-cell receptor; Th1: T helper 1 cell; Th17: T helper 17 cell)

Within 2 weeks of commencing treatment with cyclosporine, a calcineurin inhibitor, leads to suppression of Th17 activation, which in turn leads to decreased IL-17, IL-22, and downstream genes including defensin-beta 2 (DEFB-2), lipocalin-2 (LCN2), chemokine (C-X-C motif) ligand 1 (CXCL1), and chemokine (C-C motif) ligand 20 (CCL20). This might abolish self-sustaining inflammatory feedback loop. Itolizumab, an anti-CD6 monoclonal antibody, causes downregulation of priming and activation of T cells to Th1 and Th17 cells, which subsequently leads to downregulation of downstream mediators such as TNF-α, IL-17, and IL-23. Continuing inflammatory process is blocked at epidermis. This leads to the normalization of the skin architecture and long-term remission of lesions in psoriasis. However, this hypothesis has been proved only in one patient, hence larger randomized controlled studies are required to corroborate these results and to standardize the relevant guidelines.[6,7] Illustration of downstream and upstream mediators in psoriasis is shown in **Figure 3**.

LITERATURE SEARCH

Itolizumab phase 2 and 3 studies were randomized, multicentric, placebo controlled studies, which determined the efficacy of itolizumab and rest of the efficacy data is from individual case reports and series, which is mentioned in **Table 1**.

CHAPTER 10: Anti-CD6 Monoclonal Antibody: Itolizumab

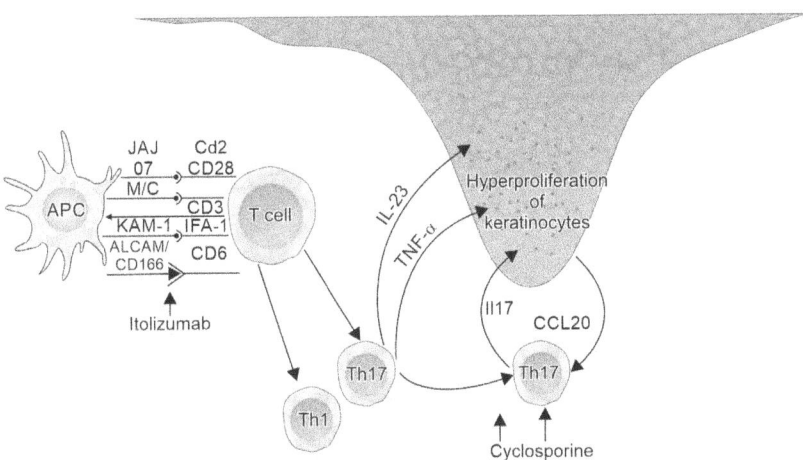

FIG. 3: Illustration of downregulation of downstream and upstream mediators in psoriasis.
[APC: antigen-presenting cell; ALCAM: activated lymphocyte cell adhesion molecule; CCL-20: chemokine (C-C motif) ligand 20; CD6: cluster of differentiation 6; IL-23: interleukin 23; Th1: T helper 1 cell; Th17: T helper 17 cell; TNF-α: tumor necrosis factor alpha]

TABLE 1: Summary of efficacy studies of itolizumab.[8-10]

Study name	Indication	Dosing schedule	Results	ADR
Phase 2	Plaque psoriasis	1.6 mg/kg body weight, once every 2 weeks for 12 weeks, followed with once in month for next 12 weeks	PASI-75 scores at 12 weeks: 45%	Chills and rigors
Phase 3	Plaque psoriasis	1.6 mg/kg body weight, once every 2 weeks for 12 weeks, followed with once in month for next 12 weeks	• PASI-75 at 45.5% at 28 weeks • PASI-90 at 21.6% at 28 weeks • 52.5% of patients maintained drug-free remission at 52 weeks	• Infusion-related reactions • Upper respiratory tract infections, pyrexia
Parthasaradhi case series of 20 patients	Plaque psoriasis	1.6 mg/kg body weight, once every 2 weeks for 12 weeks, followed with once in month for next 12 weeks	18 patients achieved PASI-75 at 24 weeks	None reported

Continued

SECTION 2: Biologics in Psoriasis

Continued

Study name	Indication	Dosing schedule	Results	ADR
Pai et al.[11] case series of five patients	Plaque psoriasis with psoriatic arthritis	1.6 mg/kg body weight, once every 2 weeks for 12 weeks, followed with once in month for next 12 weeks	• All five patients achieved PASI-75 at 24 weeks • Significant improvement in psoriatic arthropathy in one patient	None reported
Singh V case series of seven patients	Plaque psoriasis	1.6 mg/kg body weight, once every 2 weeks for 12 weeks, followed with once in month for next 12 weeks	All seven patients achieved PASI-75 at 24 weeks	None reported
Singh V case report	Pustular psoriasis	1.6 mg/kg body weight, once every 2 weeks for 12 weeks, followed with once in month for next 12 weeks	PASI-90 achieved at 24 weeks	None reported
Parasramani case series of 10 patients	Plaque psoriasis	1.6 mg/kg body weight, once every 2 weeks for 12 weeks, followed with once in month for next 12 weeks	Seven patients achieved >PASI-75 at 24 weeks and three patients achieved PASI-90 at 24 weeks	None reported
Gupta et al.	Plaque psoriasis	Cyclosporine 200 mg for first 15 days followed with itolizumab regimen	Patient achieved PASI-90 at 12 weeks and sustained remission for 15 months	None reported

(ADR: adverse drug reaction; PASI-75: Psoriasis Area and Severity Index 75; PASI-90: Psoriasis Area and Severity Index 90)

INDICATIONS

- *DCGI approved*: Moderate-to-severe chronic plaque psoriasis
- *Off-label:* Psoriatic arthritis

CONTRAINDICATIONS

Itolizumab should not be administered to patients having history of severe allergy or known hypersensitivity reaction to any component of itolizumab or any murine proteins. Additionally, itolizumab is contraindicated in patients with any active serious infection and latent tuberculosis (TB).

SIDE EFFECTS

The adverse effects of itolizumab is listed as systemwise in **Table 2**.

CHECKLIST

History of any serious infections or TB or immunocompromised conditions to be ruled out.

INVESTIGATIONS

- Complete blood count
- Screening for TB (clinical)—signs and symptoms of TB to be evaluated
- Mantoux test and chest X-ray to rule out TB before starting the therapy

VACCINATIONS

It is recommended that live/attenuated vaccines should not be given concurrently with itolizumab. The patient's vaccination record and the

TABLE 2: Adverse effects of itolizumab.

System	Adverse drug reactions
Acute infusion reactions	Nausea, flushing, urticaria, cough, hypersensitivity, pruritus, rash, wheezing, dyspnea, dizziness, headache, and hypertension
Gastrointestinal	Diarrhea, toothache, vomiting, gastritis, gastrointestinal inflammation
Infections and infestations	Abscess, folliculitis, gastroenteritis, lymphadenitis, lymph node tuberculosis, oral herpes, pyrexia, urinary tract infection, rhinitis, tooth abscess
Metabolism and nutrition disorders	Dehydration, hepatic steatosis, hypertriglyceridemia
Musculoskeletal	Musculoskeletal pain, pain in extremity, arthralgia, and back pain
Nervous system	Headache, peripheral neuropathy, cerebrovascular accident
Psychiatric disorder	Adjustment disorder with anxiety
Respiratory disorders	Cough, oropharyngeal pain, rhinorrhea

need for immunization prior to receiving itolizumab should be carefully investigated. Caution is advised in the administration of live vaccines to infants born to female patients treated with itolizumab during pregnancy, since itolizumab may cross the placenta.

DOSING

The recommended dosage of itolizumab for the treatment of plaque psoriasis is 1.6 mg/kg given as intravenous infusion once every 2 weeks for first 12 weeks, followed by 1.6 mg/kg once in 4 weeks up to 24 weeks.

MAINTENANCE REGIMENS

Once in 3 months post the 24 weeks of the therapy is advisable.

SPECIAL POPULATION

Pregnancy

As with other IgG antibodies, itolizumab may cross the placenta during pregnancy. It is not known whether itolizumab can cause fetal harm when administered to a pregnant woman, or whether it can affect reproductive capacity or fertility.

Lactation

It is not known whether itolizumab is excreted in human milk or absorbed systemically after ingestion. Because many drugs and Ig are excreted in human milk and because of the potential for serious adverse reactions in nursing infants from itolizumab, a decision should be made whether to discontinue nursing or to discontinue the drug, taking into account the importance of the drug to the mother.

MONITORING OF A PATIENT ON BIOLOGIC

Patients on itolizumab should be closely monitored for development of any infection especially TB. Patient should be asked for history of weight loss, fever, and night sweats during each visit to rule out any extrapulmonary TB.

CONCLUSION

Itolizumab is the indigenously developed biologic. It is moderately effective in the treatment of psoriasis and is given as intravenous infusion. For these reason and availability of more effective biologic, its placement in the management of psoriasis is not clear.

REFERENCES

1. India: Biocon, Inc. (2013). Alzumab™ (Itolizumab) solution for IV infusion [prescribing information]. [online] Available from https://www.biocon.com/docs/prescribing_information/immunotherapy/Alzumab_pi.pdf [Last accessed January, 2024].
2. Alonso-Ramirez R, Loisel S, Buors C, Pers JO, Montero E, Youinou P, et al. Rationale for targeting CD6 as a treatment for autoimmune diseases. Arthritis. 2010;2010:130646.
3. Nair P, Melarkode R, Rajkumar D, Montero E. CD6 synergistic co-stimulation promoting proinflammatory response is modulated without interfering with the activated leucocyte cell adhesion molecule interaction. Clin Exp Immunol. 2010;162:116-30.
4. Chappell PE, Garner LI, Yan J, Metcalfe C, Hatherley D, Johnson S, et al. Structures of CD6 and Its Ligand CD166 Give Insight into Their Interaction. Structure. 2015;23(8):1426-36.
5. Gupta A, Sharma YK, Deo K, Kothari P. Severe recalcitrant psoriasis treated with itolizumab, a novel anti-CD6 monoclonal antibody. Indian J Dermatol Venereol Leprol. 2016;82(4):459-61.
6. Alonso R, Huerta V, de Leon J, Piedra P, Puchades Y, Guirola O, et al. Towards the definition of a chimpanzee and human conserved CD6 domain 1 epitope recognized by T1 monoclonal antibody. Hybridoma (Larchmt). 2008;27(4):291-301.
7. Haider AS, Lowes AM, Suárez-Fariñas M, Zaba LC, Cardinale I, Khatcherian A, et al. Identification of cellular pathways of "type 1," Th 17 T cells and TNF alpha and inducible nitric oxide synthase-producing dendritic cells in autoimmune inflammation through pharmacogenomic study of cyclosporine A in psoriasis. J Immunol. 2008;180(3):1913-20.
8. Doral S, Uprety S, Suresh SH. Itolizumab, a novel anti-CD6 monoclonal antibody: a safe and efficacious biologic agent for management of psoriasis. Expert Opin Biol Ther. 2017;17:395-402.
9. Parthasaradhi A. Safety and Efficacy of Itolizumab in the Treatment of Psoriasis: A Case Series of 20 Patients. J Clin Diagn Res. 2016;10(11):WD01-WD03.
10. Singh V. Clinical Outcome of a Novel Anti-CD6 Biologic Itolizumab in Patients of Psoriasis with Comorbid Conditions. Dermatol Res Pract. 2016;2016:1316326.
11. Pai G, Pai AH. Itolizumab - A New Biologic for Management of Psoriasis and Psoriatic Arthritis. Case Rep Dermatol. 2017;9(2):141-5.

CHAPTER 11

Interleukin-36 Receptor Antagonist: Spesolimab

Ruchi Hemdani

INTRODUCTION

Spesolimab is an interleukin (IL)-36 receptor antagonist. It is a humanized monoclonal immunoglobulin G1 (IgG1) antibody (mAb) against human IL-36R produced by recombinant deoxyribonucleic acid (DNA) technology.[1] Spesolimab was approved by the United States Food and Drug Administration (US-FDA) in September 2022 to treat adult patients with flares of generalized pustular psoriasis (GPP).[2]

Loss-of-function mutations in the IL-36 receptor antagonist gene (*IL36RN*) and associated genes (*CARD14, AP1S3, SERPINA3,* and *MPO*),[3,4] overexpression and overactiveness of IL-36 in pustular psoriasis; all support the pathogenic role of IL-36 in GPP pathway. Dysregulated IL-36R signaling leads to a neutrophilic inflammatory response and the eruption of pustules in GPP. This is also established by advances in understanding of molecular mechanisms of GPP pathogenesis and clinical validation of novel pharmacological targets.[5] Clinical improvements with spesolimab were observed in an open-label phase 1 study involving seven patients presenting with a GPP flare.[6] Thus, spesolimab acts as selective targeted therapy for treatment of GPP flares.

PHARMACOLOGY

- Spesolimab is a humanized monoclonal antibody that selectively binds to IL-36 receptor and inhibits IL-36 signaling thereby neutralizing the downstream proinflammatory and profibrotic cytokines, although the precise mechanism linking reduced IL-36R activity and treatment of flares of GPP is unclear.[7,8] IL-36 autocrine and autoinflammatory circuit is explained in **Figure 1**.
- It is of the IgG1/κ-class produced in Chinese hamster ovary (CHO) cells.[1]
- It works by targeting IL-36R and prevents the subsequent activation of IL-36R by cognate ligands (IL-36 α, β, and γ). Its molecular weight is 146 kDa.[1,9]

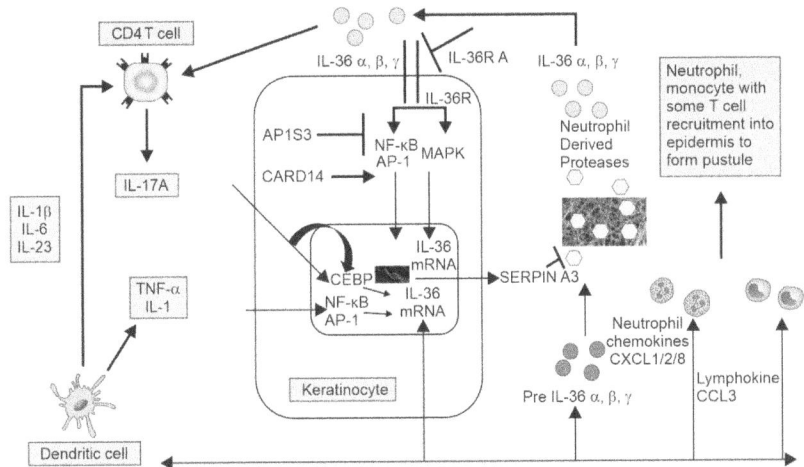

FIG. 1: Interleukin (IL)-36 autocrine and autoinflammatory circuit.
(AP-1: activating protein 1; CARD: caspase recruitment domain; MAPK: mitogen-activated protein kinase; NET: neutrophil extracellular trap; RA: receptor antagonist; NF-κβ: nuclear factor kappa-light chain enhancer of activated B cell; TNF-α: tumor necrosis factor alpha)

- Following a single intravenous dose of 900 mg in GPP patients, the estimated area under curve 0-∞ (AUC0-∞) (95% CI) and C_{max} (95% CI) were 4,750 (4,510 and 4,970) µg/day/mL and 238 (218 and 256) µg/mL, respectively.[1]
- Intravenous spesolimab exhibited target-mediated drug disposition at low doses (0.01-0.3 mg/kg) and linear kinetics at doses ≥ 0.3 mg/kg.[1,7] Bioavailability of subcutaneous spesolimab increased with increasing dose over the range of 150-600 mg and was higher when administered to the thigh than to the abdomen.[10]
- Spesolimab clearance in a typical GPP patient without antidrug antibodies (ADA), weighing 70 kg was 0.184 L/day and elimination of half-life was estimated to be 25.5 days.
- The metabolic pathway of spesolimab has not been characterized. It is expected to be degraded into small peptides and amino acids via catabolic pathways similar to endogenous IgG.[7]
- Spesolimab is not expected to undergo hepatic or renal elimination. No formal study of the effect of hepatic or renal impairment on the pharmacokinetics of spesolimab has been conducted.[1,7]
- Age, gender, and race did not affect the pharmacokinetics of spesolimab as per population pharmacokinetic analyses.[1] The clinical impact of body weight on spesolimab plasma concentrations is unknown.[1]
- No formal drug interactions studies have been conducted with spesolimab.
- *Immunogenicity:* ADA were found in 46% of patients who received at least one dose of spesolimab; median onset being 2.3 weeks after spesolimab

TABLE 1: Off-label indications of spesolimab.		
Indication	Trial	Outcome
Ulcerative colitis	Phase II trial (NCT03482635)	Lower rates of clinical remission in patients with moderate to severe UC[1]
	Phase IIa trial (NCT03123120)	Spesolimab did not induce mucosal healing in patients with mild-to-moderate UC receiving TNF-α inhibitor therapy[15]
Palmoplantar pustulosis	Phase IIa pilot study (NCT03135548)	PPP severity declined over time in all groups after the start of treatment with a faster decline in the spesolimab arms than in the placebo arm. Results indicate that spesolimab may be effective for treating PPP[16]
Atopic dermatitis	Multicenter, randomized, double-blind, and placebo-controlled, phase IIa study	Only modest improvement in AD as compared to placebo[17]
Pyoderma gangrenosum	Case report	Two cases of PG that were resistant to prednisolone, cyclosporine, adalimumab and they showed dramatic improvement with the use of spesolimab[18]

(AD: atopic dermatitis; UC: ulcerative colitis; PG: pyoderma gangrenosum; PPP: palmoplantar pustulosis; TNF: tumor necrosis factor)

administration.[1,7] Plasma concentrations of spesolimab were significantly reduced in subjects with ADA titers > 4,000. There was no indication that ADA was associated with hypersensitivity.[11]
- Carcinogenicity and mutagenicity studies have not been conducted with spesolimab.[1,7,8]

USES

Food and Drug Administration-approved Indications
Flares of GPP

Off-label Indications (Table 1)
- Ulcerative colitis (UC)
- Crohn disease (CD)
- Palmoplantar pustulosis (PPP)
- Hidradenitis suppurativa (HS)
- Atopic dermatitis
- Pyoderma gangrenosum

Generalized Pustular Psoriasis
On 1st September 2022, spesolimab was approved by the US-FDA and on 26th September 2022, it was approved in Japan, for the treatment of acute

symptoms in GPP in adult patients.[1] FDA approval was partly based on results from the 12-week pivotal phase 2 Effisayil 1 study.[11,12] Spesolimab received conditional marketing authorization on 9th December 2022 by European Medicines Agency for treatment of flares in adult patients with GPP.[13] (Conditional authorization is granted on the basis of less comprehensive data than are normally required. It is granted for medicines that fulfill an unmet medical need to treat serious diseases and when the benefits of having them available earlier outweigh any risks associated with using the medicines while waiting for further evidence). Spesolimab has received breakthrough therapy designation in China and Taiwan. Spesolimab is also in phase II/III development for GPP in multiple countries.

Clinical response (skin and pustular clearance) in patients with a GPP flare occurred rapidly with single intravenous spesolimab dose of 10 mg/kg in phase I proof of concept study compared to placebo, irrespective of *IL36RN* mutation.[1,6] Phase II Effisayil 1 trial evaluated the efficacy, safety, and tolerability of a single 900 mg dose of IV administered spesolimab, with the option of a second dose if symptoms persisted on day 8, versus placebo in 53 patients experiencing a GPP flare. At the end of 1 week, 54% of patients treated with spesolimab showed no visible pustules compared to 6% of those who received placebo.[11,12] Spesolimab thus showed superiority over placebo with higher rates of clearance.

At the end of trial, all patients were eligible to enter Effisayil ON, a 5-year open label extension trial of spesolimab for evaluation of long-term administration of spesolimab with a subcutaneous formulation.[14]

ADMINISTRATION

Dosage Form, Strength, and Preparation

Spesolimab is manufactured under brand name SPEVIGO by Boehringer Ingelheim Pharmaceuticals. SPEVIGO (spesolimab-sbzo) injection is a sterile, preservative-free, colorless to slightly brownish-yellow, clear to slightly opalescent solution supplied as single-dose glass vials for intravenous infusion. Each carton contains two single-dose 450 mg/7.5 mL (60 mg/mL).[7] Each 7.5 mL vial contains 450 mg spesolimab-sbzo, arginine hydrochloride (39.5 mg), glacial acetic acid (2.4 mg), polysorbate 20 (3.0 mg), sodium acetate (24.5 mg), sucrose (386 mg), and water for injection, USP with a pH of 5.0–6.0 vials and must be refrigerated at 2–8°C (36–46°F); however, unopened SPEVIGO vials may be stored at room temperature, 20–25°C (68–77°F), for up to 24 hours in the original carton to protect from light.[7,8]

Two vials (15 mL) are mixed in 85 mL sterile 0.9% sodium chloride injection to prepare solution for intravenous administration ensuring aseptic technique. The prepared solution should be used immediately. If not administered immediately, diluted solution may be refrigerated at 2–8°C (36–46°F) for up to 4 hours.[7]

Dosage

Spesolimab is administered as single-dose injection. The recommended dose is 900 mg by intravenous infusion over 90 minutes (maximum 180 minutes in case the infusion is slowed or stopped temporarily). An additional intravenous 900 mg dose (over 90 minutes) may be administered 1 week after the initial dose if symptoms persist.[1,7,8]

*In case a preexisting intravenous line is being used for administration of spesolimab, it must be flushed with sterile 0.9% sodium chloride injection prior to and at the end of infusion. No other infusion should be administered in parallel via the same intravenous access.

Tests to be done Prior to Administration

Limited data exists on specific investigations to be carried out but investigations for active and latent tuberculosis (TB) must be done along with other baseline investigations usually done prior to administration of biologics to rule out any other active infection.[1,7]

MONITORING DURING THERAPY

Patients should be closely monitored for development of active infection specifically for signs and symptoms of active TB during and after spesolimab treatment.[1,7]

ADVERSE EFFECTS

Spesolimab was generally well tolerated in patients with GPP. The adverse effects (AEs) as reported with treatment during Effisayil 1 trial[11,12] are tabulated in **Table 2**:

Additionally, Guillain–Barré syndrome was reported in three patients during clinical development.
- Spesolimab-associated hypersensitivity reactions may include immediate reactions such as anaphylaxis and DRESS.[11,12] If an anaphylactic or other serious allergic reaction occurs, administration of spesolimab is to be discontinued immediately and appropriate therapy should be initiated. In cases of mild or moderate infusion-related reactions, infusion must be stopped and appropriate medical therapy (e.g., systemic antihistamines and/or corticosteroids) are to be initiated. The infusion may be restarted at a slower infusion rate with gradual increase to complete the infusion once the reaction has settled.[1,7]

CONTRAINDICATIONS

- Severe or life-threatening hypersensitivity reactions to the active substance or to any of the excipients
- Active TB

TABLE 2: Adverse effects reported with treatment with spesolimab.		
AEs through week 1 (66% reported): Mostly mild AEs	AEs through week 12: Few serious AEs	AEs through week 12 and 17: Mild to moderate AEs
Asthenia and fatigue, nausea, and vomiting, headache, pruritus and prurigo, infusion site hematoma and bruising, dyspnea, eye edema, and urticaria	Drug reaction with eosinophilia and systemic symptoms (DRESS), drug-induced hepatic injury, urinary tract infection, arthritis, worsening of chronic plaque psoriasis, influenza, and cutaneous squamous cell carcinoma	Device-related infection, subcutaneous abscess, furuncle, and influenza, otitis externa, vulvovaginal candidiasis, vulvovaginal mycotic infection, latent tuberculosis, diarrhea, and gastritis

(AEs: adverse effects)

SPECIAL SITUATIONS

- *Pregnancy:* Limited data regarding use of this biologic in pregnancy are insufficient to inform a drug-associated risk of adverse pregnancy-related outcomes. Animal studies do not indicate direct or indirect harmful effects with respect to pregnancy, embryonic/fetal development, parturition, or postnatal development with this agent.[7]
- *Breastfeeding:* There are no data on the presence of spesolimab in human milk, the effects on the breastfed infant, or the effects on milk production.[1,7] Spesolimab, being a monoclonal antibody, is expected to be present in human milk as immunoglobulins are excreted in human milk. Therefore, caution is to be exercised when spesolimab is administered to a woman who is breastfeeding. The developmental and health benefits of breastfeeding should be considered along with the mother's clinical need for spesolimab and any potential adverse effects on the breastfed infant from spesolimab or from the underlying maternal condition.
- *Fertility:* The effect of spesolimab on human fertility has not been evaluated.[7] Animal studies do not indicate direct or indirect harmful effects with respect to fertility.
- *Vaccinations:* Use of live vaccines is to be avoided in patients treated with spesolimab. No specific studies have been conducted in spesolimab treated patients who have recently received live viral or live bacterial vaccines.[1,7] Spesolimab may pass through the placenta (human IgG is known to cross placental barrier) and live vaccines therefore should be avoided in neonates whose mothers have been given spesolimab during pregnancy.
- *Pediatric age group:* Safety and effectiveness of spesolimab in pediatric patients have not been established.[7]
- *Geriatric age group:* Clinical studies did not include enough subjects aged 65 years and over to determine whether they respond differently from younger adult subjects.[1,7,11]

- *Tuberculosis:* All patients are to be screened for TB infection prior to initiating treatment with spesolimab. It is not to be administered to patients with active TB infection. In patients with latent TB or a history of TB in whom an adequate course of treatment cannot be confirmed, anti-TB therapy must be considered prior to initiating spesolimab.[7]
- *Infections:* Spesolimab may increase the risk of infections (Effisayil-1 trial).[12] In patients with a chronic infection or recurrent infection, the potential risks and expected clinical benefits of treatment must be considered prior to administration. It is not recommended for use in patients with any clinically important active infection until the infection resolves or is adequately treated. There is no data on the use of spesolimab in patients with HIV and hepatitis B and C infection.[7]

SPESOLIMAB STATUS IN INDIA AS ON 27 FEBRUARY 2023

The Subject Expert Committee (SEC) under the Central Drugs Standard Control Organization (CDSCO) has recommended to the drug regulator to grant permission to Boehringer Ingelheim India for import and marketing of spesolimab formulation for the rare disease of GPP subject to conditions.[19]

CONCLUSION

Spesolimab is first in class IL-36R antagonist manufactured by Boehringer Ingelheim for treatment of flares of GPP in adults. US-FDA approved on 1st September 2022, making it the first approved drug for GPP flare.

REFERENCES

1. Blair HA. Spesolimab: first approval. Drugs. 2022;82(17):1681-6.
2. FDA. (2022). New Drug Therapy Approvals 2022. [online] Available from https://www.fda.gov/drugs/ new drugs at fda: CDER's new molecular entities and new therapeutic biological products/new drug therapy approvals 2022 [Last accessed, January, 2024].
3. Frey S, Sticht H, Wilsmann-Theis D, Gerschütz A, Wolf K, Löhr S, et al. Rare Loss-of-Function Mutation in SERPINA3 in Generalized Pustular Psoriasis. J Invest Dermatol. 2020;140(7):1451-5.e13.
4. Vergnano M, Mockenhaupt M, Benzian-Olsson N, Paulmann M, Grys K, Mahil SK, et al. Loss-of-function myeloperoxidase mutations are associated with increased neutrophil counts and pustular skin disease. Am J Hum Genet. 2020;107:539-43.
5. Sugiura K. Role of Interleukin 36 in Generalised Pustular Psoriasis and beyond. Dermatol Ther (Heidelb). 2022;12(2):315-28.
6. Bachelez H, Choon SE, Marrakchi S, Burden AD, Tsai TF, Morita A, et al. Inhibition of the interleukin-36 pathway for the treatment of generalized pustular psoriasis. N Engl J Med. 2019;380:981-3.
7. SPEVIGO® [package insert]. Ridgefield, CT: Boehringer Ingelheim Pharmaceuticals, Inc; 2022.

CHAPTER 11: Interleukin-36 Receptor Antagonist: Spesolimab

8. Drug bank online. Spesolimab: uses, interactions, mechanism of action. [online] Available from https://go.drugbank.com/drugs/DB15626 [Last accessed January, 2024].
9. Morita A, Tsai TF, Yee EYW, Okubo Y, Imafuku S, Zheng M, et al. Efficacy and safety of spesolimab in Asian patients with a generalized pustular psoriasis flare: Results from the randomized, double-blind, placebo-controlled Effisayil™ 1 study. J Dermatol. 2023;50(2):183-94.
10. Joseph D, Thoma C, Haeufel T, Li X. Assessment of the Pharmacokinetics and Safety of Spesolimab, a Humanised Anti-interleukin-36 Receptor Monoclonal Antibody, in Healthy Non-Japanese and Japanese Subjects: Results from Phase I Clinical Studies. Clin Pharmacokinet. 2022;61(12):1771-87.
11. Bachelez H, Choon SE, Marrakchi S, Burden AD, Tsai TF, Morita A, et al. Trial of spesolimab for generalized pustular psoriasis. N Engl J Med. 2021;385:2431-40.
12. Choon SE, Lebwohl MG, Marrakchi S, Burden AD, Tsai TF, Morita A, et al. Study protocol of the global Effisayil 1 Phase II, multicentre, randomised, double-blind, placebo-controlled trial of spesolimab in patients with generalized pustular psoriasis presenting with an acute flare. BMJ Open. 2021;11(3):e043666-e043666.
13. European Medicines Agency (europa.eu). (2023). Spevigo. [online] Available from https://www.ema.europa.eu/en/medicines/human/EPAR/spevigo [Last accessed January, 2024].
14. Morita A, Choon SE, Bachelez H, Anadkat MJ, Marrakchi S, Zheng M, et al. Design of Effisayil™ 2: A Randomized, Double-Blind, Placebo-Controlled Study of Spesolimab in Preventing Flares in Patients with Generalized Pustular Psoriasis. Dermatol Ther (Heidelb). 2023;13(1):347-59.
15. Ferrante M, Irving PM, Selinger CP, D'Haens G, Kuehbacher T, Seidler U, et al. Safety and tolerability of spesolimab in patients with ulcerative colitis. Expert Opin Drug Saf. 2023;22(2):141-52.
16. Mrowietz U, Burden AD, Pinter A, Reich K, Schäkel K, Baum P, et al. Spesolimab, an Anti-Interleukin-36 Receptor Antibody, in Patients with Palmoplantar Pustulosis: Results of a Phase IIa, Multicenter, Double-Blind, Randomized, Placebo-Controlled Pilot Study. Dermatol Ther (Heidelb). 2021;11(2):571-85.
17. Bissonnette R, Abramovits W, Saint-Cyr Proulx É, Lee P, Guttman-Yassky E, Zovko E, et al. Spesolimab, an anti-interleukin-36 receptor antibody, in patients with moderate-to-severe atopic dermatitis: Results from a multicentre, randomized, double-blind, placebo-controlled, phase IIa study. J Eur Acad Dermatol Venereol. 2023;37(3):549-57.
18. Guénin SH, Khattri S, Lebwohl MG. Spesolimab use in treatment of pyoderma gangrenosum. JAAD Case Rep. 2023;34:18-22.
19. Policy and regulations. (2023). SEC recommends approval for Boehringer Ingelheim's spesolimab to treat GPP. [online] Available from: https://www.pharmabiz.com/news details.aspx/aid=156552 [Last accessed January, 2024].

CHAPTER 12

Newer Biologics in Psoriasis

Siddharth Mani, Abir Saraswat

INTRODUCTION

Psoriasis is a systemic chronic inflammatory and immunogenetic disorder with unknown intrinsic and extrinsic triggers. Extensive research into its inflammatory and immune-mediated pathways in recent times has led to uncovering of many cytokines and receptors, which in turn has helped us in using various biologics that work at different levels of inflammatory pathways **(Fig. 1)**. These biologics may be upstream or downstream inhibitors depending on the level of immunosuppression. Though the invention and use of biologics in dermatology date back a few decades ago,

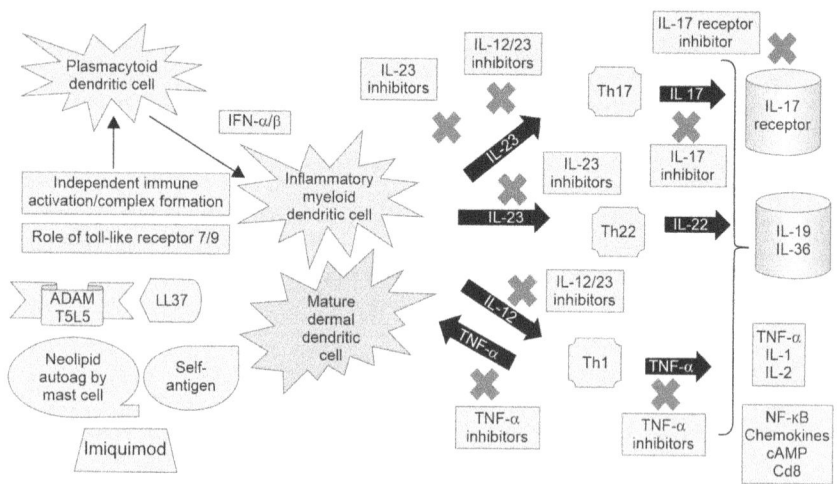

FIG. 1: Site and mechanism of action of various biologics.
(cAMP: cyclic adenosine monophosphate; IFN: interferon; IL: interleukin; NF-κB: nuclear factor-kappa B; Th: T helper; TNF: tumor necrosis factor)

there has always been a rising need for the development of newer biologics with better pharmacological properties, receptor-specific actions, and better safety profiles. In this chapter, we have briefly discussed the upcoming and newer biologics, either approved recently for their use in psoriasis or which are awaiting approval and would be available for use soon. A list of biologics and their Food and Drug Administration (FDA) approval status is mentioned in **Table 1**.

Biologic	Indication	FDA Approval
TABLE 1: Newer biologics and their FDA approval status.		
TNF-α inhibitors:		
• Golimumab • Certolizumab (pegylated)	• Psoriatic arthritis • Psoriatic arthritis • Moderate-to-severe plaque psoriasis	• June 2008 • September 2013 • May 2018
IL-12/23 inhibitors:		
• Ustekinumab	• Plaque psoriasis • Psoriatic arthritis • Plaque psoriasis (adolescent) • Plaque psoriasis (pediatric) • Psoriatic arthritis (pediatric)	• September 2009 • September 2013 • September 2017 • July 2020 • August 2022
• Briakinumab • Ebdarokimab	• Not approved for psoriasis/psoriatic arthritis • Not approved for psoriasis/psoriatic arthritis	• – • –
IL-23 inhibitors:		
• Tildrakizumab • Guselkumab	• Plaque psoriasis • Plaque psoriasis • Psoriatic arthritis	• May 2018 • July 2017 • July 2020
• Risankizumab	• Plaque psoriasis • Psoriatic arthritis	• April 2019 • January 2022
• Mirikizumab • Brazikumab	• Not approved for psoriasis/psoriatic arthritis • Not approved for psoriasis/psoriatic arthritis	• – • –
IL-17 inhibitors:		
• Ixekizumab	• Plaque psoriasis • Psoriatic arthritis • Pediatric plaque psoriasis	• May 2016 • December 2017 • March 2020
• Brodalumab • Bimekizumab • Netakimab • Sonelokimab	• Plaque psoriasis • Plaque psoriasis • Not approved for psoriasis/psoriatic arthritis • Not approved for psoriasis/psoriatic arthritis	• February 2017 • October 2023 • – • –
IL-36 inhibitor:		
Spesolimab	Generalized pustular psoriasis	September 2022

(FDA: Food and Drug Administration; IL: interleukin; TNF-α: tumor necrosis factor alpha)

TUMOR NECROSIS FACTOR-ALPHA INHIBITORS

Golimumab

Golimumab is a tumor necrosis factor-alpha (TNF-α) inhibitor that is FDA approved for psoriatic arthritis. It is given in subcutaneous (SC) form in the dose of 50 mg/4 weeks. It works on both soluble and transmembrane TNF receptors. In particular, activation of TNF receptor 1 (TNFR1) (especially with soluble TNF) activates the nuclear factor-kappa B (NFκB) receptor pathway, which in turn translocates to the nucleus and this leads to activation of transcription of several proinflammatory cytokine genes as interleukin (IL)-8, IL-1, IL-6, cyclooxygenase-2 (COX2), and TNF-α.[1] It is supposed to be one of the least immunogenic TNF-α inhibitors.[2] The drug has also been tried off-label in other forms of psoriasis, details of which are mentioned further.

Observations

- *GO VIBRANT study*: Even though the study was conducted with intravenous (IV) infusion of golimumab with primary focus on psoriatic arthritis, other characteristics such as improvement in skin and nail disease were also recorded. The drug showed significant improvement in psoriasis area and severity index (PASI) 75/90/100 at 24 weeks as compared to placebo and the same was maintained at week 52. PASI 75 response was 64.8% and 71.9% at weeks 24 and 52, respectively; PASI 90 was 42.9% and 56.1%, respectively; and PASI 100 was 25.5% and 28.6%, respectively. In patients who crossed over from placebo to golimumab at week 24, PASI responses increased numerically from weeks 24–52; PASI 75 response increased from 13.1% at week 24 to 60.6% at week 52; PASI 90 increased from 7.6 to 41.9%, respectively; and PASI 100 increased from 5.6 to 18.7%, respectively. For nail involvement, modified nail psoriasis severity index (mNAPSI) was seen and it was observed that there was significant improvement in mNAPSI scores in golimumab group as compared to placebo.[3]
- *Kudsi et al.*: They reported successful management of erythrodermic psoriasis with golimumab.[4]

Pegylated Certolizumab

Pegylated certolizumab is recombinant humanized antibody fragment that acts against both soluble and transmembrane TNF-α. It is different from conventional TNF-α blockers in two ways with absence of Fc region leading to lack of antibody-dependent cell-mediated cytotoxicity and minimal passage through placenta.[5,6] It is used in the dosage of 400 mg every 2 weeks. 200 mg every 2 weeks can be considered in patients who are less than 90 kg and have taken an initial loading dose of 400 mg at week 0, 2, and 4. The drug was approved by the United States FDA (US FDA) for chronic plaque psoriasis in May 2018.

Observations
- *CIMPACT trial*: The trial was conducted with 559 enrolled patients of psoriasis. The PASI 75 at week 12 was 5%, 61.3%, and 66.7% in placebo, certolizumab 200 mg, and certolizumab 400 mg group, respectively. At week 16, the PASI score was 3.85%, 68.2%, and 74.7% in placebo, certolizumab 200 mg, and certolizumab 400 mg group, respectively. The PASI 90 response for placebo, certolizumab 200 mg, and certolizumab 400 mg group at week 16 was 0.3%, 39.8%, and 49% respectively.[7]
- *CIMPASI-1 and CIMPASI-2 trials*: These multinational phase III trials also showed efficacy of pegylated certolizumab in psoriasis with better PASI 75 score in 400 mg group (75.8%/82.6%) as compared to 200 mg group (66.5%/81.4%) and placebo (6.5%/11.6%) at week 16.[8]
- *Dattola et al.*: In the retrospective study involving 11 Italian sites, 153 patients were enrolled. Significant improvement was noted in disease activity score (DAS-44), tender joint count (TJC), swollen joint count (SJC), mNAPSI scores, and pain-visual analog scale (VAS). Mean PASI decrease at weeks 24 and 52 were 6.30 and 7.58, respectively.[9]
- *Umezawa et al.*: In the Japanese study where 26/53/48 patients were randomized into placebo, certolizumab 400 mg, and certolizumab 200 mg groups, significant improvement was observed in PASI 75 and PASI 90 in certolizumab 200 mg and 400 mg group with 400 mg group showing some additional benefits. The PASI 75/90/100 in certolizumab 400 mg and 200 mg were 83.0%/81.1%/41.5% and 72.9%/60.4%/18.8%, respectively. The benefits were maintained till week 52 in both the certolizumab groups.[10]

INTERLEUKIN-12/23 INHIBITORS

Ustekinumab
Ustekinumab is a humanized monoclonal antibody against the p40 subunit of IL-23 and IL-12 **(Fig. 2)**. The p40 subunit binds to the IL-12Rβ1 subunit. However, ustekinumab blocks the interaction of p40 with the IL-12Rβ1 receptor and thus neutralizes IL-12 and IL-23.[11-15] The standard dosing for weight less than 100 kg is 45 mg SC initially and 4 weeks later, then every 12 weeks. For weight more than 100 kg, the dosing is doubled to 90 mg SC initially and 4 weeks later, then every 12 weeks. The drug has been approved by the US FDA for adult, adolescent, and pediatric (6–11 years) plaque psoriasis along with pediatric and adult psoriatic arthritis.

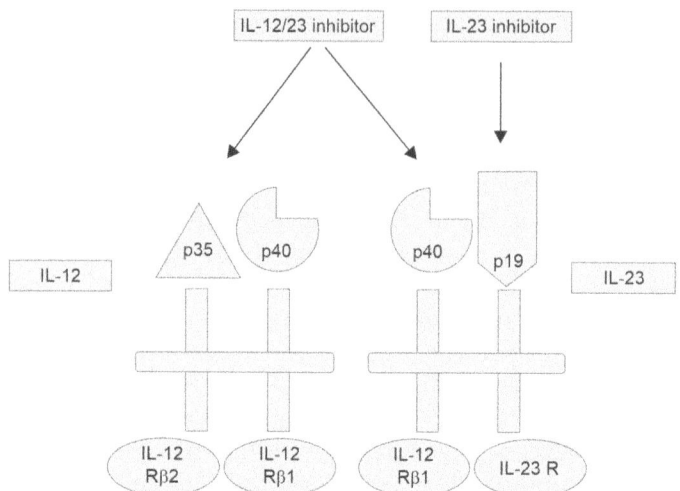

FIG. 2: Mechanism of action of interleukin-12 (IL-12)/23 and IL-23 inhibitors.

Observations

- *Krueger et al.*: In a phase II clinical trial comparing ustekinumab and placebo, percentage of patients achieving PASI 75 and PASI 90 at 12th week and percentage of patients achieving static physicians global assessment (sPGA) of "clear" or "minimal" was significantly better in the group receiving ustekinumab. The three most common adverse effects were upper respiratory tract infection, headache, and pain, but this was not statistically significant.[16]
- *Leonardi et al. and Papp et al.*: Two phase III trials (PHOENIX 1 and 2) compared the effectiveness, safety, and tolerability of ustekinumab versus placebo in psoriatic patients. The number of patients achieving PASI 75 and PASI 90 at 4th and 12th week was significantly higher, who received ustekinumab. The cumulative data showed that patients on ustekinumab maintained PASI 75 better (for a minimum of 12 months) than those who were withdrawn from treatment at week 40.[17,18]
- *ACCEPT trial*: This study compared the efficacy of ustekinumab vis-à-vis etanercept. PASI 75 was attained at week 12 in 67.5% of patients receiving 45 mg ustekinumab, 73.8% of patients receiving 90 mg ustekinumab, and 56.8% of patients receiving etanercept. Physician global assessment (PGA) was also better in the ustekinumab group.[19]
- *CADMUS study*: In this study, 110 adolescent (12–17 years) patients with plaque psoriasis were studied. The patients were divided into three groups: Ustekinumab standard dosing [SD; 0.75 mg/kg (< 60 kg), 45 mg (60–100 kg), and 90 mg (>100 kg)], ustekinumab half-standard dosing [HSD; 0.375 mg/kg (<60 kg), 22.5 mg (60–100 kg), and 45 mg (>100 kg)], or placebo with crossover to ustekinumab at week 12. While PASI 75 at week

12 was achieved in 80.6% of SD patients, 78.4% of HSD patients, and 10.8% of patients on placebo, 61.1% of SD, 54.1% of HSD patients, and 5.4% of patients on placebo achieved PASI 90 at week 12.[20,21]
- *CLEAR trial*: The study compared ustekinumab with secukinumab and secukinumab was found to have better results in terms of PASI 90 at week 16.[22]
- *AMAGINE 2 and AMAGINE 3 studies*: Brodalumab was superior in efficacy as compared to ustekinumab in both the trials.[23]

Due to inhibition of both T helper 1 (Th1) and Th17 pathways, there was prior concern of increased risk of infection with ustekinumab. However, Psoriasis Longitudinal Assessment and Registry (PSOLAR) results have demonstrated that ustekinumab was not associated with an increased risk of serious infection compared with nonbiologic therapies.[24]

The development of antibodies has been reported in various studies.[16-18] Concomitant immunosuppressive therapy, multiple dosing at induction phase, and systematic maintenance therapy are some of the ways by which this phenomenon can be reduced.

Briakinumab

Briakinumab is another IL-12/23 inhibitor. However, the approval application for psoriasis withdrawn from the USA and Europe by the manufacturers due to increased risk of major adverse cardiovascular event (MACE) was defined as nonfatal myocardial infarction, nonfatal stroke, and cardiovascular death.[25]

Observations

- *Kimball et al.*: In a phase II clinical trial, 180 patients were tested for 36 weeks. PASI 75 was achieved at week 12 in 63% of the patients receiving 200 mg once, 93% of the patients receiving 100 mg every other week for 12 weeks, 90% of patients receiving 200 mg weekly for 4 weeks, 93% of patients receiving 200 mg every other week for 12 weeks, 90% of patients receiving 200 mg weekly for 12 weeks, and 3% of patients receiving placebo.[26]
- *Gordon et al. and Papp et al.*: Following the success of the trial conducted by Kimball et al., phase III clinical trials were conducted and it was concluded that briakinumab 100 mg (every 4 weeks) in psoriasis patients led to better improvement of lesions in comparison to those who received 100 mg every 12 weeks and of course, in placebo group. Rare serious adverse events (AEs) included infections, nonmelanoma skin cancers, cardiac events, etc.[25,27]
- In two studies, briakinumab, etanercept, and placebo were compared to determine their efficacy and safety in treating psoriasis (12 weeks). Briakinumab was found to be superior to both etanercept and placebo.[28,29]

- Another study compared briakinumab to methotrexate over 52 weeks and the authors concluded that briakinumab was more efficacious than methotrexate.[30]

Ebdarokimab[31]

The new IL-12/23 inhibitor has been approved by the National Center for Drug Evaluation of the State Drug Administration of the People's Republic of China [National Medical Products Administration Centre for Drug Evaluation (NMPA CDE)] for adults with moderate-to-severe psoriasis. It is not yet approved by the US FDA. In a randomized, double-blind, placebo-controlled phase III clinical study, the response rates of PASI 75 and sPGA 0/1 in AK101 group were 79.4% (239/300) and 64.0% (193/300), respectively, at week 16 ($p < 0.0001$), which were higher than those in placebo group [16.5% (25/150) and 11.7% (18/150), $p < 0.0001$]. At the same time, AK101 showed improved response rate in terms of PASI 90 at week 16 (51.8% in the AK101 group and 7.7% in the placebo group, $p < 0.0001$), and improved dermatology life quality index (DLQI) score of those subjects as well.

INTERLEUKIN-23 INHIBITORS

Tildrakizumab

Tildrakizumab is a humanized immunoglobulin G1 (IgG1) antibody targeted against the p19 subunit of IL-23. The drug was FDA approved for use in moderate-to-severe plaque psoriasis in March 2018.[32] It is given in the dose of 100 mg SC at week 0, 4, and then 12 weekly.[33]

Observations

- *reSURFACE I*: It was a major phase III clinical trial for efficacy of tildrakizumab in psoriasis. The biologic was found to be superior to placebo in terms of PASI 75 and PGA. At week 12, 64% of patients on 100 mg and 62% of patients on 200 mg achieved PASI 75 with maximum efficacy at 22 weeks. The secondary endpoint at week 28 showed 80% of patients achieving PASI 75 in both 100 mg and 200 mg groups. The participants who were regrouped from placebo to drug group also achieved PASI 75 (78% in 200 mg group and 64% in 100 mg group).[34]
- *reSURFACE II*: In this multicentric trial, tildrakizumab was found to be more effective than placebo and etanercept in terms of PASI 75 and PGA scores.[34]

Guselkumab

Guselkumab was approved in July 2017 for the management of moderate-to-severe plaque psoriasis. It is administered in the dosing of 100 mg SC at week 0, 4, and then every 8 weeks thereafter.[13,14]

Observations
Three major phase III multicentric trials have been done for guselkumab in which its efficacy was noted against placebo and adalimumab. The details of these studies are mentioned further:
- *VOYAGE I*: A total of 837 patients were enrolled in this study. Guselkumab 100 mg was compared with adalimumab (week 0–48) and a placebo-controlled period (week 0–16), respectively, after which patients taking placebo crossed over to receive guselkumab through week 48. 91.2% of patients receiving guselkumab achieved PASI 90 compared with 73.1% in the adalimumab group and 5.7% in the placebo group at the end of the placebo-controlled period at week 16. Significantly, higher rates of response were maintained in guselkumab group as compared to adalimumab and placebo at weeks 24 and 48. The investigator's global assessment (IGA) was also better in the guselkumab group.[35]
- *VOYAGE II*: A total of 992 patients were studied in this group. The study consisted of three periods—placebo-controlled period (weeks 0–16), an active comparator-controlled period (weeks 0–28), and a randomized withdrawal and retreatment period (weeks 28–72). Guselkumab showed superior efficacy in terms of both PASI 90 and IGA.[36]
- *NAVIGATE*: 837 patients were studied in this group. Guselkumab showed better PASI 90 and 100 responses as compared to ustekinumab.[37]

Risankizumab
Risankizumab was approved in April 2019 for the treatment of moderate-to-severe plaque psoriasis with recommended dosing of 150 mg at week 0, 4, and every 12 weeks thereafter.

Observations
- *Krueger et al.*: The phase I study showed 87%, 58%, and 16% patients achieving PASI 75, 90, and 100, respectively, at 12 weeks.[38]
- *Papp et al.*: 166 patients were enrolled in this phase II trial where risankizumab was compared with ustekinumab. At 12 weeks, 77% of patients in risankizumab group achieved PASI 75 as compared to 40% in ustekinumab group. The patients' response was well maintained till week 36.[39]
- *UltIMMa 1 and 2*: In these phase III trials, patients were randomized into risankizumab, ustekinumab, and placebo group. 75%, 42%, and 5% in risankizumab, ustekinumab, and placebo group, respectively, reached PASI 75 at week 16 in UltIMMa 1. In UltIMMa 2, the percentage of patients achieving PASI 75 at week 16 was 75% (risankizumab), 48% (ustekinumab), and 2% (placebo).[40]
- *IMMvent*: Risankizumab was found to be significantly more effective than adalimumab in terms of PASI 75.[41]
- *IMMhance*: At week 16, 73% patients achieved PASI 90 as compared to 2% in placebo group.[42]

Mirikizumab

Mirikizumab is a new IL-23 inhibitor that has been approved by the FDA for ulcerative colitis but is yet to be approved for psoriasis.

Mirikizumab, a humanized monoclonal IgG4 variant antibody designed to target the p19 subunit of IL-23, was developed by Eli Lilly. In an initial phase II randomized controlled trial conducted in 2019, various doses of mirikizumab (30, 100, or 300 mg) were administered at 0 and 8 weeks. The trial revealed that 59% and 67% of patients treated with mirikizumab at doses of 100 mg and 300 mg, respectively, achieved PASI 90.[43]

Subsequent results from the phase III randomized, double-blind, placebo-controlled study known as OASIS-1 (NCT03482011) demonstrated that 64% of patients receiving mirikizumab at a dosage of 250 mg every 4 weeks achieved PASI 90 at 16 weeks, compared to 6.5% in the placebo group. Additionally, 69% of the mirikizumab-treated patients achieved an IGA score of 0–1, in contrast to 6.5% in the placebo group.[43]

Preliminary findings from the OASIS-2 (NCT03535194), a multicenter randomized, double-blind, placebo-controlled study comparing mirikizumab to placebo and secukinumab, indicated that mirikizumab met the primary and all key secondary endpoints versus placebo at week 16 (demonstrating superiority) and achieved all key secondary endpoints versus the active comparator at both week 16 (noninferiority) and week 52 (superiority).[44]

Currently, mirikizumab is under investigation in the phase III study OASIS-3.[22] The incidence of AEs was comparable between patients treated with placebo and mirikizumab, with the most common AEs being viral infections, hypertension, respiratory tract infections, injection-site pain, and diarrhea.

Brazikumab

Brazikumab is an IL-23 inhibitor which is yet to be studied for psoriasis.

INTERLEUKIN-17 INHIBITORS

Ixekizumab

Ixekizumab is a humanized IgG4 monoclonal antibody that selectively binds and neutralizes IL-17. It is US FDA approved for patients above 6 years of age having moderate-to-severe plaque psoriasis. It is given 160 mg (two 80 mg injections) SC at week 0, followed by 80 mg at weeks 2, 4, 6, 8, 10, and 12, and then 4 weekly.[13]

Observations

The safety and efficacy of ixekizumab were evaluated in three randomized, double-blind, placebo-controlled clinical trials.

- *UNCOVER I*: In this study, ixekizumab was studied against placebo. A total of 433 patients participated in the trial. 82.6% of patients receiving ixekizumab 4 weekly, 89% of patients receiving ixekizumab 2 weekly, and 3.2% in placebo group achieved PASI 75 at week 12. PASI 90 was achieved by 70.9% in ixekizumab 2-weekly group and 64.6% in ixekizumab 4-weekly group.[45]
- *UNCOVER II*: In this study, the patients were grouped into ixekizumab, etanercept, and placebo. The percentage of patients achieving PASI 75/90/100 is mentioned in **Table 2**.[46]
- *UNCOVER III*: The result is mentioned in **Table 3**.[47]

In both the studies, ixekizumab showed better efficacy than etanercept and placebo.

Brodalumab

Brodalumab selectively binds to IL-17 receptor A (IL-17RA) acting as antagonist. By binding IL-17RA, brodalumab inhibits interactions with

TABLE 2: Ixekizumab efficacy outcome at week 12.

	PASI 75	PASI 90	PASI 100
Ixekizumab 2 weekly ($n = 351$)	89.7%	70.7%	40.5%
Ixekizumab 4 weekly ($n = 347$)	77.5%	59.7%	30.8%
Etanercept ($n = 358$)	41.6%	18.7%	4.3%
Placebo ($n = 168$)	2.4%	0.6%	0.6%

(PASI: psoriasis area and severity index)

TABLE 3: Ixekizumab efficacy outcome at week 12.

	PASI 75	PASI 90	PASI 100
Ixekizumab 2 weekly ($n = 385$)	87.3%	68.1%	37.7%
Ixekizumab 4 weekly ($n = 386$)	84.2%	65.3%	35.0%
Etanercept ($n = 382$)	53.4%	25.7%	7.3%
Placebo ($n = 193$)	7.3%	3.1%	0

(PASI: psoriasis area and severity index)

TABLE 4: Results of safety and efficacy of brodalumab.				
		PASI 75	PASI 90	PASI 100
AMAGINE 1	Brodalumab 210 mg (n = 222)	83.3%	70.3%	41.9%
	Brodalumab 140 mg (n = 219)	60.3%	42.5%	23.3%
	Placebo (n = 220)	2.7%	0.9%	0.5%
AMAGINE 2	Brodalumab 210 mg (n = 612)	86%	–	44%
	Brodalumab 140 mg (n = 610)	67%	–	26%
	Ustekinumab (n = 300)	70%	–	22%
	Placebo (n = 309)	8%	–	1%
AMAGINE 3	Brodalumab 210 mg (n = 624)	89%	–	37%
	Brodalumab 140 mg (n = 620)	69%	–	27%
	Ustekinumab (n = 313)	69%	–	19%
	Placebo (n = 315)	0.3%	–	0.3%

(PASI: psoriasis area and severity index)

cytokines IL-17A, IL-17A/F, heterodimer IL-17C, IL-17E (IL-25 same as IL-17E), and IL-17F.[13]

The safety and efficacy of brodalumab were assessed in three randomized, double-blind, controlled trials. The results of the trial are mentioned in **Table 4**.[48,49]

In all the three studies, brodalumab was found to be superior in efficacy than ustekinumab and placebo.

Brodalumab has also been studied in generalized pustular psoriasis (GPP). In a phase III study, the biologic has shown to be effective in 12 patients with GPP with 75% patient showing improvement at week 2 and 83% showing remission at week 12.[50]

Bimekizumab

Bimekizumab, a monoclonal humanized IgG1 antibody developed by UCB, functions as a dual inhibitor of IL-17F and IL-17A. This sets it apart from secukinumab and ixekizumab, which selectively inhibit IL-17A, and brodalumab, an IL-17 receptor inhibitor. The biologic was approved by the US FDA on October 23 for moderate-to-severe psoriasis.

Initial phase II studies indicate that bimekizumab delivers rapid and sustained clinical improvements for patients with moderate-to-severe psoriasis, accompanied by an anticipated safety profile.[51] Recently published results from two phase III clinical trials, BE VIVID and BE READY, provide further insights.

The BE VIVID trial, a multicenter, double-blind trial spanning 52 weeks, compared the efficacy and safety of bimekizumab to placebo and ustekinumab. At week 16, 85% of bimekizumab-treated patients achieved PASI 90, compared to 50% on ustekinumab and 5% on placebo. Additionally, bimekizumab demonstrated superiority in achieving clear or almost clear skin (IGA score of 0-1) and complete clearance (PASI 100 or IGA = 0) at week 16.[52]

The BE READY trial, another multicenter, double-blind trial lasting 56 weeks, investigated bimekizumab withdrawal and two maintenance dosing schedules. Results showed sustained efficacy, with 91% achieving PASI 90 and 93% attaining an IGA score of 0-1 on bimekizumab, compared to minimal responses on placebo.[53]

Phase III trials BE SURE (NCT03412747) and BE RADIANT (NCT03536884) compared bimekizumab to adalimumab and secukinumab, respectively. At week 16, BE SURE demonstrated a PASI 90 response of 86.2% with bimekizumab versus 47.2% with adalimumab. BE RADIANT, at week 48, showed a PASI 100 rate of 67.0% with bimekizumab versus 46.2% with secukinumab. The safety profile aligned with previous studies, with nasopharyngitis and upper respiratory tract infections being more common.[54]

Across these studies, treatment-emergent adverse events (TEAEs) occurred in 61% of bimekizumab-treated patients, compared to 36% in the placebo arm. Oral candidiasis was observed in 19% of bimekizumab-treated patients versus 3% on secukinumab. In BE VIVID and BE READY, one patient developed inflammatory bowel disease and one case of new-onset ulcerative colitis occurred in either the bimekizumab or secukinumab group.

A randomized proof-of-concept trial investigating bimekizumab for psoriatic arthritis demonstrated promising results, with an 80% ACR20 response at week 8 for the top three doses.

Ongoing phase II clinical trials are exploring the efficacy of bimekizumab in the treatment of hidradenitis suppurativa.

Netakimab

Netakimab, an injectable humanized IgG1 nanobody developed by BIOCAD, specifically targets IL-17A. In netakimab, the VH domain is substituted with the VHH domain of Lama, featuring an extended complementarity determining region (CDR-H3) in its heavy chain, exhibiting a high affinity for IL-17A. Nanobodies, a novel class of drugs derived from single-domain heavy-chain-only antibodies, offer enhanced stability and improved tissue penetration.

Currently registered in Russia as Efleira® for the treatment of moderate-to-severe psoriasis in adults, netakimab has undergone initial phase II trials. These trials demonstrated that 93% of subjects achieved PASI 75 within 3 months and netakimab maintained efficacy, a favorable safety profile, and low immunogenicity throughout 1 year of treatment.

Results from the BCD-085-7/PLANETA study (NCT03390101), a comparative, randomized, double-blind, placebo-controlled phase III clinical study, indicate that at week 12, PASI 75 was achieved by 83.3% and 77.7% of patients treated with netakimab at doses of 120 mg every 4 and every 4 weeks, respectively, compared to 0% in the placebo arm.[55,56]

The drug demonstrated a safety profile consistent with expectations for the IL-17 inhibitor class, coupled with low immunogenicity. Additionally, results from phase III clinical trial (PATERA study), investigating netakimab's efficacy and safety compared to placebo in patients with active psoriatic arthritis, revealed that netakimab at a dose of 120 mg significantly outperformed placebo in patients with active psoriatic arthritis. 94.9% of patients in the netakimab group achieved ACR20 while 89.5% achieved PASI 75 response at week 54.[57]

Sonelokimab

Sonelokimab (IL17MS3086) is a trivalent camelid nanobody currently in the phase II stage, designed to bind to IL-17A and F. They offer the advantages of small proteins while retaining the properties of monoclonal antibodies.

In a multicenter, randomized, placebo-controlled, phase IIb study, 300 patients were randomized into sonelokimab 30/60/120 mg, secukinumab 300 mg, and placebo group.[58] Treatment with sonelokimab doses of 120 mg or less showed significant clinical benefit over placebo, with rapid onset of treatment effect, durable improvements, and an acceptable safety profile (incidence of *Candida* infection was higher with sonelokimab as compared to secukinumab).

INTERLEUKIN-36R INHIBITOR

Spesolimab

Spesolimab is IL-36 receptor inhibitor which was approved by the US FDA for GPP in September 2022.

- In a phase I, proof-of-concept study, the safety and efficacy of a single IV dose of spesolimab was assessed in seven patients with an acute GPP flare. This study provided the first evidence for targeting the IL-36 pathway.[59]
- The phase II Effisayil clinical trial program assessing spesolimab in GPP consists of three key studies, including Effisayil 1 (NCT03782792), which assessed the efficacy and safety of spesolimab in GPP flares; the phase IIb Effisayil 2 (NCT04399837), which has been conducted to evaluate the effectiveness of the maintenance treatment with spesolimab in preventing recurrence of flares; and the long-term extension of both these trials, Effisayil ON (NCT03886246). The results are summarized in **Table 5**.[60-63]

TABLE 5: Results of Effisayil clinical trial.

Trial	Study design	Endpoints	Main results
Phase I	• Single-arm, open-label, proof-of-concept • n = 7 adults • Ongoing moderate-to-severe GPP flare • SD of spesolimab 10 mg/kg IV at baseline • Follow-up 20 weeks	*Primary:* • Safety and tolerability (% AE) *Secondary:* • Percentage change in GPPGA, FACIT-F, and Pain-VAS at week 2 • GPPGA 0/1 at week 2	• GPPGA 0 in 43% of patients within 48 hours • GPPGA 0/1 achieved in 71% of patients by week 1 and in 100% of patients by week 4, sustained up to week 20 • Mean percentage change in GPPASI of 73.2% at week 2, sustained up to week 20 • Improvement in Pain-VAS (−46%) and FACIT-F (−12%) at week 2, sustained at week 4 • Rapid reduction in CRP and absolute neutrophil count

Phase II Effisayil 1	• Randomized, placebo-controlled, double-blind
	• n = 53 adults
	• Ongoing moderate-to-severe GPP flare 2:1 (Spesolimab 900 mg IV SD placebo)
	• Rescue SD 900 mg IV of spesolimab allowed by day 8 in both groups if persistent symptoms, and after day 8 if recurrence of a flare 12 weeks
		Primary:
		• GPPGA pustulation subscore 0 at week 1
		Secondary:
		• Week 1
		  ○ GPPGA score of 0 or 1
		  ○ GPPASI 50
		  ○ Percentage change in GPPASI from baseline
		• Week 4
		  ○ GPPASI 75
		  ○ Change from baseline in Pain-VAS, FACIT-F, and PSS
		  ○ Percentage change in GPPASI from baseline
		  ○ GPPGA pustulation subscore 0
			Significant:
			• GPPGA pustulation subscore 0 at week 1 versus placebo (54% vs. 6%; $p < 0.001$), sustained over 12 weeks
			• GPPGA total 0/1 higher than placebo (43% vs. 11%) at week 1 ($p = 0.02$), sustained over 12 weeks
			• Improvements from baseline (median) in pain VAS (−21.3) FACIT-F (7.0), DLQI (−2.5), and PSS (−4.0) within 1 week after spesolimab, sustained over 12 weeks

Continued

Continued

Trial	Study design	Endpoints	Main results
Phase IIb Effisayil 2	• Randomized, placebo-controlled, double-blind • n = 123 adults and adolescents • No active flare at baseline 1:1:1:1 • Spesolimab LD 600 mg, followed by maintenance 300 mg q4w • Spesolimab LD 600 mg, followed by maintenance 300 mg q12w • Spesolimab LD 300 mg, followed by maintenance 150 mg q12w • Placebo • Subcutaneous administration • 48 weeks	*Primary:* • Time to first GPP flare *Secondary:* • Occurrence of ≥1 GPP flare • Time to first worsening of PSS and DLQI • GPPGA score of 0 or 1 up to week 48 (sustained remission) • Occurrence of TEAE	• Non-flat dose-response relationship for the three arms of spesolimab versus placebo • High-dose spesolimab showed statistically significant superiority on time to GPP flare versus placebo ($p = 0.0005$) • *Risk of DLQI worsening versus placebo (HR): 0.58 ($p = 0.043$) for low-dose spesolimab; 0.60 ($p = 0.048$) for medium-dose spesolimab; 0.26; and ($p = 0.001$) for high-dose spesolimab* • *Patients with IL36RN mutation:* 0% of patients had a flare on high-dose spesolimab versus 75% on placebo

(AE: adverse event; CRP: C-reactive protein; DLQI: dermatology life quality index; FACIT-F: functional assessment of chronic illness therapy–fatigue; GPP: generalized pustular psoriasis; GPPASI: psoriasis area and severity index for generalized pustular psoriasis; GPPGA: generalized pustular psoriasis physician global assessment; GPPASI: generalized pustular psoriasis area and severity index; HR: hazard ratio; IL36RN: interleukin 36 receptor; IV: intravenous; LD: loading dose; pain-VAS: pain-visual analog scale; PSS: psoriasis symptom scale; q4w: every 4 weeks; q12w: every 12 weeks; SD: single dose; TEAE: treatment-emergent adverse event)

CONCLUSION

The advent of newer biologics has revolutionized the landscape of psoriasis treatment, offering unprecedented hope to patients with this chronic and often debilitating condition. The diverse mechanisms of action exhibited by these biologics target specific pathways involved in the pathogenesis of psoriasis, providing more targeted and effective therapeutic options. The clinical success observed in trials and real-world settings underscore the remarkable progress in understanding the immunological basis of psoriasis.

While the efficacy of these newer biologics is impressive, challenges such as long-term safety, cost, and accessibility remain. Ongoing research aims to address these issues and further refine treatment strategies. As we continue to unravel the complexities of psoriasis, the integration of newer biologics into clinical practice represents a promising step forward, offering not only relief for patients but also paving the way for a more personalized and holistic approach to managing this multifaceted dermatological condition.

REFERENCES

1. Nestorov I. Clinical pharmacokinetics of TNF antagonists: how do they differ? Semin Arthritis Rheum. 2005;34:12-8.
2. Thomas SS, Borazan N, Barroso N, Duan L, Taroumian S, Kretzmann B, et al. Comparative immunogenicity of TNF inhibitors: impact on clinical efficacy and tolerability in the management of autoimmune diseases. a systematic review and meta-analysis. BioDrugs. 2015;29:241-58.
3. Mease P, Elaine Husni M, Chakravarty SD, Kafka S, Parenti D, Kim L, et al. Evaluation of Improvement in Skin and Nail Psoriasis in Bio-naïve Patients With Active Psoriatic Arthritis Treated With Golimumab: Results Through Week 52 of the GO-VIBRANT Study. ACR Open Rheumatol. 2020;2:640-7.
4. Kudsi M, Alzabibi MA, Shibani M. Two cases of Erythrodermic psoriasis treated with Golimumab. Ann Med Surg. 2022;78:103961.
5. Mariette X, Förger F, Abraham B, Flynn AD, Moltó A, Flipo RM, et al. Lack of placental transfer of certolizumab pegol during pregnancy: results from CRIB, a prospective, postmarketing, pharmacokinetic study. Ann Rheum Dis. 2018;77:228-33.
6. Delgado Frías E, Díaz González JF. Certolizumab pegol. Rheumatol Clin. 2011;6 (Suppl 3):7-11.
7. Warren RB, Lebwohl M, Sofen H, Piguet V, Augustin M, Brock F, et al. Three-year efficacy and safety of certolizumab pegol for the treatment of plaque psoriasis: results from the randomized phase 3 CIMPACT trial. J Eur Acad Dermatol Venereol. 2021;35:2398-408.
8. Gottlieb AB, Blauvelt A, Thaçi D, Leonardi CL, Poulin Y, Drew J, et al. Certolizumab pegol for the treatment of chronic plaque psoriasis: results through 48 weeks from 2 phase 3, multicenter, randomized, double-blinded, placebo-controlled studies (CIMPASI-1 and CIMPASI-2). J Am Acad Dermatol. 2018;79:302-14.e6.
9. Dattola A, Balato A, Megna M, Gisondi P, Girolomoni G, De Simone C, et al. Certolizumab for the treatment of psoriasis and psoriatic arthritis: a real-world multicentre Italian study. J Eur Acad Dermatol Venereol. 2020;34:2839-45.
10. Umezawa Y, Asahina A, Imafuku S, Tada Y, Sano S, Morita A, et al. Efficacy and safety of certolizumab pegol in Japanese patients with moderate to severe plaque psoriasis: 52-week results. Dermatol Ther. 2021;11:943-60.

11. Yeilding N, Szapary P, Brodmerkel C, Benson J, Plotnick M, Zhou H, et al. Development of the IL-12/23 antagonist ustekinumab in psoriasis: past, present, and future perspectives. Ann N Y Acad Sci. 2011;1222:30-9.
12. Toichi E, Torres G, McCormick TS, Chang T, Mascelli MA, Kauffman CL, et al. An anti-IL-12 p40 antibody down-regulates type 1 cytokines, chemokines, and IL-12/IL-23 in psoriasis. J Immunol. 2006;177:4917-26.
13. Tausend W, Downing C, Tyring S. Systematic review of interleukin-12, interleukin-17, and interleukin-23 pathway inhibitors for the treatment of moderate-to-severe chronic plaque psoriasis: ustekinumab, briakinumab, tildrakizumab, guselkumab, secukinumab, ixekizumab, and brodalumab. J Cutan Med Surg. 2014;18:156-69.
14. Gaspari AA, Tyring S. New and emerging biologic therapies for moderate-to-severe plaque psoriasis: mechanistic rationales and recent clinical data for IL-17 and IL-23 inhibitors. Dermatol Ther. 2015;28:179-93.
15. Stinco G, Errichetti E. Erythrodermic psoriasis: current and future role of biologicals. BioDrugs. 2015;29:91-101.
16. Krueger GG, Langley RG, Leonardi C, Yeilding N, Guzzo C, Wang Y, et al. A human interleukin-12/23 monoclonal antibody for the treatment of psoriasis. N Engl J Med. 2007;356:580-92.
17. Leonardi CL, Kimball AB, Papp KA, Yeilding N, Guzzo C, Wang Y, et al. Efficacy and safety of ustekinumab, a human interleukin-12/23 monoclonal antibody, in patients with psoriasis: 76-week results from a randomised, double-blind, placebo-controlled trial (PHOENIX 1). Lancet. 2008;371:1665-74.
18. Papp KA, Langley RG, Lebwohl M, Krueger GG, Szapary P, Yeilding N, et al. Efficacy and safety of ustekinumab, a human interleukin-12/23 monoclonal antibody, in patients with psoriasis: 52-week results from a randomized, double-blind, placebo-controlled trial (PHOENIX 2). Lancet. 2008;371:1675-84.
19. Griffiths CE, Strober BE, van de Kerkhof P, Ho V, Fidelus-Gort R, Yeilding N, et al. Comparison of ustekinumab and etanercept for moderate-to-severe psoriasis. N Engl J Med. 2010;362(2):118-28.
20. Landells I, Marano C, Hsu MC, Li S, Zhu Y, Eichenfield LF, et al. Ustekinumab in adolescent patients age 12 to 17 years with moderate-to-severe plaque psoriasis: results of the randomized phase 3 CADMUS study. J Am Acad Dermatol. 2015;73(4):594-603.
21. Kellen R, Silverberg NB, Lebwohl M. Efficacy and safety of ustekinumab in adolescents. Pediatr Health Med Ther. 2016;7:109-20.
22. Thaci D, Blauvelt A, Reich K, Tsai TF, Vanaclocha F, Kingo K, et al. Secukinumab is superior to ustekinumab in clearing skin of subjects with moderate to severe plaque psoriasis: CLEAR, a randomized controlled trial. J Am Acad Dermatol. 2015;73:400-9.
23. Papp KA, Gordon KB, Langley RG, Lebwohl MG, Gottlieb AB, Rastogi S, et al. Impact of previous biologic use on efficacy and safety of brodalumab and ustekinumab in patients with moderate-to-severe plaque psoriasis: integrated analysis of AMAGINE-2 and AMAGINE-3. Br J Dermatol. 2018;179:320-8.
24. Kalb RE, Fiorentino DF, Lebwohl MG, Toole J, Poulin Y, Cohen AD, et al. Risk of serious infection with biologic and systemic treatment of psoriasis: results from the psoriasis longitudinal assessment and registry (PSOLAR). JAMA Dermatol. 2015;151:961-9.
25. Gordon KB, Langley RG, Gottlieb AB, Papp KA, Krueger GG, Strober BE, et al. A phase III, randomized, controlled trial of the fully human IL-12/23 mAb briakinumab in moderate-to-severe psoriasis. J Invest Dermatol. 2012;132:304-14.
26. Kimball AB, Gordon KB, Langley RG, Menter A, Chartash EK, Valdes J; ABT-874 Psoriasis Study Investigators. Safety and efficacy of ABT-874, a fully human interleukin 12/23 monoclonal antibody, in the treatment of moderate to severe chronic plaque psoriasis. Arch Dermatol. 2008;144:200-7.

27. Papp KA, Sundaram M, Bao Y, Williams DA, Gu Y, Signorovitch JE, et al. Effects of briakinumab treatment for moderate to severe psoriasis on health-related quality of life and work productivity and activity impairment: results from a randomized phase III study. J Eur Acad Dermatol Venereol. 2014;28(6):790-8.
28. Gottlieb AB, Leonardia C, Kerdel F, Mehlis S, Olds M, Williams DA. Efficacy and safety of briakinumab vs. etanercept and placebo in patients with moderate to severe chronic plaque psoriasis. Br J Dermatol. 2011;165:652-60.
29. Strober BE, Crowley JJ, Yamauchi PS, Olds M, Williams DA. Efficacy and safety results from a phase III, randomized controlled trial comparing the safety and efficacy of briakinumab with etanercept and placebo in patients with moderate to severe chronic plaque psoriasis. Br J Dermatol. 2011;165:661-8.
30. Reich K, Langley RG, Papp KA, Ortonne JP, Unnebrink K, Kaul M, et al. A 52-week trial comparing briakinumab with methotrexate in patients with psoriasis. N Engl J Med. 2011;365:1586-96.
31. ClinicalTrials.gov. (2021). A Phase 3 Study of Efficacy and Safety of AK101 in Subjects With Psoriasis. [online] Available from https://classic.clinicaltrials.gov/ct2/show/NCT05120297 [Last accessed January, 2024].
32. U.S. Food and Drug Administration. (2018). Novel Drug Approvals for 2018. [online] Available from https://www.fda.gov/drugs/new-drugs-fda-cders-new-molecular-entities-and-new-therapeutic-biological-products/novel-drug-approvals-2018 [Last accessed January, 2024].
33. Sun Pharmaceuticals Inc. Ilumya (tildrakizumab) [package insert]. Cranbury, NJ: Sun Pharmaceuticals Inc.; 2018.
34. Reich K, Papp KA, Blauvelt A, Tyring SK, Sinclair R, Thaçi D, et al. Tildrakizumab versus placebo or etanercept for chronic plaque psoriasis (reSURFACE 1 and reSURFACE 2): results from two randomised controlled, phase 3 trials. Lancet. 2017;390:276-88.
35. Blauvelt A, Papp KA, Griffiths CE, Randazzo B, Wasfi Y, Shen YK, et al. Efficacy and safety of guselkumab, an anti-interleukin-23 monoclonal antibody, compared with adalimumab for the continuous treatment of patient with moderate to severe psoriasis: results from the phase III, double-blinded, placebo- and active comparator-controlled VOYAGE 1 trial. J Am Acad Dermatol. 2017;76(3):405-17.
36. Reich K, Armstrong AW, Foley P, Song M, Wasfi Y, Randazzo B, et al. Efficacy and safety of guselkumab, an anti-interleukin-23 monoclonal antibody, compared with adalimumab for the treatment of patients with moderate to severe psoriasis with randomized withdrawal and retreatment: results from the phase III, double-blind, placebo and active comparator-controlled VOYAGE 2 trial. J Am Acad Dermatol. 2017;76:418-31.
37. Langley RG, Tsai TF, Flavin S, Song M, Randazzo B, Wasfi Y, et al. Efficacy and safety of guselkumab in patients with psoriasis who have an inadequate response to ustekinumab: results of the randomized, double-blind, phase 3 NAVIGATE trial. Br J Dermatol. 2018;178:114-23.
38. Krueger JG, Ferris LK, Menter A, Wagner F, White A, Visvanathan S, et al. Anti IL-23A mAB BI655066 for treatment of moderate-to-severe plaque psoriasis: safety, efficacy, pharmacokinetics, and biomarker results of a single-rising dose, randomized, double-blind, placebo-controlled trial. J Allergy Clin Immunol. 2015;136(1):116-24.e7.
39. Papp KA, Blauvelt A, Bukhalo M, Gooderham M, Krueger JG, Lacour JP, et al. Risankizumab versus ustekinumab for moderate-to-severe plaque psoriasis. N Engl J Med. 2017;376:1551-60.
40. Gordon KB, Strober B, Lebwohl M, Augustin M, Blauvelt A, Poulin Y, et al. Efficacy and safety of risankizumab in moderate-to-severe plaque psoriasis (UltIMMa-1 and UltIMMA-2): results from tow double-blind, randomised, placebo-controlled and ustekinumab-controlled phase 3 trials. Lancet. 2018;392:650-61.

41. Reich K, Gooderham M, Thaçi D, Crowley JJ, Ryan C, Krueger JG, et al. Risankizumab compared with adalimumab in patients with moderate-to-severe plaque psoriasis (IMMvent): a randomised, double-blind, active-comparator-controlled phase 3 trial. Lancet. 2019;394:576-86.
42. Blauvelt A, Papp KA, Gooderham M, Langley RG, Leonardi C, Lacour JP, et al. Efficacy and safety of risankizumab, an interleukin-23 inhibitor, in patients with moderate-to-severe chronic plaque psoriasis: 16-week results from the phase III IMMhance trial. Br J Dermatol. 2017;177:E248.
43. Blauvelt A, Kimball AB, Augustin M, Okubo Y, Witte MM, Capriles CR, et al. Efficacy and safety of mirikizumab in psoriasis: results from a 52-week, double-blind, placebo-controlled, randomized withdrawal, phase III trial (OASIS-1). Br J Dermatol. 2022;187:866-77.
44. Papp K, Warren RB, Green L, Reich K, Langley RG, Paul C, et al. Safety and efficacy of mirikizumab versus secukinumab and placebo in the treatment of moderate-to-severe plaque psoriasis (OASIS-2): a phase 3, multicentre, randomised, double-blind study. Lancet Rheumatol. 2023;5:e542-52.
45. Gordon KB, Blauvelt A, Papp KA, Langley RG, Luger T, Ohtsuki M, et al. Phase 3 trials of ixekizumab in moderate-to-severe plaque psoriasis. N Engl J Med. 2016;375(4):345-56.
46. Griffiths CE, Reich K, Lebwohl M, van de Kerkhof P, Paul C, Menter A, et al. Comparison of ixekizumab with etanercept or placebo in moderate-to-severe psoriasis (UNCOVER-2 and UNCOVER-3): results from two phase 3 randomised trials. Lancet. 2015;386:541-51.
47. Blauvelt A, Papp KA, Sofen H, Augustin M, Yosipovitch G, Katoh N, et al. Continuous dosing versus interrupted therapy with ixekizumab: an integrated analysis of two phase 3 trials in psoriasis. J Eur Acad Dermatol Venereol. 2017;31:1004-13.
48. Lebwohl M, Strober B, Menter A, Gordon K, Weglowska J, Puig L, et al. Phase 3 studies comparing brodalumab with ustekinumab in psoriasis. N Engl J Med. 2015;373:1318-28.
49. Papp KA, Reich K, Paul C, Blauvelt A, Baran W, Bolduc C, et al. A prospective phase III, randomized, double-blind, placebo-controlled study of brodalumab in patients with moderate-to-severe plaque psoriasis. Br J Dermatol. 2016;175:273-86.
50. Yamasaki K, Nakagawa H, Kubo Y, Ootaki K; Japanese Brodalumab Study Group. Efficacy and safety of brodalumab in patients with generalized pustular psoriasis and psoriatic erythroderma: results from a 52-week, open-label study. Br J Dermatol. 2017;176:741-51.
51. Papp KA, Merola JF, Gottlieb AB, Griffiths CEM, Cross N, Peterson L, et al. Dual neutralization of both interleukin 17A and interleukin 17F with bimekizumab in patients with psoriasis: results from BE ABLE 1, a 12-week randomized, double-blinded, placebo-controlled phase 2b trial. J Am Acad Dermatol. 2018;79:277-86.e10.
52. Reich K, Papp KA, Blauvelt A, Langley RG, Armstrong A, Warren RB, et al. Bimekizumab versus ustekinumab for the treatment of moderate to severe plaque psoriasis (BE VIVID): efficacy and safety from a 52-week, multicentre, double-blind, active comparator and placebo controlled phase 3 trial. Lancet. 2021;397:487-98.
53. Gordon KB, Foley P, Krueger JG, Pinter A, Reich K, Vender R, et al. Bimekizumab efficacy and safety in moderate to severe plaque psoriasis (BE READY): a multicentre, double-blind, placebo-controlled, randomised withdrawal phase 3 trial. Lancet. 2021;397:475-86.
54. Glatt S, Baeten D, Baker T, Griffiths M, Ionescu L, Lawson ADG, et al. Dual IL-17A and IL-17F neutralisation by bimekizumab in psoriatic arthritis: evidence from preclinical experiments and a randomised placebo-controlled clinical trial that IL-17F contributes to human chronic tissue inflammation. Ann Rheum Dis. 2018;77:523-32.

55. Kubanov AA, Bakulev AL, Samtsov AV, Khairutdinov VR, Sokolovskiy EV, Kokhan MM, et al. Netakimab—new IL-17a inhibitor: 12-week results of phase III clinical study BCD-085-7/PLANETA in patients with moderate-to-severe plaque psoriasis. Vestn Dermatol Venerol. 2019;95(2):15-28.
56. Bakulev AL, Samtsov AV, Kubanov AA, Khairutdinov VR, Kokhan MM, Artemyeva AV. Long-term efficacy and safety of netakimab in patients with moderate-to-severe psoriasis. Results of phase II open-label extension clinical study BCD-085-2-ext. Vestn Dermatol Venerol. 2019;95:56-64.
57. Korotaeva TV, Mazurov VI, Lila AM, Gaydukova IZ, Bakulev AL, Samtsov AV, et al. The efficacy and safety of netakimab in patients with psoriatic arthritis: results from the Phase III clinical study PATERA. Sci Pract Rheumatol. 2020;58:480-8.
58. Papp KA, Weinberg MA, Morris A, Reich K. IL-17A/F nanobody sonelokimab in patients with plaque psoriasis: a multicentre, randomised, placebo-controlled, phase 2b study. Lancet. 2021;397(10284):1564-75.
59. Bachelez H, Choon S-E, Marrakchi S, Burden AD, Tsai TF, Morita A, et al. Inhibition of the Interleukin-36 pathway for the treatment of generalized pustular psoriasis. N Engl J Med. 2019;380:981-3.
60. Navarini AA, Prinz JC, Morita A, Tsai TF, Viguier MA, Li L, et al. Spesolimab improves patient-reported outcomes in patients with generalized pustular psoriasis: results from the Effisayil 1 study. J Eur Acad Dermatol Venereol. 2023;37(4):730-6.
61. Morita A, Choon SE, Bachelez H, Anadkat MJ, Marrakchi S, Zheng M, et al. Design of Effisayil™ 2: a randomized, double-blind, placebo-controlled study of spesolimab in preventing flares in patients with generalized pustular psoriasis. Dermatol Ther (Heidelb). 2023;13(1):347-59.
62. Morita A, Strober B, Burden AD, Choon SE, Anadkat MJ, Marrakchi S, et al. Efficacy and safety of subcutaneous spesolimab for the prevention of generalised pustular psoriasis flares (Effisayil 2): an international, multicentre, randomised, placebo-controlled trial. Lancet. 2023;402(10412):1541-51.
63. Choon SE, Lebwohl MG, Marrakchi S, Burden AD, Tsai TF, Morita A, et al. Study protocol of the global Effisayil 1 Phase II, multicentre, randomised, double-blind, placebo-controlled trial of spesolimab in patients with generalized pustular psoriasis presenting with an acute flare. BMJ Open. 2021;11(3):e043666.

SECTION 3

Biologics in Immunobullous Disorders

CHAPTER 13

Biologics in the Management of Pemphigus—Anti-CD20 Monoclonal Antibody: Rituximab

Dipankar De, Hitaishi Mehta, Muhammed Razmi T

INTRODUCTION

Rituximab is a chimeric murine/human monoclonal immunoglobulin G1 (IgG1) kappa antibody against the cluster of differentiation 20 (CD20) antigen. It was first approved as a cancer chemotherapy agent and subsequently found useful in various autoimmune disorders.

PHARMACOLOGY

Heavy and light chain variable regions of the molecule are from a murine antibody to CD20. The murine variable regions selectively target the CD20 antigen present on the surface of B lymphocytes. Human IgG1 and kappa-chain constant regions of rituximab bind to the Fc receptors on human effector cells and decrease its immunogenicity.

CHARACTERISTICS

- *Molecular weight*: 145 KDa
- *Half-life*: 30–400 hours
- *Excretion*: Phagocytosis and catabolism in the reticuloendothelial system

MECHANISM OF ACTION

The Fab portion of rituximab attaches particularly to the CD20 antigen which is expressed specifically on the cell membranes of B lymphocytes from the pre-B cell stage to the mature B cell stage. The immune effector cells such as natural killer (NK) cells bind to rituximab via Fc receptors and help in the destruction of the bound CD20+ B lymphocytes via three possible mechanisms, that are (1) complement-dependent cytotoxicity, (2) antibody-dependent cell-mediated cytolysis, and (3) apoptosis.

PHARMACOKINETICS

The mean half-life ($t_{1/2}$) of rituximab is around 3 weeks, similar to the other IgG1-related biological agents. Moreover, levels of serum rituximab increase with multiple infusions, since lesser antigens will be available due to depletion. B cell depletion occurs within 2–3 weeks of the initial infusion of rituximab. There is a sustained reduction of B cells over the first 6 months until the first year of treatment when the B cell numbers start returning to normal. Hematopoietic stem cells, pro-B cells, short-lived plasmablasts, and long-lived plasma cells do not express CD20 and thus are not directly affected by rituximab.

TREATMENT PROTOCOLS

There are two main protocols for rituximab administration as mentioned here:
1. *Lymphoma protocol (LP)*: Rituximab is administered weekly at a dose of 375 mg/m² body surface area for 4 weeks. Most of the initial studies of rituximab followed this protocol.
2. *Rheumatoid arthritis protocol (RAP)*: 1 g each dose of rituximab is administered at an interval of 15 days. This protocol is currently approved by the United States Food and Drug Administration (US FDA) for the management of moderate to severe pemphigus vulgaris (PV) in adults. Most other dermatological indications are also managed with this protocol.

A novel low-dose rituximab regimen (500 mg, 2 weeks apart) with immunologically targeted, ultralow-dose (200 mg) top-up infusions on immunological relapse was found to be an equally effective but more affordable alternative to conventional RAP.[1] Rituximab has also been administered intralesional, mainly for cutaneous B cell lymphomas, at a dose of 10 mg/mL, with 1 mL per lesion administered in several sessions. Rituximab has also been combined with intravenous immunoglobulin (IVIg), immunoadsorption, and dexamethasone pulse therapy in autoimmune blistering diseases.

USES

The United States Food and Drug Administration Approved Indications

- Moderate to severe PV in adults
- Follicular and diffuse large B cell non-Hodgkin lymphoma (NHL)
- Chronic lymphocytic leukemia (CLL)
- Rheumatoid arthritis (RA)
- Granulomatosis with polyangiitis (GPA), formerly Wegener's granulomatosis (WG)
- Microscopic polyangiitis (MPA)

Off-label Indications
Of these indications, the first three indications are recognized by the US FDA as "orphan designations."
- Autoimmune thrombocytopenia
- Rasmussen's encephalitis
- Other autoimmune bullous diseases
- Systemic lupus erythematosus (SLE)
- Autoimmune hemolytic anemia
- Autoimmune neuropathies
- Graft-versus-host disease (GVHD)
- Mixed cryoglobulinemia
- Dermatomyositis (DM) and polymyositis (PM)
- Sjögren's syndrome
- Cutaneous B-cell lymphomas (intralesional)
- Lymphomatoid granulomatosis

Dermatological Uses of Rituximab
Pemphigus Vulgaris and Pemphigus Foliaceus
Rituximab has emerged as a promising agent for PV. Most of the patients had rapid resolution of lesions within 2–3 weeks and an absolute clearance of the clinical disease was achieved within 6–8 weeks of starting the treatment.[2] Skin lesions respond faster than mucosal lesions and most patients have remained on a reduced dose of systemic immunosuppressive therapy.[2] The first randomized controlled trial (RCT) of rituximab in PV and foliaceus was published in 2017 in which 90 patients were studied. The patients were randomized into two groups with the first group receiving rituximab and prednisolone and the second group receiving prednisolone. The patients were followed up for 36 months and by 24 months rate of remission was three times higher and adverse effects were half in the rituximab group.[2] A systematic review and meta-analysis suggested a complete clinical remission in 76% of 578 patients with pemphigus (496 with PV and 82 with pemphigus foliaceus) after one cycle of rituximab.[3] Remission was achieved at an average duration of 5.8 months and the patients remained in remission for 14.5 months with a relapse rate of 40% over a mean follow-up period of 23 months. The meta-analysis showed that in contrast to smaller doses of rituximab (<1,500 mg/cycle), larger doses (≥2,000 mg/cycle) resulted in long-lasting remission. In other parameters, different dosing regimens such as LP and RAP or high-dose rituximab and low-dose rituximab showed comparable outcomes.[3] Rituximab was approved for the management of moderate to severe PV in adults by the FDA in 2018 and the European Commission in 2019. Rituximab (two 1,000 mg intravenous infusions at an interval of 2 weeks) in combination with systemic corticosteroids (oral prednisone 0.5–1.5 mg/kg/day) with a progressive tapering with the aim of

stopping corticosteroids within 6 months is recommended as the first-line treatment in all cases of pemphigus.[4,5] Patients with relapse, poor response, or intolerance to conventional therapies are also candidates for rituximab therapy. Initiation of treatment with rituximab early in the disease course may be associated with more favorable outcomes in terms of response rates and duration of complete remission.[6] Its use also allows for more rapid tapering of corticosteroids and has a major steroid-sparing effect.

While some studies on autoimmune bullous disorders suggest a single cycle of rituximab (either LP or RAP) can induce a complete response, the other studies suggest a need for maintenance dosing over long periods to induce a response.[7] The optimum dose, frequency of cycles, and duration of the maintenance therapy with rituximab in pemphigus is yet to be determined. An additional cycle of two 1,000 mg infusions 2 weeks apart can be considered in pemphigus patients who do not attain complete remission on or off therapy after 6 months. Patients who are in complete remission on/off therapy at 6 months can be given rituximab infusion 500 mg or 1 g at 6 months. However, for the patient without complete remission at month 6 it may be recommended for two infusions of 1 g at 2 weeks apart. In patients attaining complete remission on or off therapy at 6 months, another 500 mg or 1 g infusion can be considered at month 6 in patients who initially presented with severe disease or had a high titer of anti-desmoglein (anti-Dsg) antibodies at 3 months.[8] Additional 500 mg infusions at months 12 and 18 should be considered in patients in complete remission but serum positivity of anti-Dsg antibodies.[4] Infusions after 18 months should be considered in patients who present with reappearance of serum autoantibodies after their initial disappearance. The maintenance therapy with rituximab is as mentioned below in **Flowchart 1**.

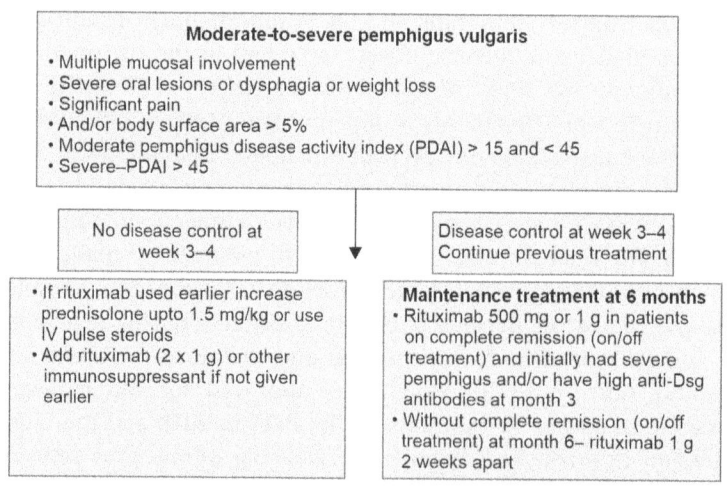

FLOWCHART 1: Maintenance therapy with rituximab.

Patients of pemphigus foliaceus treated with rituximab have response rates similar to those seen in PV. European guidelines recommend rituximab (two infusions of 1,000 mg 2 weeks apart) as the first-line management option for pemphigus foliaceus of any severity.[4]

OTHER AUTOIMMUNE BULLOUS DISEASES

Rituximab has been found to be effective in the following blistering diseases also:
- *Paraneoplastic pemphigus (PNP)*: The efficacy is less impressive. There are conflicting reports. Some reports showed improvement in the oral and cutaneous lesions,[9,10] whereas others reported minimal improvement in the mucosal lesions.[11,12]
- *Bullous pemphigoid (BP)*: A better alternative in cases that are refractory to the conventional treatment based on the evidence obtained from small case series and case reports. A recent systematic review evaluated the efficacy of rituximab in varying doses for the treatment of BP, with a mean duration of therapy of 2.6 months.[13] About 85% of patients achieved complete remission, most of whom had not responded to systemic corticosteroids before receiving biologic treatment. The recurrence rate with rituximab was 29% with an average time to recurrence of 10 months. The follow-up period ranged from 3 months to 9 years, with a mean of 33 ± 38 months.[13]
- Before the initiation of rituximab in hypertensive patients, immune status, and cardiac risk should be evaluated more vigorously considering the advanced age of this patient population and an increased risk of death due to bacterial sepsis or cardiac complications.
- *Mucous membrane pemphigoid (MMP)*: Rituximab is beneficial in severe cases unresponsive to the standard therapy. The reported clinical remission rate is 60%.[2] Rituximab is unlikely to improve the scarring sequelae.
- *Epidermolysis bullosa acquisita (EBA)*: Rituximab is beneficial in refractory cases. A review of literature assessing 20 cases of refractory EBA found that 56% of patients treated with rituximab monotherapy and 75% of those receiving rituximab in combination with immunoadsorption achieved complete remission.[14] Both lymphoma and RA protocols were used. Brazilian Society of Dermatology recommends the use of rituximab in either dosage regimen for the management of severe EBA refractory to corticosteroids.[15]

Autoimmune Connective Tissue Diseases

B cells are implicated in the pathogenesis of autoimmune connective tissue diseases. Hence, rituximab is likely to be used increasingly in these disorders.

Dermatomyositis

Rituximab is an effective treatment option for DM. Initial studies showed conflicting results on the beneficial effects of rituximab in the cutaneous manifestation of DM.[16,17] Rituximab was found to be useful as an adjunctive therapy on the skin and muscle manifestations of juvenile DM.[18] Rituximab is an appropriate second-line therapy in disease refractory to combination of systemic corticosteroid and an oral immunosuppressant,[19] and can be considered as a first-line treatment in patients with vasculopathy, calcinosis, adults with anti-melanoma differentiation-associated gene 5 (anti-MDA5) positivity and children with anti-nuclear matrix protein 2 (anti-NXP2) positivity.[20-22]

Cutaneous Lupus Erythematosus

Although there are reports of beneficial effects of rituximab in cutaneous lupus erythematosus (CLE),[23] overall data suggest poor outcomes in chronic CLE and variable outcomes in subacute CLE.[24] Its use in systemic lupus has also shown controversial results. Two randomized trials found no significant benefit when rituximab was compared with the controls (who received high doses of glucocorticoids and immunosuppressives).[25,26] Guidelines for the treatment of CLE by the European Dermatology Forum (EDF) do not recommend rituximab for the management of CLE.[27]

Systemic Sclerosis

The EUSTAR [European League Against Rheumatism (EULAR) Scleroderma Trials and Research group] study showed amelioration of skin fibrosis and prevention of further deterioration of lung function in rituximab treated systemic sclerosis (SSc) patients versus untreated matched controls, suggesting a beneficial effect of rituximab in SSc.[28] A randomized trial with 60 patients who were assigned to either receive rituximab or cyclophosphamide revealed that those who received rituximab showed better progress in percent-predicted forced vital capacity and modified Rodnan skin score (mRSS) in comparison to the cyclophosphamide group.[29] Despite these findings, further research is necessary to determine the lasting effectiveness and safety of rituximab in treating skin and lung fibrosis in SSc; therefore, its routine use cannot be suggested at this point.

Vasculitis

Rituximab was approved by the US FDA in September 2019 for GPA and MPA. The Pediatric Polyangiitis Rituximab Study was a phase IIa, international, open-label, single-arm study in which 25 pediatric patients with new-onset or relapsing disease were enrolled. During the initial 6-month remission-induction phase, patients received intravenous infusions of rituximab (375 mg/m^2 body surface area) and glucocorticoids once per week for 4 weeks. During the follow-up period, patients could receive further treatment, including rituximab, for GPA or MPA. Remission, according to the pediatric vasculitis activity score, was achieved in 56, 92, and 100% of patients by months 6, 12, and 18, respectively. In WG with polyangiitis with moderate-to-severe involvement, rituximab in combination with systemic steroids is increasingly used for induction of remission and maintenance.[30] Rituximab was found to be superior to azathioprine or cyclophosphamide for sustained remission in antineutrophil cytoplasmic antibody (ANCA)-associated vasculitides.[30,31]

Primary Cutaneous B-cell Lymphoma

Owing to its beneficial effect in nodal B cell lymphoma, rituximab has been used in primary cutaneous B-cell lymphoma (PCBCL). It was found to be effective and safe in the management of PCBCL, when used as per LP, even in combination with high-dose chemotherapy or in elderly patients. Even though recurrences were noted in those with generalized skin involvement, continuation of rituximab infusion was not indicated as these were managed effectively with other treatment measures.[32,33] Single-agent rituximab therapy may be employed for PCBCL.[34] For primary cutaneous diffuse large B-cell lymphoma, leg type (PCBCL-LT), multiagent chemotherapy should be used.[35] Intralesional rituximab at a dose of 10 mg/mL, 1 mL per lesion, three times a week was found to be useful.[36,37] PCBCL lesions in those patients with severe flu-like symptoms after intralesional injection respond better to rituximab.[38] Response was noted in lesions away from the intralesional site and a decrease in B cell count in peripheral blood was documented suggesting systemic absorption.[7] PCBCL tends to relapse and high recurrence is noted with intralesional rituximab.[39] Rituximab was found to be useful in cutaneous lymphoid hyperplasia with documented B-cell hyperplasia.[7]

Graft-versus-host Disease

Rituximab showed promising results in the management of GVHD with improvement in the mucocutaneous and musculoskeletal manifestations.[40,41] However, when it was used as a prophylactic agent along with a myeloablative conditioning regimen, it did not prevent the development of GVHD.[42]

Atopic Dermatitis

Rituximab was found to be beneficial in severe atopic dermatitis in an open study of eight patients when it was used alone.[43] In another study, six refractory atopic dermatitis patients achieved an impressive clinical improvement after a "sequential switch therapy with omalizumab and rituximab."[44] However, its failure in some patients as highlighted by McDonald et al. stresses the need for more robust studies on its use in severe atopic dermatitis.[45] Currently, rituximab cannot be recommended for management of atopic dermatitis.

GENERAL INSTRUCTIONS

- *Dosage form*: 100 mg/10 mL and 500 mg/50 mL solution in a nonreusable vial for injection. Subcutaneous formulation is available in Canada.
- To be given as intravenous infusion and not as intravenous bolus or push.
- Can be stored at 2–8°C for 24 hours (rituximab has been shown to be stable for an extra 24 hours at room temperature). Store the reconstituted solution at 2–8°C as it is free of preservatives. The prepared infusion is physically and chemically stable for 24 hours at 2–8°C and subsequently 12 hours at room temperature; hence, it should be used in < 36 hours of reconstitution.

ADMINISTRATION

- Use aseptic precautions.
- Premedication with intravenous hydrocortisone 100 mg and pheniramine maleate 22.75 mg along with oral paracetamol 500 mg.
- Rituximab can be reconstituted in an infusion bag with either 0.9% sodium chloride or 5% dextrose in water to a final strength of 1–4 mg/mL.
- Mix the solution by gently inverting the bag (no other drugs should be added).
- The rate of the initial infusion should be 50 mg/h.
- If there are no adverse reactions, the infusion rate can be slowly increased by 50 mg/h every 30 minutes up to 400 mg/h.
- Vitals are checked after every 30 minutes, before increasing the dose, in the form of blood pressure, pulse rate, respiratory rate, and temperature.
- If the initial infusion was uneventful, further infusions can be started at 100 mg/h and be increased to a maximum infusion rate of 400 mg/h.
- In case of immediate adverse reactions like infusion reactions, treatment should be discontinued temporarily.
- After waiting for 30 minutes, restart the infusion at a slower rate (half the flow rate).
- Hydrocortisone and antihistamines must be readministered.
- Discontinue the infusion if there is a serious or life-threatening cardiac complication and manage the event as per the protocol.

Tests to be done before Administration

- *Routine investigations*: Complete blood count (CBC), liver function test, renal function test, urine for routine examination
- Rule out active tuberculosis (TB) in high endemic Indian scenario
    - History of past TB, history of contact with an active case of TB.
    - History of fever, weight loss, and night sweats
    - Chest X-ray (screening for latent TB is not recommended as no increase in the incidence of TB has been observed in patients

receiving rituximab[46-48]). However, the patients are often prescribed high-dose corticosteroids along with rituximab which can result in the reactivation of TB.
- Rule out hepatitis infection/carrier status
  - Hepatitis B surface antigen (HBsAg) and total hepatitis B core antibody (anti-HBc)
  - Anti-hepatitis C antibody
- Human immunodeficiency virus (HIV) infection by enzyme-linked immunosorbent assay (ELISA) method
- Urine pregnancy test
- Electrocardiography
- Baseline assessment of IgG levels
- Anti-desmoglein 1 (anti-Dsg1) and 3 levels in pemphigus
- Flow cytometry for cluster of differentiation 19 (CD19)

MONITORING DURING RITUXIMAB THERAPY

Monitor CBC every 2 weeks during rituximab infusions and every 1–3 months, thereafter with a special focus on neutropenia. Liver and renal function tests should be done every 3 months. It is recommended to monitor IgG levels in the elderly population and in those with a low baseline IgG.[47] Peripheral blood CD19 levels, anti-Dsg1, and three titers are also useful for monitoring response to therapy in pemphigus patients. Serum autoantibodies (anti-Dsg) should be measured by ELISA at baseline, at month 3, and every 3–6 months thereafter. Periodic CD19(+) B lymphocyte monitoring may also help in predicting relapses.[49]

ADVERSE EFFECTS

Infusion Reactions

One of the most predictable and serious acute side effects of rituximab is a constellation of symptoms and signs that manifest within 2 hours of initial infusion. Incidence is up to 30–45%. Adverse effects are mild in nature and consist mainly of fever, chills, and rigors with 80–90% of the cases having National Cancer Institute (NCI) toxicity grade 1 or 2. Other symptoms include headache, flushing, nausea, dyspepsia, urticaria/rash, fatigue, sweating, throat irritation, rhinitis, pruritus, tachycardia, mild hypotension, dyspnea, and backache. About <10% of cases develop bronchospasm and/or severe hypotension. Severe (grade 3 or 4) reactions like anaphylaxis are seen in <5% of cases. Fever and muscle pain are not the features of anaphylaxis, and such complaints represent standard infusion reactions. In most patients, the standard infusion reaction is mild and brief, lacks typical symptoms of anaphylaxis, and resolves completely when drug infusion is withheld. However, some typical symptoms and signs such as throat tightness/change in voice, incessant cough, urticarial, and wheezing should alert clinicians to the possibility of anaphylaxis and should be managed vigorously.

Management
Mild reactions can be managed by holding the infusion for a while and restarting later at a slower rate as explained above. An additional dose of paracetamol and diphenhydramine can be given for the reaction to subside. Anaphylaxis should be managed by subcutaneous/intramuscular epinephrine. The intramuscular route is preferred at a dose of 0.2–0.5 mg of 1 mg/mL (1:1,000) solution every 5–15 minute until clinical improvement. Additional therapies include saline infusion, bronchodilator inhalations, and parenteral glucocorticoids. Anaphylaxis is a type 1 hypersensitivity reaction and infusion reactions are due to cytokine release. Anaphylaxis cannot be prevented by premedications, but infusion reactions can. A desensitization protocol is being devised for readministering rituximab after anaphylaxis or severe type 1 hypersensitivity.[50,51]

Tumor Lysis Syndrome
It is seen in <0.05% of patients who cannot appropriately clear the dying cells, especially in the setting of lymphomas. It is characterized by hyperuricemia, hyperkalemia, hypocalcemia, hyperphosphatemia, deranged renal function tests, and elevated lactate dehydrogenase. It usually occurs within 12–24 hours of rituximab administration. This adverse event is not directly related to pemphigus and other autoimmune dermatosis.

Cardiac Complications
Recent studies have highlighted the overall cardioprotective effects of rituximab by reducing the inflammatory burden in autoimmune diseases.[52-54] A recent cohort study reported a protective effect of rituximab against cardiovascular and metabolic complications as compared to conventional immunosuppressants, indicating that rituximab therapy may be preferred in individuals with preexisting cardiovascular and metabolic risk factors.[55] However, cardiovascular toxicities have been reported in 8% of patients with rituximab infusion.[56] Patients are advised to withhold their antihypertensive medications in the morning of the rituximab infusion given the increased frequency of mild-to-moderate hypotension occurring during rituximab infusions. Based on some case reports on adverse cardiac events such as myocardial infarctions, atrial fibrillation, and worsening of preexisting cardiac dysfunction, a thorough cardiac evaluation is indicated especially in those with cardiovascular risk factors.[57] The etiologies of acute events, such as myocarditis and arrhythmia are postulated to be due to cytokine release from dying B cells that leads to platelet activation, vasoconstriction, and plaque rupture. Cardiomyopathy may occur due to the accumulation of reticulin fibers upon multiple cycles of rituximab infusion.[58] Such a scenario

is unlikely in the setting of dermatological indications where only two doses of rituximab are given and repeated if required at the most once in a year. However, the patients receiving rituximab should be closely monitored for any cardiovascular signs or symptoms. Any chest pain during the infusion warrants an electrocardiography and the help of a cardiologist should be sought.[59] Adequate hydration before starting rituximab infusion and a slower rate of infusion may prevent these cardiovascular adverse effects.[59]

Infections

Though a single course of rituximab will not result in significant hypogammaglobulinemia, it occurs on repeated infusions. Preexisting hypogammaglobulinemia and concomitant immunosuppressant use such as cyclophosphamide are known risk factors for rituximab-induced hypogammaglobulinemia. Rheumatology literature recommends baseline assessment of IgG, immunoglobulin A (IgA), and immunoglobulin M (IgM) levels before starting rituximab. A study has shown a 56% incidence of IgG hypogammaglobulinemia after rituximab infusion.[60] Immunoglobulin G replacement was initiated in 4% of patients because of recurrent infections. Case reports of new infection or reactivation of varicella zoster, parvovirus B19, hepatitis B, and C, cytomegalovirus (CMV), John Cunningham (JC) virus [causes progressive multifocal leukoencephalopathy (PML)], West Nile virus (WNV), and herpes simplex virus (HSV) has been documented after rituximab administration.[61] Rituximab was found to increase the incidence of infectious complications in the setting of hematological malignancies and transplant recipients. However, no increase in the incidence of opportunistic infections was apparent in RA patients.[62] A recent cohort study among 963 pemphigus patients found that within the first 12 months after treatment, patients under rituximab had an elevated risk of coronavirus disease 2019 (COVID-19), parasitic, and CMV infections.[63] Rituximab was also associated with pneumonia, osteomyelitis, and viral diseases even beyond the first year after therapy. A recent retrospective study involving 409 autoimmune bullous disease patients revealed that the use of rituximab was associated with an elevated risk of COVID-19 infection, with a case-fatality ratio of 18%.[64] Additionally, advanced age, active disease, and comorbidities were identified as potential risk factors for COVID-19 mortality in patients with autoimmune blistering diseases. Rituximab has been associated with *Pneumocystis carinii* pneumonia (PCP); however, the role of prophylactic cotrimoxazole therapy in preventing PCP infection in pemphigus patients treated with rituximab remains uncertain. A retrospective study showed that prophylactic cotrimoxazole did not significantly reduce the incidence of PCP infection in this patient group, suggesting that it may not be necessary due to the low incidence of PCP.[65] However, more research is needed to evaluate its potential benefits in patients with long-term immunosuppressive therapy.

Late-onset Neutropenia after Rituximab Therapy

Late-onset neutropenia (R-LON), characterized by unexplained grade 3–4 neutropenia occurring several months after rituximab therapy, has a cumulative incidence of 9% at 1 year according to a retrospective analysis.[66] The median onset time is 3–4 months. Older age (>60 years), advanced stage of lymphoma, and purine analog or methotrexate administration were found to be significant or borderline significant risk factors for R-LON. In general, R-LON is self-limiting and rarely has significant clinical sequelae. However, treatment with granulocyte colony-stimulating factor is a good option in grade 4 R-LON patients with a high risk of infection.

Human Antichimeric Antibodies

In comparison to lymphoma patients, the occurrence of human antichimeric antibodies (HACA) to rituximab are higher in RA and SLE patients. This may be due to the autoimmune nature of primary diseases promoting the development of antidrug antibodies, lower dosages of rituximab used, and lack of use of additional immunosuppressants in autoimmune disorders compared to lymphoma. HACA may lead to an increased incidence of infusion reactions and a decrease in the therapeutic efficacy of rituximab. A recent cohort study investigated the prevalence of HACAs in patients with pemphigus undergoing treatment with rituximab and observed that HACAs are frequently detected in these patients but generally do not affect treatment outcomes.[67] However, a subset of patients with HACAs, low rituximab concentration, incomplete B-cell depletion, and persistent serum anti-DSG3 Abs had an increased risk of relapse.

Other Less Common Adverse Effects

- *Serious mucocutaneous reactions*: Stevens–Johnson syndrome, vesiculobullous dermatitis, lichenoid dermatosis, and toxic epidermal necrolysis. Rituximab carries a boxed warning for severe mucocutaneous reactions.
- *Serum sickness*: Should be suspected when the patient develops a fever, arthralgia, and characteristic urticated lesions on the palms and soles that may last days to weeks.
- No enhanced malignancy risk was reported with rituximab.

CONTRAINDICATIONS

- Contraindications to rituximab use include known anaphylaxis or immunoglobulin E (IgE) hypersensitivity to murine proteins or components of rituximab.
- Caution should be exercised in patients with active, serious infections, such as TB, sepsis, hepatitis, and opportunistic infections, and in those

with a severely immunocompromised state, severe cardiac failure, or uncontrolled cardiac disease, pregnancy, and HIV-infected patients with a cluster of differentiation 4 (CD4) count < 50/μL.

SPECIAL SITUATIONS

Pregnancy and Lactation

Pregnancy Category C Drug

Rituximab is capable of crossing the placenta and can be detected in newborns. Limited safety data are available regarding the use of rituximab during pregnancy, although available evidence suggests potential risks such as B-cell lymphocytopenia and increased susceptibility to infections in infants. A review of 231 cases of maternal rituximab exposure during pregnancy found that among 153 pregnancies with known outcomes, there were 33 spontaneous abortions and 28 elective terminations.[68] Among the 90 live births, 22 had abnormalities at birth, four had neonatal infections, and two had congenital malformations. The reported miscarriage rate may be attributed to the autoimmune nature of the treated diseases and the potential teratogenic effects of rituximab and other immunosuppressants. No specific congenital malformation pattern associated with rituximab was observed, and the malformation rate was similar to the general population. Early detection of infection in the mother and neonate is important, and monitoring for clinically significant cytopenias in neonates is recommended. Contraception is advised for 12 months after the last rituximab administration. American College of Rheumatology (ACR) advises discontinuing rituximab upon pregnancy detection in patients with rheumatic and musculoskeletal diseases, unless there is a life- or organ-threatening condition.[69] In a recent study involving 19 pregnancies in women with pemphigus treated with rituximab, the outcomes included 17 live births, one spontaneous abortion, and one termination. One neonate required hospitalization due to early-onset neonatal sepsis, and another had hydronephrosis.[70] According to the manufacturer, breastfeeding is not recommended during treatment and for 6 months after the last dose of rituximab. However, rituximab is unlikely to be absorbed by the infant's gastrointestinal tract following exposure via breast milk and is hence considered compatible with breastfeeding by some experts.[69]

Children

United States Food and Drug Administration does not recommend rituximab in patients < 18 years old due to concerns regarding the potential for prolonged immunosuppression owing to B-cell depletion in the actively developing juvenile immune system. There are reports suggesting that children with autoimmune disorders have an especially high risk of infection and rituximab toxicities, including infusion reactions, low antimicrobial antibody titers, hypogammaglobulinemia, angioedema, and fatal sepsis;[71] however, it is generally safe and effective in most of the children treated with rituximab.[72] In 2019, rituximab received its first pediatric approval for the management of GPA in children aged 2 years and older. Rituximab is being increasingly used for the management of pediatric PV, with most reports being sporadic cases or small case series.[73,74] No long-term adverse effects have been reported, infections and infusion reactions were reported in some cases in the literature.[75,76] There is no established rituximab therapy protocol for pediatric patients, but the RA protocol is commonly used. There are no established recommendations for the maintenance treatment in the pediatric population, likely because of their increased vulnerability to infections.

Latent Tuberculosis

While previous studies have demonstrated the role of B cells in host defense against *Mycobacterium tuberculosis* infection,[77] there have been no reported cases of active TB in RA patients receiving rituximab therapy in clinical trials or real-world practice. Only three cases of active TB were reported in a survey conducted by the Emerging Infections Network (EIN).[78] The ACR recommended TB screening before rituximab therapy in 2008.[79] Conversely, an international expert committee has concluded that there is no evidence supporting the systematic screening of RA patients for TB before using rituximab.[47] Additionally, the safety and efficacy of rituximab have been demonstrated in case reports of RA patients who developed TB while undergoing treatment with anti-tumor necrosis factor (anti-TNF) medications or who had a history of treatment for pulmonary TB.[80-82]

Hepatitis B Infection

The US FDA has issued a black box warning on the risk of hepatitis B virus (HBV) reactivation in those who receive rituximab. Most experts believe that the risk of HBV reactivation is highest for anti-CD20 agents among immunosuppressive therapies.[83] Reactivation of HBV is diagnosed by the detection of HBV deoxyribonucleic acid (DNA) in a previously HBV DNA-negative patient or a rise in HBV DNA by >2 $\log_{10}$ international units (IU)/mL ≥10-fold as in some studies from baseline or reverse seroconversion (previously HBsAg-negative becomes HBsAg-positive).

Screening

The risk for HBV reactivation following rituximab is particularly high in patients who are positive for HBsAg or antibody to hepatitis B core antigen (anti-HBc). Whether or not to include anti-hepatitis B surface antibodies (anti-HBs) in the screening process is still controversial. The presence of anti-HBs in unvaccinated patients could be the only marker of past HBV infection in HBsAg-negative/anti-HBc-negative patients. Reactivation of HBV is rare in such cases. However, some authors suggest "triple screening" (HBsAg, anti-HBc, and anti-HBs), because knowledge of anti-HBs status could increase vigilance during chronic therapy with high-risk biologics, such as rituximab, and may help to decide the vaccination against HBV before such therapy.

Based on the results of this initial screening, the following actions can be taken:
- HBsAg or anti-HBc-positive patients should have baseline HBV DNA levels measured.
- Patients who are nonimmune to HBV (anti-HBs < 10 IU/L) should be vaccinated.

Management Approach[84,85]
- *If HBsAg+ (chronic HBV infection)*: Start oral antiviral treatment
- *If HBsAg−, anti-HBc+, and anti-HBs ± (past HBV infection)*: Do HBV DNA levels at baseline, 6 months, and 12 months of last infusion; if present start oral antiviral treatment, if absent only regular monitoring is needed.
- *If HBsAg−, anti-HBc−, and anti-HBs− (no previous exposure)*: Consider vaccination for patients at risk.
- *If HBsAg−, anti-HBc−, and anti-HBs+ (history of HBV vaccination)*: No further action is needed.

Regular monitoring for liver enzyme derangement is recommended in all of the above categories. The most recent guidelines recommend entecavir or tenofovir as antiviral agents against HBV. Prophylactic antiviral treatment was found to be superior to "on-demand" antiviral therapy in HBV reactivation. Treatment needs to be continued for at least 12 months after the last infusion of rituximab.

Hepatitis C Infection

The association between rituximab administration and hepatitis C virus (HCV) reactivation is controversial. HCV reactivation and hepatic complications reported in lymphoma patients can be attributed to the concomitant chemotherapy administered for lymphoma. Such complications were not reported in most of the rheumatology literature where rituximab was used without concomitant chemotherapy.[86] Rituximab has also been used for extrahepatic autoimmune manifestations of HCV like cryoglobulinemic vasculitis with good safety. Given that HCV-related hepatitis is also an immune phenomenon, rituximab-associated HCV reactivation was not associated with adverse hepatic outcomes. Coadministration of rituximab and interferon-α/ribavirin in HCV-related advanced liver disease did not increase the side effects in rheumatology patients.[87] However, increased hematological side effects were noted on concomitant administration of rituximab–cyclophosphamide, doxorubicin, vincristine, and prednisolone (R-CHOP) plus anti-HCV treatment.[88] The presence of HCV infection is not a contraindication for rituximab administration. However, such patients are closely monitored for HCV viral load serially and should be managed under the supervision of a hepatologist.[86]

Human Immunodeficiency Virus

The loss of humoral immunity by rituximab in addition to the underlying destruction of the cellular immune system by HIV may further increase the risk of infection. Hence, rituximab is contraindicated in HIV infection with a CD4 cell count of <250/μL.[89]

Active Severe Infection/Sepsis

Secondary bacterial infection in pemphigus is a usual scenario in dermatology practice and is a major cause of mortality. Hence, rituximab and any immunosuppressive agent should be used judiciously in this clinical setting. Active and serious infection contraindicates rituximab use, and these infections should be ruled out by cultures of blood, urine, and pus. All patients with infection or bacteremia are potential candidates for sepsis. A modified version of the sequential (sepsis-related) organ failure assessment (SOFA) score called the quick SOFA (qSOFA) score helps to identify early sepsis.[90] The qSOFA score is easy to calculate at the bedside and has three components each weighing one point: (1) Respiratory rate ≥ 22/min, (2) altered mentation, and (3) systolic blood pressure ≤ 100 mm Hg. A score ≥ 2 indicates a poor prognosis due to sepsis and warrants prompt referral and further sepsis-related investigations. Other parameters such as fall and rise in white cell counts, thrombocytopenia, rise in C-reactive protein (CRP), rising trend of serum lactate despite correcting dehydration, deranged organ function tests, and coagulopathy also point to sepsis. Even though nonspecific, serum procalcitonin levels more than two standard deviations above the normal value help in a quick diagnosis of bacterial sepsis, even before getting culture reports.

Vaccinations

It has been consistently seen that rituximab has the most profound impact on vaccine immunogenicity compared to other immunosuppressive agents. All the patients planned for rituximab therapy should be given all indicated vaccines, such as hepatitis B vaccination for at-risk population, *Pneumococcus*, tetanus toxoid vaccinations every 10 years, and annual influenza vaccine;[91,92] though live vaccines are not routinely advocated in those who have been treated with rituximab recently, the risks need to be studied further. Ideally, vaccination should be done before starting rituximab. If the treatment has already started, vaccines can be administered at least 6 months after the last dose and at least 4 weeks before the next course. Rituximab may diminish the therapeutic effect of COVID-19 vaccines and should be administered either 2–4 weeks before the scheduled dose of rituximab or 6 months after the last infusion.

FUTURE TRENDS

Rituximab is increasingly used as a combination therapy with IVIg resulting in long-term disease-free period in autoimmune disorders. Recent clinical trials have suggested rituximab as a first-line and monotherapy agent in pemphigus.[4,8] More studies are needed in this direction. Newer anti-CD20 biologicals have been introduced to address the issue of rituximab nonresponse. Second-generation monoclonal antibodies (e.g., ofatumumab) are humanized or fully human with unmodified Fc region, thus reducing immunogenicity. Third-generation antibodies (e.g., obinutuzumab) have bioengineered Fc domains, thus improving the therapeutic activity, especially in those that express a low-affinity version of the Fc receptor on B cells.

CONCLUSION

Rituximab is approved for the management of pemphigus vulgaris. The availability of this drug has changed the outlook for pemphigus patients dramatically. The judicious use of this molecule has the potential to reduce mortality and morbidity in patients suffering from pemphigus group of disorders.

REFERENCES

1. Singh N, Handa S, Mahajan R, Sachdeva N, De D. Comparison of the efficacy and cost-effectiveness of an immunologically targeted low-dose rituximab protocol with the conventional rheumatoid arthritis protocol in severe pemphigus. Clin Exp Dermatol. 2022;47(8):1508-16.
2. Ahmed AR, Shetty S. The emerging role of rituximab in autoimmune blistering diseases. Am J Clin Dermatol. 2015;16(3):167-77.
3. Wang HH, Liu CW, Li YC, Huang YC. Efficacy of rituximab for pemphigus: a systematic review and meta-analysis of different regimens. Acta Derm Venereol. 2015;95(8):928-32.
4. Joly P, Horvath B, Patsatsi A, Uzun S, Bech R, Beissert S, et al. Updated S2K guidelines on the management of pemphigus vulgaris and foliaceus initiated by the European Academy of Dermatology And Venereology (EADV). J Eur Acad Dermatol Venereol. 2020;34(9):1900-13.
5. Harman KE, Brown D, Exton LS, Groves RW, Hampton PJ, Mohd Mustapa MF, et al. British Association of Dermatologists' guidelines for the management of pemphigus vulgaris 2017. Br J Dermatol. 2017;177(5):1170-201.
6. Lunardon L, Tsai KJ, Propert KJ, Fett N, Stanley JR, Werth VP, et al. Adjuvant rituximab therapy of pemphigus: a single-center experience with 31 patients. Arch Dermatol. 2012;148(9):1031-6.

7. España A, Ornilla E, Panizo C. Rituximab in dermatology. Actas Dermosifiliogr. 2013;104(5):380-92.
8. Joly P, Maho-Vaillant M, Prost-Squarcioni C, Hebert V, Houivet E, Calbo S, et al. First-line rituximab combined with short-term prednisone versus prednisone alone for the treatment of pemphigus (Ritux 3): a prospective, multicentre, parallel-group, open-label randomised trial. Lancet. 2017;389(10083):2031-40.
9. Heizmann M, Itin P, Wernli M, Borradori L, Bargetzi MJ. Successful treatment of paraneoplastic pemphigus in follicular NHL with rituximab: report of a case and review of treatment for paraneoplastic pemphigus in NHL and CLL. Am J Hematol. 2001;66(2):142-4.
10. Qian SX, Li JY, Hong M, Xu W, Qiu HX. Nonhematological autoimmunity (glomerulo-sclerosis, paraneoplastic pemphigus and paraneoplastic neurological syndrome) in a patient with chronic lymphocytic leukemia: Diagnosis, prognosis and management. Leuk Res. 2009;33(3):500-5.
11. Rossum MM, Verhaegen NT, Jonkman MF, Mackenzie MA, Koster A, Van Der Valk PG, et al. Follicular non-Hodgkin's lymphoma with refractory paraneoplastic pemphigus: case report with review of novel treatment modalities. Leuk Lymphoma. 2004;45(11): 2327-32.
12. Hoque SR, Black MM, Cliff S. Paraneoplastic pemphigus associated with CD20-positive follicular non-Hodgkin's lymphoma treated with rituximab: a third case resistant to rituximab therapy. Clin Exp Dermatol. 2007;32(2):172-5.
13. Kremer N, Snast I, Cohen ES, Hodak E, Mimouni D, Lapidoth M, et al. Rituximab and Omalizumab for the Treatment of Bullous Pemphigoid: A Systematic Review of the Literature. Am J Clin Dermatol. 2019;20(2):209-16.
14. Bevans SL, Sami N. The use of rituximab in treatment of epidermolysis bullosa acquisita: Three new cases and a review of the literature. Dermatol Ther. 2018;31(6): e12726.
15. Santi CG, Gripp AC, Roselino AM, Mello DS, Gordilho JO, Marsillac PF, et al. Consensus on the treatment of autoimmune bullous dermatoses: bullous pemphigoid, mucous membrane pemphigoid and epidermolysis bullosa acquisita - Brazilian Society of Dermatology. An Bras Dermatol. 2019;94(2 Suppl 1):33-47.
16. Levine TD. Rituximab in the treatment of dermatomyositis: an open-label pilot study. Arthritis Rheum. 2005;52(2):601-7.
17. Chung L, Genovese MC, Fiorentino DF. A pilot trial of rituximab in the treatment of patients with dermatomyositis. Arch Dermatol. 2007;143(6):763-7.
18. Cooper MA, Willingham DL, Brown DE, French AR, Shih FF, White AJ. Rituximab for the treatment of juvenile dermatomyositis: a report of four pediatric patients. Arthritis Rheum. 2007;56(9):3107-11.
19. Waldman R, DeWane ME, Lu J. Dermatomyositis: Diagnosis and treatment. J Am Acad Dermatol. 2020;82(2):283-96.
20. Vargas Lebrón C, Ruiz Montesino MD, Moreira Navarrete V, Toyos Sainz de Miera FJ. Treatment with rituximab in juvenile dermatomyositis: Effect on calcinosis. Reumatol Clin (Engl Ed). 2020;16(5 Pt 1):368-70.
21. de Souza FHC, Miossi R, de Moraes JCB, Bonfá E, Shinjo SK. Favorable rituximab response in patients with refractory idiopathic inflammatory myopathies. Adv Rheumatol. 2018;58(1):31.
22. So H, Wong VTL, Lao VWN, Pang HT, Yip RML. Rituximab for refractory rapidly progressive interstitial lung disease related to anti-MDA5 antibody-positive amyopathic dermatomyositis. Clin Rheumatol. 2018;37(7):1983-9.
23. Kieu V, O'Brien T, Yap LM, Baker C, Foley P, Mason G, et al. Refractory subacute cutaneous lupus erythematosus successfully treated with rituximab. Australas J Dermatol. 2009;50(3):202-6.

24. Vital EM, Wittmann M, Edward S, Md Yusof MY, MacIver H, Pease CT, et al. Brief report: responses to rituximab suggest B cell-independent inflammation in cutaneous systemic lupus erythematosus. Arthritis Rheumatol. 2015;67(6):1586-91.
25. Merrill JT, Neuwelt CM, Wallace DJ, Shanahan JC, Latinis KM, Oates JC, et al. Efficacy and safety of rituximab in moderately-to-severely active systemic lupus erythematosus: the randomized, double-blind, phase II/III systemic lupus erythematosus evaluation of rituximab trial. Arthritis Rheum. 2010;62(1):222-33.
26. Rovin BH, Furie R, Latinis K, Looney RJ, Fervenza FC, Sanchez-Guerrero J, et al. Efficacy and safety of rituximab in patients with active proliferative lupus nephritis: the Lupus Nephritis Assessment with Rituximab study. Arthritis Rheum. 2012;64(4):1215-26.
27. Kuhn A, Aberer E, Bata-Csörgő Z, Caproni M, Dreher A, Frances C, et al. S2k guideline for treatment of cutaneous lupus erythematosus - guided by the European Dermatology Forum (EDF) in cooperation with the European Academy of Dermatology and Venereology (EADV). J Eur Acad Dermatol Venereol. 2017;31(3):389-404.
28. Jordan S, Distler JH, Maurer B, Huscher D, van Laar JM, Allanore Y, et al. Effects and safety of rituximab in systemic sclerosis: an analysis from the European Scleroderma Trial and Research (EUSTAR) group. Ann Rheum Dis. 2015;74(6):1188-94.
29. Sircar G, Goswami RP, Sircar D, Ghosh A, Ghosh P. Intravenous cyclophosphamide vs rituximab for the treatment of early diffuse scleroderma lung disease: open label, randomized, controlled trial. Rheumatology (Oxford). 2018;57(12):2106-13.
30. Guillevin L, Pagnoux C, Karras A, Khouatra C, Aumaître O, Cohen P, et al. Rituximab versus azathioprine for maintenance in ANCA-associated vasculitis. N Engl J Med. 2014;371(19):1771-80.
31. Stone JH, Merkel PA, Spiera R, Seo P, Langford CA, Hoffman GS, et al. Rituximab versus cyclophosphamide for ANCA-associated vasculitis. N Engl J Med. 2010;363(3):221-32.
32. Paterno G, Zizzari A, Nasso D, Tonialini L, Angeloni C, Vaccarini S, et al. Intravenous Administration of Rituximab in the Treatment of Primary Cutaneous B-Cell Lymphomas (PCBCLs): A Retrospective Study. Blood. 2014;124(21):5470.
33. Brandenburg A, Humme D, Terhorst D, Gellrich S, Sterry W, Beyer M. Long-term outcome of intravenous therapy with rituximab in patients with primary cutaneous B-cell lymphomas. Br J Dermatol. 2013;169(5):1126-32.
34. Valencak J, Weihsengruber F, Rappersberger K, Trautinger F, Chott A, Streubel B, et al. Rituximab monotherapy for primary cutaneous B-cell lymphoma: response and follow-up in 16 patients. Ann Oncol. 2009;20(2):326-30.
35. Wilcox RA. Cutaneous B-cell lymphomas: 2016 update on diagnosis, risk-stratification, and management. Am J Hematol. 2016;91(10):1052-5.
36. Peñate Y, Hernández-Machín B, Pérez-Méndez LI, Santiago F, Rosales B, Servitje O, et al. Intralesional rituximab in the treatment of indolent primary cutaneous B-cell lymphomas: an epidemiological observational multicentre study. The Spanish Working Group on Cutaneous Lymphoma. Br J Dermatol. 2012;167(1):174-9.
37. Fink-Puches R, Wolf IH, Zalaudek I, Kerl H, Cerroni L. Treatment of primary cutaneous B-cell lymphoma with rituximab. J Am Acad Dermatol. 2005;52(2):847-53.
38. Eberle FC, Holstein J, Scheu A, Fend F, Yazdi AS. Intralesional anti-CD20 antibody for low-grade primary cutaneous B-cell lymphoma: Adverse reactions correlate with favorable clinical outcome. J Dtsch Dermatol Ges. 2017;15(3):319-23.
39. Väkevä L, Ranki A, Mälkönen T. Intralesional Rituximab Treatment for Primary Cutaneous B-cell Lymphoma: Nine Finnish Cases. Acta Derm Venereol. 2016;96(3):396-7.
40. Kim SJ, Lee JW, Jung CW, Min CK, Cho B, Shin HJ, et al. Weekly rituximab followed by monthly rituximab treatment for steroid-refractory chronic graft-versus-host disease: results from a prospective, multicenter, phase II study. Haematologica. 2010;95(11):1935-42.

41. Arai S, Pidala J, Pusic I, Chai X, Jaglowski S, Khera N, et al. A Randomized Phase II Crossover Study of Imatinib or Rituximab for Cutaneous Sclerosis after Hematopoietic Cell Transplantation. Clin Cancer Res. 2016;22(2):319-27.
42. Glass B, Hasenkamp J, Wulf G, Dreger P, Pfreundschuh M, Gramatzki M, et al. Rituximab after lymphoma-directed conditioning and allogeneic stem-cell transplantation for relapsed and refractory aggressive non-Hodgkin lymphoma (DSHNHL R3): an open-label, randomised, phase 2 trial. Lancet Oncol. 2014;15(7):757-66.
43. Simon D, Hösli S, Kostylina G, Yawalkar N, Simon HU. Anti-CD20 (rituximab) treatment improves atopic eczema. J Allergy Clin Immunol. 2008;121(1):122-8.
44. Sánchez-Ramón S, Eguíluz-Gracia I, Rodríguez-Mazariego ME, Paravisini A, Zubeldia-Ortuño JM, Gil-Herrera J, et al. Sequential combined therapy with omalizumab and rituximab: a new approach to severe atopic dermatitis. J Investig Allergol Clin Immunol. 2013;23(3):190-6.
45. McDonald BS, Jones J, Rustin M. Rituximab as a treatment for severe atopic eczema: failure to improve in three consecutive patients. Clin Exp Dermatol. 2016;41(1):45-7.
46. Alkadi A, Alduaiji N, Alrehaily A. Risk of tuberculosis reactivation with rituximab therapy. Int J Health Sci (Qassim). 2017;11(2):41-4.
47. Buch MH, Smolen JS, Betteridge N, Breedveld FC, Burmester G, Dörner T, et al. Updated consensus statement on the use of rituximab in patients with rheumatoid arthritis. Annals of the rheumatic diseases. 2011;70(6):909-20.
48. Kimby E. Tolerability and safety of rituximab (MabThera). Cancer Treat Rev. 2005;31(6): 456-73.
49. Trouvin AP, Jacquot S, Grigioni S, Curis E, Dedreux I, Roucheux A, et al. Usefulness of monitoring of B cell depletion in rituximab-treated rheumatoid arthritis patients in order to predict clinical relapse: a prospective observational study. Clin Exp Immunol. 2015;180(1):11-8.
50. Castells MC, Tennant NM, Sloane DE, Hsu FI, Barrett NA, Hong DI, et al. Hypersensitivity reactions to chemotherapy: outcomes and safety of rapid desensitization in 413 cases. J Allergy Clin Immunol. 2008;122(3):574-80.
51. Amorós-Reboredo P, Sánchez-López J, Bastida-Fernández C, do Pazo-Oubiña F, Borràs-Maixenchs N, Giné E, Valero A, et al. Desensitization to rituximab in a multidisciplinary setting. Int J Clin Pharm. 2015;37(5):744-8.
52. Gudu T, Mazilu D, Peltea A, Daniela O, Ruxandra I. Can rituximab treatment in rheumatoid arthritis patients decrease cardiovascular risk? Ann Rheum Dis (London). 2014;73:A37.
53. Provan SA, Berg IJ, Hammer HB, Mathiessen A, Kvien TK, Semb AG. The Impact of Newer Biological Disease Modifying Anti-Rheumatic Drugs on Cardiovascular Risk Factors: A 12-Month Longitudinal Study in Rheumatoid Arthritis Patients Treated with Rituximab, Abatacept and Tociliziumab. PLoS One. 2015;10(6):e0130709.
54. Hsue PY, Scherzer R, Grunfeld C, Imboden J, Wu Y, Del Puerto G, et al. Depletion of B-cells with rituximab improves endothelial function and reduces inflammation among individuals with rheumatoid arthritis. J Am Heart Assoc. 2014;3(5):e001267.
55. Kridin K, Mruwat N, Ludwig RJ. Association of Rituximab With Risk of Long-term Cardiovascular and Metabolic Outcomes in Patients With Pemphigus. JAMA Dermatology. 2023;159(1):56-61.
56. Foran JM, Rohatiner AZ, Cunningham D, Popescu RA, Solal-Celigny P, Ghielmini M, et al. European phase II study of rituximab (chimeric anti-CD20 monoclonal antibody) for patients with newly diagnosed mantle-cell lymphoma and previously treated mantle-cell lymphoma, immunocytoma, and small B-cell lymphocytic lymphoma. J Clin Oncol. 2000;18(2):317-24.
57. Passalia C, Minetto P, Arboscello E, Balleari E, Bellodi A, Del Corso L, et al. Cardiovascular adverse events complicating the administration of rituximab: report of two cases. Tumori. 2013;99(6):288e-92e.

58. Ng KH, Dearden C, Gruber P. Rituximab-induced Takotsubo syndrome: more cardiotoxic than it appears? BMJ Case Rep. 2015;2015:bcr2014208203.
59. Verma SK. Updated cardiac concerns with rituximab use: A growing challenge. Indian Heart J. 2016;68(Suppl 2):S246-s8.
60. Roberts DM, Jones RB, Smith RM, Alberici F, Kumaratne DS, Burns S, et al. Rituximab-associated hypogammaglobulinemia: incidence, predictors and outcomes in patients with multi-system autoimmune disease. J Autoimmun. 2015;57:60-5.
61. Gea-Banacloche JC. Rituximab-associated infections. Semin Hematol. 2010;47(2):187-98.
62. Kelesidis T, Daikos G, Boumpas D, Tsiodras S. Does rituximab increase the incidence of infectious complications? A narrative review. Int J Infect Dis. 2011;15(1):e2-16.
63. Kridin K, Mruwat N, Amber KT, Ludwig RJ. Risk of infections in patients with pemphigus treated with rituximab vs. azathioprine or mycophenolate mofetil: a large-scale global cohort study. Br J Dermatol. 2023;188(4):499-505.
64. De D, Ashraf R, Mehta H, Handa S, Mahajan R. Outcome of COVID-19 in patients with autoimmune bullous diseases. Indian J Dermatol Venereol Leprol. 2023;89(6):862-66.
65. Faraji H, Daneshpazhooh M, Ehsani AH, Mahmoudi H, Tavakolpour S, Aryanian Z, et al. Evaluating the risk-to-benefit ratio of using cotrimoxazole as a pneumocystis pneumonia preventative intervention among pemphigus patients treated with rituximab: A retrospective study with 494 patients. Dermatol Ther. 2022;35(2):e15257.
66. Arai Y, Yamashita K, Mizugishi K, Nishikori M, Hishizawa M, Kondo T, et al. Risk factors for late-onset neutropenia after rituximab treatment of B-cell lymphoma. Hematology. 2015;20(4):196-202.
67. Lemieux A, Maho-Vaillant M, Golinski ML, Hébert V, Boyer O, Calbo S, et al. Evaluation of Clinical Relevance and Biological Effects of Antirituximab Antibodies in Patients With Pemphigus. JAMA Dermatol. 2022;158(8):893-9.
68. Chakravarty EF, Murray ER, Kelman A, Farmer PJ. Pregnancy outcomes after maternal exposure to rituximab. Blood. 2011;117(5):1499-506.
69. Sammaritano LR, Bermas BL, Chakravarty EE, Chambers C, Clowse MEB, Lockshin MD, et al. 2020 American College of Rheumatology Guideline for the Management of Reproductive Health in Rheumatic and Musculoskeletal Diseases. Arthritis Rheumatol (Hoboken). 2020;72(4):529-56.
70. Dehghanimahmoudabadi A, Kianfar N, Akhdar M, Dasdar S, Balighi K, Mahmoudi H, et al. Pregnancy outcomes in women with pemphigus exposed to rituximab before or during pregnancy. Int J Womens Dermatol. 2022;8(3):e038.
71. Kincaid L, Weinstein M. Rituximab Therapy for Childhood Pemphigus Vulgaris. Pediatr Dermatol. 2016;33(2):e61-4.
72. Hoffman MB, Bhandari RA, Sinha AA. Rituximab Use in Pediatric Dermatology. J Drugs Dermatol. 2016;15(7):821-9.
73. Mahajan R, Handa S, Kumar S, Chatterji D, Saikia UN, De D. Pediatric autoimmune blistering disorders – a five-year demographic profile and therapy experience. International J Dermatol. 2022;61(12):1511-8.
74. Bilgic-Temel A, Özgen Z, Harman M, Kapıcıoğlu Y, Uzun S. Rituximab therapy in pediatric pemphigus patients: A retrospective analysis of five Turkish patients and review of the literature. Pediatr Dermatol. 2019;36(5):646-50.
75. Connelly EA, Aber C, Kleiner G, Nousari C, Charles C, Schachner LA. Generalized erythrodermic pemphigus foliaceus in a child and its successful response to rituximab treatment. Pediatr Dermatol. 2007;24(2):172-6.
76. Vinay K, Kanwar AJ, Sawatkar GU, Dogra S, Ishii N, Hashimoto T. Successful use of rituximab in the treatment of childhood and juvenile pemphigus. J Am Acad Dermatol. 2014;71(4):669-75.

77. Maglione PJ, Xu J, Chan J. B cells moderate inflammatory progression and enhance bacterial containment upon pulmonary challenge with Mycobacterium tuberculosis. J Immunol. 2007;178(11):7222-34.
78. Liao TL, Lin CH, Chen YM, Chang CL, Chen HH, Chen DY. Different Risk of Tuberculosis and Efficacy of Isoniazid Prophylaxis in Rheumatoid Arthritis Patients with Biologic Therapy: A Nationwide Retrospective Cohort Study in Taiwan. PLoS One. 2016;11():e0153217.
79. Saag KG, Teng GG, Patkar NM, Anuntiyo J, Finney C, Curtis JR, et al. American College of Rheumatology 2008 recommendations for the use of nonbiologic and biologic disease-modifying antirheumatic drugs in rheumatoid arthritis. Arthritis Rheum. 2008;59(6):762-84.
80. Jung N, Owczarczyk K, Hellmann M, Lehmann C, Fätkenheuer G, Hallek M, et al. Efficacy and safety of rituximab in a patient with active rheumatoid arthritis and chronic disseminated pulmonary aspergillosis and history of tuberculosis. Rheumatology (Oxford). 2008;47(6):932-3.
81. Burr ML, Malaviya AP, Gaston JH, Carmichael AJ, Ostör AJ. Rituximab in rheumatoid arthritis following anti-TNF-associated tuberculosis. Rheumatology (Oxford). 2008;47(5):738-9.
82. Pehlivan Y, Kisacik B, Bosnak VK, Onat AM. Rituximab seems to be a safer alternative in patients with active rheumatoid arthritis with tuberculosis. BMJ Case Rep. 2013;2013:bcr2012006585.
83. Perrillo RP, Gish R, Falck-Ytter YT. American Gastroenterological Association Institute Technical Review on Prevention and Treatment of Hepatitis B Virus Reactivation During Immunosuppressive Drug Therapy. Gastroenterology. 2015;148(1):221-44.e3.
84. Kusumoto S, Tobinai K. Screening for and management of hepatitis B virus reactivation in patients treated with anti-B-cell therapy. Hematology Am Soc Hematol Educ Program. 2014;2014(1):576-83.
85. Koutsianas C, Thomas K, Vassilopoulos D. Hepatitis B Reactivation in Rheumatic Diseases: Screening and Prevention. Rheum Dis Clin North Am. 2017;43(1):133-49.
86. Amber KT, Kodiyan J, Bloom R, Hertl M. The controversy of hepatitis C and rituximab: A multidisciplinary dilemma with implications for patients with pemphigus. Indian J Dermatol Venereol Leprol. 2016;82(2):182-3.
87. Petrarca A, Rigacci L, Caini P, Colagrande S, Romagnoli P, Vizzutti F, et al. Safety and efficacy of rituximab in patients with hepatitis C virus-related mixed cryoglobulinemia and severe liver disease. Blood. 2010;116(3):335-42.
88. Musto P, Dell'Olio M, La Sala A, Mantuano S, Cascavilla N. Diffuse B-Large Cell Lymphomas (DBLCL) with Hepatitis-C Virus (HCV) Infection: Clinical Outcome and Preliminary Results of a Pilot Study Combining R-CHOP with Antiviral Therapy. Blood. 2005;106:688a.
89. Hertl M, Zillikens D, Borradori L, Bruckner-Tuderman L, Burckhard H, Eming R, et al. Recommendations for the use of rituximab (anti-CD20 antibody) in the treatment of autoimmune bullous skin diseases. J Dtsch Dermatol Ges. 2008;6(5):366-73.
90. Seymour CW, Liu VX, Iwashyna TJ, Brunkhorst FM, Rea TD, Scherag A, et al. Assessment of Clinical Criteria for Sepsis: For the Third International Consensus Definitions for Sepsis and Septic Shock (Sepsis-3). Jama. 2016;315(8):762-74.
91. Friedman MA, Winthrop KL. Vaccines and Disease-Modifying Antirheumatic Drugs: Practical Implications for the Rheumatologist. Rheum Dis Clin North Am. 2017;43(1):1-13.
92. Westra J, Rondaan C, van Assen S, Bijl M. Vaccination of patients with autoimmune inflammatory rheumatic diseases. Nat Rev Rheumatol. 2015;11(3):135-45.

CHAPTER 14

Newer Biologics in the Management of Immunobullous Disorders

Surbhi Rajput

INTRODUCTION

Autoimmune bullous disorders are broadly classified as intraepidermal (pemphigus group) and subepidermal (pemphigoid group) based on the level of split. The basic pathology lies in the generation of autoantibodies against components of keratinocytes and dermoepidermal junction. The most common and well-known biologic being used for autoimmune bullous disorders is rituximab.

Recently, newer biologics targeting various inflammatory pathways have been discovered and are being explored in the field of immunobullous disorders. However, these molecules are being studied in various clinical trials for autoimmune bullous disorders and are yet to be approved by the United States Food and Drug Administration (US FDA). For the ease of understanding, this chapter has classified these molecules into four categories namely:
1. Molecules targeting B cells
2. Molecules targeting pathogenic antibodies
3. Inhibitors of chemokine, cytokines, and complement proteins
4. Miscellaneous compounds

A summary of all the newer biologics discussed in this chapter is delineated in **Table 1**.

MOLECULES TARGETING B CELLS

The pathogenesis of immunobullous disorders primarily circles around pathogenic antibodies produced by plasma cells as a result of activation of B cells. The antibodies possess cell surface receptors such as CD20, CD19, CD22, etc., which can be modulated to modify intracellular signaling causing destruction of B cells. Various novel anti-B cell therapies are being studied for immunobullous disorders.[1]

TABLE 1: A summary of biologics used in autoimmune bullous dermatoses.

Therapies targeting B cells	
Anti-CD20	• *Frist generation*: Rituximab • *Second generation*: Tositumomab, obinutuzumab, ofatumumab, ocrelizumab, and veltuzumab
Anti-CD19	Blinatumomab and inebilizumab
CD22 modulators	Epratuzumab
Anti-BAFF (B-cell-activating factor) or BlyS (B-lymphocyte stimulator)	Belimumab
Anti-APRIL (A PRoliferation-Inducing Ligand)	Atacicept
Bruton tyrosine kinase inhibitors	Ibrutinib
Therapies targeting pathogenic antibodies	
Anti-IgE antibody	Omalizumab
FcRn antagonists	Efgartigimod, rozanolixizumab, and intravenous immunoglobulins
Therapies targeting cytokines, chemokine, and complement	
Anti-IL-5 monoclonal antibody	Mepolizumab
Il-4 receptor antagonist	Dupilumab
Anti-C1s antibody	Sutimlimab
Anti-eotaxin-1 antibody	Bertilimumab
Miscellaneous	
IL-17 inhibitors	Ixekizumab
IL-12/23 inhibitors	Ustekinumab
IL-23 inhibitors	Guselkumab and tildrakizumab
Inflammasome inhibitors	AC-203
Second generation IgE antibody	Ligelizumab
Spleen tyrosine kinase inhibitor	Fostamatinib

(IgE: immunoglobulin E; IL: interleukin)

Antibodies Targeting CD20

CD20 inhibitors are classified as first-generation molecules which include rituximab and second-generation molecules including ocrelizumab, ofatumumab, veltuzumab, obinutuzumab, and tositumomab. This classification is based on the component of chimeric portion of antibodies. Second generation molecules are humanized and are less immunogenic and hence cause less adverse reactions. Another classification is based on their mechanism of action: Type I (rituximab, ofatumumab, and veltuzumab) acts via both complement-mediated cytotoxicity and antibody-dependent cell-mediated cytotoxicity and cause redistribution of CD20 molecules on lipid rafts. Type II (obinutuzumab and tositumomab) induces a stronger direct nonapoptotic, programmed cell death mediated by homotypic adhesion (adhesion of two similar types of cells to each other followed by activation of lysosomes and release of their contents), lesser degree of antibody-dependent cell-mediated cytotoxicity, and no complement-mediated cytotoxicity.[2]

Ofatumumab is the first, type I, second generation anti-CD20 monoclonal antibody which shows a greater complement-mediated cytotoxicity than rituximab. Few case reports are available which have studied its usage.[3] The drug has also been used to treat refractory pemphigus successfully. Due to its fully human nature and superior B-cell depletion, it may emerge as an option for treating pemphigus vulgaris (PV).[4,5]

Veltuzumab is also a second-generation, type I anti-CD20 monoclonal antibody which results in significantly more complement-mediated cytotoxicity than rituximab; it can be administered subcutaneously. It was reported to be effective in pemphigus and was given the status of orphan drug in 2015.[2]

Obinutuzumab and tositumomab are second generation type II anti-CD20 monoclonal antibodies. Obinutuzumab has been indicated in lupus nephritis by US FDA; however, its role in pemphigus has not yet been explored.[6]

Antibodies Targeting CD19

CD19 expression is even more common across the B-cell lineage, and it is also detected very early on pro-B cells and plasma cells. As a crucial coreceptor of the B-cell receptor (BCR), great attention has also been attached to CD19 in the context of antibody-dependent autoimmune disease.

Inebilizumab and blinatumomab are anti-CD19 cytolytic B cell depleting monoclonal antibodies which possess the capacity to destroy both memory B cells and plasma cells, since rituximab does not have the capacity to destroy plasma cells, these anti-CD19 molecules are considered more potent than rituximab. However, this is a dual-edged sword as depletion of long-lived plasma cells upon anti-CD19 antibody treatment, might lead to abolishment of vaccination-derived neutralizing antibodies. Inebilizumab was recently approved by the US FDA for treatment of neuromyelitis optica spectrum disorder.[7]

Antibodies Targeting CD22

Epratuzumab BCRs possess a coreceptor, CD22 which inhibits the overactivation of B cells. Epratuzumab is a humanized non-B-cell depleting monoclonal antibody which augments these inhibitory signals produced by CD22.[8] In addition, it also reduces expression of cell surface receptors like

CD19, CD21, and CD79b.[9] It has been used in lupus erythematous. It can be explored in pemphigus in near future.[10]

Molecules Targeting B-cell-activating Factor and B-lymphocyte Stimulator Protein

These molecules belong to tumor necrosis factor (TNF) family of cytokines. Their major role is in proliferation of B cells and plasma cells and hence maintain a T-cell independent antibody response. Their levels are positively high in patients with systemic manifestations of systemic lupus erythematosus (SLE).[11] B-cell-activating factor (BAFF), also called as B lymphocyte stimulator protein (BLyS) of the TNF family enhances B-cell survival—a function that is indispensable for B-cell maturation and enhancing immune response. Although at physiological concentrations BAFF cannot rescue B-cell apoptosis due to a strong B-cell death signal, which is transduced via the BCR stimulated by autoantigens, at higher concentrations, BAFF causes the survival of autoreactive B cells, which contributes to the pathogenesis of autoimmune diseases.

Belimumab is an anti-BAFF monoclonal antibody which is being used in SLE and received US FDA approval in 2011 for its use in SLE and lupus nephritis. B-cell-activating factor was found to be raised in bullous pemphigoid patients especially in patients with larger body surface area, refractory disease, and those not receiving corticosteroids therapy.[12]

VAY736 (Ianalumab) is a novel, de-fucosylated, human immunoglobulin G1 (IgG1) monoclonal antibody targeting BAFF-R. A randomized, placebo-controlled, and double-blind, phase II clinical trial was conducted (NCT01930175) to investigate the safety, tolerability, and efficacy of VAY736 in PV in which 16 mild-moderate PV patients were enrolled. However, it was terminated in phase II.[13]

Bruton's tyrosine kinases inhibitors (BTKIs): Bruton's tyrosine kinases are nonreceptor tyrosine kinases that mediate signal transduction inside the B cells and plasma cells leading to destruction of antibodies. Hence, inhibition of this pathway may play a substantial role in immunobullous disorders. Few studies have shown efficacy of ibrutinib in patients of chronic lymphocytic leukemia with paraneoplastic pemphigus.[14] PRN1008 was under investigation in a phase III trial for PV and other autoimmune diseases; however, the trial was suspended due to lack of efficacy (NCT03762265). Trials for various other BTKIs are underway with phase II trial of rilzabrutinib being concluded recently in which the drugs alone and with low-dose corticosteroid have shown rapid clinical improvement in PV.[15] Similarly, the efficacy and safety of tirabrutinib in patients with refractory pemphigus is under trial in a multicenter, open-label, uncontrolled, and single-arm phase II study with reports of tirabrutinib enabled remission and reduced oral corticosteroids over time without significant safety concerns in patients with

CHAPTER 14: Newer Biologics in the Management of Immunobullous Disorders

refractory pemphigus.[16] Another BTKI (PRN473) has been reported with a good response in canine pemphigus foliaceus (PF).

THERAPIES TARGETING PATHOGENIC ANTIBODIES

Neonatal Fc Receptor Antagonists

Neonatal Fc receptor (FcRn) binds to the Fc fragment of IgG antibodies in utero and increases their transport back into the cell thereby preventing their degradation and prolonging half-life of IgG and also of pathogenic antibodies.[17] FcRn-mediated IgG recycling is 40–50% more than IgG production and, hence, maintains the level of IgG in plasma. Other antibodies are not involved in FcRn-mediated recycling. These receptors are expressed on keratinocytes in skin, and it is shown that absence of these receptors in knock-out mice did not lead to acantholysis.[18] Hence, these receptors can be exploited to be used in treatment of autoimmune bullous disorders.

Efgartigimod (neonatal Fc-receptor antagonist) is an engineered Fc fraction of IgG1 which saturates the neonatal Fc receptors, and therefore causes rapid degradation and clearance of pathogenic antibodies.[19] The major advantage with this antibody is lack of infection, which was explained by the fact that these can reduce IgG amounting to 75% of total antibodies while sparing the others which are not involved in FcRn-mediated recycling like IgM. It is successfully used in myasthenia gravis and phase II study has been done in patients of pemphigus where four out of six patients showed favorable results in mild-to-moderate disease.[20]

Rozanolixizumab is a high affinity human anti-FcRn IgG4 monoclonal antibody and has shown to have favorable effects in healthy volunteers.[20]

Omalizumab is a humanized IgG antibody that binds to circulating IgE antibodies thus reducing the fraction of IgE present for binding to high affinity of FcεRI receptor on mast cells, basophils and other inflammatory cells. Recently, in bullous pemphigoid, the focus is on the presence of IgE antibodies again BPAg2 and has been shown to directly correlate with disease activity. A meta-analysis concluded that severity of bullous pemphigoid was correlated with serum IgE levels, though the disease phenotype was not.[21] Various case reports have shown an efficacy rate of up to 80% with omalizumab.[22] Some reports have studied that it is effective in rituximab refractory bullous pemphigoid and in infantile bullous pemphigoid.[23]

Ligelizumab (QGE031) is a humanized, high-affinity, and second-generation anti-IgE monoclonal antibody. This antibody demonstrated greater inhibition of IgE binding to FcεRI, basophil activation, and IgE production by B-cells as compared to omalizumab.[24] Phase II randomized controlled trial (RCT) administering ligelizumab to patients was conducted and it was seen that primary endpoint of the study was not successfully met.[25]

INHIBITORS OF CYTOKINES, CHEMOKINES, AND COMPLEMENT

It is a well-known fact that presence of eosinophils in subepidermal cleft is seen in bullous pemphigoid. Eosinophils release chemokine-like eotaxin-1 and other granular components, which causes damage to the dermoepidermal junction in presence of autoantibodies. The influx of eosinophils is mediated by IL-4 and IL-5.[26]

Bertilimumab is a fully human anti-eotaxin-1 antibody inhibiting eosinophilic migration in the skin and has been under phase II trial for moderate to extensive BP with 81% reduction in the disease, hence, it could achieve significant remission and could be used as a steroid sparing agent.[27]

Mepolizumab is a humanized IgG1 monoclonal antibody which binds to IL-5 and inhibits its binding to eosinophil surface receptor thereby preventing release of eosinophilic granules. It is being used in bronchial asthma. In patients of bullous pemphigoid, it was observed that this drug did not achieve reduction in tissue eosinophils and could not achieve disease control in bullous pemphigoid.[28]

Dupilumab is a fully human monoclonal antibody against alpha subunit of IL-4 cytokine. The alpha subunit is shared by both IL-4 and IL-13, two cytokines involved in type 2 inflammatory response. IL-4 and IL-13 are involved in upregulation of Th2 cells which thereby cause recruitment of eosinophils and also activate B cells to produce autoantibodies against BPAg2. Hence, dupilumab acts in two ways, i.e., downregulation of eosinophil chemotaxis and inhibits proliferation of B cell.[29] It was also shown to be effective in refractory bullous pemphigoid in few case reports.[30]

Complement System Inhibitors

Direct immunofluorescent studies from bullous pemphigoid suggest that there is deposition of complement proteins in perilesional skin. Complement components such as C3, C5, C1s and membrane attack complex are found in blister fluid. C5a causes granulocyte influx and tissue inflammation. C5a causes LTB4 activation leading to granulocyte chemotaxis.[31]

Sutimlimab is a monoclonal IgG4 anti-C1s antibody which has been found to be effective in bullous pemphigoid. C1s is a complement component serine protease which causes propagation of classical pathway ultimately leading to formation of pivotal C3 converts enzyme. Binding of sutimlimab to C1s, it specifically inhibits the classical pathway, preventing the enzymatic action of the C1 complex on its substrates thereby blocking formation of C3-convertase. It leaves the alternate and lectin pathway which are required for humeral response against microbes.[32] It had a good safety profile and predictable and consistent pharmacokinetics and pharmacodynamics in healthy volunteers.[33]

Nomacopan, a small recombinant protein formerly called as coversin, is an antagonist of C5a and LTB4 hence inhibiting influx of neutrophils. Phase II RCTs have shown that nomacopan was used in seven out of nine patients of mild-to-moderate relapsing bullous pemphigoid. There was improvement in quality of life of patients and no adverse effects were noticed.[34]

Avdoralimab is a specific anti-C5aR1 monoclonal antibody which mediates the C5aR1-receptor-mediated BPAg 180 pathogenicity. It has shown favorable safety profile in treatment of solid tumors and rheumatoid arthritis. Various studies have hypothesized that avdoralimab might be a safe and effective treatment in BP patients.[35]

MISCELLANEOUS AGENTS

Dimethyl fumarate is a derivative of Krebs cycle at the cellular level. It acts as an oral immunomodulator by inhibiting the aerobic glycolysis in myeloid and lymphoid cells and hence reduction of infiltration and activation of neutrophils and lymphocytes. It has been approved for neurological disorders like multiple sclerosis. It has been experimented in BP like epidermolysis bullosa in murine models, however, studies on human volunteers are awaited.[36]

IL-17 and IL-23 inhibitors: IL-17 plays a significant role in pathogenesis of bullous pemphigoid as it causes activation of neutrophilic metalloproteinases (MMP) and elastases. IL-17 levels were found to be raised in serum and blister fluid levels in BP patients. IL-23 activates IL-17 and also causes direct activation of MMP-9. Hence, this IL-17/IL-23 axis can be explored as a good therapeutic option in bullous pemphigoid. Six doses of subcutaneous injections of ixekizumab were given to patients 2 weeks apart. However, the study was interrupted due to lack of benefit.[37] Ustekinumab is an antagonist of p40 unit of IL-23 and has been studied for its role in BP. A phase II open label 8 weeks study is undergoing to see its effect in refractory BP along with topical corticosteroids.[38] Other specific IL-23 inhibitors (risankizumab, guselkumab, tildrakizumab, and mirikizumab) are also being studied for their role in autoimmune blistering disorders.[39]

Inflammasome inhibitors: The NLRP3 inflammasome is a multimeric protein complex that controls caspase-1 and promotes the release of proinflammatory cytokines. The pharmacological modulation of the same can be of interest in the treatment of blistering disorders. AC-203 is an inflammasome and IL-1B modulator and has been studied for the treatment of refractory bullous pemphigoid. It is used as an ointment preparation and has been studied in various reports in comparison to clobetasol ointment.[40]

Spleen tyrosine kinase inhibitors have emerged as an important non-receptor tyrosine kinase mediating inflammation in an in vivo mouse model of epidermolysis bullosa acquisita.

Fostamatinib is a spleen tyrosine kinase inhibitor which can be employed to reduce inflammation in pemphigoid group of disorders especially with mechanobullous component.[41]

CONCLUSION

Treatment of immunobullous disorders has shifted from global immunosuppression to targeted immunosuppression with the advent of second generation anti-CD20 antibodies. Research in the field of molecular therapy and biologics has led to the discoveries of newer therapeutic agents which are more efficacious with lesser side effects. However, it should be noted that all these treatments are off-label for these disorders and their use should be carefully considered by dermatologists and should only be limited to refractory or complicated cases for which long-term treatment with corticosteroid or immunosuppressive drug therapies is inappropriate.

REFERENCES

1. Musette P, Bouaziz JD. B cell modulation strategies in autoimmune diseases: New concepts. Front Immunol. 2018;9:622.
2. Bhattacharjee R, De D, Handa S, Minz RW, Saikia B, Joshi N. Assessment of the effects of rituximab monotherapy on different subsets of circulating T-regulatory cells and clinical disease severity in severe pemphigus vulgaris. Dermatology. 2016;232: 572-7.
3. Rapp M, Pentland A, Richardson C. Successful treatment of pemphigus vulgaris with ofatumumab. J Drugs Dermatol. 2018;17:1338-9.
4. Klufas DM, Amerson E, Twu O, Clark L, Shinkai K. Refractory pemphigus vulgaris successfully treated with ofatumumab. JAAD Case Reports. 2020;6(8):734-6.
5. Izumi K, Bieber K, Ludwig RJ. Current clinical trials in pemphigus and pemphigoid. Front Immunol. 201910:978.
6. Meyer S, Evers M, Jansen JH, Buijs J, Broek B, Reitsma SE, et al. New insights in Type I and II CD20 antibody mechanisms-of-action with a panel of novel CD20 antibodies. Br J Haematol. 2018;180:808-20.
7. Ali F, Sharma K, Anjum V, Ali A. Inebilizumab-cdon: USFDA Approved for the Treatment of NMOSD (Neuromyelitis Optica Spectrum Disorder). Curr Drug Discov Technol. 2022;19(1):e140122193419.
8. Antoniu S. Epratuzumab for systemic lupus erythematosus. Expert Opin Biol Ther. 2014;14:1045-7.
9. Rossi EA, Goldenberg DM, Michel R, Rossi DL, Wallace DJ, Chang CH. Trogocytosis of multiple B-cell surface markers by CD22 targeting with epratuzumab. Blood. 2013;122:3020-9.
10. Clowse ME, Wallace DJ, Furie RA, Petri MA, Pike MC, Leszczyński P, et al. Efficacy and safety of epratuzumab in moderately to severely active systemic lupus erythematosus: Results from two phase III randomized, double-blind, placebo-controlled trials. Arthritis Rheumatol. 2017;69:362-75.
11. Schneider P. The role of APRIL and BAFF in lymphocyte activation. Curr Opin Immunol. 2005;17:282-9.

12. Asashima N, Fujimoto M, Watanabe R, Nakashima H, Yazawa N, Okochi H, et al. Serum levels of BAFF are increased in bullous pemphigoid but not in pemphigus vulgaris. Br J Dermatol. 2006;155:330-6.
13. Ellebrecht CT, Maseda D, Payne AS. Pemphigus and Pemphigoid: From Disease Mechanisms to Druggable Pathways. J Invest Dermatol. 2022;142:907-14.
14. Lee A, Sandhu S, Imlay-Gillespie L, Mulligan S, Shumack S. Successful use of Bruton's kinase inhibitor, ibrutinib, to control paraneoplastic pemphigus in a patient with paraneoplastic autoimmune multiorgan syndrome and chronic lymphocytic leukaemia. Australas J Dermatol. 2017;58:e240-2.
15. Murrell DF, Patsatsi A, Stavropoulos P, Baum S, Zeeli T, Kern JS, et al.; BELIEVE trial investigators. Proof of concept for the clinical effects of oral rilzabrutinib, the first Bruton tyrosine kinase inhibitor for pemphigus vulgaris: the phase II BELIEVE study. Br J Dermatol. 2021;185:745-55.
16. Yamagami J, Ujiie H, Aoyama Y, Ishii N, Tateishi C, Ishiko A, et al. A multicenter, open-label, uncontrolled, single-arm phase 2 study of tirabrutinib, an oral Bruton's tyrosine kinase inhibitor, in pemphigus. J Dermatol Sci. 2021;103:135-42.
17. Kuo TT, Baker K, Yoshida M, Qiao SW, Aveson VG, Lencer WI, et al. Neonatal Fc receptor: From immunity to therapeutics. J Clin Immunol. 2010;30:777-89.
18. Didona D, Maglie R, Eming R, Hertl M. Pemphigus: Current and future therapeutic strategies. Front Immunol. 2019;10:1418.
19. Alaibac M. Biological therapy of autoimmune blistering diseases. Expert Opin Biol Ther. 2019;19:149-56.
20. Ulrichts P, Guglietta A, Dreier T, vanBragt T, Hanssens V, Hofman E, et al. Neonatal Fc receptor antagonist efgartigimod safely and sustainably reduces IgGs in humans. J Clin Invest. 2018;128:4372-86.
21. Saniklidou AH, Tighe PJ, Fairclough LC, Todd I. IgE autoantibodies and their association with the disease activity and phenotype in bullous pemphigoid: A systematic review. Arch Dermatol Res. 2018;310:11-28.
22. Yu KK, Crew AB, Messingham KA, Fairley JA, Woodley DT. Omalizumab therapy for bullous pemphigoid. J Am Acad Dermatol. 2014;71:468-74.
23. BilgiçTemel A, Bassorgun CI, Akman-Karakaş A, Alpsoy E, Uzun S. Successful treatment of a bullous pemphigoid patient with rituximab who was refractory to corticosteroid and omalizumab treatments. Case Rep Dermatol. 2017;9:38-44.
24. Gauvreau GM, Arm JP, Boulet LP, Leigh R, Cockcroft DW, Davis BE, et al. Efficacy and safety of multiple doses of QGE031 (ligelizumab) versus omalizumab and placebo in inhibiting allergen-induced early asthmatic responses. J Allergy Clin Immunol. 2016;138:1051-9.
25. National Library of Medicine (U.S.). (2012). A Randomized, Double-blind, Placebo Controlled, Parallel Group Study Evaluating the Efficacy, Safety, Pharmacokinetics and Pharmacodynamics of QGE031 in the Treatment of Patients with Bullous Pemphigoid With Disease Refractory to Oral Steroid Treatment. NCT01688882. [online] Available from https://classic.clinicaltrials.gov/ct2/history/NCT01688882?V_1=View#StudyPage Top [Last accessed January, 2024].
26. Simon D, Borradori L, Simon HU. Eosinophils as putative therapeutic targets in bullous pemphigoid. Exp Dermatol. 2017;26:1187-92.
27. Fiorino A, Baum S, Czernik A, Hall R, Zeeli T, Baniel A, et al. 570 Safety and efficacy of bertilimumab, a human anti-eotaxin-1 monoclonal antibody, in bullous pemphigoid in a phase 2a study. J Investig Dermatol. 2019;139:S98.
28. Simon D, Yousefi S, Cazzaniga S, Bürgler C, Radonjic S, Houriet C, et al. Mepolizumab failed to affect bullous pemphigoid: A randomized, placebo-controlled, double-blind phase 2 pilot study. Allergy. 2020;75:669-72.

29. Cozzani E, Gasparini G, Di Zenzo G, Parodi A. Immunoglobulin E and bullous pemphigoid. Eur J Dermatol. 2018;28:440-8.
30. Kaye A, Gordon SC, Deverapalli SC, Her MJ, Rosmarin D. Dupilumab for the treatment of recalcitrant bullous pemphigoid. JAMA Dermatol. 2018;154:1225-6.
31. Maglie R, Hertl M. Pharmacological advances in pemphigoid. Curr Opin Pharmacol. 2019;46:34-43.
32. Bartko J, Schoergenhofer C, Schwameis M, Firbas C, Beliveau M, Chang C, et al. A randomized, first-in-human healthy volunteer trial of sutimlimab, a humanized antibody for the specific inhibition of the classical complement pathway. Clin Pharmacol Ther. 2018;104:655-63.
33. Sezin T, Murthy S, Attah C, Seutter M, Holtsche MM, Hammers CM, et al. Dual inhibition of complement factor 5 and leukotriene B4 synergistically suppresses murine pemphigoid disease. JCI Insight. 2019;4:e128239.
34. Sadik CD, Rashid H, Hammers CM, Diercks GF, Weidinger A, Beissert S, et al. Evaluation of Nomacopan for Treatment of Bullous Pemphigoid: A Phase 2a Nonrandomized Controlled Trial. JAMA Dermatol. 2022;158:641-9.
35. National Library of Medicine (U.S.). (2010). Treatment of Bullous Pemphigoid with Avdoralimab (IPH5401), an Anti-C5aR1 Monoclonal Antibody, NCT04563923. [online] Available from https://clinicaltrials.gov/ct2/show/NCT04563923 [Last accessed January, 2024].
36. Müller S, Behnen M, Bieber K, Möller S, Hellberg L, Witte M, et al. Dimethyl fumarate Impairs Neutrophil Functions. J Investig Dermatol. 2016;136:117-26.
37. National Library of Medicine (U.S.). (2017). Ixekizumab in the Treatment of Bullous Pemphigoid, NCT03099538. [online] Available from https:// clinicaltrials.gov/ct2/show/NCT03099538 [Last accessed January, 2024].
38. National Library of Medicine (U.S.). (2019). Efficacy and Safety of Ustekinumab in Bullous Pemphigoid, NCT04117932. [online] Available from https://clinicaltrials.gov/ct2/show/NCT04117932 [Last accessed January, 2024].
39. National Library of Medicine (U.S.). (2020). The Effects of Tildrakizumab in Treatment of Bullous Pemphigoid, NCT04465292. [online] Available from https://clinicaltrials.gov/ct2/show/NCT04465292 [Last accessed January, 2024].
40. Kridin K, Kowalski EH, Kneiber D, Laufer-Britva R, Amber KT. From bench to bedside: Evolving therapeutic targets in autoimmune blistering disease. J Eur Acad Dermatol Venereol. 2019;33:2239-52.
41. Németh T, Virtic O, Sitaru C, Mócsai A. The Syk tyrosine kinase is required for skin inflammation in an *in vivo* mouse model of epidermolysis bullosa acquisita. J Invest Dermatol. 2017;137:2131-9.

SECTION 4

Biologics in Urticaria

CHAPTER 15

Anti-IgE Monoclonal Antibody: Omalizumab

Kiran Godse, Bhojani Amee

INTRODUCTION

Omalizumab is a recombinant humanized immunoglobulin G1 (IgG1) monoclonal antibody against human immunoglobulin E (IgE). It blocks the attachment of IgE to mast cells and basophils, thereby preventing its degranulation. It also binds with free IgE, forming immune complex and reducing serum levels of IgE.

PHARMACOLOGY

Omalizumab is derived from a murine monoclonal antibody which was humanized to produce omalizumab in its present form. The complementarity-determining regions (CDRs) form 5% of its nonhuman amino-acid residues.[1]

CHARACTERISTICS

- Route of administration—subcutaneous
- Peak serum concentration—after 7-8 days
- Half-life—around 26 days
- *Elimination:*
  - Free omalizumab—via the reticuloendothelial system
  - Omalizumab-IgE complex—via endocytosis
- Distributed in intravascular compartment
- Response to therapy—4-8 weeks

MECHANISM OF ACTION[2]

- Omalizumab binds to free IgE and forms omalizumab–IgE complex. These hexamers are nonimmunogenic, have a half-life of about 40 days, and are cleared by the reticuloendothelial system. Serum total IgE level increases after the first dose due to formation of omalizumab–IgE complexes.

- Omalizumab does not bind to the receptor-bound IgE nor to the FcεRI receptor. Thus, omalizumab neutralizes IgE-mediated immune response without causing basophil degranulation or cross-linking with basophil-bound IgE.
- Reduction in circulating free IgE levels with maximum reduction at 3 days after subcutaneous injection
- Reduction in concentration of IgE FcεRI receptors on mast cell and basophil as free IgE is required for stabilization of these receptors. Hence, in the presence of omalizumab, these are degraded faster. The decrease in free IgE also causes downregulation of these receptors.
- Decrease in mast cell sensitivity, i.e., a greater concentration of allergen, is required for mast cell to degranulate.
- Reduction in IgE basophil crosslinking. However, this is an indirect effect as decrease in free IgE and downregulation of IgE FcεRI receptors lead to less IgE–basophil linking.
- Decrease in IgG autoantibody activity

USES

Omalizumab is approved by the Food and Drug Administration (FDA).
- *Nondermatological use*: Bronchial asthma, chronic rhinosinusitis with nasal polyp
- *Dermatological use*: Chronic spontaneous urticaria (CSU) for 12 years or older individuals

Offlabel Indications
- Inducible urticaria
- Atopic dermatitis (AD)
- Bullous pemphigoid
- Systemic mastocytosis
- Hyperimmunoglobulin E syndrome (HIES)
- Latex allergy
- Food allergy
- Kimura disease
- Urticarial vasculitis

Chronic Spontaneous Urticaria

The US FDA approved omalizumab on March 21, 2014, for use in refractory CSU.[2]

The recommended dose is 300 mg by subcutaneous injection every 4 weeks. Some patients may achieve control of their symptoms with a dose of 150 mg every 4 weeks.[3]

In other cases, the dose needs to be increased to 600 mg every 2 weeks according to the European Academy of Allergy and Clinical Immunology (EAACI) guidelines. The dose is not based on body weight or serum IgE level. The appropriate duration of omalizumab therapy for CSU has not been evaluated. Periodic reassessment of the need for continued medication is recommended.[4,5]

There are three landmark studies on the use of omalizumab in CSU, namely ASTERIA 1 study, ASTERIA 2 study, and GLACIAL study. In these three studies, a total of 733 patients having CSU received omalizumab and it was found to be effective and safe in the dose of 300 mg 4-weekly subcutaneous injections.

There was 62–71% reduction in itch from baseline at 12 weeks, 34–44% of patients were itch- and hive-free at 12 weeks, and 73–78% had improvement in Dermatology Life Quality Index (DLQI) scores at 12 weeks. Common side effects observed were injection site reactions, headache, joint pain, and upper respiratory infections.[6-8]

Omalizumab is a safe and effective alternative to corticosteroids for refractory urticaria patients. It is equally effective and safe for long-term use up to 4 years.[9]

Predictors for Better Response
- Higher baseline serum IgE levels are a predictor of better response in patients with CSU. However, there are studies to suggest no correlation between serum IgE levels and response.[10,11]
- A greater than two-fold increase in IgE after 4 weeks of treatment compared to baseline IgE[10]
- Higher baseline levels of high affinity IgE receptors on blood basophils[12]

Off-label Use of Omalizumab in Other Diseases
Atopic Dermatitis
It is believed that omalizumab may be useful in the treatment of AD because it is associated with elevated serum IgE levels.[13]

There have been mixed reports about the efficacy of omalizumab in the treatment of AD with Lane et al.[14] reporting significant improvement in three patients, Vigo et al.[15] showed improvement in five out of seven patients, while Krathen and Hsu[16] described three cases of severe AD in adults who did not respond to omalizumab. Hotze et al. conducted a pilot study and found omalizumab to be effective in a subset of patient with AD, who had absent filaggrin mutation and a higher serum level of phosphatidylcholine.[17] Thus, based on these reports, it is currently difficult to make recommendations about the use of omalizumab in cases of AD and more studies are needed to validate the effectiveness of omalizumab for AD.

Bullous Pemphigoid

The standard therapy for bullous pemphigoid is systemic steroids plus a potentially steroid-sparing agent. Compared to the standard therapy, omalizumab has a relatively selective effect. Omalizumab may be an effective and relatively safe therapeutic option for patients with bullous pemphigoid who do not respond to or have contraindications to standard treatment. The onset of action is rapid, and a dose of 300 mg/month may be sufficient to suppress the blistering.[18]

Systemic Mastocytosis

Omalizumab has been reported to be safe and effective in preventing recurrent anaphylaxis in patients with systemic mastocytosis.[19]

Hyperimmunoglobulin E Syndrome

Hyperimmunoglobulin E syndrome is a heterogenous group of immune disorders characterized by very high levels of serum IgE, dermatitis, and recurrent skin and lung infections. Studies report clinical improvement in patients with high serum IgE levels and presenting with severe atopic eczema.[20,21]

ADMINISTRATION

- Available as lyophilized powder and a solvent water for injection
- One vial of omalizumab 150 mg powder and solvent for solution for injection delivers 150 mg of omalizumab
- Reconstituted solution contains 125 mg/mL of omalizumab (150 mg in 1.2 mL)
- For omalizumab 150 mg vial, 1.4 mL of water for injection is transferred into the vial.
- The vial is swirled in an upright position (do not shake) for 5–10 seconds every 5 minutes to dissolve the products.
- The lyophilized product takes 15–20 minutes to dissolve completely forming a clear viscous solution.
- The solution may have few small bubbles along the edge of the vial.
- Using a syringe equipped with an 18-gauge needle, the solution is withdrawn from the inverted vial.
- The 18-gauge needle is replaced by a 25-gauge needle for subcutaneous injection.
- The excess solution is expelled to obtain the required 1.2 mL dose.
- As the solution is viscous, the injection takes 5–10 seconds to administer.[22]

Tests to be done Prior to Administration

There are no monitoring guidelines for omalizumab. Body weight measurement and baseline serum IgE levels are not required before the administration of omalizumab for CSU.

MONITORING DURING THERAPY

Omalizumab does not necessitate hospital admission for administration.

It should only be administered by a healthcare professional or a physician, who is trained in the recognition and treatment of anaphylaxis, in a setting where the appropriate equipment is available to respond to an episode of anaphylaxis.[22]

The patient should be observed for a period of 2 hours for the first three injections and for 30 minutes for subsequent injections as an incidence of 0.2% of anaphylaxis has been reported.[23]

There are rare reports of thrombocytopenia; hence, monitoring of platelet counts at baseline and during therapy may be advisable.

All reports of thrombocytopenia have been transient and reversible. Currently, there are no guidelines available for monitoring of platelet counts.[17]

ADVERSE EFFECTS

- *Anaphylaxis*: This is a black box warning. The condition has been reported in 0.1-0.2% patients. Th US FDA reports that 39% of anaphylaxis cases occurred after the first dose, 19% after the second dose, 10% after the third dose, and 32% after subsequent doses. Patients with a prior history of anaphylaxis are at an increased risk. The time of onset of such reaction varies from few minutes to 4 days; however, 70% of reactions are thought to occur within an hour.[24]
- *Injection site reactions*: Self-resolving adverse effect, which usually resolves within a week. Most of the reactions are mild.
- Increased risk of helminthic infection
- *Cardiovascular and cerebrovascular events*: A postmarketing observational cohort study (EXCELS) which was intended for malignancy found an increased risk of arterial thromboembolic events (ATE) in patients on omalizumab. However, further studies have failed to find any significant difference in rates of thromboembolic events in the omalizumab group versus normal population.
- Serum sickness/anaphylactoid reactions

CONTRAINDICATIONS

Absolute
There is known hypersensitivity to omalizumab.

Special Situations
- *Renal or hepatic impairment*: As omalizumab is primarily degraded in the reticular endothelial system, no dose adjustment is recommended in renal or hepatic impairment.

- *Pregnancy*: There are no adequate studies of omalizumab in pregnant women, but it is a pregnancy category B drug. It should be administered only if benefit outweighs the risks.[25,26]
- *Lactation*: The presence of omalizumab in human milk and its potential harm to the infant have not been studied. Omalizumab should be administered with caution to nursing mothers.[21]
- *Geriatric patients*: No dose adjustment is required in the elderly patients.
- *Pediatric patients*: Safety and efficacy in this group have not been established. It is approved for use in children aged 12 years and older.

CONCLUSION

Omalizumab is first in class monoclonal antibody against IgE. It is effective in the management of chronic spontaneous and other forms of chronic urticaria. It is being increasingly used successfully in the management of bullous pemphigoid.

REFERENCES

1. Belliveau PP. Omalizumab: a monoclonal anti-IgE antibody. Med Gen Med. 2005;7:27.
2. Godse K, Mehta A, Patil S, Gautam M, Nadkarni N. Omalizumab—a review. Indian J Dermatol. 2015;60:381-4.
3. Kim MJ, Kim BR, Kim SH, Chang YS, Youn SW. Clinical response to low-dose omalizumab treatment in chronic spontaneous urticaria: A retrospective study of 179 patients. Acta Derm Venereol. 2023;103:adv11627.
4. Navines-Ferrer A, Serrano-Candelas E, Molina-Molina G, Martín M. IgE- related chronic diseases and anti-IgE-based treatments. J Immunol Res. 2016;2016:8163803.
5. U.S. Food and Drug Administration (2016). Xolair (Omalizumab) for injection, for subcutaneous use. Highlights of Prescribing Information. [online] Available from http://www.accessdata.fda.gov/drugsatfda_docs/label/2014/103976s5211lbl.pdf [Accessed January 2024].
6. Maurer M, Rosen K, Hsieh HJ, Saini S, Grattan C, Gimenéz-Arnau A, et al. Omalizumab for the treatment of chronic idiopathic or spontaneous urticaria. N Engl J Med. 2013;368:924-35.
7. Saini S, Rosen KE, Hsieh HJ, Wong DA, Conner E, Kaplan A, et al. A randomized, placebo-controlled, dose-ranging study of single-dose omalizumab in patients with H1-antihistamine-refractory chronic idiopathic urticaria. J Allergy Clin Immunol. 2011;128:567-73.
8. Rottem M, Segal R, Kivity S, Shamshines L, Graif Y, Shalit M, et al. Omalizumab therapy for chronic spontaneous urticaria: the Israeli experience. Isr Med Assoc J. 2014;16:487-90.
9. Godse K, Rajagopalan M, Girdhar M, Kandhari S, Shah B, Chhajed PN, et al. Position statement for the use of Omalizumab in the management of chronic spontaneous urticaria in Indian patients. Indian Dermatol Online J. 2016;7:6-11.
10. Straesser MD, Oliver E, Palacios T, Kyin T, Patrie J, Borish L, et al. Serum IgE as an immunological marker to predict response to omalizumab treatment in symptomatic chronic urticaria. J Allergy Clin Immunol Pract. 2018;6:1386.

11. Marzano AV, Genovese G, Casazza G, Fierro MT, Dapavo P, Crimi N, et al. Predictors of response to omalizumab and relapse in chronic spontaneous urticaria: a study of 470 patients. J Eur Acad Dermatol Venereol. 2019;33:918-24.
12. Deza G, Bertolín-Colilla M, Pujol RM, Curto-Barredo L, Soto D, García M, et al. Basophil FcεRI expression in chronic spontaneous urticaria: A potential immunological predictor of response to omalizumab therapy. Acta Derm Venereol. 2017;97:698-704.
13. Johansson SG, Haahtela T, O'Byrne PM. Omalizumab and the immune system: an overview of preclinical and clinical data. Ann Allergy Asthma Immunol. 2002;89:132-8.
14. Lane Je, Cheyney JM, Lane TN, Kent DE, Cohen DJ. Treatment of recalcitrant atopic dermatitis with Omalizumab. J Am Acad Dermatol. 2006;54:68-72.
15. Vigo PG, Girgis KR, Pfuetze BL, Critchlow ME, Fisher J, Hussain I. Efficacy of anti-IgE therapy in patients with atopic dermatitis. J Am Acad Dermatol. 2006;55:168-70.
16. Krathen RA, Hsu S. Failure of omalizumab for treatment of severe adult atopic dermatitis. J Am Acad Dermatol. 2005;53:338-40.
17. Hotze M, Baurecht H, Rodríguez E, Chapman-Rothe N, Ollert M, Fölster-Holst R, et al. Increased efficacy of omalizumab in atopic dermatitis patients with wild-type filaggrin status and higher serum levels of phosphatidylcholines. Allergy. 2014;69(1):132-5.
18. Gonul M, Keseroglu HO, Ergin C, Özcan I, Erdem Ö. Bullous pemphigoid successfully treated with omalizumab. Indian J Dermatol Venereol Leprol. 2016;82:577-9.
19. Douglass J, Caroll K, Voskamp A, Bourke P, Wei A, O'Hehir RE. Omalizumab is effective in treating systemic mastocytosis in a nonatopic patient. Allergy. 2010;65(7):926-7.
20. Belloni B, Ziai M, Lim A, Lemercier B, Sbornik M, Weidinger S, et al. Low dose anti-IgE therapy in patients with atopic eczema with high serum IgE levels. J Allergy Clin Immunol. 2007;120(5):1223-5.
21. Chulanrojanamontri L, Wimoolchart S, Tuchinda P, Kulthanan K, Kiewjoy N. Role of omalizumab in a patient with hyper-IgE syndrome and review dermatologic manifestations. Asian Pac J Allergy Immunol. 2009;27(4):233-6.
22. Xolair [Internet]. [cited 2024 Feb 2]. XOLAIR® (omalizumab). Available from: https://www.xolair.com
23. Kim HL, Leigh R, Becker A. Omalizumab: practical considerations regarding the risk of anaphylaxis. Allergy Asthma Clin Immunol. 2010;6:32.
24. Cox L, Platts-Mills TA, Finegold I, Schwartz LB, Simons FE, Wallace DV. American Academy of Allergy, Asthma and Immunology/American College of Allergy, Asthma and Immunology joint taskforce report on omalizumab-associated anaphylaxis. J Allergy Clin Immunol. 2007;120:1373-7.
25. Godse K. Omalizumab in severe chronic urticaria. Indian J Dermatol Venereol Leprol. 2008;74:157-8.
26. Godse K, Vasani R. Viva voce on omalizumab. Indian J Drugs Dermatol. 2016;2:121-3.

CHAPTER 16

Newer Biologics in Urticaria

Shreya Poddar, Indrashish Podder

INTRODUCTION

Urticaria is a well-established disease with limited treatment modalities. Chronic urticaria (CU), defined as lasting more than 6 weeks, has a global prevalence ranging from 0.1 to 1.4%. While various triggers can cause urticaria, about 75% of CU cases are of unknown origin, termed "chronic spontaneous urticaria" when no specific trigger is identified.[1]

The use of monoclonal antibodies (mAbs) as a treatment for chronic spontaneous urticaria (CSU) has garnered considerable attention in recent years. While omalizumab remains the only approved mAb for treating CSU, ongoing research has shown promising results for other biologics that are currently under investigation in clinical trials. This chapter provides an overview of the available evidence regarding the use of mAbs in CSU, along with the potential challenges and opportunities they present.

Mast cells play a crucial role in the development of CSU by releasing proinflammatory mediators that recruit immune cells. Several pathogenic mechanisms have been suggested, including impaired intracellular signaling pathways, type I and type II autoimmunity. Notably, a significant percentage of CSU patients produce IgG autoantibodies against IgE or its receptor [high-affinity IgE receptors (FcεRI)], leading to mast cell and basophil degranulation and histamine release. There is also evidence of type I autoimmunity, with some CSU patients showing IgG and IgE antibodies against thyroperoxidase (TPO).[2,3]

Recently, an alternative pathogenic mechanism has been proposed, involving coagulation cascade activation initiated by tissue factors expressed on eosinophils in affected skin. This results in increased vascular permeability and mast-cell degranulation.[4]

Chronic urticaria can have a substantial impact on patients' quality of life, affecting sleep, school or work performance, and mental health in the form of anxiety and depression.[5]

Traditionally, CU treatment involves avoidance of triggers and addressing underlying causes. For CSU, second-generation H1-antihistamines (H1AH) are the primary treatment. However, up to 60% of patients do not respond adequately, even with increased dosages.[6,7] Up-dosing of H1 antihistamine can have potential adverse effects, particularly in children. Consequently, in the past two decades, novel treatment approaches, including mAbs (mAbs) and immunosuppressants like cyclosporine, have been introduced to optimize symptom control and enhance quality of life.[8]

These novel treatments, particularly mAbs, target specific molecular pathways underlying CSU. They offer the potential for increased efficacy while minimizing the side effects and toxicity associated with immunosuppressants. Currently, omalizumab, an anti-IgEmAb, is the only biologic approved as an add-on treatment for CSU.[9] Omalizumab has been discussed in the previous chapter.

The various biologics and their possible site of action in CU are shown in **Figure 1**.

LIGELIZUMAB

Ligelizumab, an anti-IgE mAb, is emerging as a potential game-changer in the management of CSU. This biologic exerts its therapeutic effect by binding to IgE, thereby preventing its binding to FcεRI on mast cells and basophils. This interaction is crucial for the release of inflammatory mediators, making ligelizumab an attractive molecule for the treatment of IgE-driven diseases, including CSU.[10]

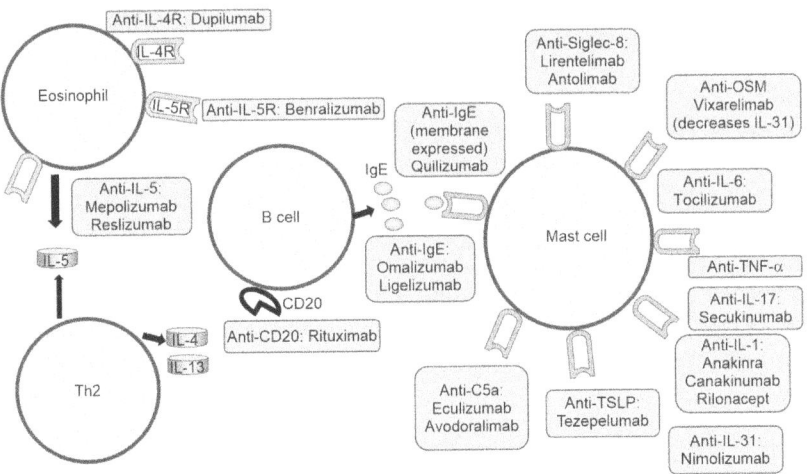

FIG. 1: Biologics and their sites of action in chronic urticaria pathogenesis pathway.
(IL: interleukin; TNF-α: tumor necrosis factor alpha)

What sets ligelizumab apart from its predecessor, omalizumab, is its remarkable in vivo affinity to IgE. In clinical trials, it demonstrated a ninefold higher affinity for IgE compared to omalizumab, with a confidence interval of 95% ranging from 6.1 to 14. This increased affinity is expected to translate into enhanced efficacy, particularly in FcεRI-driven diseases such as CSU. Unlike omalizumab, which primarily inhibits IgE binding to CD23 involved in antigen presentation, ligelizumab focuses on disrupting the IgE-FcεRI interaction at the mast cell and basophil level.

Moreover, ligelizumab has shown superiority over omalizumab in suppressing the skin prick response to allergens in atopic individuals, with statistically significant differences ($p < 0.001$) in favor of ligelizumab.[11]

It is worth noting that as of now, ligelizumab does not hold specific labeling for any disease, but multiple clinical trials are either ongoing or have been conducted to evaluate its effectiveness and safety in CSU. These trials, such as NCT03907878, NCT04210843, NCT04513548, NCT03580369, and NCT03580356, have contributed valuable insights into the potential of ligelizumab for the treatment of CSU.[12-19]

Among the notable trials conducted, a randomized, double-blind, placebo-controlled trial enrolled 382 adults with moderate-to-severe CSU who had inadequate control with H1 antihistamines alone or in combination with H2 antihistamines or leukotriene receptor antagonists. Patients were randomized into six treatment groups, including monthly doses of 240 mg, 72 mg, or 24 mg of ligelizumab, 300 mg of monthly omalizumab, a single 120 mg dose of ligelizumab followed by a placebo. At week 12, a significantly higher percentage of patients in the ligelizumab subgroups achieved a complete response to treatment (defined as a weekly hives severity score of 0) compared to the omalizumab group. The rates were particularly striking in the 72 mg and 240 mg ligelizumab groups, with 51% and 42% complete responses, respectively, versus 26% in the omalizumab group. Similar trends were observed in achieving an Urticaria Activity Score of 7 (UAS7) equal to 0. Importantly, patients treated with 240 mg of ligelizumab displayed a more sustained response even after treatment discontinuation.[12]

Extension phases of these trials further demonstrated the long-term safety and efficacy of ligelizumab. Notably, half of the patients who initially showed a poor response in the first phase reached a complete response at both week 12 and week 52, with disease control persisting even after treatment suspension. The median time to relapse was an impressive 38 weeks.[14]

Another randomized, double-blind, placebo-controlled trial, involving 49 adolescents aged 12-17 with treatment-refractory CSU, investigated the effectiveness of ligelizumab as an add-on treatment to H1 antihistamines for 24 weeks. Preliminary results indicated that all three groups experienced reductions from baseline in key urticaria-related parameters at various endpoints (week 12, 24, and 40), including UAS7, ISS7, HSS7, and Dermatology Life Quality Index (DLQI).[15]

In terms of safety, around 900 individuals treated with ligelizumab in these trials reported no serious adverse events, further underlining its potential as a safe and efficacious biologic for the treatment of CSU.[20]

These findings collectively suggest that ligelizumab may hold promise as a novel and effective therapeutic option for patients with CSU, offering superior results compared to its predecessor, omalizumab. Ongoing and upcoming trials will provide further insights into the clinical utility of this biologic in the management of CSU.

QUILIZUMAB

Quilizumab, an afucosylated monoclonal antibody targeting the M1 segment of IgE, has shown promise in reducing IgE levels, specifically surface IgE, due to its higher affinity for afucosylated IgE. In vitro studies demonstrated its ability to induce apoptosis in IgE-switched B cells, resulting in decreased IgE production.[21] Notably in patients with asthma and allergic rhinitis, quilizumab led to significant and long-lasting reductions in IgE levels.[22]

A randomized, double-blind, placebo-controlled trial on 32 patients with CSU refractory to H1 antihistamines (H1AH) assessed the impact of quilizumab on serum total IgE levels. However, at week 20, no significant changes were observed in clinical scores compared to the placebo group. It has been speculated that the ineffectiveness of quilizumab in this trial might be attributed to differences in its mechanism of action compared to omalizumab, or potential issues related to the dosage used.[23] As of now, no other clinical trials on quilizumab in urticaria are underway.

OTHER ANTI-IgE BIOLOGICS

In addition to quilizumab, other anti-IgE mAbs, such as GI-301 and UB-221, have garnered attention. An open-label, dose-escalating trial to evaluate the safety of UB-221 in CSU has been completed, while two additional trials are investigating UB-221 as an add-on treatment for CSU.[24-26]

TARGETING INTERLEUKIN-5 (ANTI-IL-5) IN URTICARIA

The interleukin-5 (IL-5) signaling pathway plays a pivotal role in eosinophil and B-cell proliferation, maturation, and survival.[27] Given that eosinophilic inflammation represents a specific endotype in conditions like asthma and other Th2-driven diseases, mAbs targeting IL-5 (mepolizumab and reslizumab) or its receptor (benralizumab) have proven successful in treating severe refractory eosinophilic asthma, offering a potential therapeutic avenue.[28]

In the context of CSU, which also exhibits a Th2 inflammation pattern, mast cells, B cells, and basophils play a central role by releasing various mediators, including IL-5. Eosinophils, in particular, have been implicated in mast cell degranulation and tissue damage mediated by the major basic protein. Interestingly, eosinophilic infiltration in both lesional and non-lesional skin of CSU patients without blood eosinophilia highlights their pathogenic role in the disease. Notably, approximately 10% of CSU patients may present with blood eosinopenia, which has been associated with more severe disease.[29]

In light of this evidence, the use of anti-IL-5 mAbs in CSU has been explored. Here are summaries of specific biologics targeting IL-5.

Mepolizumab

Mepolizumab is currently approved by the European Medicines Agency (EMA) for the treatment of severe refractory eosinophilic asthma in patients over 6 years of age, severe chronic rhinosinusitis with nasal polyps, uncontrolled eosinophilic granulomatosis with polyangiitis, and hypereosinophilic syndrome.[30] Notably, mepolizumab has shown promise in the treatment of concomitant CU induced by nonsteroidal anti-inflammatory drugs (NSAIDs). In a case report, a patient with severe eosinophilic asthma and refractory CU experienced a complete response after 16 weeks of mepolizumab treatment. However, the discontinuation of treatment due to an immune complex reaction resulted in the relapse of urticaria symptoms. An ongoing single-arm open-label trial is investigating the efficacy of mepolizumab in refractory CSU (NCT03494881).[31]

Reslizumab

Reslizumab is approved for adults with severe asthma inadequately controlled by a combination of high-dose inhaled corticosteroids and another asthma prevention medication.[32] In a 43-year-old patient with severe refractory eosinophilic asthma and refractory CSU with cold urticaria, reslizumab was found to induce a sustained improvement in symptoms during a 5-month treatment period.[33]

Benralizumab

Benralizumab, an anti-IL-5 receptor (IL-5R) monoclonal antibody, is indicated as an add-on maintenance treatment for severe uncontrolled eosinophilic asthma in patients aged 12 and older.[34] A trial involving 12 adult patients with moderate-to-severe CSU inadequately controlled by H1 antihistamines showed promising results. Following 3 months of monthly benralizumab treatment, nine patients completed the course and exhibited a significant reduction in their UAS7 score at week 20 (95% CI −6.6 to −24.8; $p < 0.001$), with no reported adverse events. Five of them achieved a complete response (UAS7 = 0) at week 24. A phase II randomized, double-blind, placebo-controlled trial on benralizumab is currently ongoing in patients with H1 antihistamine-refractory CSU (NCT04612725).

DUPILUMAB: TARGETING THE IL-4 RECEPTOR

Dupilumab is a monoclonal antibody designed to target the IL-4 receptor alpha chain (IL-4Rα), effectively blocking the actions of IL-4 and IL-13, two critical cytokines implicated in the Th2 inflammatory pathway. Of particular significance, IL-4 plays a pivotal role in driving Th2 cell differentiation and B cell class-switching to IgE, processes intimately linked to the pathogenesis of urticaria.[35]

It is noteworthy to mention that the use of dupilumab for CSU remains off-label, and the available data is limited to three case series, comprising a total of 10 patients. However, these initial findings suggest that dupilumab may be a promising therapeutic option for patients with refractory CSU.[36-38]

In one of these case series, six patients suffering from CSU, refractory to concomitant treatment with antihistamines and omalizumab, underwent treatment with dupilumab in combination with other medications, such as H1 antihistamines and/or topical tacrolimus and/or montelukast. Remarkably, five out of six patients achieved controlled disease, as evidenced by an UAS7 ≤ 6, or even the complete resolution of CSU by the third month of treatment.[36]

Staubach et al. reported the cases of two children, aged 6 and 17 years old, respectively, both struggling with CSU and previously treated with updosing omalizumab and cyclosporine. In response to dupilumab therapy, their symptoms notably improved, especially in the case of the patients with elevated IgE levels.[37]

Similar promising results were observed in two adult women with refractory CSU, one of whom was initially prescribed dupilumab for comorbid atopic dermatitis, and she experienced a complete and sustained response to the treatment.[38]

Currently, two randomized, double-blind, placebo-controlled trials (RDBPCTs), namely DUPISCU and CUPID (NCT03749135 and NCT04180488, respectively), are actively investigating the efficacy of dupilumab in a cohort of 456 individuals dealing with moderate-to-severe CSU refractory to H1 antihistamines.

ANTI-CD20: RITUXIMAB

In the context of CSU, studies have reported the efficacy of rituximab in patients refractory to conventional treatments. Notably, the long-lasting remission observed with rituximab may be attributed to B-cell depletion and subsequent reduction in IgG autoantibody synthesis. However, it is important to consider the increased risk of infections associated with reduced Ig levels.[39]

Despite these promising findings, an open-label trial assessing rituximab's efficacy in refractory CSU was prematurely stopped, leaving questions about its utility in this context.

ANTI-IL-17: SECUKINUMAB

Elevated IL-17 levels have been observed in patients with CSU, particularly those with severe disease. Secukinumab, an IL-17 neutralizing agent, is currently approved for the treatment of psoriasis and spondyloarthritis. In a study, it demonstrated significant efficacy in patients with severe CSU refractory to omalizumab, with a substantial reduction in urticaria activity scores.[40]

ANTI-IL-1: CANAKINUMAB

Canakinumab antagonizes IL-1β, a pivotal cytokine in innate immunity. A study evaluating its efficacy in CSU concluded that IL-1β is not involved in the pathogenesis of CSU, there was no significant change in urticaria activity scores.[41]

ANTI-TUMOR NECROSIS FACTOR ALPHA: INFLIXIMAB

Tumor necrosis factor alpha (TNF-α) levels have been reported to increase in the skin and serum of patients with urticaria, correlating with disease severity. Infliximab, a TNF-α inhibitor, has shown promise in treating CSU, with cases of symptom resolution for extended periods, although additional studies are warranted.[42]

ANTI-TSLP: TEZEPELUMAB

Thymic stromal lymphopoietin (TSLP), IL-25, and IL-33 play crucial roles in Th2 inflammatory responses. Tezepelumab, a monoclonal antibody inhibiting TSLP, is being evaluated for its potential to treat CSU in an ongoing clinical trial.[43]

OTHER BIOLOGICS

- *Barzolvolimab:* This agent antagonizes the tyrosine kinase receptor KIT, involved in mast-cell differentiation. Early trials are exploring its efficacy and safety in refractory CSU.[44,45]
- *MTPS9579A:* It is an anti-tryptase monoclonal antibody that aims to reduce active tryptase levels. Clinical trials are underway to evaluate its potential in the treatment of refractory CSU.[46]
- *LY3454738*: Investigated for its role in Th2 inflammation, this agent failed to demonstrate efficacy in a clinical trial on patients with refractory CSU.[47]
- *Lirentelimab:* It is an anti-sialic acid-binding agent with potential inhibitory effects on eosinophils and mast cells. Studies are ongoing to assess its safety and efficacy in refractory CU.[48]

CONCLUSION

The management of CSU has seen significant advancements with the use of omalizumab and other promising biological drugs like dupilumab and tezepelumab. These treatments offer hope for better symptom control and improved quality of life for CSU patients. However, it is important to acknowledge that our understanding of these therapies is still evolving, and further research is required.

REFERENCES

1. Giménez-Arnau AM, Manzanares N, Podder I. Recent updates in urticaria. Med Clin (Barc). 2023;161:435-44.
2. Hide M, Francis DM, Grattan CE, Hakimi J, Kochan JP, Greaves MW. Autoantibodies against the high-affinity IgE receptor as a cause of histamine release in chronic urticaria. N Engl J Med. 1993;328:1599-604.
3. Tong LJ, Balakrishnan G, Kochan JP, Kinét JP, Kaplan A. Assessment of autoimmunity in patients with chronic urticaria. J Allergy Clin Immunol. 1997;99:461-5.
4. Cugno M, Marzano AV, Asero R, Tedeschi A. Activation of blood coagulation in chronic urticaria: Pathophysiological and clinical implications. Intern Emerg Med. 2010;5: 97-101.
5. Gonçalo M, Gimenéz-Arnau A, Al-Ahmad M, Ben-Shoshan M, Bernstein JA, Ensina LF, et al. The global burden of chronic urticaria for the patient and society. Br J Dermatol. 2021;184:226-36.
6. Guillén-Aguinaga S, Jáuregui Presa I, Aguinaga-Ontoso E, Guillén-Grima F, Ferrer M. Updosing nonsedating antihistamines in patients with chronic spontaneous urticaria: A systematic review and meta-analysis. Br J Dermatol. 2016;175:1153-65.
7. Manti S, Salpietro C, Cuppari C. Antihistamines: Recommended Dosage–Divergence between Clinical Practice and Guideline Recommendations. Int Arch Allergy Immunol. 2019;178:93-6.
8. Kaplan AP. Chronic Spontaneous Urticaria: Pathogenesis and Treatment Considerations. Allergy Asthma Immunol Res. 2017;9:477-82.
9. European Medicines Agency. Omalizumab. [online] Available from https://www.ema.europa.eu/en/medicines/human/EPAR/xolair. [Last accessed February, 2024].
10. Arm JP, Bottoli I, Skerjanec A, Floch D, Groenewegen A, Maahs S, et al. Pharmacokinetics, pharmacodynamics and safety of QGE031 (ligelizumab), a novel high-affinity anti-IgE antibody, in atopic subjects. Clin Exp Allergy. 2014;44:1371-85.
11. Gasser P, Tarchevskaya SS, Guntern P, Brigger D, Ruppli R, Zbären N, et al. The mechanistic and functional profile of the therapeutic anti-IgE antibody ligelizumab differs from omalizumab. Nat Commun. 2020;11:165.
12. Maurer M, Giménez-Arnau AM, Sussman G, Metz M, Baker DR, Bauer A, et al. Ligelizumab for Chronic Spontaneous Urticaria. N Engl J Med. 2019;381:1321-32.
13. Giménez-Arnau A, Maurer M, Bernstein J, Staubach P, Barbier N, Hua E, et al. Ligelizumab improves sleep interference and disease burden in patients with chronic spontaneous urticaria. Clin Transl Allergy. 2022;12:e12121.
14. Maurer M, Giménez-Arnau A, Bernstein JA, Chu CY, Danilycheva I, Hide M, et al. Sustained safety and efficacy of ligelizumab in patients with chronic spontaneous urticaria: A one-year extension study. Allergy. 2021;77:2175-84.
15. ClinicalTrials.gov. Study to Investigate the Efficacy and Safety of QGE031 in Adolescent Patients with Chronic Spontaneous Urticaria (CSU). [online] Available from https://clinicaltrials.gov/ct2/show/NCT03437278. [Last accessed February, 2024].

16. ClinicalTrials.gov. A Safety and Efficacy Study of Ligelizumab in the Treatment of CSU in Japanese Patients Inadequately Controlled with H1-Antihistamines. [online] Available from https://www.clinicaltrials.gov/ct2/show/NCT03907878 [Last accessed February, 2024].
17. ClinicalTrials.gov. Study of Efficacy and Safety of Ligelizumab in Chronic Spontaneous Urticaria Patients Who Completed a Previous Study with Ligelizumab. [online] Available from https://clinicaltrials.gov/ct2/show/record/NCT04210843. [Last accessed February, 2024].
18. ClinicalTri-als.gov. Study of Mechanism of Action of Ligelizumab (QGE031) in Patients with Chronic Urticaria. [online] Available from https://clinicaltrials.gov/ct2/show/record/NCT04513548. [Last accessed February, 2024].
19. ClinicalTrials.gov. A Phase III Study of Efficacy and Safety of Ligelizumab in the Treatment of CSU in Adolescents and Adults Inadequately Controlled With H1-Antihistamines. [online] Available from https://clinicaltrials.gov/ct2/show/NCT03580356. [Last accessed February, 2024].
20. Wedi B. Ligelizumab for the treatment of chronic spontaneous urticaria. Expert Opin Biol Ther. 2020;20:853-61.
21. Brightbill D, Hans LL, Yuwen LZ, Tan M, Meng G, Gloria Y, et al. Quilizumab is an Afucosylated Humanized Anti-M1 Prime Therapeutic Antibody. Clin Anti-Inflamm. Anti-Allergy Drugs (Discontin). 2014;1:24-31.
22. Gauvreau GM, Harris JM, Boulet LP, Scheerens H, Fitzgerald JM, Putnam WS, et al. Targeting membrane-expressed IgE B cell receptor with an antibody to the M1 prime epitope reduces IgE production. Sci Transl Med. 2014;6:243ra85.
23. Harris JM, Cabanski CR, Scheerens H, Samineni D, Bradley MS, Cochran C, et al. A randomized trial of quilizumab in adults with refractory chronic spontaneous urticaria. J Allergy Clin Immunol. 2016;138:1730-2.
24. ClinicalTrials.gov. Evaluate the Safety, Tolerability, Pharmacokinetics, and Pharmacodynamics of UB-221 as an Add-on Therapy in CSU Patients. [online] Available from https://clinicaltrials.gov/ct2/show/record/NCT03632291?term=ub-221&draw=2&rank=3. [Last accessed February, 2024].
25. ClinicalTrials.gov. Evaluating the Safety and Tolerability and Determining the PK and PD of Single Dose UB-221 in Chronic Spontaneous Urticaria. [online] Available from https://clinicaltrials.gov/ct2/show/NCT04175704. [Last accessed February, 2024].
26. ClinicalTrials.gov. A Study to Evaluate the Pharmacodynamics, Pharmacokinetics, Safety, and Efficacy of UB-221 IV Infusion as an Add-on Therapy in Patients with Chronic Spontaneous Urticaria. [online] Available from https://clinicaltrials.gov/ct2/show/NCT05298215?term=ub-221&draw=2&rank=1. [Last accessed February, 2024].
27. Adachi T, Alam R. The mechanism of IL-5 signal transduction. Am J Physiol. 1998;275:C623-33.
28. Farne HA, Wilson A, Powell C, Bax L, Milan SJ. Anti-IL5 therapies for asthma. Cochrane Database Syst Rev. 2017;(9):CD010834.
29. Altrichter S, Frischbutter S, Fok JS, Kolkhir P, Jiao Q, Skov PS, et al. The role of eosinophils in chronic spontaneous urticaria. J Allergy Clin Immunol. 2020;145:1510-6.
30. European Medicines Agency. Mepolizumab. [online] Available from https://www.ema.europa.eu/en/medicines/human/EPAR/nucala. [Last accessed February, 2024].
31. ClinicalTrials.gov. Mepolizumab for the Treatment of Chronic Spontaneous Urticaria. [online] Available from https://clinicaltrials.gov/ct2/show/NCT03494881. [Last accessed February, 2024].
32. European Medicines Agency. Cinqaero, reslizumab [online] Available from https://www.ema.europa.eu/en/medicines/human/EPAR/cinqaero. [Last accessed February, 2024].

33. Maurer M, Altrichter S, Metz M, Zuberbier T, Church MK, Bergmann KC. Benefit from reslizumab treatment in a patient with chronic spontaneous urticaria and cold urticaria. J Eur Acad Dermatol Venereol. 2018;32:e112-3.
34. European Medicines Agency. Fasenra. [online] Available from https://www.ema.europa.eu/en/documents/productinformation/fasenra-epar-product-information_en.pdf. [Last accessed February, 2024].
35. Matsunaga K, Katoh N, Fujieda S, Izuhara K, Oishi K. Dupilumab: Basic aspects and applications to allergic diseases. Allergol Int. 2020;69:187-96.
36. Lee JK, Simpson RS. Dupilumab as a novel therapy for difficult to treat chronic spontaneous urticaria. J Allergy Clin Immunol Pract. 2019;7:1659-61.e1.
37. Staubach P, Peveling-Oberhag A, Lang BM, Zimmer S, Sohn A, Mann C. Severe chronic spontaneous urticaria in children treatment options according to the guidelines and beyond—A 10 years review. J Dermatol Treat. 2022;33:1119-22.
38. Errichetti E, Stinco G. Recalcitrant chronic urticaria treated with dupilumab: Report of two instances refractory to H1-antihistamines, omalizumab and cyclosporine and brief literature review. Dermatol Ther. 2021;34:e14821.
39. McAtee CL, Lubega J, Underbrink K, Curry K, Msaouel P, Barrow M, et al. Association of Rituximab Use With Adverse Events in Children, Adolescents, and Young Adults. JAMA Netw Open. 2021;4:2036321.
40. Sabag DA, Matanes L, Bejar J, Sheffer H, Barzilai A, Church MK, et al. Interleukin-17 is a potential player and treatment target in severe chronic spontaneous urticaria. Clin Exp Allergy. 2020;50:799-804.
41. Maul JT, Distler M, Kolios A, Maul LV, Guillet C, Graf N, et al. Canakinumab Lacks Efficacy in Treating Adult Patients with Moderate to Severe Chronic Spontaneous Urticaria in a Phase II Randomized Double-Blind Placebo-Controlled Single-Center Study. J Allergy Clin Immunol Pract. 2021;9:463-8.e3.
42. Wilson LH, Eliason MJ, Leiferman KM, Hull CM, Powell DL. Treatment of refractory chronic urticaria with tumor necrosis factor-alfa inhibitors. J Am Acad Dermatol. 2011;64:1221-2.
43. ClinicalTrials.gov. Study to Evaluate Tezepelumab in Adults with Chronic Spontaneous Urticaria (INCEPTION). [online] Available from https://clinicaltrials.gov/ct2/show/NCT04833855. [Last accessed February, 2024].
44. ClinicalTrials.gov. A Study of CDX-0159 in Patients with Chronic Spontaneous Urticaria. [online] Available from https://www.clinicaltrials.gov/ct2/show/NCT04538794. [Last accessed February, 2024].
45. ClinicalTrials.gov. A Phase 2 Study of CDX-0159 in Patients with Chronic Spontaneous Urticaria. [online] Available from https://clinicaltrials.gov/ct2/show/NCT05368285. [Last accessed February, 2024]
46. ClinicalTrials.gov. A Study of MTPS9579A in Participants with Refractory Chronic Spontaneous Urticaria. [online] Available from https://www.clinicaltrials.gov/ct2/show/NCT05129423. [Last accessed February, 2024].
47. ClinicalTrials.gov. A Study of LY3454738 in Adults with Chronic Spontaneous Urticaria. [online] Available from https://clinicaltrials.gov/ct2/show/NCT04159701. [Last accessed February, 2024].
48. ClinicalTrials.gov. A Study to Assess the Efficacy and Safety of AK002 in Subjects with Antihistamine-Resistant Chronic Urticaria. [online] Available from https://clinicaltrials.gov/ct2/show/NCT03436797?term=Siglec-8&draw=2&rank=1. [Last accessed February, 2024].

SECTION 5

Biologics in Atopic Dermatitis

CHAPTER 17

Interleukin-4 Inhibitor: Dupilumab

Sandipan Dhar, Disha Chakraborty, Abhishek De

INTRODUCTION TO ATOPIC DERMATITIS AND ITS MANAGEMENT

Atopic dermatitis (AD), also referred to as atopic eczema, is a persistent and inflammatory skin condition that affects millions of people worldwide. It presents as eczematous lesions causing severe itching, redness, and dryness. It impairs the skin barrier. Also, significantly lowers the quality of life for individuals who have it. Although there have been many different AD treatment modalities throughout the years, finding efficient and long-lasting remedies has been of utmost importance. Topical emollients, oral antihistamines, and systemic immunosuppressants have historically been used to treat AD.[1] Many patients have received symptomatic relief from these treatments, but they frequently fail to achieve persistent, all-encompassing illness control. Additionally, in mild to moderately severe AD, their use may be associated with limited efficacy and unfavorable side effects like systemic toxicity. Because of this unmet medical need, there is increasing interest in creating biologic drugs that directly target the immunological processes that underlie AD. Biologics are designed to selectively target specific molecules and pathways within the immune system, offering a more targeted and potentially safer approach to disease management. One biologic has received a lot of interest and has shown to be incredibly effective in the treatment of AD is dupilumab.[2]

This chapter focuses entirely on dupilumab for several compelling reasons. Dupilumab is the first biologic licensed for the treatment of moderate-to-severe AD in adults and adolescents. Its ground-breaking approval in 2017 represented a turning point in the treatment of AD, providing patients who had long struggled with AD with new prospects.[3] Secondly, dupilumab targets the interleukin-4 (IL-4) receptor α-subunit, resulting in a novel mode of action. By doing this, it interferes with the AD-related signaling pathways, which reduces inflammation and enhances the strength of the skin barrier. Its novel approach to treating AD has set it apart from traditional therapies and has made it a central figure in discussions about the future of AD management.[4]

MILESTONES IN THE DEVELOPMENT OF DUPILUMAB

Identification of Target Pathways and Proof of Concept

The identification of IL-4 and IL-13 as important cytokines implicated in the inflammatory cascade of AD set the groundwork for the development of dupilumab. Early preclinical studies suggested that inhibiting the IL-4 receptor, α-subunit would be useful in reducing AD symptoms. The foundation for the development of dupilumab as a biologic for AD was laid out as a result of this proof of concept.[1,2]

Clinical Trials Initiation and Breakthrough Designation

The first clinical trials on dupilumab started as early as 2011 to assess its efficacy and safety in patients with mild-to-moderate AD. Dupilumab was approved to treat adults with moderate-to-severe AD on the basis of the pivotal phase III SOLO 1 (NCT02277743), SOLO 2 (NCT02277769), and CHRONOS (NCT02260986) studies, which assessed the safety and effectiveness of the (subsequently) approved dupilumab dosage regimen in comparison to placebo.[5]

The United States Food and Drug Administration (US FDA) designated dupilumab with "breakthrough therapy" status in November 2014 for the treatment of moderate-to-severe AD in adults, and in September 2016, this indication underwent priority review. Dupilumab subsequently received the FDA's "breakthrough therapy" designation in October 2016 for the treatment of moderate-to-severe AD in patients aged 12–18 years and also for severe AD in patients aged 6 months to 12 years, when topical medications were ineffective or inappropriate.[6]

Global Approval and Ongoing Research

Dupilumab was approved in the USA on March 28, 2017, for treating moderate-to-severe AD in adults who cannot be satisfactorily controlled with topical prescription medications or when they are not recommended. Dupilumab thus became the first licensed targeted biologic therapy for AD. The biologic was authorized by regulatory bodies all over the world after the FDA gave it its approval, including the European Medicines Agency (EMA) and other national regulatory bodies. Due to the treatment's widespread acceptance, more people now have access to it globally.[7,8]

Dupilumab (Dupixent™) was developed jointly by Regeneron Pharmaceuticals and Sanofi using VelocImmune technology. Regeneron and Sanofi collaborated in 2007 to create and market completely human therapeutic antibodies.[7]

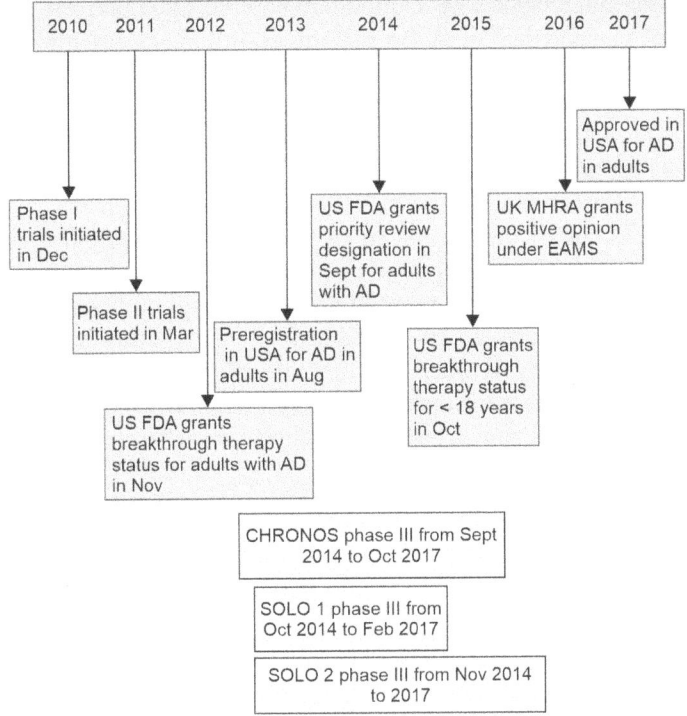

FLOWCHART 1: Milestones in the development of dupilumab.

Flowchart 1 summarizes these abovementioned milestones in the development of dupilumab.

UNDERSTANDING HOW DUPILUMAB WORKS AND ITS INDICATIONS

Mechanism of Action

Dupilumab targets the α-subunit of the IL-4 receptor and is a fully humanized immunoglobulin G4 (IgG4) monoclonal antibody. The two forms of IL-4 receptors are type I and type II. Type I is a heterodimer of the IL-4R and the common chain (C), and type II, is a heterodimer of the IL-4R and the interleukin-13 receptor alpha 1 (IL-13RA1) chain. Dupilumab suppresses the downstream signaling of IL-4 and IL-13, two essential cytokines of the Th2 pathway that are involved in B-cell activation, dendritic cell (DC) differentiation, and IgE class switching. In addition, it decreases eosinophil recruitment.[9]

Pharmacokinetics

Dupilumab exhibits nonlinear target-mediated pharmacokinetics. This is because its exposure increases more rapidly than in a dose-proportionate way. Its bioavailability is 64%. Dupilumab 600 mg subcutaneous injections take 1 week to reach their peak serum levels and 16 weeks to achieve a steady state concentration. Dupilumab's metabolic route has not been identified. Given that it is a human monoclonal IgG4 antibody, it is expected to degrade similarly to natural IgG via antibody-complex endocytosis and target-mediated clearance.

Formal clinical trials must be conducted to learn more about the pharmacokinetics of dupilumab in hepatic and renal impairment. Two hepatitis B patients receiving concurrent entecavir were reported to have significantly improved symptoms after receiving dupilumab medication for AD. There was also no trace of hepatitis or hepatitis B virus (HBV) reactivation. However, it must also be said that the FDA still does not comment on its use in renal or hepatic diseases. So, the authors advocate its use in renal or hepatic impairment should be dealt with utmost caution until clinical trials are conducted for the same.[9,10]

Pharmacodynamics

It is unclear how dupilumab's pharmacodynamic action and clinical effects are related. However, after receiving the drug, serum levels of IL-4 and IL-13 escalated, which is indicative of receptor blockade.[11]

Drug Interactions

Live vaccines are contraindicated while the patient is on dupilumab. During chronic inflammation, the levels of several cytokines, such as interleukin-1 (IL-1), IL-10, IL-6, interferon-γ (IFN-γ), and tumor necrosis factor-α (TNF-α) are elevated which might affect the level of CYP450 enzymes. Concurrent use of CYP450 substrates, particularly those with narrow therapeutic indices, is advised to be monitored for effect and drug concentration (e.g., warfarin and cyclosporine). Hence, modifying the dosage is advised if necessary since dupilumab may modify serum levels of some cytokines.[12]

Indications

The FDA approved and off-label indications are summarized in **Table 1**.[13]

CLINICAL EFFICACY BASED ON PREVIOUS DATA, RECENT CLINICAL TRIALS, REAL-WORLD EVIDENCE, AND OUTCOMES

The results of the previously conducted trials on dupilumab in atopic dermatitis are summarized in **Table 2**.[14-18]

TABLE 1: FDA approved and off-label indications of dupilumab.	
FDA approved	**Off label**
March 2017: Moderate-to-severe AD in adults and adolescents at least 12 years-old refractory to topical treatments or when those therapies are not advisable. *June 2022*: Approved for moderate-to-severe AD in *age of 6 month to 5-year-old* refractory to topical treatments or when those therapies are not advisable	Alopecia areata
Prurigo nodularis: Approved in 2022 by US FDA	Chronic hand eczema
Asthma	Nummular eczema
Chronic rhinosinusitis with nasal polyposis	Pemphigus vulgaris and pemphigus foliaceus
Eosinophilic esophagitis	Bullous pemphigoid
	Idiopathic chronic eczematous eruption of aging
	Allergic contact dermatitis
	Chronic spontaneous urticaria
	Cholinergic urticaria

(AD: atopic dermatitis; FDA: Food and Drug Administration)

Recent Trial Results

R668-AD-1652 LIBERTY AD PEDS was a randomized, double-blinded, placebo-controlled, parallel-group, phase III clinical trial conducted by Siegfried et al. on children of age between 6 and 11 years with severe AD. They were treated with either dupilumab or placebo for 16 weeks and the treatment group showed significant improvement from as early as 2 weeks till the end of the study period. Improvement was assessed not only in terms of AD signs and symptoms but also in terms of quality of life improvement.[19]

A phase 3 double-blind, placebo-controlled trial assessed the safety and efficacy of dupilumab in 133 adolescents and adults with moderate-to-severe atopic hand and foot dermatitis who had an insufficient response or intolerance to topical corticosteroids. The results showed that 40% of patients achieved clear or almost clear skin in terms of Investigator Global Assessment (IGA) scale on hands and feet as the primary endpoint compared to 17% with placebo. Again, 52% of patients saw a clinically meaningful reduction in itch on hands and feet and there was a 69% average reduction in signs of hand and foot lesions from baseline compared to 31% with placebo. There was significant improvement in the overall appearance of hand and foot skin, reduction in pain, improved sleep, and thereby a better quality of life.[20]

TABLE 2: Studies on dupilumab in atopic dermatitis.

Type of study and level of evidence	Efficacy and results of study	Safety profile	Conclusion and comments	Reference
Retrospective chart analysis on 25 patients of AD treated with dupilumab from three centers in India Level of Evidence 4	After 6 months of treatment, 68% of the patients achieved EASI-75, indicating near-complete remission in the majority of our patients	The safety profile was favorable, with two reported cases of mild conjunctivitis	First Indian data for safety and efficacy on real-world use of dupilumab	Dhar, De, and Srinivas 2021[14]
Open-label phase IIa study and subsequent phase III Open-label extension study on 37 children of age between 6 and 12 years Level of Evidence 2	• Sustained improvements were also seen in EASI-50, EASI-90, SCORAD, and percentage body surface area affected by AD in the phase IIa and OLE study up to week 52 • AD symptoms and QoL as assessed by POEM and CDLQI showed improvement from baseline to week 48 of the OLE	• The majority of reported TEAEs were of mild or moderate severity • The overall incidence of serious TEAEs was low	First Indian data for safety and efficacy on real-world use of dupilumab. Approved by US FDA for prolonged treatment in children aged ≥6 to <12 years with uncontrolled severe atopic dermatitis on May 26th 2020	Cork et al. 2021[15]
Two randomized, placebo-controlled, phase 3 trials (SOLO 1 and SOLO 2) Level of Evidence 2	• Enrolled 671 patients in SOLO 1 and 708 in SOLO 2. • Dupilumab improved the signs and symptoms of atopic dermatitis, including pruritus, symptoms of anxiety and depression, and quality of life, as compared with placebo	Injection-site reactions and conjunctivitis were more frequent in the dupilumab groups than in the placebo groups		Simpson et al. 2016[16]

Continued

Continued

Type of study and level of evidence	Efficacy and results of study	Safety profile	Conclusion and comments	Reference
Randomized, double-blind, placebo-controlled, parallel-group, phase 3 trial was conducted in 31 hospitals, clinics, and academic institutions in Europe and North America	6 months to <6 years, moderate-to-severe atopic dermatitis by IGA score 3–4 and an inadequate response to TCS given dupilumab for 16 weeks	Showed significant improvement for dupilumab treated patients	Approved by US FDA as first biologic medicine for children aged 6 months to 5 years with moderate-to-severe atopic dermatitis on 7th June 2022 (Sanofi 2022)	Paller et al. 2022[17]
Level of Evidence 1	Six trials involving 2,447 patients were identified. Pooled analysis revealed significant improvements in Eczema Area and Severity Index (EASI) score	Acceptable safety profile	Systematic review and meta-analysis	Wang et al. 2018[18]

(AD: atopic dermatitis; IGA: Investigator Global Assessment; TCS: topical corticosteroid; TEAEs: treatment-emergent adverse events)

TABLE 3: Clinical trials of dupilumab in patients with prurigo nodularis.

Disease	Trial name	Primary and secondary endpoints	Result
Prurigo nodularis	LIBERTY-PN PRIME (randomized double-blind placebo controlled trial) 300 mg dupilumab 2 weekly with placebo in the ratio of 1:1 Adults with ≥20 nodules and severe itch uncontrolled with topical therapies enrolled N = 151	• Primary endpoint was pruritus improvement, measured by proportion of patients with a ≥4-point reduction in Worst Itch Numeric Rating Scale (WI-NRS) from baseline at week 24. • Key secondary endpoints included nodule number reduction to ≤5 at week 24	≥4-point WI-NRS reduction at week 24 in the dupilumab and placebo arms was achieved by 60.0% and 18.4% of patients
	Adults with ≥20 nodules and severe itch uncontrolled with topical therapies enrolled N = 160	• Primary endpoint was pruritus improvement, measured by proportion of patients with a ≥4-point reduction in WI-NRS from baseline at week 12 • Key secondary endpoints included nodule number reduction to ≤5 at week 24	≥4-point WI-NRS reduction at week 12 in the dupilumab and placebo arms was achieved by 37.2% and 22% of patients

Recent trials have shown its efficacy in patients of 2 to <18 years of age suffering from uncontrollable AD. A single-center retrospective study was conducted on 39 patients and efficacy was evaluated on the basis of scores like SCORAD, P-NRS, CDLQI, and POEM calculated at baseline and weeks 4, 10, and 16. Eight patients were aged 2 to <6 years, 15 were 6 to <12 years, and 16 were 12 to <18 years. At the end of the study, there was a statistically significant improvement in terms of all the scoring systems across maximum patients of all age groups. Two patients reported conjunctivitis. The most significant conclusion from this study was that dupilumab was efficacious in 2 to <6 years age group.[21]

RECENT CLINICAL TRIALS IN PRURIGO NODULARIS

The results are summarized in **Table 3**.[22]

DRUG DOSAGE AND MONITORING

The single-dose prefilled syringe strengths (**Fig. 1**) of dupilumab injection are 300 mg/2 mL and 200 mg/1.14 mL, respectively. The medication is sterile

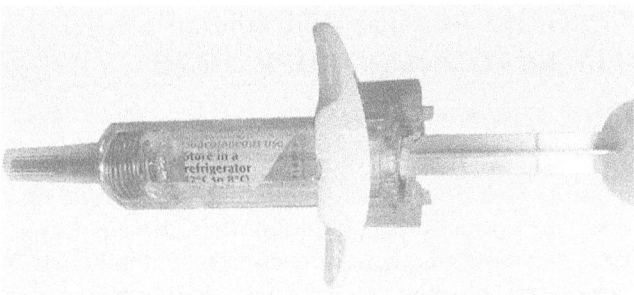

FIG. 1: Dupilumab device.

TABLE 4: Age- and weight-wise dosage of dupilumab.		
Body weight (dosage in pediatric patients 6 months to 5 years of age)	**Initial and subsequent dosage**	
5 to <15 kg	200 mg (one 200 mg injection) every 4 weeks (Q4W)	
15 to <30 kg	300 mg (one 300 mg injection) every 4 weeks (Q4W)	
Body weight (dosage in pediatric patients 6 years to 17 years of age)	**Initial dose**	**Subsequent doses**
15 to <30 kg	600 mg (two 300 mg injections)	300 mg Q4W
30 to <60 kg	400 mg (two 200 mg injections)	200 mg Q2W
60 kg or more	600 mg (two 300 mg injections)	300 mg Q2W

and free of preservatives. It is kept in the original carton in the refrigerator between 36 and 46°F (2 and 8°C) to protect it from light. Subcutaneous injections of dupilumab are given (preferred sites: thigh or belly, excluding the two inches surrounding the navel). Adult patients should start with a 600 mg dosage of dupilumab (two 300 mg injections, given at separate locations), then receive 300 mg once every 15 days. It should be continued for 16 weeks in order to have sufficient therapeutic results.[1,2]

Dose in pediatric age group is summarized in **Table 4**.

Monitoring

As per clinical trials, laboratory monitoring is not necessary for dupilumab which makes it an even better choice for uncontrolled moderate-to-severe AD.[1,2]

SAFETY PROFILE ACROSS AGE GROUPS AND CONTRAINDICATIONS OF DUPILUMAB

Documented Adverse Effects

According to a meta-analysis of seven randomized, double-blinded, placebo-controlled clinical trials, dupilumab was found to be more tolerable and had a superior safety profile than the majority of systemic medications. The most frequent side effects of dupilumab are ocular adverse reactions and injection-site responses like tenderness and bruising. Common ocular adverse effects include conjunctivitis, keratitis, pruritus, dry eyes, and blepharitis. These conditions can be managed with topical steroid drops or artificial tears. The most frequent opportunistic infection encountered with dupilumab therapy is herpes simplex virus infection. In clinical trials, urticaria and responses resembling serum sickness were only seen by <1% of individuals. Headache, nasopharyngitis, arthralgia, myalgia, helminth infections, oropharyngeal discomfort, gastritis diarrhea, toothache, eosinophilia, and sleeplessness are further unusual side effects of dupilumab therapy. Antidrug neutralizing antibodies may possibly develop which might lead to decreased efficacy. After using dupilumab, a single case of IgA nephropathy exacerbation has been documented.[23]

Recently documented facial skin responses known as dupilumab facial redness (DFR) include erythema, scaling, papules, itching, rash, and burning with overall discomfort in the face and neck. Topical calcineurin inhibitors, topical corticosteroids, and antifungal medications were the most frequently utilized therapy for DFR. The contraindication of dupilumab is hypersensitivity to the drug or any of its contents like L-arginine hydrochloride, L-histidine, polysorbate, and sodium acetate.[23]

Use in Pregnancy and Lactation

Dupilumab for severe AD in pregnancy has not been shown to cause adverse effects on mothers or fetuses. Dupilumab may impair newborn immunity, which needs additional study. Dupilumab has not been well investigated for nursing. Due to its enormous molecular weight, dupilumab is unlikely to transfer into breastmilk; however, limited data advises against using it in breastfeeding mothers.[24,25]

Several studies highlight that dupilumab not only treats the physical symptoms of AD, such as itching, redness, and skin lesions but also improves the quality of life by addressing emotional and psychological difficulties. Clinical trials and real-world studies show that patients experience less intense symptoms, improved sleep, and enhanced emotional and mental health. The authors have earlier shown in their study the treatment's ability to improve the appearance of skin lesions and decrease the postinflammatory hyperpigmentation.[14,26]

Table 5 shows GRADE scoring of AD-related outcomes.

TABLE 5: GRADE scoring of AD-related outcomes.

Outcome	Importance
SCORAD, EASI 50, 75, pruritus measured by peak pruritus numerical scale, safety or adverse effects	Critical (7–9)
IGA, resource utilization, pain control, rescue medication use, sleep disturbance, symptoms of anxiety, depression, quality of life	Important (4–6)
Cutaneous microbiome, skin barrier, T cell profile	Low importance (1–3)

(AD: atopic dermatitis; EASI: Eczema Area and Severity Index; IGA: Investigator Global Assessment)

COMBINATION OF DUPILUMAB WITH OTHER MONOCLONAL ANTIBODIES IN PATIENTS WITH COEXISTING DERMATOLOGICAL OR NONDERMATOLOGICAL CONDITIONS

Gisondi et al. reported a case series of 24 patients who were receiving dupilumab for AD except two patients who were receiving it for bullous pemphigoid and asthma respectively. Out of them, seven patients were receiving guselkumab and one was receiving secukinumab for psoriasis. Three patients had coexisting Crohn's disease treated with adalimumab, three of chronic urticaria treated with omalizumab and two of primary familial hypercholesterolemia with evolocumab. Also, there were two hidradenitis suppurativa patients receiving adalimumab one with psoriatic arthritis on secukinumab and one with rheumatoid arthritis on abatacept, one with ankylosing spondylitis on secukinumab and one with colorectal carcinoma with cetuximab. It was noted that combination therapy did not lead to significant adverse reactions other than mild injection site reactions. Also, dupilumab did not exhibit any immunosuppressive effects or any interactions with CYP450 enzymes.[27]

APPROVAL IN INDIA

Mumbai, July 11, 2023. Sanofi Healthcare India Pvt. Ltd. announced that it has received marketing authorization for Dupixent® (dupilumab), in India as the first biologic medicine for the treatment of moderate-to-severe AD in adults whose disease is not adequately controlled with topical prescription therapies or when those therapies are not advisable. Dupixent® can be used along with or without topical therapy.[28]

CONCLUSION

The introduction of dupilumab has undeniably transformed the landscape of AD management, offering a beacon of hope for individuals burdened by this chronic skin condition. This monoclonal antibody has not only demonstrated its remarkable efficacy in alleviating the physical symptoms of AD but has also exhibited a profound positive impact on the quality of life for patients. Through the relief of itching, the restoration of restful sleep, the enhancement of emotional well-being, and the facilitation of social engagement, dupilumab has provided a holistic approach to AD care.

In essence, dupilumab's journey in the field of AD is an exemplary illustration of the intersection between medical innovation and patient-centered care. The profound impact it has had on the lives of those living with AD underscores the importance of not only addressing the physical manifestations of the disease but also recognizing the emotional and social dimensions that are intertwined with it.

As we move forward, a collaborative effort between healthcare providers, researchers, and pharmaceutical companies will be pivotal in surmounting the challenges and seizing the opportunities that lie ahead. By doing so, we can continue to improve the lives of individuals affected by AD, offering them not only relief from physical discomfort but also the promise of a brighter, more fulfilling future.

REFERENCES

1. Paller A, Jaworski JC, Simpson EL, Boguniewicz M, Russell JJ, Block JK, et al. Major Comorbidities of Atopic Dermatitis: Beyond Allergic Disorders. Am J Clin Dermatol. 2018;19(6):821-38.
2. Giavina-Bianchi M, Giavina-Bianchi P. Systemic Treatment for Severe Atopic Dermatitis. Arch Immunol Ther Exp (Warsz). 2019;67(2):69-78.
3. Shirley M. Dupilumab: First Global Approval. Drugs. 2017;77(10):1115-21.
4. Harb H, Chatila TA. Mechanisms of Dupilumab. Clin Exp Allergy. 2020;50(1):5-14.
5. Beck LA, Thaçi D, Hamilton JD, Graham NM, Bieber T, Rocklin R, et al. Dupilumab treatment in adults with moderate-to-severe atopic dermatitis. N Engl J Med. 2014;371(2):130-9.
6. Regeneron Pharmaceuticals. (2016). Regeneron reports third quarter 2016 financial and operating results (media release). [online] Available from https://regeneronpharmaceuticalsinc.gcs-web.com/news-releases/news-release-details/regeneron-reports-third-quarter-2016-financial-and-operating [Last accessed January, 2024].
7. Regeneron Pharmaceuticals. (2017). Regeneron and Sanofi Announce FDA Approval of Dupixent® (Dupilumab), The First Targeted Biologic Therapy for Adults with Moderate-to-Severe Atopic Dermatitis (media release). [online] Available from https://investor.regeneron.com/news-releases/news-release-details/regeneron-and-sanofi-announce-fda-approval-dupixentr-dupilumab [Last accessed January, 2024].
8. Regeneron Pharmaceuticals. (2016). Regeneron and Sanofi Announce Marketing Authorization Application for Dupixent® (Dupilumab) Accepted for Review by the EMA (media release). [online] Available from https://newsroom.regeneron.com/news-releases/news-release-details/regeneron-and-sanofi-announce-marketing-authorization [Last accessed January, 2024].
9. van der Schaft J, Thijs JL, de Bruin-Weller MS, Balak DMW. Dupilumab after the 2017 approval for the treatment of atopic dermatitis: what's new and what's next? Curr Opin Allergy Clin Immunol. 2019;19(4):341-9.
10. Ly K, Smith MP, Thibodeaux Q, Beck K, Bhutani T, Liao W. Dupilumab in patients with chronic hepatitis B on concomitant entecavir. JAAD case reports. 2019;5(7):624-6.

11. Li Z, Radin A, Li M, Hamilton JD, Kajiwara M, Davis JD, et al. Pharmacokinetics, Pharmacodynamics, Safety, and Tolerability of Dupilumab in Healthy Adult Subjects. Clin Pharmacol Drug Dev. 2020;9(6):742-55.
12. D'Ippolito D, Pisano M. Dupilumab (Dupixent): An Interleukin-4 Receptor Antagonist for Atopic Dermatitis. P T. 2018;43(9):532-5.
13. Nutten S. Atopic Dermatitis: Global Epidemiology and Risk Factors. Ann Nutr Metab. 2015;66(Suppl. 1):8-16.
14. Dhar S, De A, Srinivas SM. Real-World Effectiveness and Safety of Dupilumab for the Treatment of Moderate to Severe Atopic Dermatitis in Indian Patients: A Multi Centric Retrospective Study. Indian J Dermatol. 2021;66(3):297-301.
15. Cork MJ, Thaçi D, Eichenfield LF, Arkwright PD, Sun X, Chen Z, et al. Dupilumab provides favourable long-term safety and efficacy in children aged ≥6 to <12 years with uncontrolled severe atopic dermatitis: results from an open-label phase IIa study and subsequent phase III open-label extension study. Br J Dermatol. 2021;184(5):857-70.
16. Simpson EL, Bieber T, Guttman-Yassky E, Beck LA, Blauvelt A, Cork MJ, et al. SOLO 1 and SOLO 2 Investigators. Two Phase 3 Trials of Dupilumab versus Placebo in Atopic Dermatitis. N Engl J Med. 2016;375(24):2335-48.
17. Paller AS, Simpson EL, Siegfried EC, Cork MJ, Wollenberg A, Arkwright PD, et al. Dupilumab in children aged 6 months to younger than 6 years with uncontrolled atopic dermatitis: A randomised, double-blind, placebo-controlled, phase 3 trial. Lancet. 2022;400(10356):908-19.
18. Wang FP, Tang XJ, Wei CQ, Xu LR, Mao H, Luo FM. Dupilumab treatment in moderate-to-severe atopic dermatitis: A systematic review and meta-analysis. J Dermatol Sci. 2018;90(2):190-8.
19. Siegfried EC, Cork MJ, Katoh N, Zhang H, Chuang CC, Thomas RB, et al. Dupilumab Provides Clinically Meaningful Responses in Children Aged 6-11 Years with Severe Atopic Dermatitis: Post Hoc Analysis Results from a Phase III Trial. Am J Clin Dermatol. 2023;24(5):787-98.
20. Cather J, Young M, DiRuggiero DC, Tofte S, Williams L, Gonzalez T. A Review of Phase 3 Trials of Dupilumab for the Treatment of Atopic Dermatitis in Adults, Adolescents, and Children Aged 6 and Up. Dermatol Ther (Heidelb). 2022;12(9):2013-38.
21. Wang Y, Shen C, Liu D, Yang L, Huang C, Tao J. Dupilumab Improves Clinical Scores in Pediatric Patients Aged 2 to <18 Years with Uncontrolled Atopic Dermatitis: A Single-Center, Real-World Study. Dermatol Ther. 2023;2023:5626410.
22. Yamamoto M, Kawase Y, Nakajima E, Matsuura Y, Akita W, Aoki R, et al. Exacerbation of IgA nephropathy in a patient receiving dupilumab. JAAD Case Rep. 2022;21:150-3.
23. Muzumdar S, Skudalski L, Sharp K, Waldman RA. Dupilumab Facial Redness/Dupilumab Facial Dermatitis: A Guide for Clinicians. Am J Clin Dermatol. 2022;23(1):61-7.
24. Kage P, Simon JC, Treudler R. A case of atopic eczema treated safely with dupilumab during pregnancy and lactation. J Eur Acad Dermatol Venereol. 2020;34:e256-e257.
25. Treudler R, Kage P, Simon JC. A case of atopic eczema treated safely with dupilumab during pregnancy and lactation. Allergy. 2020;75(Suppl 109):432.
26. Tsianakas A, Luger TA, Radin A. Dupilumab treatment improves quality of life in adult patients with moderate-to-severe atopic dermatitis: results from a randomized, placebo-controlled clinical trial. Br J Dermatol. 2018;178(2):406-14.
27. Gisondi P, Maurelli M, Costanzo A, Esposito M, Girolomoni G. The Combination of Dupilumab with Other Monoclonal Antibodies. Dermatol Ther (Heidelb). 2023;13(1):7-12.
28. Sanofi. (2023). Dupixent® (dupilumab) is now approved in India for the treatment of adults with moderate-to-severe atopic dermatitis. [online] Available from https://www.sanofi.in/dam/jcr:2bee5e28-ca06-4dc9-9e7c-9b52d82b3323/Dupixent%C2%AE-moderate-to-severe.pdf [Last accessed January, 2024]

CHAPTER 18

Newer Biologics in the Management of Atopic Dermatitis

Disha Chakraborty, Abhishek De

INTRODUCTION

Atopic dermatitis (AD) is a T cell-mediated disorder of unknown etiology that occurs in individuals with genetic predisposition. It has a chronic course with remission and relapses. It has a complicated pathophysiological profile and is linked to a number of causes. Its clinical manifestation varies widely in terms of the signs and symptoms as well as the age of presentation. It is marked by severe itching and dry skin, which reflects a change in barrier performance and immune system dysfunction. There is mainly type 2 helper T cell (Th2)-mediated dysfunction although other pathways like Th17, Th22, and Th1 may also be involved.[1]

Atopic dermatitis is triggered by environmental factors in those who are genetically predisposed. Whether AD is a disease that is pathogenically conditioned by a change in barrier function and that leads to an insufficient immune response or, primarily an immune dysfunction that also ends up changing barrier function, has been the subject of debate for decades. However, the observed clinical variability prohibits us from completely excluding the possibility that both triggers may play a separate and synergistic role in certain patient profiles and subpopulations. In this sense, AD is now viewed as an imbalance between Th1- and Th2-type inflammatory responses, with a predominance of the Th2/Th22 response in both acute and chronic forms, as well as participation from the Th17 pathway and a contribution from the Th1 axis, especially in its more chronic forms. This hypothesis is oversimplified, and depending on the clinical profile, additional inflammatory pathways may contribute considerably.[1,2]

RATIONALE FOR BIOLOGIC THERAPY IN ATOPIC DERMATITIS

Ineffectiveness of Conventional Therapy

Traditional treatments, such as calcineurin inhibitors and topical corticosteroids (TCS), target inflammation and symptom relief. Despite the fact that they can be helpful for mild to moderate AD, long-term use is linked to a risk of systemic absorption, striae formation, and skin thinning, particularly in young patients. Systemic immunosuppressants, such as cyclosporine and methotrexate, are only used in severe cases because of systemic toxicity, the necessity for ongoing monitoring, and the risk of relapse after stopping treatment.[3]

Biologics as Precision Medicine

Through the targeting of particular immune response components, biologic treatments present a promising avenue for the treatment of AD. Since they are intended to be more targeted and selective, they pose less of a threat of systemic adverse effects. In biologics, the main cytokines and pathways involved in the pathophysiology of AD are targeted. Drugs like tralokinumab, lebrikizumab, and nemolizumab, for example, specifically target interleukin 4 (IL-4), IL-13, and IL-31, respectively, with the goal of preventing the inflammatory cascade that leads to AD.[4]

Potential Benefits of Biologics in Terms of Efficacy, Safety, Maintenance of Skin Barrier, and Reduction in Topical Steroid Dependency

Biologics can considerably reduce pruritus, the degree of dermatitis, and improve quality of life in AD patients. Patients with moderate to severe disease who have not responded well to prior therapies are a candidate for biologic therapy. Biologics are generally well tolerated and have a lower risk of systemic side effects. They are appropriate for both adults and children with severe AD, because they provide a longer term therapy alternative that is safer overall. Biologics may assist in restoring the skin barrier function by lowering inflammation and modifying immunological responses, addressing one of the core issues with AD. They reduce the requirement for long-term application of topical steroids, which would reduce the risk of steroid-related side effects.[5]

    The purpose of this chapter is to give a thorough overview of the biologics in the treatment of AD, except dupilumab as it has been covered in a separate chapter. Biologics have become a potential and revolutionary class of drugs as dermatologists look for new ways to treat the complex nature of AD. The purpose of this chapter is to discuss mechanisms of action, clinical effectiveness, and practical issues related to the use of biologics in AD. We

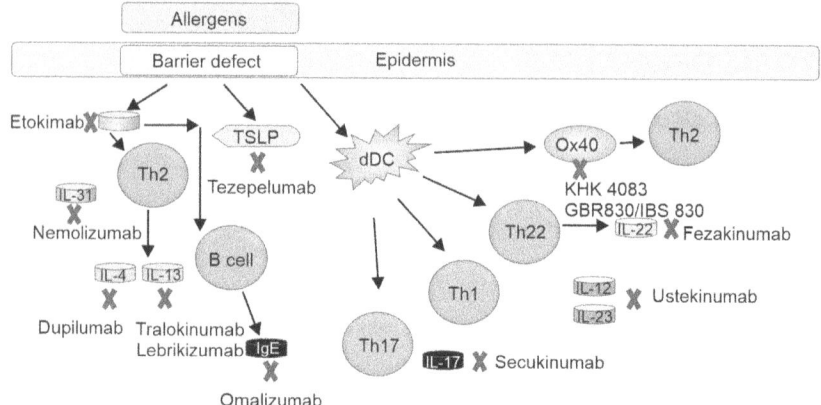

FIG. 1: Possible sites of action in atopic dermatitis.
(IgE: immunoglobulin E; IL: interleukin; Th2: type 2 helper T cell; TSLP: thymic stromal lymphopoietin)

aim to provide readers with a background on changing landscape of AD treatment by going into the nuances of approved biologics like tralokinumab, lebrikizumab, and nemolizumab, as well as highlighting upcoming biologics. Possible sites at which biologics might act in AD have been mentioned in **Figure 1**.

SELECTIVE INTERLEUKIN-13 INHIBITORS

The development of medications that target IL-13 may maximize therapeutic efficacy while minimizing side effects as it is a key mediator in the pathophysiology of AD. This has led to the development of new targeted therapies, such as the selective IL-13 inhibitors *lebrikizumab and tralokinumab*.

Tralokinumab

Since 2021, both the United States Food and Drug Administration (FDA) and the European Union have approved tralokinumab, a completely humanized immunoglobulin G4 (IgG4) monoclonal antibody (mAb) that targets IL-13 for the treatment of moderate-to-severe AD.[6]

Mechanism of Action

Tralokinumab competitively inhibits the binding of IL-13 to two distinct receptors, interleukin 13 receptor alpha 1 (IL-13Rα1) and IL-13Rα2, which act as a decoy receptor to regulate IL-13 in the body.[7]

Dosage, Forms, and Administration

An initial dose of 600 mg [four 150 mg subcutaneous (SC) injections] of tralokinumab (ADBRY) is advised, followed by 300 mg (two 150 mg injections) given every other week. Patients under 100 kg who get clear or nearly clear skin after 16 weeks of treatment may be given a dose of 300 mg every 4 weeks.[8]

Injection: 150 mg/mL solution in a single-dose prefilled syringe with a needle guard.[7,8]

Warning, Precautions, and Contraindications
- *Hypersensitivity*: Anaphylaxis and angioedema have been reported following the use of tralokinumab.
- Conjunctivitis and keratitis
- *Parasitic (helminth) infections*: Before beginning treatment, individuals who already have helminth infections must be treated.
- Live vaccines should be avoided because of the risk of infection.

Adverse Reactions
Upper respiratory tract infections, conjunctivitis, injection-site responses, and eosinophilia are the most frequent adverse effects (incidence < 1%).

Concomitant Topical Therapies
Tralokinumab can be combined with TCS. It is possible to use topical calcineurin inhibitors (TCIs), but they should only be applied to problematic locations, such as the face, neck, intertriginous, and vaginal regions.[8,9]

Missed Doses
The missed dose should be administered as soon as possible and then the regular dosing can be continued thereafter in scheduled time.[8,9]

Preparation for Use
Prefilled syringes may be kept at room temperature up to 25°C (77°F) after being removed from the refrigerator, but they must be used within 14 days or discarded. Before injection, tralokinumab-prefilled syringes must be removed from the refrigerator and allowed to reach room temperature (30 minutes for the 150 mg/mL prefilled syringes).

Before using the drug, it should be visually checked for impurities and color changes. The injection is a colorless to light yellow, transparent to opalescent solution. If the liquid is hazy, discolored, or visible particulate matter (other than clear to opalescent, colorless to pale yellow), it should not be used. Because tralokinumab does not include preservatives, any unused product should be thrown away.[8,9]

Pharmacokinetics
Tralokinumab concentrations at steady-state were attained after 16 weeks of treatment with a 600 mg beginning dose and 300 mg every 2 weeks. Tralokinumab has an absolute bioavailability of about 76%. After dosing, it takes 5-8 days for it to reach its peak (Tmax). Tralokinumab has a 3-week half-life.[9]

Pharmacodynamics

Blood levels of Th2 and Th22 immune indicators, such as lactate dehydrogenase (LDH) and serum immunoglobulin E (IgE), as well as periostin, IL-22, and thymus and activation-regulated chemokine (TARC/CCL17), were found to be lower in people on tralokinumab. In AD skin, the drug enhanced the protein expression of loricrin while downregulating the expression of keratin 16 and Ki-67. In lesional skin, it reduced the expression of genes involved in the Th2 pathway, including as CCL17, CCL18, and CCL26, as well as indicators of genes regulated by Th17 and Th22. It is unclear how clinically significant these biomarkers are.[9]

Results of Clinical Trials

Three randomized, double-blind, placebo-controlled trials [ECZema TRAlokinumab trial no. 1 (ECZTRA 1) (NCT03131648), ECZTRA 2 (NCT03160885), and ECZTRA 3 (NCT03363854)] were used to evaluate the effectiveness of tralokinumab. A total of 1,934 patients aged 18 and older with moderate-to-severe AD that had not been sufficiently managed by topical medication(s) were included. The severity of the disease was determined by the following criteria: An Eczema Area and Severity Index (EASI) score of 16 on a scale of 0 to 72; an Investigator's Global Assessment (IGA) score of 3; and a minimum body surface area (BSA) involvement of 10%. At baseline, 50% of individuals had an IGA score of 3 (moderate AD), 50% had an IGA score of 4 (severe AD), and 58% of subjects were male and 69% of subjects were white. The baseline weekly averaged Worst Daily Pruritus Numeric Rating Scale (NRS) was 8 on a scale from 0 to 10, while the baseline mean EASI score was 32. In all three trials, participants were given SC injections of tralokinumab at a dose of 600 mg on day 0 and 300 mg every other week for a total of 16 weeks. IGA 0 or 1 ("clear" or "almost clear") or EASI-75 ("improvement of at least 75% in EASI score from baseline") were used to classify respondents at the end of the study, i.e., week 16.[10]

Subjects responding to initial treatment with 300 mg every other week were re-randomized to receive 300 mg every other week and 300 mg every 4 weeks, or placebo every other week for another 36 weeks following first-dose administration in order to assess maintenance of response in the monotherapy trials (ECZTRA 1 and ECZTRA 2). For a further 36 weeks, subjects who first received a placebo and saw a clinical response by week 16 received placebo every other week. Subjects on open-label treatment with 300 mg every other week and optional TCS use were those who did not respond at week 16 and those who lost clinical response throughout the maintenance period.[10]

The ECZTRA 3 trial randomized patients to receive tralokinumab 300 mg on alternate weeks with TCS or placebo with TCS and topical TCI as per requirement till week 16. Patients in the tralokinumab 300 mg with TCS group who showed a clinical response at week 16 were re-randomized to receive the drug every other week or every 4 weeks for 16 weeks after the initial dosage. Patients in the placebo with TCS group who showed clinical improvement at week 16 continued for an additional 16 weeks. Subjects, who did not show clinical response at week 16 got 300 mg of tralokinumab every other week for 16 weeks. A mid-potency TCS (mometasone furoate 0.1% cream) was administered at each visit. Patients were directed to apply a thin film of TCS daily to active lesions from week 0 to week 32 and stop treatment when control was established. The investigator utilized a lesser potency TCS or TCI in regions with thin skin where the supplied TCS is not recommended.[11]

All three trials measured the percentage of individuals with IGA 0 or 1 at week 16 and the percentage with EASI-75 at week 16. Secondary endpoints saw a minimum 4-point decrease in Worst Daily Pruritus NRS (weekly average) from baseline to week 16 on the 11-point itch NRS.

In the three pivotal studies, a higher percentage of participants in the tralokinumab 300 mg every other week arm than in the placebo arm attained EASI-90.[10,11]

Table 1 summarizes the results of these trials.

TABLE 1: Summary of results of various trials.						
	ECZTRA 1		ECZTRA 2		ECZTRA 3	
	ADBRY 300 mg every other week	Placebo	ADBRY 300 mg every other week	Placebo	ADBRY 300 mg every other week + TCS	Placebo + TCS
Number of subjects randomized and dosed	60	197	577	193	243	123
IGA 0 or 1	16%	7%	21%	9%	38%	27%
• EASI-75 • Difference from placebo (95% CI)	25%	13%	33%	10%	56%	37%
• Number of subjects with baseline • Worst Daily Pruritus NRS (weekly average) score ≥4	594	194	563	192	240	123
Worst Daily Pruritus NRS (≥4 point reduction)	20%	10%	25%	9%	46%	35%

(CI: confidence interval; EASI: Eczema Area and Severity Index; ECZTRA 1: ECZema TRAlokinumab trial no. 1; IGA: Investigator's Global Assessment; NRS: Numeric Rating Scale; TCS: topical corticosteroids)

Lebrikizumab

Mechanism of Action
A humanized IgG4 mAb called lebrikizumab binds to soluble IL-13 with high affinity to an epitope that does not interfere with its binding to the receptor but instead hinders IL-4R/IL-13Rα1 heterodimerization, hence inhibiting downstream signaling. Lebrikizumab, unlike tralokinumab, allows IL-13 to continue to bind to the IL-13Rα2 decoy receptor, maintaining the hypothesized endogenous regulation mechanism.[12]

Pharmacology
The first treatment with lebrikizumab was for asthma. Lebrikizumab's pharmacokinetics were examined in a meta-analysis of more than 2,000 individuals who received it for moderate-to-severe asthma. Lebrikizumab is injected subcutaneously and has consistently demonstrated linear dose-proportional pharmacokinetics, high bioavailability (estimated at 85%), and a half-life of 19–26 days.[13]

Clinical Efficacy as per Trials
Phase II Trials
TREBLE trial (NCT02340234) was a randomized, placebo-controlled, double-blind, phase IIa (proof of concept) multicenter study that assessed lebrikizumab's efficacy and safety as an add-on therapy to TCS in individuals with moderate-to-severe AD. Patients ($n = 209$) aged 18–75 with moderate-to-severe AD (EASI ≥ 14, IGA ≥ 3, BSA ≥ 10%, and visual analog scale for pruritus ≥ 3) inadequately controlled with TCS and emollients were randomly assigned (1) lebrikizumab 125 mg single dose at baseline, (2) lebrikizumab 250 mg single dose at baseline.[13]

To prevent study dropouts, all patients received medium-potency TCS twice daily. The primary endpoint, a 50% reduction in EASI score (EASI 50) from baseline to week 12, was achieved by 82.4% of lebrikizumab 125 mg Q4W patients compared to 62.3% of placebo patients ($p = 0.026$). Single-dose groups did not respond. The 125 mg Q4W group also had more patients achieving secondary endpoints, including an EASI 75 response (54.9% vs. 34.0% placebo; $p = 0.036$), a 50% SCORAD (SCORing Atopic Dermatitis) reduction (SCORAD 50; 51.0% vs. 26.4% placebo; $p = 0.012$), and an IGA score of 0 (clear) or 1 (almost clear; 33.3% vs. 18.9% placebo; $p = 0.098$).[13]

A phase IIb randomized, placebo-controlled, double-blind, dose-ranging clinical trial (NCT03443024) examined lebrikizumab's efficacy, dose–response, and safety. In a 3:3:3:2 ratio, 280 adult patients with chronic moderate-to-severe AD (defined as EASI ≥ 16, IGA ≥ 3, and affected BSA ≥ 10%) who were not controlled by standard topical treatment were randomized into four arms: (1) Lebrikizumab loading dose (LD) of 250 mg, followed by 125 mg Q4W; (2) 500 mg LD, followed by 250 mg Q4W; (3) 500 mg LD at baseline and week 2, followed by 250 mg Q2W; and (4) placebo Q2W.

Lebrikizumab was evaluated as monotherapy in that trial, with TCS being allowed as per requirement. Compared to placebo, all lebrikizumab groups showed significant dose-dependent changes in EASI score from baseline to week 16 [−62.3% ($p = 0.02$) in 125 mg Q4W, −69.2% ($p = 0.002$) in 250 mg Q4W, and −72.1% ($p < 0.001$) in 250 mg Q2W]. Lebrikizumab 250 mg groups' secondary endpoint response rates were also significantly higher, including IGA 0/1, EASI 50, 75, and 90.[14]

By week 4, placebo and lebrikizumab groups differed dose-dependently. Lebrikizumab improved pruritus NRS scores in all groups (−35.9% in 125 mg Q4W, −49.6% in 250 mg Q4W, and −60.6% in 250 mg Q2W) compared to placebo (mean worsening of 4.3%). The high-dose group showed a minimum 4-point reduction in NRS score as early as day 2 (15.3% vs. 4.3% in placebo group). In placebo-treated patients, rescue TCS use was threefold higher, sooner, and longer than in lebrikizumab-treated individuals. TCS use does not appear to confound study results.[14]

Phase III Trials

Phase III studies for lebrikizumab consist of five important international studies, including two pivotal duplicate monotherapy studies (ADvocate 1 and 2), a combination trial (ADhere), a long-term extension study (ADjoin), and pediatric studies.

The pivotal studies ADvocate 1 (NCT04146363) and ADvocate 2 (NCT04178967) are randomized, double-blind, placebo-controlled, parallel-group phase III trials evaluating lebrikizumab as monotherapy in moderate-to-severe AD patients (12 years or older, weighing at least 40 kg) with an EASI ≥ 16, IGA ≥ 3, and affected BSA ≥ 10%. The induction period lasts 16 weeks, followed by a 36-week maintenance period.[15]

In the induction phase, patients ($n = 424$ in ADvocate 1 and $n = 427$ in ADvocate 2) were randomized 2:1 to receive 500 mg of lebrikizumab at baseline and week 2 and 250 mg Q2W from weeks 4–14, or placebo Q2W. TCS might be used as rescue therapy, but lebrikizumab was stopped if systemic therapy was needed. Lebrikizumab improved the primary outcome response, defined as an IGA score of 0 or 1 with a 2-point reduction from baseline at week 16, in 43% of ADvocate 1 and 33% of ADvocate 2, compared to 13% and 11%, respectively.

Lebrikizumab treatment led to significant improvements in skin clearance, pruritus, and itch interference on sleep and quality of life, as measured by secondary efficacy endpoints (EASI 75, EASI 90, pruritus NRS ≥ 4 points improvement, Sleep-loss Scale Score ≥ 1 point improvement, and DLQI). Patients in the lebrikizumab group showed a higher EASI 75 response at week 16 (59% in ADvocate 1; 52% in ADvocate 2) compared to the placebo group (16% and 18%, respectively; $p < 0.001$). Both studies reached statistical significance for IGA 0/1, EASI 90, and pruritus NRS at week 4. Lebrikizumab improved pruritus NRS compared to placebo in week 2 of trial 1 (but not trial 2).[15]

Adverse Reactions as Reported in Clinical Trials

Lebrikizumab-treated individuals reported the same number of adverse events (AE) as placebo patients (67% vs. 66%) in the phase II TREBLE trial, including major AE, discontinuation rates, and overall infections. The median AE lasted 1–3 days and was mild to moderate. A dose–response relation was absent. Conjunctivitis occurred in 15 lebrikizumab patients (9.6%) and 4 placebo individuals (7.5%). In lebrikizumab-treated patients, herpetic infections and peripheral eosinophilia were rare (3.8% and 3.2%, respectively) and minor. All eosinophil-related episodes were asymptomatic.[16]

Lebrikizumab patients had a lower rate of AE in both ADvocate 1 (45%, placebo: 52%) and ADvocate 2 (53%, placebo: 66%) during the induction period, but there were no significant differences in AE-related discontinuation rates (1.4%) and placebo (1.7%). Lebrikizumab-treated individuals reported conjunctivitis more often than placebo (7.4% vs. 2.8% in trial 1; 7.5% vs. 2.1% in trial 2). However, lebrikizumab reduced skin infections (2.8% vs. 5.7% in trial 1 and 1.4% vs. 6.2% in trial 2).[13]

Over 52 weeks, 63% of lebrikizumab patients reported treatment-emergent side effects. In ADvocate 1 and 2, conjunctivitis (8%), nasopharyngitis (7% and 10%), headache (3% and 6%), herpes infection (5%), injection-site reactions (1.8% and 2.9%), and eosinophilia were the most prevalent AEs among lebrikizumab users.[13]

In ADhere, lebrikizumab + TCS caused 43% more AEs than placebo plus TCS (35%). Most were mild or moderate in nature and did not require therapy cessation. The most common AEs in lebrikizumab patients were headache (5%), conjunctivitis (5%), injection-site reactions (3%), herpes infection (3%) and hypertension (3%).[13]

NEW INVESTIGATIONAL INTERLEUKIN-13 BLOCKER

Different binding epitopes distinguish lebrikizumab and tralokinumab as selective IL-13 inhibitors. Cendakimab, another phase II IL-13 antibody, works similarly to tralokinumab. Lebrikizumab, unlike tralokinumab and cendakimab, blocks downstream signaling through the IL-4Rα/IL-13Rα1 heterodimeric receptor, allowing for potential neutralization of excessive IL-13 through the IL-13Rα2 decoy receptor. Lebrikizumab binds and inhibits IL-13 better than tralokinumab or cendakimab in vitro. Clinical efficacy consequences of these discrepancies are unclear.[17]

Combination of Lebrikizumab with Other Drugs

It can be tough to directly compare lebrikizumab with other targeted therapies such as dupilumab, tralokinumab, and Janus kinase (JAK) inhibitors, because no head-to-head studies have been conducted and because each study has a different design, duration, population size, participant selection process, and concurrent TCS use. Future research should compare the effectiveness and safety of lebrikizumab with these drugs in head-to-head studies and network meta-analyses.[18]

Nemolizumab

Interleukin 31, a proinflammatory cytokine, is known as a perpetrator of the itch-scratch cycle that leads to disruption of the skin barrier in AD through overexpression of IL-31 receptors on sensory nerves.[19]

Mechanism of Action

Nemolizumab is a humanized IgG2 mAb that acts by blocking the IL-31R.[19]

Approval

In Japan, nemolizumab (Mitchga) was initially approved in 2022 to treat severe AD in patients 13 years of age and older. Galderma received a Breakthrough Therapy designation from the United States FDA in 2019 to evaluate nemolizumab's potential to alleviate pruritus brought on by prurigo nodularis. Studies on safety and efficacy are currently being conducted.[20]

Dosage and Administration

Nemolizumab is subcutaneously administered. In Japan, it has been approved at a dose of a 60-mg SC injection to be given at intervals of 4 weeks for the treatment of AD.[21]

Pharmacokinetics

Sidbury et al. conducted a study to evaluate the pharmacokinetics, safety, efficacy, and biomarker profile on adolescents treated with nemolizumab for AD. At the end of treatment (week 16), nemolizumab was eliminated from the serum with an average half-life of 16.7 ± 4.1 days.[22]

Results of Clinical Trials

In a 16-week phase III trial, Japanese AD patients with moderate-to-severe pruritus and poor response to topical medicines and antihistamines were randomized to SC nemolizumab (60 mg) or placebo Q4W with topical medications. The primary endpoint was pruritus Visual Analog Scale (VAS) score mean percent change. At baseline, pruritus median VAS score was 75 and EASI score varied from 22.7 (placebo) to 24.2 (nemolizumab). The VAS score was decreased by 42.8% in the nemolizumab group and 21.4% in the placebo group at week 16 ($p < 0.001$). For the secondary effectiveness endpoints, including the change in EASI score and the time course of VAS score change for pruritus up to 4 weeks, no adjustments were made for multiple comparisons; hence, no clinical inferences can be drawn. The mean EASI score change was −45.9% with nemolizumab and −33.2% with placebo. A decrease in daily mean VAS score for pruritus was recorded as early as day 2 (−10.3% nemolizumab vs. −4.4% placebo) by day 15. Overall, nemolizumab was well tolerated with mild-to-moderate AEs. Nemolizumab caused more injection-site responses than placebo (8% vs. 3%).[23]

A phase IIb study on moderate-to-severe AD patients with severe AD-associated pruritus uncontrolled by topical therapies to 10 mg, 30 mg, or 90 mg SC nemolizumab Q4W or placebo until week 20, with a 12-week follow-up until week 32. Treatment and placebo groups used TCS and moisturizers. EASI scores at baseline were 24.2–25.9 for all nemolizumab groups and 27 for placebo. The 30 mg group demonstrated the greatest improvement in the primary endpoint (mean percentage change in baseline EASI at 24 weeks vs. placebo; −68.8% vs. −52.1%; $p = 0.016$). As early as week 1, all nemolizumab doses demonstrated significant reductions in peak pruritus NRS ($p < 0.05$), with the most effective response in the 30 mg treatment group (67.3% vs. 35.8% placebo at week 24, $p < 0.001$). Additionally, the 30 mg group outperformed placebo in secondary endpoints, such as EASI-50, EASI-75, and EASI-90 ($p < 0.05$).[24]

Adverse Events

The most frequent AEs associated with nemolizumab were nasopharyngitis, upper respiratory tract infection, and worsening of AD. Additionally, patients with a history of asthma experienced a dose-dependent rise in asthma-related incidents. Some of these incidents may have happened because nemolizumab-effective therapy enhanced activity levels and general well-being, which in turn exacerbated asthma symptoms. Every asthma-related incident was minor and controllable.[23,24]

Tezepelumab

Tezepelumab is a fully human IgGλ2 mAb-binding thymic stromal lymphopoietin (TSLP), an epidermal keratinocyte-derived cytokine that stimulates dendritic cells to produce type 2 cytokines like IL-4, IL-5, IL-13, and tumor necrosis factor (TNF). It causes pruritus in AD by stimulating cutaneous sensory neurons. Patients with acute or chronic AD have been observed to have an overexpression of TSLP in keratinocytes. Children with AD have also been found to have high serum levels of TSLP.[25]

Clinical Trials

Patients were randomized to receive either 280 mg of tezepelumab SC or a placebo Q2W with concurrent TCS in a phase IIa trial. However, at week 12, the primary endpoint, EASI-50 versus placebo, failed to attain statistical significance. Similar to this, at week 12, there was just a numerical difference between the two groups in terms of IGA response rates. Other secondary objectives, such as the EASI-75, EASI-90, SCORAD, and NRS scores at week 12, did not show statistically significant improvements in tezepelumab-treated individuals compared to placebo. Additionally, exploratory biomarker subgroup analysis did not reveal any significant changes. AEs were mild to severe and equivalent between groups. Except for injection-site erythema, the majority of AEs were not thought to be treatment related. Nasopharyngitis, upper respiratory tract infections, diarrhea, and headache were additional frequent AEs.[25,26] Tezepelumab has been approved for the treatment for severe asthma but not for AD.

ISB 830 (PREVIOUSLY KNOWN AS GBR 830)

ISB 830 is a humanized IgG1 anti-OX40 mAb. Antigen-presenting cells produce OX40L, which enhances effector T-cell responses. In a phase IIa trial, ISB 830 was tested for safety and efficacy in adults with moderate-to-severe AD with inadequate topical therapy. On day 1 (baseline) and day 29, patients were randomized in a 3:1 ratio to receive either 10 mg/kg intravenous (IV) ISB 830 or placebo. Biopsies were taken on days 1, 29, and 71. Treatment-emergent adverse events (TEAEs), baseline epidermal hyperplasia, and lesional biomarker gene expression were the primary objectives. SCORAD, IGA, BSA, and EASI percent improvement from baseline were secondary objectives. The study solely evaluated treatment group differences in primary endpoints. TEAEs were similar between treatment groups (63.0% vs. 63.0%) for ISB 830. Nasopharyngitis (8.7%) was the only treatment-related AE. Biomarker analysis showed a significant decrease in OX40+ T cells and OX40L+ dendritic cells in ISB 830-treated lesional skin. ISB 830 patients had a higher EASI-50 rate than placebo (76.9% vs. 37.5%). IGA responses were 23.1% in ISB 830-treated groups and 12.5% in placebo-treated participants at day 71. Two IV doses of ISB 830 given 4 weeks apart improved tissue and clinical assessments even 42 days later, suggesting it may offer a new treatment for moderate-to-severe AD. The drug is currently in phase IIb stage for AD.[27,28]

OTHER DRUGS USED FOR ATOPIC DERMATITIS WITH VARIABLE RESULTS

Anti-IL-17 Therapy for Atopic Dermatitis

In a phase I trial, MOR106, a mouse and human IgG1 anti-IL-17C mAb, demonstrated promising outcomes. At week 4, 83% of AD patients receiving MOR106 achieved the EASI-50, compared to 20% in the placebo group, and improvements persisted in the treatment group for the course of the subsequent 10 weeks. However, two phase II trials (NCT03568071 and NCT03864627) evaluating the safety, effectiveness, and tolerability of MOR106 in patients with moderate-to-severe AD were stopped early, because they did not show promising results in terms of their primary endpoints. The phase II trial for secukinumab, a human IgG1 anti-IL-17A mAb, just ended (NCT02594098), with no appreciable improvements in EASI or IGA scores. Another phase II trial (NCT03568136) testing secukinumab for moderate-to-severe AD just ended with undetermined results.[29,30]

Omalizumab and Ligelizumab

Omalizumab, a recombinant anti-IgE mAb, has shown mixed effectiveness in treating AD. In an AD systematic review and meta-analysis, fewer than 50% of patients treated with omalizumab showed significant clinical improvement (SCORAD-50, EASI-75, or IGA 0- or 2-point reduction). In a phase IV trial in children with severe AD, omalizumab dramatically reduced disease severity and topical steroid use. A 2013 phase II trial of ligelizumab (QGE031), a mAb with stronger IgE affinity than omalizumab, was completed without findings, suggesting lack of effectiveness in AD (NCT01552629).[31,32]

Fezakinumab—not Under Trial Currently

Fezakinumab is a human IgG1λ anti-IL-22 mAb. Th22 cells release IL-22, which causes epidermal hyperplasia and barrier abnormalities in AD patients. AD severity and treatment response are linked to IL-22 levels. A small study of 60 moderate-to-severe AD patients treated for 10 weeks with fezakinumab SC Q2W, with a primary goal at week 12 and a secondary endpoint at week 20, revealed clinical benefit in severe patients but not moderate patients. A follow-up mechanistic research found that patients with high IL-22 levels responded, while those with low levels did not and possibly even worsen. This study suggests molecular mechanisms-based adjusted medication according to a patient-specific genetic profile.[33]

FUTURE DIRECTIONS

Ongoing Research and Clinical Trials

Biologic therapy for AD is rapidly developing and evolving. In order to assess the effectiveness and safety of innovative biologics that target various components of the disease, many clinical trials are now being conducted. To improve treatment outcomes, researchers are looking into combination medicines and alternative routes including IL-22 and IL-17.

Personalized Medicine

The idea of individualized medicine is a promising future direction. Treatment choices may be influenced by genetic profiling, biomarker discovery, and other patient-specific characteristics, enabling more specialized and precise approaches to AD care.

Long-term Safety and Maintenance Therapy

It is critical to evaluate biologics in terms of long-term safety and efficacy as more patients receive prolonged biologic treatment. Studies examining the long-term advantages and hazards of biologic treatments will offer insightful data.

Use in Pediatric Population
Further research is needed to expand the use of biologics in pediatric patients. Understanding the safety and efficacy profiles of these drugs in children and adolescents will enhance treatment options for this vulnerable population.

CHALLENGES
Cost and Access
For many patients, the price of biologic medicines might be a barrier to access. It is a big problem to guarantee inexpensive and equal access to these medicines, particularly in healthcare systems with constrained resources.

Safety Concerns
Despite the generally positive safety profiles of biologics, continual care is required to track and handle any possible concerns, such as infections and cancer. Dermatologists need to be up to date on the most recent safety information and suggestions.

Patient Adherence
Since biologics frequently call for repeated injections or infusions, patient compliance can be difficult. Healthcare professionals must inform patients about the value of compliance and provide assistance to overcome any obstacles.

CONCLUSION
Biologic treatments have become a potential new area of research in the constantly changing therapy of AD. Recognizing biologics' potential to improve the lives of individuals with moderate to severe disease is crucial as we navigate the future of AD treatment. Clinical trials and ongoing research raise the possibility of new therapy alternatives and individualized strategies, but they also need strict safety oversight. To ensure that patients benefit from these ground-breaking medicines, problems like cost, access, and long-term safety must be addressed with creative solutions. Dermatologists and other medical professionals may deliver the best care and enhance the quality of life for people with AD by addressing these issues and being on the cutting edge of AD research. We may look forward to a time when biologic medicines are crucial to providing AD patients with long-lasting relief through sustained research, collaboration, and a patient-centered approach.

REFERENCES
1. Bieber T. Atopic dermatitis. Ann Dermatol. 2010;22(2):125-37.
2. Williams H, Flohr C. How epidemiology has challenged 3 prevailing concepts about atopic dermatitis. J Allergy Clin Immunol. 2006;118:209-13.

3. Huang A, Cho C, Leung DYM, Brar K. Atopic Dermatitis: Early Treatment in Children. Curr Treat Options Allergy. 2017;4(3):355-69.
4. Guttman-Yassky E, Dhingra N, Leung DY. New era of biologic therapeutics in atopic dermatitis. Expert Opin Biol Ther. 2013;13(4):549-61.
5. Del Rosso JQ, Cash K. Topical corticosteroid application and the structural and functional integrity of the epidermal barrier. J Clin Aesthet Dermatol. 2013;6(11):20-7.
6. Duggan S. Tralokinumab: First Approval. Drugs. 2021;81(14):1657-63.
7. Tollenaere MAX, Molck C, Henderson I, Pollack S, Addis P, Petersen HH, et al. Tralokinumab Effectively Disrupts the IL-13/IL-13Rα1/IL-4Rα Signaling Complex but not the IL-13/IL-13Rα2 Complex. JID Innov. 2023;3(5):100214.
8. Wollenberg A, Weidinger S, Worm M, Bieber T. Tralokinumab in atopic dermatitis. J Dtsch Dermatol Ges. 2021;19(10):1435-42.
9. Simpson EL, Guttman-Yassky E, Eichenfield LF, Boguniewicz M, Bieber T, Schneider S, et al. Tralokinumab therapy for moderate-to-severe atopic dermatitis: Clinical outcomes with targeted IL-13 inhibition. Allergy. 2023;78(11):2875-91.
10. Wollenberg A, Blauvelt A, Guttman-Yassky E, Worm M, Lynde C, Lacour JP, et al. ECZTRA 1 and ECZTRA 2 study investigators. Tralokinumab for moderate-to-severe atopic dermatitis: results from two 52-week, randomized, double-blind, multicentre, placebo-controlled phase III trials (ECZTRA 1 and ECZTRA 2). Br J Dermatol. 2021;184(3):437-49.
11. Silverberg JI, Adam DN, Zirwas M, Kalia S, Gutermuth J, Pinter A, et al. Tralokinumab Plus Topical Corticosteroids as Needed Provides Progressive and Sustained Efficacy in Adults with Moderate-to-Severe Atopic Dermatitis Over a 32-Week Period: An ECZTRA 3 Post Hoc Analysis. Am J Clin Dermatol. 2022;23(4):547-59.
12. Okragly AJ, Ryuzoji A, Wulur I, Daniels M, Van Horn RD, Patel CN, et al. Binding, Neutralization and Internalization of the Interleukin-13 Antibody, Lebrikizumab. Dermatol Ther (Heidelb). 2023;13(7):1535-47.
13. Bernardo D, Bieber T, Torres T. Lebrikizumab for the Treatment of Moderate-to-Severe Atopic Dermatitis. Am J Clin Dermatol. 2023;(5):753-64.
14. Guttman-Yassky E, Blauvelt A, Eichenfield LF, Paller AS, Armstrong AW, Drew J, et al. Efficacy and Safety of Lebrikizumab, a High-Affinity Interleukin 13 Inhibitor, in Adults with moderate to severe atopic dermatitis: A Phase 2b Randomized Clinical Trial. JAMA Dermatol. 2020;156(4):411-20.
15. Silverberg JI, Guttman-Yassky E, Thaçi D, Irvine AD, Stein Gold L, Blauvelt A, et al. ADvocate1 and ADvocate2 Investigators. Two Phase 3 Trials of Lebrikizumab for Moderate-to-Severe Atopic Dermatitis. N Engl J Med. 2023;388(12):1080-91.
16. Simpson EL, Flohr C, Eichenfield LF, Bieber T, Sofen H, Taïeb A, et al. Efficacy and safety of lebrikizumab (an anti-IL-13 monoclonal antibody) in adults with moderate-to-severe atopic dermatitis inadequately controlled by topical corticosteroids: a randomized, placebo-controlled phase II trial (TREBLE). J Am Acad Dermatol. 2018;78(5):863-71.e11.
17. A study to evaluate safety and effectiveness of cendakimab (CC-93538) in participants with moderate to severe atopic dermatitis (AD). [online] Available from https://ctv.veeva.com/study/a-study-to-evaluate-safety-and-effectiveness-of-cendakimab-cc-93538-in-participants-with-moderate [Last accessed January, 2024].
18. Gonçalves F, Freitas E, Torres T. Selective IL-13 inhibitors for the treatment of atopic dermatitis. Drugs Context. 2021;10:1-7.
19. Kabashima K, Matsumura T, Komazaki H, Kawashima M; Nemolizumab-JP01 Study Group. Nemolizumab Improves Patient-Reported Symptoms of Atopic Dermatitis with Pruritus: Post Hoc Analysis of a Japanese Phase III Randomized Controlled Trial. Dermatol Ther (Heidelb). 2023;13(4):997-1011.
20. Keam SJ. Nemolizumab: First Approval. Drugs. 2022;10(10):1143-50.
21. Kabashima K, Matsumura T, Komazaki H, Kawashima M; Nemolizumab JP01 andJP02 Study Group. Nemolizumab plus topical agents in patients with atopic dermatitis

(AD) and moderate-to-severe pruritus provide improvement in pruritus and signs of AD for up to 68 weeks: results from two phase III, long-term studies. Br J Dermatol. 2022;186(4):642-51.
22. Sidbury R, Alpizar S, Laquer V, Dhawan S, Abramovits W, Loprete L, et al. Pharmacokinetics, Safety, Efficacy, and Biomarker Profiles During Nemolizumab Treatment of Atopic Dermatitis in Adolescents. Dermatol Ther (Heidelb). 2022;12(3):631-42.
23. Kabashima K, Matsumura T, Komazaki H, Kawashima M; Nemolizumab-JP01 Study Group. Trial of Nemolizumab and Topical Agents for Atopic Dermatitis with Pruritus. N Engl J Med. 2020;383(2):141-50.
24. Silverberg JI, Pinter A, Pulka G, Poulin Y, Bouaziz JD, Wollenberg A, et al. Phase 2B randomized study of nemolizumab in adults with moderate-to-severe atopic dermatitis and severe pruritus. J Allergy Clin Immunol. 2020;145(1):173-82.
25. Simpson EL, Parnes JR, She D, Crouch S, Rees W, Mo M, et al. Tezepelumab, an anti-thymic stromal lymphopoietin monoclonal antibody, in the treatment of moderate to severe atopic dermatitis: A randomized phase 2a clinical trial. J Am Acad Dermatol. 2019;80(4):1013-21.
26. Indra AK. Epidermal TSLP: a trigger factor for pathogenesis of atopic dermatitis. Expert Rev Proteomics. 2013;10(4):309-11.
27. Guttman-Yassky E, Pavel AB, Zhou L, Estrada YD, Zhang N, Xu H, et al. GBR 830, an anti-OX40, improves skin gene signatures and clinical scores in patients with atopic dermatitis. J Allergy Clin Immunol. 2019;144(2):482-93.e7.
28. Webb GJ, Hirschfield GM, Lane PJ. OX40, OX40L and Autoimmunity: a Comprehensive Review. Clin Rev Allergy Immunol. 2016;50(3):312-32.
29. Galapagos NV, MorphoSys AG. MorphoSys and Galapagos Present Results from a Phase 1 Study with MOR106 in Atopic Dermatitis as Late-Breaking Abstract at the American Academy of Dermatology (AAD) Meeting in San Diego (news with additional features). [online] Available from https://www.morphosys.com/en/news/morphosys-and-galapagos-present-results-phase-1-study-mor106-atopic-dermatitis-late-breaking [Last accessed January, 2024].
30. Galapagos NV, MorphoSys AG. MOR106 Clinical Development in Atopic Dermatitis Stopped (news with additional features). [online] Available from https://www.morphosys.com/en/news/morphosys-ag-mor106-clinical-development-atopic-dermatitis-stopped-news-additional-features [Last accessed January, 2024].
31. Wang HH, Li YC, Huang YC. Efficacy of omalizumab in patients with atopic dermatitis: A systematic review and meta-analysis. J Allergy Clin Immunol. 2016;138(6):1719-22.
32. Chan S, Cornelius V, Cro S, Harper JI, Lack G. Treatment Effect of Omalizumab on Severe Pediatric Atopic Dermatitis: The ADAPT Randomized Clinical Trial. JAMA pediatrics. 2019;174(1):29-37.
33. Guttman-Yassky E, Brunner PM, Neumann AU, Khattri S, Pavel AB, Malik K, et al. Efficacy and safety of fezakinumab (an IL-22 monoclonal antibody) in adults with moderate-to-severe atopic dermatitis inadequately controlled by conventional treatments: A randomized, double-blind, phase 2a trial. J Am Acad Dermatol. 2018;78(5):872-81.

SECTION 6

Biologic Approach to Management of Various Diseases

CHAPTER 19

Psoriasis

*Murlidhar Rajagopalan, Shekhar Neema,
Ankan Gupta, Manish Khandare, Manas Chatterjee*

INTRODUCTION

Psoriasis is a common disease affecting approximately 2-3% of general population. Approximately 30-40% of affected individuals require systemic therapy. Choice of systemic therapy depends on factors, such as availability, affordability, comorbidities, ease of administration, tolerability, rapidity of response desired, adverse effect profile, and previous treatment administered and comfort level of the physician with the available treatment. The advent of biological therapy in psoriasis has increased our armamentarium in management of psoriasis and they yield a more targeted therapy, result in rapid improvement, and are associated with less adverse effects in comparison to the conventional systemic therapy. This chapter will deal with the practical aspects of choosing a biologic in a psoriasis patient reporting to the outpatient department (OPD). Also, an algorithm on what all investigations are required before initiating a patient on biologics will be briefly discussed here. The discussion is based on available literature and the clinical experience of the authors. The focus on chapter is on biologics available in our country so that the information is practically useful.

There are three scenarios in which one needs to initiate biologics:

Scenario 1: These are the most common presentations where a physician thinks about initiating biologics.
- Failure, intolerance, or toxicity of conventional systemic therapy
- Comorbidities precluding use of conventional therapy
- Comorbidities like psoriatic arthritis
- When rapid control is desired because of social or economic pressure—this is especially when psoriasis affects high impact areas. This could include the face, palms, soles, and genitals.

Scenario 2: As a first-line therapy, especially when rapid control and complete clearance are desirable and there are no financial constraints. This could depend on the patient's choice too as some patients do want a faster clearance. Studies have shown that most patients who are treated for psoriasis are not very happy with the treatment approach when complete clearance is not achieved. It is not practical to expect a patient to be philosophical about his disease, especially when he himself suffers and the disease, through comorbidities, could affect his lifespan, mental, and social health.

Scenario 3: When patient has failed the conventional systemic therapy. This happens when patients are indefinitely on conventional therapy and patient stops responding to conventional therapy. One must be compassionate and not lead a patient to believe that being on a biological leads to cure of the disease. The cure has not been demonstrated with any therapy for psoriasis so far.

SYSTEMIC THERAPY IN PSORIASIS[1]

Systemic therapy in psoriasis should be initiated when topical therapy and phototherapy has failed. Indications to start systemic therapy are:
- Psoriasis Area and Severity Index (PASI) >10, Dermatology Life Quality Index (DLQI) >10, and body surface area >10%
- Involvement of high impact sites, such as palm, soles, nails, and genitalia
- Associated psoriatic arthritis
- Significant cosmetic or psychosocial impact

This supposes that we are treating severe psoriasis. However, the definition of moderate psoriasis is in flux today with a lot of discussion going on about what is moderate disease and how do we really classify moderate disease. A linking of disease extent to the quality-of-life score seems to be a better method to decide on when to escalate therapy for a psoriasis patient.

WHEN TO START BIOLOGICALS?

To answer the first question, when to start biologic therapy in a patient who presents to us with severe psoriasis, most of the current literature complies with the fact that biologicals should be used when conventional therapy fails. However, biologics may be offered as first-line therapy, if the clinical situation demands. Some examples have been stated above. People who fulfill the disease severity criteria have disease at high impact site, failure of conventional therapy, or toxicity resulting from conventional systemic therapy should be offered biologic therapy. Patient with large impact on social functioning should be offered biologic therapy if their disease is not well controlled with conventional therapy.[2]

Scenario 1: We will be discussing chronic plaque psoriasis in general. Other variants of psoriasis shall be dealt with separately.

Methotrexate is most commonly used systemic agent for management of psoriasis and often is first line for its management. It is started in the dose of 5–10 mg/week and dose can be escalated to maximum of 25 mg/week.

Limitations of methotrexate are gastrointestinal intolerance, hepatotoxicity in long-term use, and ineffectiveness in many cases. We should also understand that many methotrexate-naïve patients of psoriasis already have metabolic dysfunction-associated steatotic liver disease (MASLD); this makes use of methotrexate riskier. When on methotrexate, we do not have dependable algorithms to predict hepatic damage as normal enzyme levels do not always correlate with structural damage to the liver. Cyclosporine is another systemic option for management of psoriasis especially when rapid control of disease is desired. Cyclosporine is initiated in the dose of 2.5–3 mg/kg and increased up to 5 mg/kg in case of poor response after 4 weeks. Cyclosporine cannot be continued for more than a year at a time. Acitretin can also be used for management of plaque psoriasis. It is not very effective as monotherapy in 25 mg daily dose and associated with unacceptable mucocutaneous adverse effects with 50 mg daily dose. This drug takes time to act and the action is unpredictable. The patient who is prone for the metabolic syndrome due to psoriasis may well have his dyslipidemia unmasked once acitretin is started. There is a shortage of good studies to document what happens to the dyslipidemia once the acitretin is stopped. Apremilast is a phosphodiesterase-4 (PDE4) inhibitor and is used in the dose of 30 mg twice a day for the management of psoriasis. The drug is not very effective as a monotherapy. However, it has an important role in the management of moderate psoriasis since it does not require any monitoring and is not immunosuppressive. It can be used as maintenance therapy. Tofacitinib is approved for use in psoriatic arthritis; however, it is increasingly being used in the management of chronic plaque psoriasis due to ease of administration. It should only be used as second- or third-line therapy.

In case, where patient has not been able to tolerate conventional systemic therapy, developed unacceptable adverse effect like hepatotoxicity with methotrexate or did not respond to conventional systemic therapy; which biologic should be offered? The available biologics for management of psoriasis as of now in India are etanercept, infliximab, adalimumab, itolizumab, secukinumab, and ixekizumab. Spesolimab is an interleukin-36 (IL-36) inhibitor and is likely to be available in Indian markets soon. The specific indication for spesolimab is generalized pustular psoriasis (GPP) and it has been discussed in a separate chapter. Etanercept and infliximab are available both as originator and biosimilar molecule while adalimumab is available only as biosimilar. However, none of these molecules have been recognized by the United States Food and Drug Administration (US FDA) as a true biosimilar. Etanercept and infliximab are only intended biosimilar and it is incorrect to term their Indian versions as true biosimilars. Immunogenicity studies for these molecules are also lacking. Mechanism of action of various biologics and prebiologic investigations has been dealt in detail in separate chapters and we will only deal with the concept of administering biologic in this chapter.

Once patient is ready for biologic, the choice of biologic depends on many factors. The most important factor in our setting is economic as majority of our patients are self-financed and finally choice of biologic depends much more on economics than science. Notwithstanding these factors, we will try to understand why we choose one biologic over another in a particular scenario for benefit of the patient. Does it really make a difference or is it just a matter of familiarity with the particular drug? We have tried to deal with the matter of cost-effectiveness of various biologics in detail in a separate chapter and will not discuss that part here.

STEPS WHILE STARTING THE PATIENT ON A BIOLOGIC AGENT

1. Counseling patient about the need for biologic, economic impact, and understanding that despite being expensive therapy, it is not a cure for your disease.
2. *Pretreatment history and investigations*:
    a. History suggestive of multiple sclerosis, congestive cardiac failure, inflammatory bowel disease, or tuberculosis
    b. Complete blood count, urine examination, blood urea, serum creatinine, blood sugar fasting, and postprandial
    c. Liver function test, hepatitis B surface antigen, hepatitis B core total antibody, antihepatitis C virus, and immunoglobulin M (IgM)
    d. Chest X-ray, interferon gamma release assays (IGRAs) for latent tuberculosis (details in separate chapter).
3. Planning vaccination (details in separate chapter)
4. *Choosing biologic*:
    a. Rapidity of response desired
    b. Comorbidities
    c. Facilities available
5. Administering biologic
6. Follow-up

Choosing Biologic in Chronic Plaque Psoriasis

With the availability of multiple biologics and majority of the dermatology practice being an outpatient practice, use of infliximab for management of chronic plaque psoriasis is limited to institutions and in crisis situations. Both infliximab and itolizumab are given by infusion and require hospital visit or admission, which is a big hindrance for their use in daily practice. Infliximab is reserved for patients who require rapid control of disease or have failed other biologics and will be discussed somewhere else. So, the choice is between etanercept, adalimumab, secukinumab, and ixekizumab **(Table 1)**.

TABLE 1: Psoriasis Area and Severity Index (PASI) response of available biologics.

Drug	Dose	PASI-75	PASI-90	PASI-100	Remarks
Etanercept[3,4]	50 mg twice a week	49%	20.7%	4.3%	After 12 weeks
	25 mg twice a week	34%			
	25 mg once a week	14%			
Adalimumab[5]	80 mg day 0, 40 mg week 1 and every other week	71%	45%	20%	After 16 weeks (trial data for 12 weeks not available)
	40 mg every week	80%	–		After 12 weeks (PASI-90 and PASI-100 data not available in this study)
Infliximab[6]	300 mg 0–4 weeks and monthly	80%	57%		After 10 weeks
Secukinumab[3]	300 mg	77%	54%	24%	After 12 weeks
	160 mg week 0, 80 mg week 2, 4, 6, 8, 10, 12 and 80 mg thereafter	67%	42%	14%	
Ixekizumab[7]	160 mg	90%	72%	57%	After 16 weeks

These results are from trial data and include originator molecule. We should remember that clinical trial data do not mimic real life experience. The similar studies from biosimilars, biomimics, and intended copies are lacking and these issues have been discussed in detail in separate chapters. Real world experience differs from trial data in various ways because in real world majority of patients are not treatment naive and expect faster improvement because of cost involved in treatment as compared to trials where treatment is generally offered free of cost.

- When rapid control of skin disease is desired, IL-17 inhibitors, such as secukinumab and ixekizumab appear to be the best option. Real world experience suggests rapid and sustained clearance of disease even in therapy experienced patients. PASI-75 is achieved as early as 6 weeks of treatment.
- Adalimumab biosimilar is a cost-effective option for management of psoriasis. In case where patient can wait, it is an excellent choice because of its cost-effectiveness. It achieves clearance in reasonable number of patients.

- Etanercept in a standard dose of 50 mg twice a week appears to be more expensive than adalimumab, which is also administered subcutaneously. Adalimumab is more effective as compared to etanercept. Only benefit of using etanercept is its safety profile, it can be used in children and has been used in pregnant women and human immunodeficiency virus (HIV) patients. Etanercept can also be used as an add-on therapy when patient is not responding adequately to methotrexate. The risk of infections and tuberculosis is highest with infliximab and adalimumab.

Comorbidities

Psoriasis is a chronic disease and many of the patients with psoriasis have other comorbidities. The presence of comorbidities can alter the choice of biologic in a particular patient. Absolute and relative contraindications of various biologics have been discussed in detail in various chapters, here we shall discuss about how to approach patients with psoriasis using biologic in presence of these comorbidities **(Table 2)**.

Presence of other concomitant diseases, such as pyoderma gangrenosum, hidradenitis suppurativa, or inflammatory bowel disease which may benefit from treatment with the use of tumor necrosis factor alpha (anti-TNF-α) therapy and can reduce the threshold for using biologics. Biologic during pregnancy and lactation has been discussed in detail in separate chapter.

Choosing a Biologic: Based on the Facilities Available and Preferred Route of Administration

While it is a reasonable assumption that patient will prefer subcutaneous injections over infusions as patients need to come to hospital or daycare center to take infusion, there are studies which suggest that lot of patients prefer intravenous therapy over subcutaneous therapy because of reasons like interactions with staff during injection, dislike for self-injection, and less frequent injections.[17]

Most of the physicians prefer the use of subcutaneous route as these can be injected in a clinic-based setting and subsequent injections can be administered by the caregiver or patient himself. Schedule of treatment can also determine the choice of biologic. Ustekinumab requires injection once in 12 weeks for maintenance and has become first-line biologic therapy for management of plaque psoriasis in western world. Infliximab has dosing schedule of 0, 2, 6 weeks, and 8 weekly thereafter; however, it is given as infusion and most of the physicians do not prefer to use it for this indication. Etanercept has initial dosing of 50 mg twice a week or once a week for 12 weeks and patient or caregiver should be ready to learn to self-inject. Adalimumab has once in fortnightly maintenance dosing and secukinumab has once-in-a-month maintenance dosing; however, secukinumab requires weekly injections for initial 5 weeks as induction therapy. Ixekizumab needs to be administered every 2 weeks for the first 12 weeks and 4 weekly thereafter.

TABLE 2: Choice of biologic with comorbidities.		
Infection	How to screen?	What to do?
Tuberculosis:[8]		
Active tuberculosis	History, clinical examination, investigations such as chest X-ray and sputum for AFB	Initiate biologic after completion of therapy in consultation with the pulmonologist
Latent tuberculosis	• Screening with tuberculin skin test or IGRA (IGRA preferred) • Annual screening in patients on biologics	• Treat with INH monotherapy for 9 months or INH and rifampicin for 3 months—current recommendation is to avoid monotherapy and uses combination of INH and rifampicin for 2 months • Initiate or resume biologic after 1 month of therapy • Secukinumab, ixekizumab, and etanercept have lowest risk of reactivation of latent tuberculosis infection and are preferred biologic
Hepatitis B[9-11]	HbsAg, hepatitis B core antibody	• Secukinumab is the first choice as per expert opinion • Use of TNF-α inhibitor can lead to viral reactivation • Anti-TNF-α therapy can be used in combination with oral antivirals • Oral antivirals should be started 2–4 weeks before starting biologics • Frequent monitoring of LFT and viral load in consultation with the hepatologist • Data with ixekizumab is sparse
Hepatitis C[12,13]	Anti-hepatitis C virus, immunoglobulin M	• Etanercept used as a second-line therapy • Secukinumab is considered safe in patients with hepatitis C infection The data on ixekizumab is scant • Frequent monitoring of LFT and viral load in consultation with the hepatologist
HIV infection	HIV serology	• Etanercept preferred • Secukinumab has been used successfully in various case reports • In combination with antiretroviral, monitor CD4 count and viral load

Continued

Continued

Comorbidities	Screening	What to do?
Psoriatic arthropathy	History, examination, X-ray joints, ultrasound of tendo-Achilles, MRI—spine	• Adalimumab as first-line biologic therapy when psoriatic arthritis is predominant • Secukinumab or ixekizumab as first-line biologic therapy when psoriasis is more extensive • Secukinumab or ixekizumab when patient does not respond to TNF-α inhibitors
Multiple sclerosis	History, examination, and neurologist consultation	• IL-17 inhibitors preferred • Anti-TNF-α inhibitors contraindicated
Congestive heart failure	History, examination, 2D echocardiography, and cardiologist consultation	• IL-17 inhibitors preferred • New York Heart Association (NYHA) class I/II—anti-TNF-α therapy (with caution) recommended • NYHA class III/IV—IL-17 inhibitors recommended
Coronary artery disease	History and examination	Anti-TNF-α therapy preferred
Inflammatory bowel disease	History and examination	• Anti-TNF-α therapy—adalimumab and infliximab preferred • IL-17 inhibitors—contraindicated
Autoimmune diseases[14]	ANA and ANA profile	• Antinuclear antibodies may develop while patient is on infliximab • Anti-dsDNA and drug-induced lupus may develop rarely, but the severity of symptoms is not bad • Development of ANA is associated with treatment failure • Prospective studies are available in which ANA was determined before starting anti-TNF-α therapy and patients were followed up on treatment • Though development of drug-induced lupus in patient treated with anti-TNF-α therapy is rare, it is prudent to consider biologic therapy in this scenario with caution

Continued

Continued

Comorbidities	Screening	What to do?
Chronic liver disease of noninfectious etiology	Liver function test	• Pharmacokinetic data of biologics in presence of liver disease is not available • Various case reports of successful use of TNF-α inhibitors in presence of chronic liver disease exist • Etanercept or adalimumab preferred • Secukinumab or ixekizumab may also be used in compensated liver disease • Most TNF-α blockers can induce changes in liver enzymes and even worsening of liver disease • However, literature is scant
Chronic renal failure	Renal function test	• Metabolized by proteolysis • Etanercept preferred • *Caution*: Risk of infection
Cancer[15]		• Data is scant • Possible increase risk of recurrence of solid organ malignancy • Should be used with caution, avoid, if possible. Use when disease is in remission for 5 years or more
Obesity[16]		• Secukinumab or ixekizumab preferred • TNF-α inhibitors can be used, associated with mean weight gain of 1–4 kg • Use biologic with lifestyle modification • Weight reduction is associated with better efficacy of biologic therapy

(AFB: acid-fast bacillus; ANA: antinuclear antibody; HBsAg: hepatitis B virus surface antigen; HIV: human immunodeficiency virus; IGRA: interferon gamma release assay; INH: isoniazid; LFT: liver function test; MRI: magnetic resonance imaging; TNF-α: tumor necrosis factor alpha)

Thus, choosing a biologic not only depends on science of pathogenesis and targeted therapy of psoriasis but it also depends on numerous other factors, which requires consideration by physicians before prescribing biologic else best of the science can fail because of the circumstances.

Combination with Biologics

Biologics can be either used as monotherapy or can be combined with other form of systemic therapy. Combination therapy can enhance efficacy of treatment, decrease the side effects by allowing dose reductions, and increase the onset of remission. Combination therapy can be used in following settings:

- *Synergistic mechanism of action*:
    - Rescue therapy: Use of additional conventional systemic agent at the initiation of biologic therapy for <120 days
    - Bridging therapy: Initiation of conventional systemic therapy before starting biologic therapy and used concomitantly with biologics for <120 days
    - Concomitant therapy: Systemic therapy used for >120 days along with biologics
- *Rotational therapy*: Faster action of biologic and continued action of second drug can reduce cost of therapy
- *To reduce adverse effect of biologics*: Use of methotrexate for prevention of development of human antichimeric antibody while using infliximab

It is not possible to combine all forms of systemic therapy with biologics as it may lead to unacceptable immunosuppression in some cases. There are no approved indications for combining biologic with conventional systemic agents in psoriasis; however, in real world adding conventional systemic agents offers multiple advantages, such as better efficacy, improved pharmacoeconomics, and improved long-term disease management. We shall discuss briefly regarding the systemic therapies that can be combined safely with biologics in the scenarios given in **Table 3**.

TABLE 3: Systemic therapies combined with biologics.

Biologic therapy	Systemic therapy	Efficacy				Literature
		Baseline (biologic)		Combination		
		PASI-75	PASI-90	PASI-75	PASI-90	
Etanercept	Phototherapy (NBUVB)	55%	23%	85%	58%	Kircik et al.[18]

- Etanercept is used in dose of 50 mg twice weekly and NBUVB given thrice weekly
- 26% patients also achieved PASI-100
- Caution should be exercised as there is higher risk of development of cutaneous malignancy and combination should be limited to shortest period of time
- Phototherapy has been used with standard dosing of etanercept for faster clearance, reduced dosing of etanercept (50 mg weekly), or as rescue therapy in patients not responding adequately after 12 weeks of etanercept

Continued

Continued

	Methotrexate	55%	23%	70.2%	34%		Gottlieb AB[19]

- Methotrexate was used in the dose of 7.5–15 mg/week
- Patients who can tolerate and do not have any contraindications to the use of methotrexate should be given a combination of low-dose methotrexate with etanercept
- There are no safety issues in this combination and faster clearance can be achieved

	Acitretin	55%	23%	57.9%			Lee JH[20]

- In this randomized controlled trial, acitretin 10 mg twice a day and etanercept 25 mg twice weekly was compared with etanercept 50 mg twice weekly
- Similar PASI score could be achieved even at half the etanercept dose

	Cyclosporine	55%	23%	–	–		Cohen Barak E[21]

- No guidelines for combination, risk of infection, and malignancy prevents combined use of these drugs. It has been used safely in many difficult cases. It has role in the following scenarios:
  - Patient already on anti-TNF-α therapy and has exacerbation and needs a rescue therapy
  - Patient on cyclosporine for long and requires transition from cyclosporine, should be slowly tapered to prevent rebound
  - May be used as a combination therapy rarely in severe recalcitrant psoriasis

Adalimumab	Phototherapy	71%	45%	95%	75%		Bagel J[22]

- Adalimumab was given in approved dose and NBUVB was given three times a week, 55% patients also achieved PASI-100 in combination group as compared to 20% with monotherapy
- Erythema is the only adverse effect encountered. It can be used as rescue therapy, bridge therapy, concomitant, or maintenance therapy. Caution as already been discussed

	Methotrexate	71%	45%	–	–		–

- There are no studies in clinical efficacy of combination of adalimumab and methotrexate in psoriasis
- Studies in rheumatoid arthritis found combination to be safe and effective

	Acitretin	71%	45%	–	–		–

- There are no studies showing clinical efficacy of combination of adalimumab and acitretin
- Case reports of safe and efficacious combination exist. Combination can be used safely as bridging therapy or as maintenance therapy in case one wants to reduce the maintenance dose of biologics

	Cyclosporine	71%	45%	–	–		Cohen Barak E[21]

No guidelines for combinations; issues are same as it has been discussed with etanercept and cyclosporine combination

Continued

Continued

Infliximab	Phototherapy	80%	57%	–	–	–
No guidelines for combination, combination can be used as rescue therapy when biologic is losing its efficacy or as maintenance therapy							
	Methotrexate	80%	57%	–	–	Spertino J[23]
Minor increase in efficacy on combining low-dose methotrexate to infliximab; however, it improves drug survival (duration for which infliximab is effective), decreases infusion reactions, and development of antidrug antibodies. Thus, low-dose methotrexate should always be combined with infliximab						
	Acitretin	80%	57%	–	–	–
No studies in plaque psoriasis. It has been combined in erythrodermic psoriasis as maintenance therapy and found to be safe and effective. It can be used as a rescue therapy or maintenance therapy						
	Cyclosporine	80%	57%	–	–	–
No guidelines for combination. Avoid combination as risk of infection is high						
Itolizumab	Cyclosporine	45%	21%	–	–	Gupta et al.[24]
• In this case report, treatment was initiated with cyclosporine 100 mg twice a day for 2 weeks followed by standard dosing of itolizumab, this resulted in PASI-90 response in 12 weeks • Studies of combination therapy of itolizumab with other systemic therapy, such as methotrexate, acitretin, and phototherapy is lacking						
Secuki-numab	–	81%	60%	–	–	–
Ixekizumab		90%	72%	–	–	–
• Reports of combination therapy with secukinumab and ixekizumab with other systemic therapy are scant, possibly because it achieves clearance of disease in majority of patients when used as monotherapy • It is reasonable to assume that it can be combined with acitretin, apremilast, and phototherapy safely if required						

(NBUVB: narrowband ultraviolet B; PASI: Psoriasis Area and Severity Index)

Combining Biologics with Biologics

We have come to a point where multiple biologics of different class with different mechanism of actions are available. Since, biomarker for efficacy of particular biologic in a subset of patients is not available; we have some percentage of patients who do not respond to a biologic in a desired manner. When a patient does not achieve desirable response with one biologic, there is a scope for using combination biologic. However, there is a fear that blocking multiple immune pathways by using multiple biologics can lead to severe immune suppression and can be counter-productive. There are reports of use of combination of IL-12/23 monoclonal antibody with anti-TNF-α therapy for the management of recalcitrant psoriasis.[25] Combining different classes of biologics should be avoided unless there is a strong clinical need and patient should be closely followed-up for the risk of infection.

Scenario 2: As a first-line therapy, especially when rapid control and complete clearance is desirable and there are no financial constraints.
- Patient who wants rapid control and complete clearance of disease because of social reasons often comes to dermatologist in distress. What can be done in this scenario? Secukinumab and ixekizumab are biologic which are FDA-approved as first line for the management of chronic plaque psoriasis and provide rapid clearance in this scenario. Infliximab is another option to gain rapid control of disease; however, safety should not be compromised and all investigations should be conducted prior to the initiation of biologics.

Scenario 3: When patient has failed conventional systemic therapy and at least one biologic therapy.

When patient does not respond to one biologic therapy, how to use another biologic therapy?

SWITCHING BIOLOGICS

Patient may be required to switch from one biologic to another because of various reasons, such as primary failure, secondary failure, adverse effects like infusion reactions or other factors like patients request and cost of therapy.

When switching is performed for safety reasons, a washout period should be allowed to normalize the safety parameter. However, when a switch is performed for inadequate response, washout period is not necessary. A switch should be considered when patient does not achieve PASI-50 at the end of induction phase (in real world, if patient does not achieve PASI-75, switch should be considered as PASI-75 which is considered as the meaningful response).

Switching for Inefficacy

If switching is done for inefficacy, switching can be done between same classes of biologic or a new class of biologic can be introduced. Inefficacy in biologics is not a class action unlike adverse effects and they can be interchanged within the same class. For example, patient not responding to etanercept can be given adalimumab or infliximab, similarly patient not responding to infliximab can be given a trial of adalimumab or etanercept. Patient not responding to secukinumab can be offered ixekizumab. There is no pecking order or hierarchy in anti-TNF-α inhibitor or IL-17 inhibitor, a patient who shows poor response to one drug can be offered another drug in same class. In general, response in biologic-experienced patient is not as

good as biologic-naive patient.[23,26] Biologic within same class can be used in patient with secondary failure to biologic (loss of PASI-50 response); however, those with primary failure (not able to achieve PASI-50) are likely to fail other biologic in same class and class switch should be preferred over molecule switching.
- Switching from etanercept—switch to adalimumab, infliximab, secukinumab, or ixekizumab, start 1 week after last dose (when next dose is due)
- Switching from adalimumab—switch to etanercept, adalimumab, infliximab, secukinumab, or ixekizumab, start 2 weeks after last dose (when next dose is due)
- Switching from infliximab—switch to adalimumab, etanercept, secukinumab, or ixekizumab, start 2–4 weeks after last dose
- Switching from secukinumab—switch to any of the anti-TNF-α inhibitors or ixekizumab, start between 2 and 4 weeks
- Switching from ixekizumab—switch to any of the anti-TNF-α inhibitors or secukinumab, start between 2 and 4 weeks

Switching for Adverse Effects

If a patient develops adverse effects while on biologic, one needs to switch biologic. This switch depends on whether adverse effect is due to the class effect or it is due to the specific adverse effect of the biologic.
- Antidrug antibodies (ADAs) to TNF-α inhibitors do not cross react. Patient who develops ADA and develops loss of response can be started on another anti-TNF-α inhibitor.
- Patients who develop infectious complications like reactivation of latent tuberculosis or hepatitis B infection require stoppage of drug and institution of appropriate therapy. Since, this reactivation is a class action of anti-TNF-α inhibitor; it should be restarted only after clinical evaluation. Ideally, a different class of biologic like IL-17 inhibitor should be used.
- Patients who develop other class action adverse effects of anti-TNF-α inhibitors like worsening of congestive heart failure or precipitation of multiple sclerosis in a rare event, these drugs should be avoided for future use.
- Patients who develop worsening or new onset inflammatory bowel disease while on IL-17 inhibitors should not be restarted on same class of drug, while patients who develop mucosal candidiasis can be treated for candidiasis and treatment can be continued.

Switching of biologic in this scenario can be better understood by knowing the use of biologic in presence of comorbidities and contraindications of various biologics discussed in previous sections and earlier chapters.

BIOLOGICS FOR LESS COMMON FORMS OF PSORIASIS

Nail Psoriasis

Nail involvement occurs in up to 50% of patients with psoriasis. Nail psoriasis is associated with more severe disease, duration of skin lesions, and arthropathy. Involvement of nail even without arthritis has negative impact on functioning and quality of life. Patient can have constant pain, which can result in restriction of day-to-day activities. Nail involvement is objectively measured using Nail Psoriasis Severity Index (NAPSI). Topical therapies are not very effective for the management of nail psoriasis. A systematic review compared efficacy of available biologics for the treatment of nail psoriasis.[27] The highest mean NAPSI improvement at 24 weeks was seen with brodalumab, followed by etanercept and ixekizumab. The highest probability of complete resolution of nail at 24 weeks was seen with adalimumab (44.6%), followed by ixekizumab (41%), brodalumab (31.6%), etanercept (31%), infliximab (26.2%), and ustekinumab (19.4%). IL-23 inhibitors were not part of this systematic review.[27]

TRANSFIGURE trial demonstrated sustained efficacy of secukinumab in the treatment of nail psoriasis. Secukinumab has also been used as intramatricial injection in the dose of 7.5 mg/mL and 15 mg/mL every 2 weeks for 12 weeks. It resulted in significant improvement in nail involvement at 12 weeks.[28] Ixekizumab shows greater efficacy in nail psoriasis as compared to ustekinumab, etanercept, adalimumab, and guselkumab in head-to-head studies. Ixekizumab was also found to be effective in patient who has secondary failure to secukinumab.[29-31] Ixekizumab showed complete clearance in 60% patients suffering from nail psoriasis in pooled data from various trials.[32] Infliximab and adalimumab have also been used successfully for the management of nail psoriasis.[33,34]

Approach to Treatment

Isolated nail psoriasis should be first treated with topical calcipotriol and steroid combination therapy and intramatricial steroid injection. Involvement of more than 3 nails and/or impairment of quality of life are indications of systemic treatment of nail psoriasis. TNF inhibitors as well as IL-17 inhibitors work well for nail psoriasis.

The choice of biologic should depend on other factors, such as cutaneous involvement, associated arthritis, comorbidities, and economic factors.

Palmoplantar Psoriasis, Scalp Psoriasis, and Other Variants of Psoriasis

Psoriasis involving palms and soles and other difficult-to-treat areas like genital and scalp can be quite disabling and can severely impair the quality of life despite involving less body surface area. Biologics can be used for these areas when conventional systemic therapy does not work adequately; however, biologics have not been studied rigorously for these forms of psoriasis. A network meta-analysis of controlled trial concluded that secukinumab had highest probability of complete resolution. Ixekizumab and TNF inhibitors are also effective for the management of palmoplantar psoriasis.[35] There are many case reports of successful management of palmoplantar psoriasis using TNF-α inhibitors and same can be tried in recalcitrant cases.[36]

Secukinumab has been studied in double-blind, randomized, placebo-controlled trial for management of palmoplantar psoriasis and found to be very effective in 300 mg dose. At week 16, Palmoplantar Psoriasis Area and Severity Index (ppPASI) reduced by 54% and almost 33% patients achieved clear palms.[37] We suggest using secukinumab for the management of palmoplantar psoriasis not responding to conventional systemic treatment.

Scalp psoriasis not responding to topical and systemic therapy may require treatment with biologic agents. Secukinumab, ixekizumab, etanercept, and adalimumab have shown efficacy in scalp psoriasis. However, secukinumab and ixekizumab has shown to be most efficacious biologics in the management of scalp psoriasis.[38]

Erythrodermic Psoriasis

Psoriatic erythroderma can occur de novo or it can occur as an extension of chronic plaque psoriasis. Erythrodermic flare of psoriasis is associated with chills, edema, weight loss, and altered temperature regulation. Untreated disease is associated with serious morbidity and even mortality in some cases.[39] As erythrodermic psoriasis is an uncommon disease, high quality scientific data is lacking and treatment is based on the experience and expert opinions.

Erythroderma causes severe physiological disturbance; hence drugs which act faster should be used so that physiology can be restored at the earliest. National Psoriasis Foundation guidelines for management of erythrodermic psoriasis recommended cyclosporine and infliximab as first-line agent. Etanercept can also be used as second-line agent along with methotrexate.[40]

Secukinumab and ixekizumab have also been successfully used recently by various authors for the management of erythrodermic psoriasis.[41,42]

Infliximab, secukinumab, ixekizumab, brodalumab, guselkumab, risankizumab, certolizumab pegol, and bimekizumab have been approved for erythrodermic psoriasis in Japan.[43]

Infliximab, secukinumab, and ixekizumab are good biologic options for treating erythrodermic psoriasis in our country as they result in rapid response.

Generalized Pustular Psoriasis

Generalized pustular psoriasis is a rare form of life-threatening psoriasis, characterized by the development of sterile pustules with widespread erythema. GPP variants include childhood GPP, von Zumbusch type, and impetigo herpetiformis (GPP in pregnant women). Extensive GPP can be life-threatening and needs faster control of the disease. Robust evidence-based data for treatment of this variant is lacking and guidelines are based on limited data and expert recommendations.

National Psoriasis Foundation recommends acitretin, methotrexate, cyclosporine, and infliximab as the first-line therapy.[44] However, many experts believe that in extensive disease, infliximab should be used as first-line option because of its rapid onset of action. Secukinumab and ixekizumab are good alternatives to infliximab in the management of GPP.[43,45] Spesolimab is an IL-36 inhibitor and is approved for the management of GPP flare in adults. When available it can become the first-line agent in the management of GPP in adults.

Infliximab, adalimumab, secukinumab, ixekizumab, brodalumab, guselkumab, risankizumab, certolizumab pegol, and bimekizumab are approved for GPP in Japan.[43]

Secukinumab and ixekizumab should be used as a first-line biologic drug for the management of childhood GPP. Etanercept and adalimumab can also be used.

Generalized pustular psoriasis in pregnancy is difficult to manage as it can be life-threatening for both mother and child. Cyclosporine and oral steroids are traditionally considered first-line therapy for management of GPP in pregnancy. Infliximab has been used safely for management of GPP in pregnancy; care should be taken about vaccination of neonate postdelivery (details have been discussed in the Section on Biologics in Special Situation). Secukinumab has also been used in the management of GPP of pregnancy.[46]

HOW LONG TO USE BIOLOGICS?

Physician who counsels patients to start biologic is always faced with this question by patients and sometimes by himself. How long can we use them continuously? Should we use them continuously once we start using them to maintain remission or we can use them as on required basis, thus reducing the cost of therapy? There are multiple studies, which have been done that have looked at efficacy of various biologics in continuous or intermittent manner.

Study involving intermittent and continuous therapy of infliximab had to be terminated because of higher adverse effects in intermittent group and most of the experts agree that infliximab should be used in continuous manner.[47] Long-term safety and efficacy in real world practice for infliximab have been studied for up to 98 weeks.[48]

Etanercept has been studied as continuous and intermittent therapy. Patient with interrupted therapy had longer survival of biologic. Another study found that retreatment requires almost 4 weeks more than initial treatment to achieve remission.[49]

Adalimumab results in PASI-75 response in 80% patients. Study done by Papp et al. found that patient in whom treatment was withdrawn after remission was achieved and reinitiated on relapse, 69% patient achieved PASI-75. There were no safety issues in intermittent and continuous therapy groups. In real world, patient stops therapy in-between and it is reassuring that majority of these patients regain control of the disease without any major safety issues.[50] Adalimumab has been used continuously for 3 years safely and its efficacy has been maintained in a phase III trial.[51]

Secukinumab has also been studied in as needed versus fixed interval maintenance regime in a randomized, double-blind trial. Study concluded that fixed interval dosing is much more efficacious as compared to as needed basis; however, safety in both groups was found to be comparable. However, an extension of the ERASURE and FIXTURE trials by Blauvelt et al. showed that intermittent treatment with secukinumab brought down the efficacy of the drug. Long-term safety data from various trials is available for up to 2 years of continuous use in psoriasis and psoriatic arthritis.[52,53] Long-term integrated pooled clinical trial and postmarketing-surveillance data suggests safety up to 5 years.[54]

Studies have shown that ixekizumab also maintained efficacy over 3 years period and no new safety signals were detected.[55]

CONCLUSION

Successful use of biologics for management of psoriasis requires basic understanding of the pathogenesis of disease, availability of conventional systemic therapy, comorbid diseases, and financial constraints of patient.

REFERENCES

1. National Institute for Health and Care Excellence. (2012). Psoriasis: assessment and management. Clinical Guideline [CG153]. [online] Available from https://www.nice.org.uk/guidance/cg153 [Last accessed January, 2024].
2. Smith CH, Jabbar-Lopez ZK, Yiu ZZ, Bale T, Burden AD, Coates LC, et al. British Association of Dermatologists guidelines for biologic therapy for psoriasis 2017. Br J Dermatol. 2017;177(3):628-36.
3. Langley RG, Elewski BE, Lebwohl M, Reich K, Griffiths CE, Papp K, et al. Secukinumab in plaque psoriasis results of two phase 3 trials. N Engl J Med. 2014;371(4):326-38.
4. Leonardi CL, Powers JL, Matheson RT, Goffe BS, Zitnik R, Wang A, et al. Etanercept as monotherapy in patients with psoriasis. N Engl J Med. 2003;349(21):2014-22.
5. Menter A, Tyring SK, Gordon K, Kimball AB, Leonardi CL, Langley RG, et al. Adalimumab therapy for moderate to severe psoriasis: a randomized, controlled phase III trial. J Am Acad Dermatol. 2008;58(1):106-15.
6. Reich K, Nestle FO, Papp K, Ortonne JP, Evans R, Guzzo C, et al. Infliximab induction and maintenance therapy for moderate-to-severe psoriasis: a phase III, multicentre, double-blind trial. Lancet. 2005;366(9494):1367-74.

7. Lebwohl MG, Gordon KB, Gallo G, Zhang L, Paul C. Ixekizumab sustains high level of efficacy and favourable safety profile over 4 years in patients with moderate psoriasis: results from UNCOVER-3 study. J Eur Acad Dermatol Venereol. 2020;34(2):301-9.
8. Cantini F, Nannini C, Niccoli L, Iannone F, Delogu G, Garlaschi G, et al. Guidance for the management of patients with latent tuberculosis infection requiring biologic therapy in rheumatology and dermatology clinical practice. Autoimmun Rev. 2015;14(6):503-9.
9. Vassilopoulos D, Apostolopoulou A, Hadziyannis E, Papatheodoridis GV, Manolakopoulos S, Koskinas J, et al. Long-term safety of anti-TNF treatment in patients with rheumatic diseases and chronic or resolved hepatitis B virus infection. Ann Rheum Dis. 2010;69(7):1352-5.
10. Amin M, No DJ, Egeberg A, Wu JJ. Choosing first-line biologic treatment for moderate-to-severe psoriasis: what does the evidence say? Am J Clin Dermatol. 2018;19(1):1-13.
11. Kishimoto M, Komine M, Kamiya K, Sugai J, Kuwahara A, Morimoto N, et al. Case of psoriasis with hepatitis B virus infection during tumor necrosis factor inhibitor treatment successfully treated with ixekizumab and tenofovir alafenamide fumarate. J Dermatol. 2022;49(6):e193-e194.
12. Di Nuzzo S, Boccaletti V, Fantini C, Cortelazzi C, Missale G, Fabrizi G, et al. Are anti-TNF-a agents safe for treating psoriasis in hepatitis C virus patients with advanced liver disease? Case reports and review of the literature. Dermatology. 2016;232(1):102-6.
13. Megna M, Patruno C, Bongiorno MR, Gambardella A, Guarneri C, Romita P, et al. Hepatitis Virus Reactivation in Patients with Psoriasis Treated with Secukinumab in a Real-World Setting of Hepatitis B or Hepatitis C Infection. Clin Drug Investig. 2022;42(6):525-31.
14. Silvy F, Bertin D, Bardin N, Auger I, Guzian MC, Mattei JP, et al. Antinuclear antibodies in patients with psoriatic arthritis treated or not with biologics. PloS One. 2015;10(7):e0134218.
15. Majewksi S, Kheterpal M, Nardone B, Sable K, West DP, Lacouture ME, et al. First line biologic agent therapy for moderate-to-severe psoriasis in cancer survivors. J Am Acad Dermatol. 2016;74(5):AB250.
16. Briot K, Garnero P, Le Henanff A, Dougados M, Roux C. Body weight, body composition, and bone turnover changes in patients with spondyloarthropathy receiving anti-tumour necrosis factor a treatment. Ann Rheum Dis. 2005;64(8):1137-40.
17. Scarpato S, Antivalle M, Favalli EG, Nacci F, Frigelli S, Bartoli F, et al. Patient preferences in the choice of anti-TNF therapies in rheumatoid arthritis. Results from a questionnaire survey (RIVIERA study). Rheumatology (Oxford). 2010;49:289-94.
18. Kircik L, Bagel J, Korman N, Menter A, Elmets CA, Koo J, et al. Utilization of narrow-band ultraviolet light b therapy and etanercept for the treatment of psoriasis (UNITE): efficacy, safety, and patient-reported outcomes. J Drugs Dermatol. 2008;7(3):245-53.
19. Gottlieb AB, Langley RG, Strober BE, Papp KA, Klekotka P, Creamer K, et al. A randomized, double-blind, placebo-controlled study to evaluate the addition of methotrexate to etanercept in patients with moderate to severe plaque psoriasis. Br J Dermatol. 2012;167(3):649-57.
20. Lee JH, Youn JI, Kim TY, Choi JH, Park CJ, Choe YB, et al. A multicenter, randomized, open-label pilot trial assessing the efficacy and safety of etanercept 50 mg twice weekly followed by etanercept 25 mg twice weekly, the combination of etanercept 25 mg twice weekly and acitretin and acitretin alone in patients with moderate to severe psoriasis. BMC Dermatol. 2016;16(1):11.
21. Cohen Barak E, Kerner M, Rozenman D, Ziv M. Combination therapy of cyclosporine and anti-tumor necrosis factor a in psoriasis: a case series of 10 patients. Dermatol Ther. 2015;28(3):126-30.
22. Bagel J. Adalimumab plus narrowband ultraviolet-B light phototherapy for the treatment of moderate to severe psoriasis. J Drugs Dermatol. 2011;10(4):366-71.
23. Spertino J, López-Ferrer A, Vilarrasa E, Puig L. Long-term study of infliximab for psoriasis in daily practice: drug survival depends on combined treatment, obesity and infusion reactions. J Eur Acad Dermatol Venereol. 2014;28(11):1514-21.

24. Gupta A, Sharma YK, Deo K, Kothari P. Severe recalcitrant psoriasis treated with itolizumab, a novel anti-CD6 monoclonal antibody. Indian J Dermatol Venereol Leprol. 2016;82(4):459-61.
25. Gniadecki R, Bang B, Sand C. Combination of anti-tumour necrosis factor-a and anti-interleukin-12/23 antibodies in refractory psoriasis and psoriatic arthritis: a long-term case-series observational study. Br J Dermatol. 2016;174(5):1145-6.
26. Kerdel F, Zaiac M. An evolution in switching therapy for psoriasis patients who fail to meet treatment goals. Dermatol Ther. 2015;28(6):390-403.
27. Khan M, Wallace CE, Ahmed F, Rahman SM, Memon N, Haque A. Assessing Comparative Efficacy of Biologics for the Treatment of Psoriasis with Nail Involvement: A Systematic Review. J Psoriasis Psoriatic Arthritis. 2023;1-8.
28. Reich K, Sullivan J, Arenberger P, Mrowietz U, Jazayeri S, Augustin M, et al. Effect of secukinumab on the clinical activity and disease burden of nail psoriasis: 32-week results from the randomized placebo-controlled TRANSFIGURE trial. Br J Dermatol. 2019;181(5):954-66.
29. Wasel N, Thaçi D, French LE, Conrad C, Dutronc Y, Gallo G, et al. Ixekizumab and ustekinumab efficacy in nail psoriasis in patients with moderate-to-severe psoriasis: 52-week results from a phase 3, head- to-head study (IXORA-S). Dermatol Ther (Heidelb). 2020;10(4):663-70.
30. van de Kerkhof P, Guenther L, Gottlieb AB, Sebastian M, Wu JJ, Foley P, et al. Ixekizumab treatment improves fingernail psoriasis in patients with moderate-to-severe psoriasis: results from the randomized, controlled and open-label phases of UNCOVER-3. J Eur Acad Dermatol Venereol. 2017;31(3):477-82.
31. Blauvelt A, Leonardi C, Elewski B, Crowley JJ, Guenther LC, Gooderham M, et al. A head-to-head comparison of ixekizumab vs. guselkumab in patients with moderate-to-severe plaque psoriasis: 24-week efficacy and safety results from a randomized, double-blinded trial. Br J Dermatol. 2020;182(6):1348-58.
32. Egeberg A, Kristensen LE, Vender R, Zaheri S, El Baou C, Gallo G, et al. Sustained resolution of nail psoriasis through 5 years with ixekizumab: a post hoc analysis from UNCOVER-3. Acta Derm Venereol. 2022;102:adv00787.
33. Fabroni C, Gori A, Troiano M, Prignano F, Lotti T. Infliximab efficacy in nail psoriasis. A retrospective study in 48 patients. J Eur Acad Dermatol Venereol. 2011;25(5):549-53.
34. Elewski BE, Okun MM, Papp K, Baker CS, Crowley JJ, Guillet G, et al. Adalimumab for nail psoriasis: efficacy and safety from the first 26 weeks of a phase 3, randomized, placebo-controlled trial. J Am Acad Dermatol. 2018;78(1):90-99.e1.
35. Tsiogkas SG, Grammatikopoulou MG, Kontouli KM, Minopoulou I, Goulis DD, Zafiriou E, et al. Efficacy of biologic agents for palmoplantar psoriasis: a systematic review and network meta-analysis. Expert Rev Clin Immunol. 2023;19(12):1485-98.
36. Weinberg JM. Successful treatment of recalcitrant palmoplantar psoriasis with etanercept. Cutis. 2003;72(5):396-8.
37. Gottlieb A, Sullivan J, van Doorn M, Kubanov A, You R, Parneix A, et al. Secukinumab shows significant efficacy in palmoplantar psoriasis: results from GESTURE, a randomized controlled trial. J Am Acad Dermatol. 2017;76(1):70-80.
38. Kivelevitch D, Amin S, Menter A. Clinical utility of secukinumab in moderate-to-severe scalp psoriasis: evidence to date. Clin Cosmet Investig Dermatol. 2019;12:249-53.
39. Boyd AS, Menter A. Erythrodermic psoriasis: precipitating factors, course, and prognosis in 50 patients. J Am Acad Dermatol. 1989;21(5 Pt 1):985-91.
40. Rosenbach M, Hsu S, Korman NJ, Lebwohl MG, Young M, Bebo BF Jr, et al. Treatment of erythrodermic psoriasis: from the medical board of the National Psoriasis Foundation. J Am Acad Dermatol. 2010;62(4):655-62.

41. Mugheddu C, Atzori L, Lappi A, Pau M, Murgia S, Rongioletti F. Successful secukinumab treatment of generalized pustular psoriasis and erythrodermic psoriasis. J Eur Acad Dermatol Venereol. 2017;31(9):e420-e421.
42. Avallone G, Cariti C, Dapavo P, Ortoncelli M, Conforto L, Mastorino L, et al. Real-life comparison between secukinumab and ixekizumab in the treatment of pustular and erythrodermic psoriasis. J Eur Acad Dermatol Venereol. 2022;36(7):e574-e576.
43. Saeki H, Mabuchi T, Asahina A, Abe M, Igarashi A, Imafuku S, et al. English version of Japanese guidance for use of biologics for psoriasis (the 2022 version). J Dermatol. 2023;50(2):e41-e68.
44. Robinson A, Van Voorhees AS, Hsu S, Korman NJ, Lebwohl MG, Bebo BF Jr, et al. Treatment of pustular psoriasis: from the Medical Board of the National Psoriasis Foundation. J Am Acad Dermatol. 2012;67(2):279-88.
45. Imafuku S, Honma M, Okubo Y, Komine M, Ohtsuki M, Morita A, et al. Efficacy and safety of secukinumab in patients with generalized pustular psoriasis: a 52-week analysis from phase III open-label multicenter Japanese study. J Dermatol. 2016;43(9):1011-7.
46. Neema S, Shrestha S, Sathu S, Vasudevan B. Excellent Response to Secukinumab in Treatment Resistant Impetigo Herpetiformis. Indian Dermatol Online J. 2022;14(1):118-9.
47. Menter A, Feldman SR, Weinstein GD, Papp K, Evans R, Guzzo C, et al. A randomized comparison of continuous vs. intermittent infliximab maintenance regimens over 1 year in the treatment of moderate-to-severe plaque psoriasis. J Am Acad Dermatol. 2007;56(1):31.e1-15.
48. Shear NH, Hartmann M, Toledo-Bahena M, Katsambas A, Connors L, Chang Q, et al. Long-term efficacy and safety of infliximab maintenance therapy in patients with plaque-type psoriasis in real-world practice. Br J Dermatol. 2014;171(3):631-41.
49. Ortonne JP, Taieb A, Ormerod AD, Robertson D, Foehl J, Pedersen R, et al. Patients with moderate-to-severe psoriasis recapture clinical response during re-treatment with etanercept. Br J Dermatol. 2009;161(5):1190-5.
50. Papp K, Crowley J, Ortonne JP, Leu J, Okun M, Gupta SR, et al. Adalimumab for moderate to severe chronic plaque psoriasis: efficacy and safety of retreatment and disease recurrence following withdrawal from therapy. Br J Dermatol. 2011;164(2):434-41.
51. Gordon K, Papp K, Poulin Y, Gu Y, Rozzo S, Sasso EH. Long-term efficacy and safety of adalimumab in patients with moderate to severe psoriasis treated continuously over 3 years: results from an open-label extension study for patients from REVEAL. J Am Acad Dermatol. 2012;66(2):241-51.
52. Kavanaugh A, Mease PJ, Reimold AM, Tahir H, Rech J, Hall S, et al. Secukinumab for Long-term Treatment of Psoriatic Arthritis: A Two-Year Followup from a Phase III, Randomized, Double-Blind Placebo-Controlled Study. Arthritis Care Res (Hoboken). 2017;69(3):347-55.
53. Mrowietz U, Leonardi CL, Girolomoni G, Toth D, Morita A, Balki SA, et al. Secukinumab retreatment-as-needed versus fixed-interval maintenance regimen for moderate to severe plaque psoriasis: a randomized, double-blind, noninferiority trial (SCULPTURE). J Am Acad Dermatol. 2015;73(1):27-36.e1.
54. Gottlieb AB, Deodhar A, Mcinnes IB, Baraliakos X, Reich K, Schreiber S, et al. Long-term Safety of Secukinumab Over Five Years in Patients with Moderate-to-severe Plaque Psoriasis, Psoriatic Arthritis and Ankylosing Spondylitis: Update on Integrated Pooled Clinical Trial and Post-marketing Surveillance Data. Acta Derm Venereol. 2022;102:adv00698.
55. Burlando M, Salvi I, Castelli R, Herzum A, Cozzani E, Parodi A. Long-term clinical efficacy and safety of ixekizumab for psoriatic patients: a single-center experience. Eur Rev Med Pharmacol Sci. 2023;27(9):4060-4.

CHAPTER 20

Immunobullous Disorders

Himadri, Ankan Gupta

INTRODUCTION

Immunobullous disorders are a group of autoimmune disorders, characterized by vesicobullous lesions over the skin and mucosa. These include pemphigus group of disorders, bullous pemphigoid (BP), mucous membrane pemphigoid, epidermolysis bullosa acquisita, dermatitis herpetiformis, and other rare disorders.

Pemphigus is characterized by flaccid vesiculobullous lesions over skin and mucosae. Pemphigus vulgaris and pemphigus foliaceus are the most common types and are fatal if not treated. Management of both the types is similar with most experts believing treating pemphigus foliaceus in general is more difficult.

Systemic steroids have been the cornerstone of therapy and continue to be the most common drug used to attain clinical remission. The role of steroid-sparing agents (SSAs) is for maintenance and assisting in decreasing the cumulative dose of systemic steroids. The SSAs traditionally employed, in decreasing order of preference, include azathioprine (AZA), mycophenolate mofetil (MMF), and dapsone. Cyclophosphamide (CYC) is a common SSA used in India with steroids, orally and as pulse dosing, but western literature supports its use in only refractory cases. Rituximab has been a revelation in the last decade for treating autoimmune vesiculobullous disorders. We suggest rituximab to be the first-line SSA in all fresh cases. It is essential for readers to know the definitions of disease process and therapy before proceeding further.[1]

INITIAL MANAGEMENT[2]

Rituximab has now become the first-line SSA for the management of pemphigus.
- For mild cases (body surface area < 5% and limited oral lesions not impairing oral intake or requiring analgesia), the first-line therapy options include:
  ○ Rituximab and/or systemic steroids (prednisone 0.5 mg/kg/day), or
  ○ Systemic steroids (prednisone 0.5–1 mg/kg/day with or without SSA like AZA or MMF)

- For moderate and severe pemphigus:
  - Rituximab along with systemic steroids (prednisone 1-1.5 mg/kg/day) with progressive tapering to stop steroids after 6 months or maintenance at the physiological dose
  - Rituximab is administered alone in patients with absolute contraindication to systemic steroids.
  - Systemic steroids (prednisone 1-1.5 mg/kg/day) with or without SSA with slow tapering of steroids over 20-24 weeks
- In refractory cases, intravenous immunoglobulin (IVIg) (2 g/kg/cycle), intravenous corticosteroid pulses (methylprednisolone 0.5-1 g/day or dexamethasone 100 mg/day for 3 consecutive days), or immunoadsorption are the other options to bring control. These are in addition to the therapy suggested for moderate and severe pemphigus.

Our experience with CYC and pulse dosing is limited and its use will not be discussed further in this chapter. Use of pyridostigmine and tetracyclines as adjunctive options in management are not part of the guidelines and will not be discussed.

The role of adequate antibiotic coverage proactively, skin cleansing and oral care, antiseptic baths, and compresses, and topical and intralesional steroids cannot be overemphasized. Early recognition of bacterial infection and/or superadded herpetic infection is foremost and helps in decreasing the cumulative steroid dosing and early disease control. The management would also include:

- Bone protection with vitamin D correction, calcium, and bisphosphonate therapy
- Gut protection with H2 antihistamines or proton pump inhibitors
- Analgesia before dressings
- Requisite glycemic control, and management of hypertension
  Initial management of pemphigus should be done in an inpatient setting.

MAINTENANCE AND STEROID TAPERING

It is important for the clinician to recognize the markers of disease activity in a patient with pemphigus. Tapering the steroid dose before achieving clinical inactivity is erroneously labeled as recalcitrant and leads to incorrect decisions. The speed of tapering steroids does not have a consensus with decreasing the dose by 10-25% every 2-3 weeks till 15-25 mg/day and slower tapering thereafter being an acceptable approach.[2] In patients who show renewed activity on tapering of steroids, it is suggested that the dose be increased to the last recognized dose where there was clinical remission which is then followed by either tapering by small amount, e.g., 2.5-5 mg every fortnight or tapering monthly rather than fortnightly. We prefer to increase the steroid dose to "2-step-back" dose and tapering by 2.5 mg fortnightly. If disease continues to be active despite this step, we restart at the initial dose and then taper the steroid at a slower rate from the beginning. In refractory cases where disease flares up with tapering of steroids at a very high dose of steroids, adding IVIg or pulse steroids are recommended.

INTRODUCTION OF STEROID-SPARING AGENT

The aim in management of pemphigus is to have a long remission period completely off therapy.[1] SSAs are the drugs to maintain remission, and rituximab has proved to be a boon in this regard.[2-6] Most clinicians institute SSA along with steroids at the initial stage itself with the rationale of SSA taking over the mantle on disease control as the steroids are tapered. The guidelines also recommend to start rituximab or the traditional SSAs at the time of presentation which is different from the previously popular practice where they were introduced much later in the treatment or in a recalcitrant disease. Also, early introduction of rituximab is found to be more effective if the disease is of recent onset.

With more data emerging of superior efficacy and improved quality of life with rituximab, prescribing the traditional SSA should now be restricted to patients who have a contraindication for rituximab or refuse to take rituximab for one or the other reason. A negative viral screening including the core antibody of hepatitis B, eliminating the possibility of latent and active tuberculosis, antinuclear antibodies (ANAs) negativity, cardiac clearance, and normal immunoglobulin levels are fundamental requisites before planning for rituximab. Most of these investigations take a few weeks to show up and can be planned sequentially to allay the cost. Any contradictory result deters the use of rituximab and warrants a discussion with the concerned specialist physician regarding the feasibility of using rituximab or opting for an alternative SSA. AZA is the conventional SSA that may be considered as first line if rituximab cannot be administered. It requires an initial thiopurine methyltransferase (TPMT) enzyme level to decide on its use and dosing; if the TPMT assay is not available, starting with 1 mg/kg of AZA and stringent monitoring of blood counts and hepatic profile is required. MMF is another option, which is safer than AZA but not as effective as AZA.[3]

DISCONTINUATION OF THERAPY

After rituximab infusion, the steroid dose can be tapered and stopped after 3–4 months in mild cases and 6 months in moderate and severe cases. Some clinicians prefer maintaining the patient on a physiological steroid dose for prolonged periods, but there is no evidence to support this practice.

With other SSAs, there is a controversy where few physicians taper and discontinue the steroids and start tapering the SSA after 6–8 weeks. We prefer tapering the steroid to the physiological dose and start tapering of SSA within 4–8 weeks, depending upon the clinical remission. AZA can be tapered by 50 mg and MMF by 500 mg every 8 weeks and discontinued over a period of 6–12 months after achieving complete remission on therapy. Steroids at physiological dose are continued till immunological remission. Occasional flares can be managed in a similar way by "2-step-back" method if required. Additional dose of rituximab is given at 6, 12, and 18 months. Further infusion may be required if there is an increase in anti-Dsg antibodies, which should be monitored every 6 months.[2]

TIMING FOR VACCINATION

The timing for vaccination with use of rituximab in pemphigus is tricky. For vaccines to be effective maximally, the ideal timing should be such that the disease activity is minimal and iatrogenic immunosuppression should be in "low-dose immunosuppression" range as discussed in the chapter on vaccines. The other important aspect is to vaccinate prior to using a biological agent. It is important to be patient while using rituximab in pemphigus as the risk of acquiring infections can be fatal and outweigh the benefits of its use.

DOSING OF RITUXIMAB

The "rheumatoid arthritis" protocol of infusing 1,000 mg of rituximab 2 weeks apart is the standard regimen used by most dermatologists.[5] The lymphoma protocol is not superior and uses a higher amount of total rituximab. The lower dose rituximab protocol employs 500 mg rituximab 2 weeks apart and is proving to be effective, but the duration of remission might be lower.[6,7] Patients who initially had severe pemphigus and/or have high levels of anti-Dsg antibodies at month 3, may benefit with a repeat infusion of 500 or 1,000 mg of rituximab at month 6, if they have achieved remission on/off therapy. If they have not achieved complete remission, two infusions of 1,000 mg 2 weeks apart (2 g in total) should be given. Further infusion of 500 mg of rituximab is recommended at month 12 and 18 in patients in complete remission, and additional infusions as maintenance if there is an increase in anti-Dsg antibodies. An ultra-low-dose rituximab infusion of a single dose of 200 mg has recently been tried, wherein all eight patients improved clinically; however, only partial control was achieved in 3/8 patients.[8] A low-dose or ultra-low-dose rituximab infusion may be a better option for inducing remission, especially during a pandemic, such as COVID-19; however, 3 monthly repeat infusions may be required since relapse rate is higher with these regimens.[9]

RITUXIMAB FOR PEMPHIGUS IN CHILDREN

Pemphigus is rare in children and data of use of rituximab in children is scarce. Though the long-term effects of rituximab are yet to be seen, it does appear to be a safe SSA for use.[10,11]

RITUXIMAB FOR PEMPHIGUS IN PREGNANCY

Pemphigus is an uncommon disease in pregnancy and can be mostly managed with steroids alone or steroids and IVIg. Severe pemphigus requiring biologic therapy for management is rare. Rituximab is a pregnancy category C drug. Its prescribing information states that contraception should be advised during and after 12 months of rituximab use in women in reproductive age group. The British Society for Rheumatology (BSR) guidelines recommend rituximab should be stopped 6 months prior to conception; however, pregnant patients who were exposed to rituximab have had uneventful pregnancy outcomes.[12,13] Rituximab can cause neonatal cytopenia or B-cell depletion and can increase the risk of infections in neonate.[14] The vaccination of neonate needs to be discussed with the neonatologists and avoidance of live vaccines is advised.

ADVERSE EFFECTS WITH USE OF RITUXIMAB

The adverse events with use of rituximab are mostly infusion reactions, which can be minimized with premedication. Rituximab desensitization protocols are also available if rituximab therapy is highly desired.[15] Infections, though definitely a risk, remain incalculable because of the concomitant use of steroids. Other rare idiosyncratic side effects include thromboembolic phenomenon, long-term persistent hypogammaglobulinemia, and progressive multifocal leukoencephalopathy.[16,17]

ALTERNATIVE TREATMENT OPTIONS FOR PEMPHIGUS

Rarely, patients do not respond to most standard therapies or may have contraindications to their use. Other drugs in our arsenal with proven efficacy include dapsone, methotrexate,[18] cyclosporine,[19] and tetracyclines.[20] CYC, immunoadsorption, and plasmapheresis are reserved for most refractory cases.

PROPOSED PROTOCOL FOR USE OF RITUXIMAB IN A PATIENT WITH MODERATE TO SEVERE PEMPHIGUS (ADULT WEIGHING 60 KG)

- *Step I (control of disease activity)*:
  - Establish the diagnosis with biopsy, direct immunofluorescence, and enzyme-linked immunosorbent assay (ELISA) for desmogleins.
  - Do a presteroid investigation and discuss with patient the options of SSA with benefits of using rituximab over other SSA.
  - Start the patient on steroid equivalent to 1 mg/kg (up to 2 mg/kg as required).

- *Step II (maintenance)*:
  - Taper the steroids after new lesions stop appearing and older lesions start epithelializing.
  - Taper steroids every fortnightly as discussed above. Slower tapering may be required as described in the text.
- *Step III (introduction of rituximab)*:
  - After meticulously ruling out all contraindications for rituximab, plan for the first infusion.
  - Complete vaccination 2 weeks prior to infusion of rituximab.
- *Step IV (premedication and infusion)*:
  - Regular vital and cardiac monitoring must be done. Make sure that the resuscitation kit is available and accessible.
  - Withhold the steroid dose and antihypertensives on the day of infusion.
  - Premedicate 1 hour prior to the infusion with:
    - Injection methylprednisolone 100 mg as intravenous infusion in 100 mL of normal saline over 30 minutes
    - Tablet paracetamol 1 g
    - Injection pheniramine (Avil) 22.75 mg intravenously
  - Monitor vitals every 30 minutes during infusion
  - Speed of infusion:
    - 25 mL/h for the first 30 minutes
    - 50 mL/h for the next 30 minutes
    - Increase by 50 mL/h every 30 minutes thereafter to a maximum 200 mL/h.
    - Rate of infusion can be doubled for subsequent infusions if no infusion reaction occurs in the first infusion.
- *Step V (surveillance)*:
  - Immunological recovery takes at least 6 months and steroids are tapered and maintained at physiological dose till immunological remission.
  - Continue the vaccination protocol for the rest of their lives with annual influenza shots, 5-yearly pneumococcal shots, and hepatitis B boosters.

PARANEOPLASTIC PEMPHIGUS[21]

Besides treatment of the underlying neoplasm, immunosuppressants are often used for clinical improvement similar to pemphigus vulgaris. Oral prednisolone (1 mg/kg/day) is given with rituximab (375 mg/m weekly for 4 weeks or two doses of 1 g given 2 weeks apart. The dose can be repeated every 3–6 months). Other SSAs such as CYC, MMF, AZA, and cyclosporine may also be used.

BULLOUS PEMPHIGOID

Traditionally, the aim of treatment in BP has been to control acute disease activity with minimum immunosuppression required to achieve remission, which is unlike pemphigus group, where the target is prolonged remission of disease and protocols use higher doses of steroids even if not warranted for acute control. This is because BP affects the elderly, and it is observed that morbidity due to use of immunosuppressives can sometimes override that due to the disease itself. Restricting the treatment to topical therapy and nonimmunosuppressive drugs like dapsone and tetracyclines is recommended in mild cases.[22] Oral steroids form the mainstay of treatment in patients not responding to nonimmunosuppressive drugs and in patients with widespread or very symptomatic disease. Biologicals are fast becoming a go-to option, their main advantage being selective function and favorable adverse effect profile as compared to systemic steroids.

Drug-induced BP is not rare and common drugs that are incriminated include gliptins, anti-programmed-death (PD-1 inhibitors) drugs, and loop diuretics. It is not clear whether the prognosis changes on discontinuation of these drugs, especially the gliptins but for the benefit of doubt, authors prefer replacing these drugs with safer options. Herein again, theoretically once the drug is discontinued, biologics could be employed to suppress the inflammatory cascade without risking adverse effects of steroids.

MANAGEMENT OF BULLOUS PEMPHIGOID[22-26]

- High potency topical corticosteroid, tetracyclines, and antineutrophilic agents (in patients with neutrophil-rich BP) are first-line agents.
- Oral corticosteroids (prednisolone 0.5–1 mg/kg or equivalent) with the least required dose for minimum required period is employed and effort is made to revert to drug therapy mentioned in point 1, which is maintained for few months after the disease is completely controlled.
- Patients relapsing on tapering of steroids require other SSA (methotrexate, AZA, and mycophenolate) to facilitate tapering of the steroid dose. The choice of SSA is generally made with consideration of risk for adverse effects, and patient preference. Rituximab, dupilumab, and omalizumab are other considerations here.
  - Rituximab, both the lymphoma protocol and RA protocol, has been employed successfully for management of BP. The current data is not strong enough to suggest rituximab as a first-line agent in management of BP because of the age group it affects and concerns of higher immunosuppression with rituximab. Instead, the focus has been on nonimmunosuppressive biologicals. Low-dose rituximab is also successful as seen in literature and authors' practice where two doses of 500 mg rituximab is employed 2 weeks apart.[27]

- Dupilumab has been used at an initial dose of 600 mg followed by 300 mg weekly or on alternate weeks with success.
- Omalizumab acts against the anti-BP180 immunoglobulin E (IgE) antibodies binding to FcεRI on mast cells and eosinophil. It is usually given at a dose of 300 mg subcutaneously every 4 weeks.
- Recently anti-IL-17A biologics have also been shown to be effective in management of BP.[26]
- JAK inhibitors—baricitinib, upadacitinib, and tofacitinib—have been successfully used anecdotally in BP.[28,29]

• IVIg is used in refractory cases, not responding to steroids where acute control is warranted and other immunosuppressives are risky to use.

The response to treatment is assessed clinically and with serial monitoring of antibodies. Patients should not develop any new lesions, and there should be cessation of pruritus. Eosinophilia and IgE levels are considered surrogate markers for BP activity in several centers. Tapering of treatment is tried at the earliest and best individualized.

OTHER IMMUNOBULLOUS DISEASES

Besides the above, rituximab and IVIg are also being used in other immunobullous disorders, such as mucous membrane pemphigoid and epidermolysis bullosa acquisita. As our understanding of biological agents is ever expanding, this knowledge must be transferred to our clinical practice for the betterment of our patients.

CONCLUSION

The availability of targeted therapy has changed the way we treat immunobullous disorders. Rituximab is a cost effective treatment for the management of pemphigus group of disorders. Omalizumab is a very promising agent for the management of bullous pemphigoid. The treating physicians should utilize these drugs optimally for the better management of patients.

REFERENCES

1. Murrell DF, Dick S, Ahmed AR, Amagai M, Barnadas MA, Borradori L, et al. Consensus statement on definitions of disease, end points, and therapeutic response for pemphigus. J Am Acad Dermatol. 2008;58(6):1043-6.
2. Joly P, Horvath B, Patsatsi A, Uzun S, Bech R, Beissert S, et al. Updated S2K guidelines on the management of pemphigus vulgaris and foliaceus initiated by the european academy of dermatology and venereology (EADV). J Eur Acad Dermatol Venereol. 2020;34(9):1900-13.
3. Chams-Davatchi C, Esmaili N, Daneshpazhooh M, Valikhani M, Balighi K, Hallaji Z, et al. Randomized controlled open-label trial of four treatment regimens for pemphigus vulgaris. J Am Acad Dermatol. 2007;57(4):622-8.
4. Joly P, Maho-Vaillant M, Prost-Squarcioni C, Hebert V, Houivet E, Calbo S, et al. First-line rituximab combined with short-term prednisone versus prednisone alone for the

treatment of pemphigus (Ritux 3): a prospective, multicentre, parallel-group, open-label randomised trial. The Lancet. 2017;389(10083):2031-40.
5. Leshem YA, Hodak E, David M, Anhalt GJ, Mimouni D. Successful treatment of pemphigus with biweekly 1-g infusions of rituximab: a retrospective study of 47 patients. J Am Acad Dermatol. 2013;68(3):404-11.
6. Horváth B, Huizinga J, Pas HH, Mulder AB, Jonkman MF. Low-dose rituximab is effective in pemphigus. Br J Dermatol. 2012;166(2):405-12.
7. Singh N, Handa S, Mahajan R, Sachdeva N, De D. Comparison of the efficacy and cost-effectiveness of an immunologically targeted low-dose rituximab protocol with the conventional rheumatoid arthritis protocol in severe pemphigus. Clin Exp Dermatol. 2022;47(8):1508-16.
8. Russo I, Miotto S, Saponeri A, Alaibac M. Ultra-low dose rituximab for refractory pemghigus vulgaris: a pilot study. Expert Opin Biol Ther. 2020;20(6):673-8.
9. Tavakolpour S, Aryanian Z, Seirafianpour F, Dodangeh M, Etesami I, Daneshpazhooh M, et al. A systematic review on efficacy, safety, and treatment-durability of low-dose rituximab for the treatment of Pemphigus: special focus on COVID-19 pandemic concerns. Immunopharmacol Immunotoxicol. 2021;43(5):507-18.
10. Vinay K, Kanwar AJ, Sawatkar GU, Dogra S, Ishii N, Hashimoto T. Successful use of rituximab in the treatment of childhood and juvenile pemphigus. J Am Acad Dermatol. 2014;71(4):669-75.
11. Tavakolpour S, Mahmoudi H, Balighi K, Abedini R, Daneshpazhooh M. Sixteen-year history of rituximab therapy for 1085 pemphigus vulgaris patients: A systematic review. Int Immunopharmacol. 2018;54:131-8.
12. De Cock D, Birmingham L, Watson KD, Kearsley-Fleet L, Hyrich KL; BSRBR Control Centre Consortium, Symmons DP. Pregnancy outcomes in women with rheumatoid arthritis ever treated with rituximab. Rheumatol Oxf Engl. 2017;56(4):661-3.
13. Chakravarty EF, Murray ER, Kelman A, Farmer P. Pregnancy outcomes after maternal exposure to rituximab. Blood. 2011;117(5):1499-506.
14. Soh MC, MacKillop L. Biologics in pregnancy - for the obstetrician. Obstet Gynaecol. 2016;18(1):25-32.
15. Abadoglu O, Epozturk K, Atayik E, Kaptanoglu E. Successful rapid rituximab desensitization for hypersensitivity reactions to monoclonal antibodies in a patient with rheumatoid arthritis: a remarkable option. J Investig Allergol Clin Immunol. 2011;21(4):319-21.
16. Clifford DB, Ances B, Costello C, Rosen-Schmidt S, Andersson M, Parks D, et al. Rituximab-associated progressive multifocal leukoencephalopathy in rheumatoid arthritis. Arch Neurol. 2011;68(9):1156-64.
17. Chakraborty S, Tarantolo SR, Treves J, Sambol D, Hauke RJ, Batra SK. Progressive Multifocal Leukoencephalopathy in a HIV-Negative Patient with Small Lymphocytic Leukemia following Treatment with Rituximab. Case Rep Oncol. 2011;4(1):136-42.
18. Tran KD, Wolverton JE, Soter NA. Methotrexate in the treatment of pemphigus vulgaris: experience in 23 patients. Br J Dermatol. 2013;169(4):916-21.
19. Vardy DA, Cohen AD. Cyclosporine therapy should be considered for maintenance of remission in patients with pemphigus. Arch Dermatol. 2001;137(4):505-6.
20. McCarty M, Fivenson D. Two decades of using the combination of tetracycline derivatives and niacinamide as steroid-sparing agents in the management of pemphigus: defining a niche for these low toxicity agents. J Am Acad Dermatol. 2014;71(3):475-9.
21. Wieczorek M, Czernik A. Paraneoplastic pemphigus: a short review. Clin Cosmet Investig Dermatol. 2016;9:291-5.
22. Joly P, Roujeau JC, Benichou J, Picard C, Dreno B, Delaporte E, et al. A comparison of oral and topical corticosteroids in patients with bullous pemphigoid. N Engl J Med. 2002;346(5):321-7.

23. Williams HC, Wojnarowska F, Kirtschig G, Mason J, Godec TR, Schmidt E, et al. Doxycycline versus prednisolone as an initial treatment strategy for bullous pemphigoid: a pragmatic, non-inferiority, randomised controlled trial. Lancet Lond Engl. 2017;389(10079):1630-8.
24. Cao P, Xu W, Zhang L. Rituximab, Omalizumab, and Dupilumab Treatment Outcomes in Bullous Pemphigoid: A Systematic Review. Front Immunol. 2022;13:928621.
25. Czernik A, Toosi S, Bystryn JC, Grando SA. Intravenous immunoglobulin in the treatment of autoimmune bullous dermatoses: an update. Autoimmunity. 2012;45(1):111-8.
26. Bakirtzi K, Sotiriou E, Papadimitriou I, Vakirlis E, Delli FS, Ioannides D. Anti-interleukin-17A biologics for the long-term treatment of bullous pemphigoid: A prospective, cohort study. J Eur Acad Dermatol Venereol. 2023;37(6):e749-e751.
27. Suárez-Carantoña C, Jiménez-Cauhé J, González-García A, Fernández-Guarino M, Asunción Ballester M. Low-Dose Rituximab for Bullous Pemphigoid. Protocol and Single-Center Experience. Actas Dermosifiliogr. 2023;114(1):62-8.
28. Youssef S, Gallitano S, Bordone LA. Two cases of bullous pemphigoid effectively treated with oral tofacitinib. JAAD Case Rep. 2022;32:77-80.
29. Nash D, Kirchhof MG. Bullous pemphigoid treated with janus kinase inhibitor upadacitinib. JAAD Case Rep. 2023;32:81-3.

CHAPTER 21

Hidradenitis Suppurativa

Sharmila Patil, Aarti Zope

INTRODUCTION

Hidradenitis suppurativa (HS) (derived from the Greek word *hidros* = sweat; *aden* = glands) is a chronic recurrent painful progressive debilitating inflammatory condition; a.k.a Acne inversa; affecting apocrine gland bearing skin in buttocks, axillae, groin, and submammary region.[1] The exact pathogenesis of this disease is not known; however, currently it is considered an autoinflammatory disease with the involvement of the Th17 and Th1 pathways. Follicular hyperkeratosis and subsequent follicular occlusion play a role in the pathogenesis of HS.[2] It affects 0.5–4% of the global population. It generally starts around puberty and is more common in females. The primary lesions are tender, deep-seated follicular papules, and pustules, which may enlarge to become nodules or pus discharging abscesses and ultimately leading to nodular scars and interconnected sinuses. It is associated with significant morbidity and poor quality of life. The etiopathogenesis is multifactorial; with immunological, genetic, and hormonal factors along with smoking and obesity playing some role in the causation of the disease.

DISEASE STAGING

Staging of the disease is important to know the extent of the disease and plan treatment for the patient. Hurley's and modified Sartorius staging system (mSS) are most commonly used. Hurley's staging system is simpler and hence more commonly used in clinical settings. The Dermatology Life Quality Index (DLQI) can also be used to know the impact of disease on the quality of life of the patient. Other scores used to assess disease activity and severity are Hidradenitis Suppurativa Physician Global Assessment (HS-PGA), Hidradenitis Suppurativa Clinical Response (HiSCR), HS Severity Index (HSSI), Sonographic Scoring of HS (SOS-HS), Acne Inversa Severity Index, Refined Hurley Classification (AISI), International HS Severity Scoring System (IHS4), Severity Assessment of HS (SAHS), and HS Area and Severity Index (HASI).

Hurley's Staging System (Figs. 1A to C)[3]
- *Stage I*: Abscess formation without sinus tracts.
- *Stage II*: Recurrent abscess with sinus tract and scar formation.
- *Stage III*: Multiple interconnected tracts and abscess.

Modified Sartorius Staging System[4]
It is a more objective staging system in which numerical scoring is done in the following manner to assess disease severity **(Table 1)**.

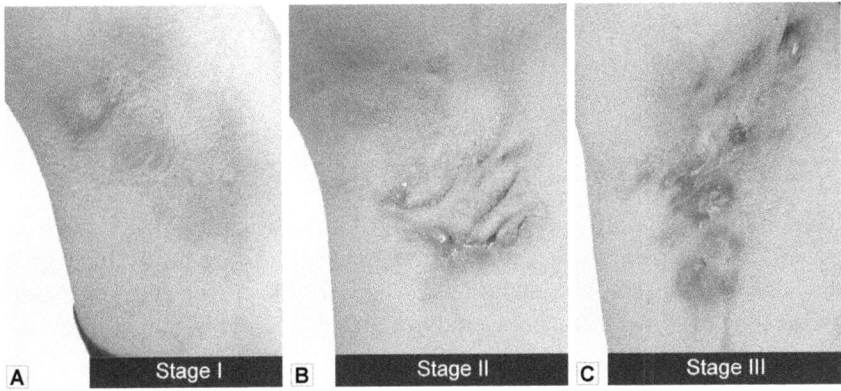

FIGS. 1A TO C: Hurley staging system.

TABLE 1: Modified Sartorius staging system.									
Parameters		**Score**							
Anatomic regions involved		*Three points per region*: (1) Axilla, (2) groin, gluteal, and (3) other							
Number and scores of lesions; for each region		One point for nodules, six points for fistula/sinus tract, and one point for scars							
Longest distance between two lesions (or size of lesion if single) for each region		One point if <5 cm; three points if 5–10 cm; nine points if >10 cm							
Lesions clearly separated by normal skin		Zero points if yes (Hurley I and II), nine points if no (= Hurley III)							
Modified Sartorius staging system		Right axilla	Left axilla	Right groin	Left groin	Right gluteal region	Left gluteal region	Other
Number of nodules and number of fistulas	One point per nodule Six point per fistula								

Continued

Continued

Parameters		Score					
Distance	<5 cm = 1 point						
	5–10 cm = 3 points						
	>10 cm = 9 points						
Hurley III	Yes = 9 point						
	No = 0 point						
Sum/total score							

MANAGEMENT OF HIDRADENITIS SUPPURATIVA

It is a multidisciplinary approach involving dermatologists, plastic surgeons, psychiatrists, nutritionists, and dieticians. The approach to treatment depends on the severity of lesions in HS. It also involves appropriate management of wounds, pain, and comorbidities. An important part of management includes counseling of the patient regarding the nature of the disease, the need for long-term follow-up and keeping realistic goals. Lifestyle modifications involving weight reduction and smoking cessation; zero dairy, and low carbohydrate diet; cessation of smoking; loose clothing, boxer type of underwear, avoiding picking or squeezing also play an important role. Additionally, surgical interventions can be planned for long-term remission of the disease.

Goals of Treatment
- To reduce the formation of new inflammatory lesions, sinus tracts, and scarring.
- To treat existing lesions and reduce associated symptoms (e.g., pain and suppuration).
- To minimize associated psychological morbidity.

Conventional therapy in HS is enumerated in **Table 2**.

In spite of patients being on long-term oral and topical antibiotics and retinoids, clinical outcomes are not satisfactory; recurrences and relapses are common. If antibiotics are not sufficient or no longer effective, newer systemic therapies like biologics can be used in patients with refractory disease. Hence, with the further understanding of pathogenesis of HS and availability of biologics, we have now shifted to include biologics in management of HS.

TABLE 2: Conventional therapy in HS.	
Topical	Systemic
1% clindamycin gel	Antibiotics (clindamycin, rifampicin, tetracycline, minocycline, dicloxacillin, erythromycin, amoxicillin + clavulanic acid, cephalexin, and trimethoprim)
5% benzoyl peroxide gel	Hormonal therapy (cyproterone acetate, ethinyl estradiol, norgestrel, desogestrel, spironolactone, and finasteride)
0.1% adapalene	Corticosteroids (prednisolone)
Silver sulfadiazine	Azathioprine
15% azelaic acid	Cyclosporine
Intralesional corticosteroids (triamcinolone)	Dapsone
Botulinum toxin A	Methotrexate
15% resorcinol peel	Retinoids (isotretinoin and acitretin)
Perilesional GM-CSF	Human immunoglobulin
Radiotherapy	Biologics (infliximab, adalimumab, anakinra, etanercept, ustekinumab, and secukinumab)
Cryosurgery	NSAIDs
Laser (CO$_2$, neodymium-doped yttrium aluminum garnet, and pulsed dye)	Mycophenolate mofetil
Surgical excision	Tacrolimus
Photodynamic therapy	Metformin
	Apremilast

Note: Nd:YAG laser is applicable for Hurley stage II-III disease; CO$_2$ laser excision can be considered in patients with Hurley stage II-III with fibrotic sinus tracts.
(GM-CSF: granulocyte-macrophage colony stimulating factor; HS: hidradenitis suppurativa; NSAIDs: nonsteroidal anti-inflammatory drugs)

IMMUNOPATHOGENESIS AND BASIS OF TREATMENT WITH BIOLOGICS

The exact immunopathogenesis of HS has not been delineated. Tumor necrosis factor alpha (TNF-α) levels were found to be higher in the skin and serum of patients with HS.[5] This finding is consistent with the effectiveness of anti-TNF-α drugs in its management. Interleukin (IL-1b) receptors are upregulated in affected and perilesional skin in HS patients.[6] Th17 cells and IL-17, IL-23 were also found to be raised in HS skin, which also implicates the Th17 pathway in causation and opens newer targets in the management of this chronic, debilitating condition.[7]

TABLE 3: Biologics used in HS.		
Monoclonal antibodies	**TNF-α inhibitors**	**Adalimumab (ADA) and infliximab (INF)**
	Fusion antibody proteins	Etanercept (ETN)
IL-12/23 inhibitors		Ustekinumab
IL-17 inhibitors		Secukinumab (SEC)
IL-1 receptor antagonist		Anakinra
IL-1-β inhibitor		Canakinumab

(HS: hidradenitis suppurativa; TNF: tumor necrosis factor)

Biologicals are mainly used for recalcitrant HS either as monotherapy or to supplement surgical excision. In 2001, infliximab was first described as effective in HS patients with concomitant Crohn's disease.[8] First reports of the use of adalimumab (ADA) in HS dates back to 2006, leading to the United States Food and Drug Administration (USFDA) approval in 2015.[9]

Biologics used in HS are enumerated in **Table 3**.

Biologics can be considered for patients with HS presenting with inflammatory lesions, skin tunnels, and scarring who do not achieve satisfactory sustained disease control with conventional therapy, such as oral doxycycline, oral retinoids, apremilast, methotrexate, hormonal therapy, and a combination of these.

The choice of systemic therapy depends on various factors, such as availability of the drug, affordability of the patient, associated comorbidities, ease of administration, tolerability, rapidity of response desired, severity of disease, adverse effect profile, and previous treatment administered.

Steps while starting the patient on biologics are discussed in **Box 1**.

We will discuss biologicals available and used in India for the management of HS in detail. Detailed descriptions of individual biologics have been given elsewhere in this book. Our aim is to discuss biologics usage specifically in HS.

SPECIFIC BIOLOGIC AGENTS

Adalimumab

Adalimumab is a monoclonal antibody against TNF-α which is indicated for Hurley stage II and III disease. The dosing in HS consists of 160 mg (four injections of 40 mg in 1 day or two injections of 40 mg on 2 consecutive days) loading dose on day 0; followed by 80 mg after 2 weeks and 40 mg every week afterward.

Clinical Trials

Two trials of the efficacy of ADA in HS worth mentioning are PIONEER I and II trials.[10] These are similarly designed phase 3 multicenter randomized

BOX 1	**Steps for incorporating biologics into the treatment of hidradenitis suppurativa.**

When to use?
 Moderate to severe hidradenitis suppurativa (Hurley stage II and III)
 Which all to choose?
 • Adalimumab
 • Infliximab
 • Secukinumab
 • Etanercept
 How to choose?
 Step 1: Check the suitability for an individual: know the safety profile of each biologic.
 TNF-α antagonists:
 • Serious infection
 • Malignancy
 • Demyelinating disease
 • Congestive heart failure
 • Hepatitis B
 • Hematologic
 • Lupus-like syndrome
 • Live vaccines
 Step 2:
 • Evaluate for comorbidities
 • Inflammatory bowel diseases especially Crohn's disease—favor adalimumab/infliximab
 • Pyoderma gangrenosum—adalimumab/infliximab
 • Behçet's disease, Psoriasis—TNF inhibitor/secukinumab
 • Metabolic syndrome
   ◦ Obesity—disfavor TNF antagonist
   ◦ Cardiovascular disease (CVD)
 • Coronary artery disease—favor TNF-α antagonists
   ◦ Arthropathies spondyloarthropathy (joint disease)
 • Favor—TNF-α antagonists > IL-17 blocker
   ◦ Squamous cell carcinoma—disfavor TNF-α antagonists	

Step 3:
 • Consider concomitant medical issues
 • Serious infections
 • *Caution*: All biologicals
 • Tuberculosis
 • *Caution*: All biologicals
 • Hepatitis
 • *Hepatitis B*: Caution—TNF-α antagonists
 • Hepatitis C:
   ◦ Favor—TNF-α antagonists-etanercept
   ◦ Deep fungal infections
 • *Caution*: TNF-α antagonists
 Congestive heart failure (moderate to severe): Caution TNF-α antagonists
	Multiple sclerosis
	 Caution: TNF-α antagonist
	 Prior malignancy
	 Caution: All biological
	 Cutaneous SCC
	 Caution: TNF-α antagonists
	 Solid tumors
	 Depends upon type, severity and duration, and the risk-benefit ratio

Continued

Continued

Step 4: Choose best method of administration and frequency of administration
Adalimumab is the biologic of choice as it is approved for the management of HS. If the patient does not respond to adalimumab; secukinumab can be used

Self-administration/subcutaneous:	In-office administration/infusion:
• *Adalimumab*: Every other week or every week • *Etanercept*: Every week or twice a week	• *Infliximab*: 0, 2, 6, and every 8 weeks • *Secukinumab*: 300 mg—0, 1, 2, 3, 4 weeks, and every 4 weeks

clinical trials (I, $n = 307$; II, and $n = 326$) with two double-blinded placebo-controlled periods. Patients with moderate to severe HS were randomly assigned in 1:1 ratio to either ADA (40 mg once a week) or placebo for initial 12 weeks (period 1); followed by 24 weeks phase (period 2) in which patients were reassigned to ADA weekly or every other week or placebo. Patients in PIONEER II were allowed to continue oral tetracycline therapy at stable doses. The primary endpoint assessed was clinical response defined as a 50% reduction from baseline in abscess and inflammatory-nodule count, with no increase in the abscess or draining-fistula counts, at week 12. Clinical response rates were higher for the group receiving ADA weekly than for the placebo group (41.8% vs. 26.0%; $p = 0.003$) in PIONEER I and (58.9% vs. 27.6%; $p < 0.001$) in PIONEER II trials. Patients receiving ADA had significantly greater improvement in secondary outcomes (lesions, pain, and modified Sartorius score for disease severity) at week 12 in PIONEER II only. Rates of serious adverse events were found to be similar in the study groups.

A 3-year open-label extension study that followed PIONEER trials suggest long-term efficacy and safety of ADA.[11] Zouboulis et al., studied long-term ADA efficacy in patients with moderate to severe HS. They assessed the response to and tolerability of long-term administration of ADA in HS in an open-label extension study for 52 weeks or more. At week 12, 52.3% of those receiving ADA weekly and 73% of partial responders (PRRs) achieved HiSCR (Hidradenitis Suppurativa Clinical Response). Achievement of HiSCR was maintained through week 168 (~39 months) in 52.3% of the weekly ADA group and 57.1% of PRRs. Sustained improvement in lesion counts, skin pain, and Dermatology Life Quality Index (DLQI) scores was also observed. Safety profiles throughout long-term extension study were similar to those in the PIONEER studies.

Miller et al. performed a double-blind placebo-controlled randomized trial, in 21 patients; of whom 15 patients received ADA 80 mg at baseline followed by 40 mg every other week for 12 weeks, and six received placebo. A significant reduction was seen in the Sartorius score after 6 weeks and an almost significant reduction was seen after 12 weeks in the ADA group (−10.7 vs. 7.5; $p = 0.024$ and −11.3 vs. 5.8; $p = 0.07$) as compared to placebo group.[12]

Side Effects
Side effects of ADA include injection site reaction, reactivation of tuberculosis, infections (URTI), rash, fever, antibody formation, ANA positivity, and lupus-like syndrome. Adalimumab is pregnancy category B; it can be continued safely till the second trimester. Shifting to certolizumab (no placental transfer), in the third trimester can be considered; but there are no studies or published reports with the use of certolizumab in HS. If a patient develops antibodies against ADA, shifting to other biologic can be considered.

Infliximab
Infliximab is a chimeric monoclonal antibody against TNF-α. It is used as second-line therapy for moderate to severe HS patients unresponsive to ADA and has the advantage of weight-based dosing. It is the preferred drug in patients with systemic disease, associated GIT involvement (HS associated with IBD), or syndromic HS. The dose used is 5 mg/kg at weeks 0, 2, 6, and then every 8 weeks, as an infusion over 2 hours with close monitoring for an infusion reaction. Side effects include infusion reactions and increased risk of infections. It is not preferred by dermatologists in view of the need for intravenous infusion and the risk of anaphylaxis. A small, randomized placebo, controlled trial of infliximab 5 mg/kg for HS showed improvement in disease severity.[13]

Etanercept
Etanercept is a recombinant fully human dimeric fusion protein comprising of the human TNF-α p75 receptor and the Fc portion of human IgG1 molecule that can bind to two TNF molecules, thereby effectively removing them from circulation. It functions as a TNF-α inhibitor, thereby preventing interaction with its cell surface receptors on target cells and blocking its proinflammatory effects. Since trials studying the efficacy of Etanercept in HS have yielded variable results, around 30–50% in HiSCR, it is not a preferred agent in HS.[14,15]

Ustekinumab
Ustekinumab is a monoclonal antibody against the p40 subunit of IL-12/IL-23. As we know, Th1 and Th17 response is mediated by IL-12 and IL-23. It is used to treat patients with moderate to severe recalcitrant plaque psoriasis and psoriatic arthritis. IL-23 was also found to be raised in HS skin, which also implicates the Th17 pathway in the causation of HS. This involvement of Th17 pathway might explain the observed therapeutic effect of ustekinumab in HS. It is not available in India as of now. The dose of ustekinumab used is 45 mg (or 90 mg; if the weight > 100 kg) subcutaneous injections are administered at weeks 0, 4, and 12 weekly thereafter (dose in children is 0.75 mg/kg).

Clinical Trials

Blok et al. in an open-label study of 17 patients of HS who received 45 or 90 mg ustekinumab at weeks 0, 4, 16, and 28; found out that there was a statistically significant improvement in modified Sartorius score (mSS). The mean mSS of patients in the treatment group reduced from 112.12 at baseline to 60.18 at week 40 (46.33% improvement; $p < 0.01$). Also mean mHSLASI (modified Hidradenitis Suppurative Lesional Area Severity Index) of treated patients reduced significantly from 26.29 at baseline to 19.59 at week 40 (25.5% improvement; $p = 0.01$).[16]

Side Effects

Nasopharyngitis, increased infection risk, reactivation of tuberculosis, and increased risk of nonmelanoma skin cancers.

Secukinumab

Secukinumab (SEC) is a fully humanized monoclonal antibody against IL-17A. It is used in the treatment of moderate to severe HS. It has been approved by US FDA in October 2023 for the management of moderate-to-severe HS.

Clinical Trials

Kimball et al. assessed the efficacy of secukinumab in patients with moderate to severe HS in two randomized trials.[17] SUNSHINE and SUNRISE were identical multicenter randomized placebo controlled double blind phase 3 trials. Patients were randomly assigned (1:1:1) to receive subcutaneous SEC 300 mg every 2 weeks, 300 mg every 4 weeks, or placebo. The primary endpoint was the proportion of patients with HiSCR at week 16. Safety was assessed by evaluating adverse events and serious adverse events. In SUNSHINE trial, patients receiving SEC every 2 weeks had better responses compared with placebo (45% vs. 34%, odds ratio 1.8; $p = 0.007$). There was no statistically significant difference between the group receiving SEC every 4 weeks and the placebo group. In the SUNRISE trial, compared with the placebo group (31%), every 2 weeks SEC group (42%), and every 4 weeks SEC group (46%) had better HiSCR (p values being 0.015 and 0.0022 respectively). Patient responses were sustained till the end of the trial up to 52 weeks. Long-term efficacy of secukinumab and recurrences of HS while on SEC needs further evaluation.

Other IL-17 inhibitors studied in HS are bimekizumab, brodalumab, and ixekizumab. Brodalumab showed 100% improvement in HiSCR in an open-label trial done by Frew et al.[18,19] Ixekizumab showed improvement in a few case reports; while exacerbation of HS was seen in a case report published by Gordon et al.[20]

Side Effects
Injection site reactions, nasopharyngitis, increased risk of infections, reactivation of tuberculosis.

INTERLEUKIN-1 RECEPTOR ANTAGONIST/SECOND-LINE BIOLOGIC THERAPIES

Interleukin-1 is a proinflammatory cytokine that plays an important role in the regulation of inflammation and immune response. Interleukin-1 receptor antagonist (IL-1Ra) is a naturally occurring antagonist that competes with IL-1a and IL-1b for the IL-1 receptor. The relative amounts of IL-1a, IL-1b, and IL-1Ra influence the severity of inflammation.

Anakinra
It is a recombinant nonglycosylated form of the human IL-1R-α; competitively inhibiting the biologic activity of IL-1a and IL-1b. The US FDA and the European Medical Agency have approved the use of anakinra for the treatment of moderate to severe rheumatoid arthritis. It is not available in India and is prohibitively expensive. It is used as a third-line treatment option for HS unresponsive to TNF-α inhibitors. The dose used is daily subcutaneous injection of 100 mg (children: 1–2 mg/kg) initially; may increase by 0.5–1 mg/kg increments to control active inflammation, not to exceed 8 mg/kg. The daily dosing schedule of anakinra is a major disadvantage over other biologics. Side effects of anakinra include serious infections and neutropenia.

Clinical Trials
Tzanetakou et al., investigated the safety and efficacy of anakinra in HS, in a double-blind randomized placebo-controlled clinical trial with 12 weeks treatment phase and 12 weeks follow-up phase. Among 20 patients, 10 were randomized to either the placebo group or the anakinra group. The disease activity score was reduced at week 12 in 78% in anakinra arm versus in 20% in the placebo arm ($p = 0.02$).[21]

The dose of biologics in the long term can be modified according to the needs of the patient and disease activity. Biologics can be combined with apremilast, tofacitinib and other newer therapies. It is also used in combination with surgical intervention and/or laser hair removal. Most of laser therapies have been focused on modification of disease activity in the groin and axillae because the destruction of pilosebaceous apparatus might prevent the extension of the disease. Most biologics are well-tolerated and show a favorable safety profile in the short-medium term. However, long-term safety concerns, including infection risks, development of malignancy, and demyelinating diseases should be assessed.

PEDIATRIC HIDRADENITIS SUPPURATIVA

Hidradenitis suppurativa is a rare and poorly described disease in children. Actual prevalence and incidence is not known. There are no therapeutic trials published in pediatric HS. The treatment recommendations are based on case reports and interpretation of therapies in adults.[22] In males, it is more common in prepubertal period; while in females in the postpubertal period. History of HS in family members, presence of other elements of follicular occlusion tetrad (acne conglobata, dissecting cellulitis of the scalp, or pilonidal sinus), and increased body mass index (BMI) are risk factors for pediatric HS. Pediatric patients with HS should also be examined for possible endocrine comorbidities [premature adrenarche, precocious puberty, polycystic ovary syndrome (PCOS), metabolic syndrome, hypothyroidism, and diabetes].[23] Options in childhood HS management include topical therapy (clindamycin and benzoyl peroxide), or systemic therapy (clindamycin, rifampicin, finasteride, dapsone, steroids, and TNF-α blockers), or surgery or nonablative laser treatment depending on severity of the disease. Early recognition and treatment are important to minimize the life-course effects of this disease. The goal of treatment in children should be to minimize scarring, progression, and need for surgery.

Biologics in Pediatric Hidradenitis Suppurativa

Biologics commonly used in pediatric HS are infliximab and ADA. The recommended dosing regimen for ADA in HS for adolescents 12 years of age and older who weigh < 60 kg differs from adult dosing. Adolescents weighing 30–60 kg are treated with 80 mg on day 1 and 40 mg on day 8, followed by 40 mg every other week. Adolescents weighing at least 60 kg are treated with the same regimen as adults. Long-term efficacy and safety trials of biologic use in pediatric cases are lacking.

SUMMARY

Successful management of HS is challenging and at times requires comprehensive care. There is no uniformly effective therapy for HS; it requires a basic understanding of the pathogenesis of the disease, availability of conventional systemic therapy, comorbid disease, and financial constraints of the patient. Management is patient-based and the choice of drug depends on clinical severity, patient profile, and risk-benefit ratio. Biologics seem to represent an effective therapeutic option for HS, but complete and persistent resolution is rarely achieved. Flares of disease usually develop regardless of the prescribed treatment.

Trials demonstrating the efficacy of biologic therapy for moderate to severe HS have inspired new multidisciplinary treatment strategies especially combined biologic and surgical therapy for recalcitrant HS. Lower rates of recurrence and disease progression, as well as a longer disease-free interval, may be achieved with the use of adjuvant biologic therapy including infliximab ($n = 8$) and ustekinumab ($n = 3$) which were initiated 2–3 weeks after closure and were continued for an average of 10.5 months after radical resection for recalcitrant HS.[24]

Hidradenitis suppurativa is a rare paradoxical adverse effect of biologics exposure observed in 25 patients treated with these five biologics (ADA, infliximab, etanercept, rituximab, and tocilizumab).[25,26] Median duration of biologics exposure before HS onset was 12 months (range 1–120). There was a trend toward a better outcome when the biologics were discontinued or switched. Reintroducing the same biologics resulted in HS relapse in three patients.

CONCLUSION

The short-term side effects of biologics are usually minimal with regard to the risk–benefit ratio. The long-term effects ultimately determine the utility of each biologic therapy and the most appropriate disease–therapeutic pairing. A higher response rate could be associated with higher doses and several authors have suggested the use of biological drugs with higher doses in HS than those used in psoriasis. Not all biologics are equally effective, but finding the optimal biological to achieve optimal control is the goal in the biologic treatment of HS.

REFERENCES

1. Sellheyer K, Krahl D. "Hidradenitis suppurativa" is acne inversa! An appeal to (finally) abandon a misnomer. Int J Dermatol. 2005;44(7):535-40.
2. Attanoos RL, Appleton MA, Douglas-Jones AG. The pathogenesis of hidradenitis suppurativa: a closer look at apocrine and apoeccrine glands. Br J Dermatol. 1995;133(2):254-8.
3. Hurley HJ. Axillary hyperhidrosis, apocrine bromhidrosis, hidradenitis suppurativa, and familial benign pemphigus: surgical approach. In: Roenigk RK, Roenigk HH Jr (Eds). Roenigk and Roenigk's Dermatologic Surgery: Principles and Practice, 2nd edition. New York, NY: Marcel Dekker; 1996. pp. 623-45.
4. Revuz J. [Modifications to the Sartorius score and instructions for evaluating the severity of suppurative hidradenitis]. Ann Dermatol Venereol. 2007;134(2):173-4.
5. Mozeika E, Pilmane M, Nürnberg BM, Jemec GB. Tumour necrosis factor-alpha and matrix metalloproteinase-2 are expressed strongly in hidradenitis suppurativa. Acta Derm Venereol. 2013;93(3):301-4.
6. van der Zee HH, de Ruiter L, van den Broecke DG, Dik WA, Laman JD, Prens EP. Elevated levels of tumour necrosis factor (TNF)-α, interleukin (IL)-1β and IL-10 in hidradenitis suppurativa skin: a rationale for targeting TNF-α and IL-1β. Br J Dermatol. 2011;164(6):1292-8.
7. Schlapbach C, Hänni T, Yawalkar N, Hunger RE. Expression of the IL-23/Th17 pathway in lesions of hidradenitis suppurativa. J Am Acad Dermatol. 2011;65(4):790-8.
8. Martínez F, Nos P, Benlloch S, Ponce J. Hidradenitis suppurativa and Crohn's disease: response to treatment with infliximab. Inflamm Bowel Dis. 2001;7(4):323-6.
9. Moul DK, Korman NJ. The cutting edge. Severe hidradenitis suppurativa treated with adalimumab. Arch Dermatol. 2006;142(9):1110-2.

10. Kimball AB, Okun MM, Williams DA, Gottlieb AB, Papp KA, Zouboulis CC, et al. Two Phase 3 Trials of Adalimumab for Hidradenitis Suppurativa. N Engl J Med. 2016;375(5):422-34.
11. Zouboulis CC, Okun MM, Prens EP, Gniadecki R, Foley PA, Lynde C, et al. Long-term adalimumab efficacy in patients with moderate-to-severe hidradenitis suppurativa/acne inversa: 3-year results of a phase 3 open-label extension study. J Am Acad Dermatol. 2019;80(1):60-9.e2.
12. Miller I, Lynggaard CD, Lophaven S, Zachariae C, Dufour DN, Jemec GB. A double-blind placebo-controlled randomized trial of adalimumab in the treatment of hidradenitis suppurativa. Br J Dermatol. 2011;165(2):391-8.
13. Grant A, Gonzalez T, Montgomery MO, Cardenas V, Kerdel FA. Infliximab therapy for patients with moderate to severe hidradenitis suppurativa: a randomized, double-blind, placebo-controlled crossover trial. J Am Acad Dermatol. 2010;62(2):205-17.
14. Pelekanou A, Kanni T, Savva A, Mouktaroudi M, Raftogiannis M, Kotsaki A, et al. Long-term efficacy of etanercept in hidradenitis suppurativa: results from an open-label phase II prospective trial. Exp Dermatol. 2010;19(6):538-40.
15. Adams DR, Yankura JA, Fogelberg AC, Anderson BE. Treatment of hidradenitis suppurativa with etanercept injection. Arch Dermatol. 2010;146(5):501-4.
16. Blok JL, Li K, Brodmerkel C, Horvátovich P, Jonkman MF, Horváth B. Ustekinumab in hidradenitis suppurativa: clinical results and a search for potential biomarkers in serum. Br J Dermatol. 2016;174(4):839-46.
17. Kimball AB, Jemec GBE, Alavi A, Reguiai Z, Gottlieb AB, Bechara FG, et al. Secukinumab in moderate-to-severe hidradenitis suppurativa (SUNSHINE and SUNRISE): week 16 and week 52 results of two identical, multicentre, randomised, placebo-controlled, double-blind phase 3 trials. Lancet. 2023;401(10378):747-61.
18. Frew JW, Navrazhina K, Grand D, Sullivan-Whalen M, Gilleaudeau P, Garcet S, et al. The effect of subcutaneous brodalumab on clinical disease activity in hidradenitis suppurativa: An open-label cohort study. J Am Acad Dermatol. 2020;83(5):1341-8.
19. Frew JW, Navrazhina K, Sullivan-Whalen M, Gilleaudeau P, Garcet S, Krueger JG. Weekly administration of brodalumab in hidradenitis suppurativa: an open-label cohort study. Br J Dermatol. 2021;184(2):350-2.
20. Gordon KB, Leonardi CL, Lebwohl M, Blauvelt A, Cameron GS, Braun D, et al. A 52-week, open-label study of the efficacy and safety of ixekizumab, an anti-interleukin-17A monoclonal antibody, in patients with chronic plaque psoriasis. J Am Acad Dermatol. 2014;71(6):1176-82.
21. Tzanetakou V, Kanni T, Giatrakou S, Katoulis A, Papadavid E, Netea MG, et al. Safety and Efficacy of Anakinra in Severe Hidradenitis Suppurativa: A Randomized Clinical Trial. JAMA Dermatol. 2016;152(1):52-9.
22. Sachdeva M, Kim P, Mufti A, Maliyar K, Sibbald C, Alavi A. Biologic Use in Pediatric Patients With Hidradenitis Suppurativa: A Systematic Review. J Cutan Med Surg. 2022;26(2):176-80.
23. Liy-Wong C, Kim M, Kirkorian AY, Eichenfield LF, Diaz LZ, Horev A, et al. Hidradenitis Suppurativa in the Pediatric Population: An International, Multicenter, Retrospective, Cross-sectional Study of 481 Pediatric Patients. JAMA Dermatol. 2021;157(4):385-91
24. DeFazio MV, Economides JM, King KS, Han KD, Shanmugam VK, Attinger CE, et al. Outcomes After Combined Radical Resection and Targeted Biologic Therapy for the Management of Recalcitrant Hidradenitis Suppurativa. Ann Plast Surg. 2016;77(2):217-22.
25. Harvin G, Kasarala G. Two Cases of Paradoxical Hidradenitis Suppurativa while on Adalimumab. Case Rep Gastroenterol. 2016;10(1):88-94.
26. Faivre C, Villani AP, Aubin F, Lipsker D, Bottaro M, Cohen JD, et al. Hidradenitis suppurativa (HS): An unrecognized paradoxical effect of biologic agents (BA) used in chronic inflammatory diseases. J Am Acad Dermatol. 2016;74(6):1153-9.

CHAPTER 22

Use of Biologics in Dermatological Aspects of Autoimmune Rheumatic Diseases

Shivraj Padiyar, Prathyusha Manikuppam

INTRODUCTION

Connective tissue disorders (CTDs) are characterized by heterogeneity in immunopathogenesis, clinical and laboratory features, and prognosis. Several immunological pathways across the adaptive and innate immune systems interact and result in various specific and nonspecific clinical features seen in CTDs. Cutaneous involvement in CTDs has varied manifestations, and responses to available immunosuppressants are also different. It is a challenge for the physician to balance between the desired response to treatment and the undesired adverse effects of immunosuppression. The availability of biological disease-modifying antirheumatic drugs (bDMARDs) has heralded novel possibilities in the field of therapeutics in autoimmune disorders.

The available literature on the clinical efficacy of bDMARDs on cutaneous manifestations of CTDs is limited due to many reasons. The biologics have been introduced in clinical practice in the recent past. The cost of treatment has been a major hurdle for its use across patients of different socioeconomic statuses. In the majority of the clinical trials on the efficacy of biologics in CTDs, composite disease activity scoring and response criteria have been used rather than skin-specific measures. The aim of this chapter is to analyze the available data and interpret them to make clinical decisions on pharmacotherapy of cutaneous manifestation of CTDs.

SYSTEMIC LUPUS ERYTHEMATOSUS

The first-line systemic therapies for cutaneous lupus erythematosus (CLE) are hydroxychloroquine, corticosteroids, methotrexate, mycophenolate mofetil, and calcineurin inhibitors like cyclosporine and tacrolimus. However, despite these therapies, a proportion of them may have refractory cutaneous manifestations **(Table 1)**.

Figure 1 depicts the various sites of action of biologics in systemic lupus erythematosus (SLE).

TABLE 1: Dosage, adverse events, and prebiological workup of various biologicals.

Drug	Dosage and administration	Adverse events	Prebiological workup
Rituximab	IV: 1,000 mg, 2 doses, 2 weeks apart, intravenous	• Infusion reactions, late-onset neutropenia, hypogammaglobulinemia • Infections (bacterial, hepatitis B reactivation, and PML)	Blood-borne virus screen (hepatitis B/C/HIV), hepatitis B core antigen, immunoglobulin G, chest X-ray, and urine routine
Belimumab	• IV: 10 mg/kg every 4 weeks • SC: 200 mg once weekly	Infusion reactions, infections (bacterial, viral, and PML), depression, and suicidal tendencies	Blood-borne virus screen (hepatitis B/C/HIV), hepatitis B core antigen, immunoglobulin G, chest X-ray, and urine routine
Anifrolumab	IV: 300 mg every 4 weeks	Respiratory tract infections, herpes zoster, infusion reactions	Rule out active infections, blood-borne virus screen, Quantiferon TB gold, and CT chest
Tocilizumab	• IV: 8 mg/kg every month • SC: 162 mg every 2 weeks	• Herpes zoster • Transaminitis, infections, neutropenia, thrombocytopenia, and diverticulitis	Blood-borne virus screen (hepatitis B/C/HIV), Quantiferon TB gold, CT chest, and urine routine

(CT: computed tomography; HIV: human immunodeficiency virus; IV: intravenous; PML: progressive multifocal leukoencephalopathy; SC: subcutaneous; TB: tuberculosis)

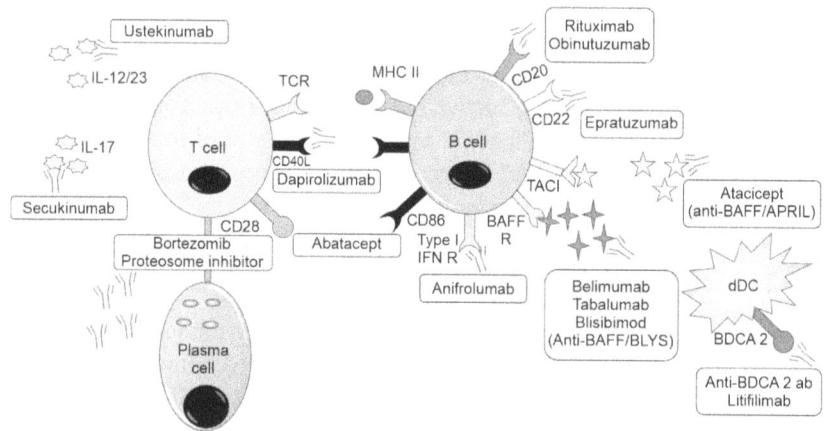

FIG. 1: Sites of action of biologics in SLE.

(IFN: interferon; IL: interleukin; MHC: major histocompatibility complex; SLE: systemic lupus erythematosus; TCR: T-cell receptor)

B cells play a major role in SLE pathogenesis through the formation of autoantibodies and immune complexes, activation of dendritic and T cells, cytokine production, and chemokine-mediated reactions. However, their role in CLE pathogenesis is still not very clear. A recent study done by Abernathy-Close et al. demonstrated significant transcriptional B-cell signatures in discoid lesions, followed by acute CLE (ACLE) and subacute CLE (SCLE) lesions.[1] A similar study done by Jenks et al., in primary chronic CLE (CCLE), showed that around 38% of patients demonstrated a highly activated SLE-like B-cell profile.[2] Considering the multifunctional role of B cells, the use of B-cell-targeted therapies looks promising.

Rituximab is an anti-CD20 monoclonal antibody. The landmark study for rituximab in extrarenal manifestations (EXPLORER trial) did not show significant responses in the cutaneous endpoints. However, one must realize that this trial had many fallacies like significant background immunosuppression, use of stricter outcome measures, and heterogenous population, and the efficacy of this agent in real-world scenario is different. A number of cohort studies have shown the efficacy of rituximab in severe CLE, but the results are variable. Complete response rates with rituximab in CLE vary between 28 and 50% and partial response rates vary between 23 and 76% as per the previous prospective and retrospective cohort studies.[3-6] However, relapses were seen in around 40% of patients. The response to various types of CLE is also variable. Although the study done by Vital et al.[5] showed a favorable response in ACLE patients (43%) with no response in CCLE lesions, further larger study[4] showed a good response in all three types of CLE lesions. Rituximab may also be used to reduce the overall steroid burden in patients with relapsing CLE.

Thus, summarizing, rituximab is efficacious in CLE, with variable responses across the subtypes. It can be used as an agent of choice in severe refractory CLE.

Belimumab, on the other hand, blocks the binding of soluble human B lymphocyte stimulator (BLyS) to its B cell receptors, thus reducing the B-cell survival. In 2020, the Food and Drug Administration (FDA) approved Benlysta® (belimumab) for both the intravenous (IV) and subcutaneous (SC) administration routes for the treatment of adult patients with active lupus nephritis (LN) who are receiving standard therapy. Post hoc analysis of phase III randomized trials of belimumab (BLISS 52 and 76) showed overall improvements in terms of Systemic Lupus Erythematosus Disease Activity Index (SLEDAI) score; however, cutaneous specific outcomes were not studied.[7] In a multicenter retrospective study of 16 patients with CLE, belimumab showed that 50% of patients achieved CLASI 50 (CLE Disease Area and Severity Index activity), and a complete response was seen in 19%. A higher proportion of patients with Fitzpatrick skin phototypes IV to VI than II and III.[8] A systematic review and meta-analysis of more than six published studies demonstrated that belimumab use in CLE was associated with a cutaneous clinical response ranging from 44 to 55%, with a 50% lower flare risk over 1 year of treatment, regardless of whether or not patients had SLE.[9] A recently done large multicenter study from Italy, BeRLiSS (Belimumab in Real-Life Setting Study), showed significant improvements in CLASI score of 4 (2-7.5) at baseline to 0 (0-3) ($p < 0.001$) at 6 months in the IV belimumab group.[10] Early disease and low baseline damage were considered significant predictors of response. Belimumab has also been shown to be useful in recalcitrant disease. Vashisht et al. reported a series of five cases that showed significant improvements in CLASI scores (median 17, 9-31) to (3, 2-14); ($p = 0.043$) with a median time to clinical response was 8-12 weeks. Thus, belimumab appears as a promising agent for treatment in CLE with limited data on its success in refractory cases.

Anifrolumab is a human monoclonal antibody that binds to type I interferon (IFN) receptor subunit 1. Anifrolumab is the second biologic, which has been approved by the FDA for the management of active lupus. The phase III TULIP-1 (Treatment of Uncontrolled Lupus via the Interferon Pathway) trial,[11] although it did not meet the primary endpoints, showed CLASI 50 response in 24 (42%) of 58 patients in the anifrolumab 300 mg group and 14 (25%) of 54 in the placebo group [difference 17.0 (95% CI −0.3 to 34.3)]. Similarly in the TULIP 2 (trial CLASI 50 week 12 was achieved in 49.0% of the patients (24 of 49) receiving anifrolumab and in 25.0% (10 of 40) receiving placebo (95% CI 4.3-43.6; adjusted $p = 0.04$).[12] Anifrolumab was also tried in refractory cutaneous lupus. A multicenter prospective study conducted in France, in 11 patients, concluded that there was a significant reduction in the median CLASI 50 activity from 15 (4-35) at baseline to 2 (0-13) at week 16 ($p < 0.001$), with a median time to achieve CLASI 50 being 1 month.[13] Sifalimumab on the other hand is a human IgG1κ monoclonal antibody targeting IFN-α molecule, leaving other IFN molecules to bind to the IFN receptor. There is a paucity of data for sifalimumab in SLE. A phase IIB trial done in the UK showed that sifalimumab at doses between 200 and 1,200 mg showed meaningful reductions in CLASI in 70-90% of the patients[14] at week 52. However, given FDA approval for anifrolumab in 2021, the company announced that it would not develop sifalimumab further.[15]

Aligning with earlier findings, a subsequent analysis of a phase II randomized controlled trial (RCT) involving ustekinumab, an IL-12/23 monoclonal antibody, revealed a decrease in the skin disease activity among SLE patients with elevated CLASI scores. The percentage of patients experiencing a ≥50% improvement in CLASI activity score plateaued at week 28 (67.7%) and persisted through week 48 (68.6%) within the ustekinumab group.[16]

In a phase II trial,[17] adults with histologically confirmed CLE, with or without systemic manifestations, were randomly assigned in a 1:1:1:1 ratio to receive SC litifilimab (at doses of 50, 150, or 450 mg) or placebo at weeks 0, 2, 4, 8, and 12. A dose-response model was employed to evaluate responses across the four groups based on the primary endpoint, which measured the percent change from baseline to 16 weeks in the CLASI-A (Cutaneous Lupus

Erythematosus Disease Area and Severity Index Activity score; scores range from 0 to 70, with higher scores indicating more widespread or severe skin involvement). Treatment with litifilimab was found to be superior to placebo with regard to a measure of skin disease activity over a period of 16 weeks.

SYSTEMIC SCLEROSIS

Systemic sclerosis or scleroderma is a rare CTD of the skin and internal organs. The pathogenesis of this is complex, usually a combination of autoimmunity, endothelial damage, and fibrosis. B cells play an important role in the production of profibrotic cytokines and subsequent fibrosis. A multicentric study from the EUSTAR group[18] was conducted in 63 patients of severe diffuse systemic sclerosis with mRSS (modified Rodnan Skin score) as the primary outcome. Rituximab showed significant improvement in mean mRSS from baseline to follow-up (26.6 ± 1.4 vs. 20.3 ± 1.8; $p = 0.0001$). Subsequently, a large RCT from India also replicated similar findings with the improvement of mean mRSS from baseline to follow-up at 6 months [21.77 (9.86) to 12.10 (10.14)].[19]

Calcinosis is a bothersome refractory manifestation of scleroderma. Although multiple therapies have been tried, optimal treatment in refractory cases still remains a challenge. Rituximab has found a promising role in the management of scleroderma-associated calcinosis. In a series of eight patients, 50% of patients achieved complete response in calcinosis.[20]

Interleukin-6 (IL-6) is an important driver of fibroblast transformation to myofibroblast via the Janus kinase/signal transducer and activator of transcription-3 (JAK/STAT3) signaling pathway.[21] Tocilizumab is a humanized IL-6 receptor antagonist (IL-6Ra). Many studies have dwelled on the efficacy of this drug for skin tightening in systemic sclerosis. The earliest phase II trial of tocilizumab (fascinate study) showed no significant change in mRSS as compared to the placebo (change of −2.70, 95% CI −5.85 to 0.45; $p = 0.0915$).[22] Subsequently, a phase III trial multicenter study was conducted in 210 participants, with mRSS as the primary outcome. The mean mRSS reduction was −6.14 for SC tocilizumab group as compared to −4.41 for placebo [difference −1.73 (95% CI −3.78 to 0.32); $p = 0.10$].[23] Thus summarizing, tocilizumab has not seen light of the day on the efficacy of cutaneous manifestations in systemic sclerosis and may need further evidence to justify its use solely for skin tightening.

Abatacept is a human fusion protein that blocks the costimulatory CD80–CD86 molecule. In a small RCT,[24] seven patients with Diffuse Cutaneous Systemic Sclerosis (DcSSc) were randomly assigned to receive abatacept, while three were assigned to the placebo group. Abatacept dosing was based on body weight, with 500 mg/dose for patients weighing ≤60 kg, 750 mg/dose for those between 60 and 100 kg, and 1,000 mg/dose for those weighing over 100 kg. Infusions were administered every 28 days, following the standard dosage interval in rheumatoid arthritis. The primary endpoint of the study was the improvement of mRSS after 24 weeks. Significantly, the mRSS showed notable differences between the intervention and placebo groups.

Riociguat is soluble guanylate cyclase (sGC) stimulator and has antiproliferative as well as vasorelaxing action.[25] It has been tried in patients with early DcSSc [Riociguat Safety and Efficacy in Patients with Diffuse Cutaneous Systemic Sclerosis (RISE-SSc)] in a randomized, double-blind, placebo-controlled multicenter trial. Even though mRSS decreased in this trial, the fall was not statistically significant.

Romilkimab is a bispecific monoclonal (immunoglobulin-G4) antibody that binds and neutralizes both IL-4 and IL-13. A randomized, double-blind, placebo-controlled, 24-week, phase II, proof-of-concept study of romilkimab in early DcSSc was conducted in which significant change in mRSS scores were noticed.[26]

INFLAMMATORY MYOSITIS

Cutaneous manifestations of dermatomyositis (DM) vary from the pathognomonic Gottron's papules and heliotrope rash to nonspecific lesions like calcinosis, panniculitis, photosensitivity, and others. Cutaneous manifestations, especially calcinosis and vasculopathy can be a source of considerable morbidity and may pose a difficult challenge in management.

The post hoc analysis of the landmark Rituximab in Myositis (RIM) trial[27] done on refractory DM patients, shed light on the utility of rituximab in cutaneous manifestations of DM. Rituximab showed a significant decrease in the frequency of erythroderma, erythematous rashes without secondary changes, heliotrope rash, Gottron sign and papules, periungual erythema, and mechanics hands. However, it did not show significant improvements in cutaneous ulcerations, panniculitis, calcinosis, lipodystrophy, and scarring. A retrospective study done later, on refractory DM, showed a 72.2% improvement in skin response with rituximab with a significant steroid-sparing effect.[28]

Rituximab has also found a potential role in reversing small vessel vasculopathy changes demonstrated by its effect on nailfold capillaries. A retrospective study demonstrated normal capillary density in 80% of patients at 6 months, and 100% of patients at 2 years, in patients treated with rituximab.[29]

Although larger studies have not shown significant benefits in panniculitis, multiple case reports have demonstrated its usefulness in refractory cases.[30,31]

CUTANEOUS VASCULITIS

Cutaneous vasculitis can be either primary cutaneous vasculitis or systemic manifestation of connective tissue disease or systemic vasculitis. The common CTDs that present with cutaneous vasculitis are Sjögren syndrome, SLE, rheumatoid arthritis, and mixed CTD. Sjögren syndrome can cause small vessel vasculitis either due to the disease per se or can be associated with cryoglobulinemic vasculitis (CV). CV is an immune complex-mediated disease characterized by arthralgia, fatigue, and purpura with systemic involvement in the form of neuropathy and nephropathy. It could be either seen in association with hepatitis C virus or underlying CTD. Rituximab has been studied in various studies and has demonstrated a complete response in 50–62% of cases.[32-34] IgA vasculitis on the other hand is characterized by palpable purpura, arthritis, and renal involvement. Although self-limiting in the pediatric population, it can be refractory in adults requiring biologicals. The usage of rituximab is mainly for renal involvement, and its utility in cutaneous lesions is limited to individual case reports.[35]

LIVEDOID VASCULOPATHY

It is a rare disease of multiple etiologies, culminating in recurrent painful ulcers in the lower extremities, which heal with white stellate scars. There is thrombotic occlusion of cutaneous microcirculation leading to ischemia and ulcers. This can occur secondary to inherited or acquired thrombophilia, connective tissue diseases, malignancies, or vasculitis, just to name a few. There is a potential contribution of both prothrombotic factors and inflammatory pathways, as there is evidence for both anticoagulation and immunosuppressive agents.[36] Antiplatelet agents and anticoagulation may be the first line of treatment and immunosuppressive agents are given in unresponsive or refractory cases. Biological agents that have been tried in refractory cases are rituximab and tumor necrosis factor inhibitors. Most of the evidence comes from case reports and case series.[37,38]

CONCLUSION

The use of biologics in the management of cutaneous manifestation of autoimmune connective tissue disease is increasing. It improves the clinical outcome and quality of life in difficult to treat disease.

REFERENCES

1. Abernathy-Close L, Lazar S, Stannard J, Tsoi LC, Eddy S, Rizvi SM, et al. B Cell Signatures Distinguish Cutaneous Lupus Erythematosus Subtypes and the Presence of Systemic Disease Activity. Front Immunol. 2021;12:775353.
2. Jenks SA, Wei C, Bugrovsky R, Hill A, Wang X, Rossi FM, et al. B cell subset composition segments clinically and serologically distinct groups in chronic cutaneous lupus erythematosus. Ann Rheum Dis. 2021;80(9):1190-200.
3. Quelhas da Costa R, Aguirre-Alastuey ME, Isenberg DA, Saracino AM. Assessment of Response to B-Cell Depletion Using Rituximab in Cutaneous Lupus Erythematosus. JAMA Dermatol. 2018;154(12):1432-40.

4. Md Yusof MY, Shaw D, El-Sherbiny YM, Dunn E, Rawstron AC, Emery P, et al. Predicting and managing primary and secondary non-response to rituximab using B-cell biomarkers in systemic lupus erythematosus. Ann Rheum Dis. 2017;76(11):1829-36.
5. Vital EM, Wittmann M, Edward S, Md Yusof MY, MacIver H, Pease CT, et al. Brief report: responses to rituximab suggest B cell-independent inflammation in cutaneous systemic lupus erythematosus. Arthritis Rheumatol. 2015;67(6):1586-91.
6. Hofmann S, Leandro M, Morris S, Isenberg D. Effects of rituximab-based B-cell depletion therapy on skin manifestations of lupus erythematosus – report of 17 cases and review of the literature. Lupus. 2013;22(9):932-9.
7. Navarra SV, Guzmán RM, Gallacher AE, Hall S, Levy RA, Jimenez RE, et al. Efficacy and safety of belimumab in patients with active systemic lupus erythematosus: a randomised, placebo-controlled, phase 3 trial. Lancet Lond Engl. 2011;377(9767):721-31.
8. Salle R, Chasset F, Kottler D, Picard-Dahan C, Jannic A, Mekki N, et al. Belimumab for refractory manifestations of cutaneous lupus: A multicenter, retrospective observational study of 16 patients. J Am Acad Dermatol. 2020;83(6):1816-9.
9. Kneeland R, Montes D, Endo J, Shields B, Bartels CM, Garg S. Improvement in Cutaneous Lupus Erythematosus After Twenty Weeks of Belimumab Use: A Systematic Review and Meta-Analysis. Arthritis Care Res (Hoboken). 2023;75(8):1838-48.
10. Zen M, Gatto M, Depascale R, Regola F, Fredi M, Andreoli L, et al. Early and Late Response and Glucocorticoid-Sparing Effect of Belimumab in Patients with Systemic Lupus Erythematosus with Joint and Skin Manifestations: Results from the Belimumab in Real Life Setting Study—Joint and Skin (BeRLiSS-JS). J Pers Med. 2023;13(4):691.
11. Furie RA, Morand EF, Bruce IN, Manzi S, Kalunian KC, Vital EM, et al. Type I interferon inhibitor anifrolumab in active systemic lupus erythematosus (TULIP-1): a randomised, controlled, phase 3 trial. Lancet Rheumatol. 2019;1(4):e208-19.
12. Morand EF, Furie R, Tanaka Y, Bruce IN, Askanase AD, Richez C, et al. Trial of Anifrolumab in Active Systemic Lupus Erythematosus. N Engl J Med. 2020;382(3):211-21.
13. Chasset F, Jaume L, Mathian A, Abisror N, Dutheil A, Barbaud A, et al. Rapid efficacy of anifrolumab in refractory cutaneous lupus erythematosus. J Am Acad Dermatol. 2023;89(1):171-3.
14. Khamashta M, Merrill JT, Werth VP, Furie R, Kalunian K, Illei GG, et al. Sifalimumab, an anti-interferon-α monoclonal antibody, in moderate to severe systemic lupus erythematosus: a randomised, double-blind, placebo-controlled study. Ann Rheum Dis. 2016;75(11):1909-16.
15. Isenberg DA, Merrill JT. Why, why, why de-lupus (does so badly in clinical trials). Expert Rev Clin Immunol. 2016;12(2):95-8.
16. Van Vollenhoven RF, Hahn BH, Tsokos GC, Lipsky P, Fei K, Gordon RM, et al. Maintenance of Efficacy and Safety of Ustekinumab Through One Year in a Phase II Multicenter, Prospective, Randomized, Double-Blind, Placebo-Controlled Crossover Trial of Patients With Active Systemic Lupus Erythematosus. Arthritis Rheumatol. 2020;72(5):761-8.
17. Werth VP, Furie RA, Romero-Diaz J, Navarra S, Kalunian K, Vollenhoven RF van, et al. Trial of Anti-BDCA2 Antibody Litifilimab for Cutaneous Lupus Erythematosus. N Engl J Med. 2022;387(10):894-904.
18. Jordan S, Distler JHW, Maurer B, Huscher D, Laar JM van, Allanore Y, et al. Effects and safety of rituximab in systemic sclerosis: an analysis from the European Scleroderma Trial and Research (EUSTAR) group. Ann Rheum Dis. 2015;74(6):1188-94.
19. Sircar G, Goswami RP, Sircar D, Ghosh A, Ghosh P. Intravenous cyclophosphamide vs rituximab for the treatment of early diffuse scleroderma lung disease: open label, randomized, controlled trial. Rheumatology. 2018;57(12):2106-13.
20. Narváez J, Pirola JP, LLuch J, Juarez P, Nolla JM, Valenzuela A. Effectiveness and safety of rituximab for the treatment of refractory systemic sclerosis associated calcinosis: A case series and systematic review of the literature. Autoimmun Rev. 2019;18(3):262-9.

21. Li Y, Zhao J, Yin Y, Li K, Zhang C, Zheng Y. The Role of IL-6 in Fibrotic Diseases: Molecular and Cellular Mechanisms. Int J Biol Sci. 2022;18(14):5405-14.
22. Khanna D, Denton CP, Jahreis A, Laar JM van, Frech TM, Anderson ME, et al. Safety and efficacy of subcutaneous tocilizumab in adults with systemic sclerosis (faSScinate): a phase 2, randomised, controlled trial. The Lancet. 2016;387(10038):2630-40.
23. Khanna D, Lin CJF, Furst DE, Goldin J, Kim G, Kuwana M, et al. Tocilizumab in systemic sclerosis: a randomised, double-blind, placebo-controlled, phase 3 trial. Lancet Respir Med. 2020;8(10):963-74.
24. Chakravarty EF, Martyanov V, Fiorentino D, Wood TA, Haddon DJ, Jarrell JA, et al. Gene expression changes reflect clinical response in a placebo-controlled randomized trial of abatacept in patients with diffuse cutaneous systemic sclerosis. Arthritis Res Ther. 2015;17(1):159.
25. Khanna D, Allanore Y, Denton CP, Kuwana M, Matucci-Cerinic M, Pope JE, et al. Riociguat in patients with early diffuse cutaneous systemic sclerosis (RISE-SSc): randomised, double-blind, placebo-controlled multicentre trial. Ann Rheum Dis. 2020;79(5):618-25.
26. Allanore Y, Wung P, Soubrane C, Esperet C, Marrache F, Bejuit R, et al. A randomised, double-blind, placebo-controlled, 24-week, phase II, proof-of-concept study of romilkimab (SAR156597) in early diffuse cutaneous systemic sclerosis. Ann Rheum Dis. 2020;79(12):1600-7.
27. Aggarwal R, Loganathan P, Koontz D, Qi Z, Reed AM, Oddis CV. Cutaneous improvement in refractory adult and juvenile dermatomyositis after treatment with rituximab. Rheumatol Oxf Engl. 2017;56(2):247-54.
28. Kuye IO, Smith GP. The Use of Rituximab in the Management of Refractory Dermatomyositis. J Drugs Dermatol. 2017;16(2):162-6.
29. Argobi Y, Smith GP. Tracking changes in nailfold capillaries during dermatomyositis treatment. J Am Acad Dermatol. 2019;81(1):275-6.
30. Ambooken B, Balakrishnan PP, Asokan N, Krishnan J, Ambooken B, Balakrishnan PP, et al. Ulcerated lobular panniculitis: An unusual initial presentation of anti-Mi-2-alpha positive dermatomyositis. Indian J Dermatol Venereol Leprol. 2022;88(3):381-4.
31. Sable KA, Rosenfeld D, Speiser J, Lake E. Juvenile Dermatomyositis–Associated Panniculitis. Cutis. 2022;110(6):E8-E10.
32. Wink F, Houtman PM, Jansen TLTA. Rituximab in cryoglobulinaemic vasculitis, evidence for its effectivity: a case report and review of literature. Clin Rheumatol. 2011;30(2):293-300.
33. Saadoun D, Resche-Rigon M, Sene D, Perard L, Karras A, Cacoub P. Rituximab combined with Peg-interferon-ribavirin in refractory hepatitis C virus-associated cryoglobulinaemia vasculitis. Ann Rheum Dis. 2008;67(10):1431-6.
34. Treatment with rituximab in patients with mixed cryoglobulinemia syndrome: Results of multicenter cohort study and review of the literature. Autoimmun Rev. 2011;11(1):48-55.
35. Fenoglio R, Sciascia S, Naretto C, De Simone E, Del Vecchio G, Ferro M, et al. Rituximab in severe immunoglobulin-A vasculitis (Henoch-Schönlein) with aggressive nephritis. Clin Exp Rheumatol. 2020;38 Suppl 124(2):195-200.
36. Vasudevan B, Neema S, Verma R. Livedoid vasculopathy: A review of pathogenesis and principles of management. Indian J Dermatol Venereol Leprol. 2016;82:478.
37. Gao Y, Jin H. Efficacy of an anti-TNF-alpha agent in refractory livedoid vasculopathy: a retrospective analysis. J Dermatol Treat. 2022;33(1):178-83.
38. Huang XW, Zheng HX, Wang ML, He WM, Feng MX, Zeng K, et al. Adalimumab in Treating Refractory Livedoid Vasculopathy. Vaccines. 2022;10(4):549.

> # SECTION 7

Biologics and Chronic Infections

CHAPTER 23

Management of Latent Tuberculosis Infection

Bhushan Madke, Swetalina Pradhan

INTRODUCTION

Anti-tumor necrosis factor alpha (anti-TNF-α) agents are being increasingly used in the management of moderate-to-severe psoriasis. Therapy with anti-TNF-α agents is fraught with risk of reactivation of latent tuberculosis infection (LTBI). This chapter addresses the intricate relation between LTBI and anti-TNF-α agents and provides working guidelines for screening of LTBI and its management before prescribing anti-TNF-α therapy in patients with psoriasis.

Tuberculosis (TB) affects all age groups and is present worldwide. In 2021, an estimated 10.6 million people fell ill with TB worldwide out of which six million were men, 3.4 million were women, and 1.2 million were children. Among all TB cases, 6.7% were among people living with HIV. Geographically, most TB cases in 2021 were in the World Health Organization (WHO) regions of Southeast Asia (45%), Africa (23%), and the Western Pacific (18%), with smaller shares in the Eastern Mediterranean (8.1%), the Americas (2.9%), and Europe (2.2%). There has been 4.5% hike in the number of people who fell ill due to TB in 2021 compared to 2020 which is reverse to the data over many years. Similarly, the TB incidence rate (new cases per 100,000 population per year) is estimated to have increased by 3.6% between 2020 and 2021, following declines of about 2% per year for most of the past two decades. In 2021, eight countries accounted for more than two-thirds of global TB cases: India (28%), Indonesia (9.2%), China (7.4%), the Philippines (7.0%), Pakistan (5.8%), Nigeria (4.4%), Bangladesh (3.6%), and Democratic Republic of the Congo (2.9%).

In 2021, 82% of global TB deaths among human immunodeficiency virus (HIV)-negative people occurred in the WHO African and Southeast Asia regions out of which India alone accounted for 36%. The African and Southeast Asia regions accounted for 82% of the combined total of TB deaths in HIV-negative and HIV-positive people; India accounted for 32%.[1]

PATHOGENESIS OF TUBERCULOUS INFECTION

Mycobacterium tuberculosis (*M. tuberculosis*)/tubercle bacilli are carried in airborne particles, called droplet nuclei, of 1–5 µ sized in diameter generated from the person having active respiratory TB (lung or laryngeal). After inhalation of the droplet nuclei containing *M. tuberculosis*, the infectious bacilli traverse the mouth or nasal passages, upper respiratory tract, and bronchi to reach the alveoli of the lungs.

Within 2–8 weeks, special immune cells called macrophages ingest and surround the tubercle bacilli. The cells form a barrier shell, called a granuloma, that keeps the bacilli contained and under control leading to establishment of LTBI.

Persons with LTBI have *M. tuberculosis* in their bodies, but do not have TB disease and cannot spread the infection to another susceptible host. However, in some infected individuals, the tubercle bacilli overcome the cellular immune system and multiply, resulting in progression from LTBI to TB disease. The progression from LTBI to TB disease may occur at any time, from soon to many years later. Hence, detection of LTBI is of utmost important in cases where chance of iatrogenic immunosuppression persists. Currently, LTBI can be screened by using either tuberculin skin test (TST) or an interferon gamma release assay (IGRA). It usually takes about 2–8 weeks interval period for the body's immune system to be able to react to tuberculin and for the infection to be detected by the TST or IGRA. Within weeks after infection, the immune system is usually able to halt the multiplication of the tubercle bacilli, preventing further progression.

Biologics are protein molecules, which target the specific points in the immunopathogenesis of the diseases. They are produced by recombinant DNA technology. These molecules target specific pathogenetic pathways in a disease. Because of this specific action on immune system, they have fewer side effects compared to other immunosuppressives having broader action. In the current era, biologics have revolutionized the treatment of various diseases and specifically dermatological conditions.

The biological drugs are divided into three groups:[2]
1. Recombinant human cytokines and growth factors
2. Monoclonal antibodies
3. Fusion antibody proteins

Out of these three groups, monoclonal antibodies have been used frequently in various dermatological diseases. Out of monoclonal antibodies anti-TNF-α drugs, such as infliximab, adalimumab, certolizumab, and golimumab have been used commonly in various autoimmune and inflammatory conditions, i.e., psoriasis vulgaris, psoriatic arthropathy, pustular psoriasis, sarcoidosis, Crohn's disease, ulcerative colitis, rheumatoid arthritis, ankylosing spondylitis, hidradenitis suppurativa, subcorneal pustular dermatosis, pyoderma gangrenosum, toxic epidermal necrolysis, Behçet's syndrome, and SAPHO syndrome. Monoclonal antibodies, such as omalizumab, efalizumab, and rituximab have been found useful in various other conditions like atopic dermatitis, urticaria, dermatomyositis, discoid lupus erythematosus (DLE), lichen planus, CD20+ non-Hodgkin B-cell lymphoma, paraneoplastic pemphigus, urticarial vasculitis, systemic lupus erythematosus (SLE), cutaneous B-cell lymphoma, epidermolysis bullosa acquisita (EBA), and recalcitrant pemphigus.[3-5]

After monoclonal antibodies next commonly, used biologicals are fusion proteins among which etanercept is Food and Drug Administration (FDA) approved for treatment of rheumatoid arthritis, ankylosing spondylitis, psoriatic arthropathy, and plaque psoriasis (moderate to severe).[4,5]

Though there are several indications of different biological drugs in dermatological diseases, out of them anti-TNF-α agents have been widely used and psoriasis has been the most common disease to be studied as an indication.

PSORIASIS, ANTI-TNF THERAPY, AND LATENT TUBERCULOSIS INFECTION

The prevalence of psoriasis is 2–3% of the world's population.[6] The pathogenesis of psoriasis is multifactorial and is considered to be the result of combination of genetic susceptibility, immune dysregulation, and environmental factors.[7] Key cytokines involved in the pathogenesis of psoriasis are TNF-α and interleukins (IL-12, IL-17, IL-22, and IL-23).[8] Due to advances in the understanding of the immunopathogenesis of psoriasis, more specific/targeted drugs are being used for the treatment of the same. In the last three decades, anti-TNF-α biological therapy has revolutionized the treatment of moderate-to-severe plaque psoriasis. There are 11 biologicals approved for moderate-to-severe plaque psoriasis currently approved by the US FDA. These include TNF-α antagonist (adalimumab, etanercept, infliximab, and certolizumab), one IL-12/IL-23 p40 inhibitor (ustekinumab), IL-17 inhibitors (secukinumab, brodalumabb, and ixekizumab), and IL-23 inhibitors (guselkumab, tildrakizumab, and risankizumab).[9]

However, various studies have confirmed that anti-TNF-α therapy is associated with 25 times risk of activation of LTBI, depending on the clinical setting and the anti-TNF agent used.[10,11]

Therefore, it is logical that psoriatic patients planned for anti-TNF-α therapy should be proactively screened for LTBI and if found to be positive preemptive antituberculosis treatment should be instituted prior to the initiation of biological treatment.

Interleukin-17 Inhibitors and Latent Tuberculosis Infection

Secukinumab, an interleukin-17 inhibitor, has been proved to be effective in psoriasis, psoriatic arthritis, and ankylosing spondylitis. A pooled analysis of 21 clinical trials of secukinumab (15 trials in psoriasis, 3 in psoriatic arthritis, and 3 in ankylosing spondylitis) including 7,355 patients with an overall exposure of 16,227 patient-years showed no case of TB reactivation.[12] However, given the high prevalence of TB in our country and role of IL-17 in defense against mycobacteria latent TB should be ruled out before starting treatment with these agents.

Rituximab and Latent Tuberculosis Infection

Rituximab is a chimeric monoclonal antibody directed against CD20 protein on B lymphocytes. Rituximab has been approved for pemphigus vulgaris and shown promising clinical efficacy. Being an anti-B lymphocytes agent, rituximab does not affect the immune response of T-cell. A study of 54 patients in whom rituximab was used for various rheumatologic conditions showed no increased risk of reactivation of latent TB.[13] However, rituximab is used along with steroids and other immunosuppressant in the management of pemphigus. It is advisable to rule out latent TB in this subset of patients.

Latent Tuberculosis Infection: Who Needs Investigation?

Latent TB infection, defined as a state of persistent immune response to prior-acquired *M. tuberculosis* antigens without evidence of clinically manifest active TB, affects about one-third of the world's population. Approximately 10% of people with LTBI will develop active TB disease in their lifetime.[14] Risk of reactivation depends on immunological status of the host. Testing for LTBI should be performed only in individuals who have high-risk of reactivation of TB and those who will benefit from treatment.

These high-risk groups as per current WHO guidelines are:
- People living with HIV
- Children < 5 years who are in close contact with people suffering from TB
- Patients initiating anti-TNF-α treatment
- Patients receiving dialysis
- Patient preparing for organ or hematologic transplantation
- Patients with silicosis[15]

Testing for LTBI should be performed only after clinical evaluation has ruled out active TB.

Screening for Latent Tuberculosis Infection

Tuberculin skin test and IGRAs are being currently done for diagnosis of LTBI. The diagnosis of LTBI is traditionally based on TST positivity in the absence of active TB.[16] However, TST has a low sensitivity and specificity in patients with prior *Mycobacterium bovis* infection and bacillus Calmette-Guérin (BCG) vaccination and hence loses its relevance. Therefore, IGRAs have been introduced to compensate for the drawback of TST in detecting LTBI.[17,18] It must be borne in mind that IGRAs are to be used for screening of LTBI and not for diagnosis of active TB.[19] Diagnosis of active TB requires different set of investigations. All patients with psoriasis who are considered

CHAPTER 23: Management of Latent Tuberculosis Infection

as a potential candidate for receiving anti-TNF-α therapy should receive HIV testing independent of screening for LTBI.

Tuberculin Skin Test

Tuberculin skin test is one of the widely used investigations used for diagnosis of TB since the 19th century. Targeted tuberculin testing for LTBI has been considered as a strategic component of TB control by the Centers for Disease Control and Prevention (CDC, Atlanta, USA) which specifically identifies individuals at high risk for developing TB and would benefit by the treatment of LTBI, if detected.

Tuberculin skin test administration: Tuberculin skin test is commonly done by intradermal injection, called the Mantoux technique (after Charles Mantoux), who described the technique in the early part of the 20th century. A standardized product called PPD-S (purified protein derivative-standardized) prepared from *M. tuberculosis* is used for this purpose. There are also various types of PPD of nontuberculous (i.e., atypical) *Mycobacterium,* such as PPD-A (*Mycobacterium avium*), PPD-G (Gause strain of scotochromogen), PPD-B (nonphotochromogen Battey bacilli), PPD-F (rapid grower *Mycobacterium fortuitum*), and PPD-Y (yellow photochromogen *Mycobacterium kansasii*).

Tuberculin skin test is performed by injecting 0.1 mL of PPD into the inner surface of the forearm. The injection is given intradermally with a tuberculin syringe (plastic body with a less-than-half-inch needle, either 26 or 27 gauge), with the needle bevel facing upward. The injection should produce a pale elevation of the skin (a wheal) 6–10 mm in diameter when placed correctly. Subcutaneous administration will result in rapid "washout" from the area without time for the development of a reaction while very superficial placement will result into leakage of reagent through the skin. Hence, a trained laboratory professional should be delegated the task of TST administration. If the injection is unsuccessful and not able to raise a desired wheal, it may be repeated immediately, usually on the other forearm.

Reading of tuberculin skin test: The reaction should be read between 48 and 72 hours after administration.

The reaction is measured in millimeters of the induration (palpable, raised, hardened area, or swelling) across the forearm (perpendicular to the long axis). The induration and not the erythema measurement is done in the test.[20,21] The physician should particularly stress on measurement of the indurated area rather than accepting the reading as "positive" or "negative" as this will allow any future comparisons **(Box 1 and Table 1)**.

Interpretation of tuberculin skin test: Skin test interpretation depends on the below-mentioned two factors:
1. Measurement in millimeters of the induration.
2. Person's risk of being infected with TB and of progression to disease if infected.

> **BOX 1** **Classification of the tuberculin skin test reaction.**
>
> *An induration of 5 mm or more is considered positive in:*
> - HIV-infected persons
> - A recent contact of a person with TB disease
> - Persons with fibrotic changes on chest radiograph consistent with prior TB
> - Patients with organ transplants
> - Persons who are immunosuppressed due to other reasons (e.g., taking the equivalent of > 15 mg/day of prednisone for 1 month or longer, taking TNF-α antagonists, etc.)
>
> *An induration of 10 mm or more is considered positive in:*
> - Recent immigrants (< 5 years) from high-prevalence countries
> - Injection drug users
> - Residents and employees of high-risk congregate settings
> - Mycobacteriology laboratory personnel
> - Persons with clinical conditions that place them at high-risk
> - Children < 4 years of age
> - Infants, children, and adolescents exposed to adults in high-risk categories
>
> *An induration of 15 mm or more is considered positive in:* Any person, including persons with no known risk factors for TB. However, targeted skin testing programs should only be conducted among high-risk groups
>
> (HIV: human immunodeficiency virus; TB: tuberculosis; TNF-α: tumor necrosis factor alpha)

TABLE 1: Comparison between false-positive and false-negative reactions.

False-positive reactions	False-negative reactions
• Infection with nontuberculous mycobacteria • Previous BCG vaccination • Incorrect method of TST administration • Incorrect interpretation of reaction • Incorrect antigen bottle used	• Cutaneous anergy (anergy is the inability to react to skin tests because of a weakened immune system) • Recent TB infection (within 8–10 weeks of exposure) • Very old TB infection (many years) • Very young age infection (< 6 months old) • Recent live virus vaccination (e.g., measles and smallpox) • Overwhelming TB disease • Some viral illnesses (e.g., measles and chicken pox) • Incorrect method of TST administration • Incorrect interpretation of reaction

(BCG: bacillus Calmette–Guérin; TST: tuberculin skin test; TB: tuberculosis)

Boosted reaction: The ability to react to tuberculin may decrease over time in some persons infected with *M. tuberculosis* leading to a false-negative reaction. In such cases, two-step testing is done where second TST is given after an initial negative test. The initial TST may stimulate the immune system, causing a positive or boosted reaction to subsequent tests. The

CHAPTER 23: Management of Latent Tuberculosis Infection

second boosted reading is the correct one, i.e., the result that should be used for decision-making or future comparison. Boosting is maximal if the second test is placed between 1 and 5 weeks after the initial test, and it may continue to be observed for up to 2 years.

Mantoux conversion: Conversion is defined as a change (within a 2-year period) of Mantoux reactivity, which meets either of the following criteria:[22]
- A change from a negative to a positive reaction
- An increase of ≥10 mm
- Conversion has been associated with an annual incidence of TB disease of 4% in adolescents or 6% in contacts of smear-positive cases.

Conversion is the development of new or enhanced hypersensitivity due to infection with tuberculous or nontuberculous mycobacteria, including BCG vaccination which is opposite of boosting that occurs due to recall of the hypersensitivity response in the absence of new infection.

Therefore, when testing TB contacts for conversion, the second tuberculin test is done 8 weeks after the date of last contact with the source case.

Bacillus Calmette–Guérin vaccine and the Mantoux test: According to the US recommendation, TST is not contraindicated for BCG-vaccinated persons and also prior BCG vaccination should not influence the interpretation of the test.

A diagnosis of LTBI and treatment for the same is considered for any BCG-vaccinated person whose skin test is 10 mm or greater, under any of the following circumstances:
- History of contact with another person with infectious TB.
- He was born or has lived in a high TB prevalence country.
- Continuous exposure to populations where TB prevalence is high.

Disadvantages of tuberculin skin test: The disadvantages are mentioned below:
- Poor inter-reader reliability
- False-positives/specificity (nontuberculous mycobacterial infection or prior BCG vaccination)
- Poor positive predictive value in low prevalence region

Interferon Gamma Release Assay

Background of IGRA: Various subsets of immune cells (e.g., macrophages and T lymphocytes) are involved in the immune response directed against the bacilli after being infected with *M. tuberculosis*. These cells do not fully eradicate the bacilli, but rather contain the infection.[23] Macrophages have an important role in the first-line of defense against the infection by ingesting and subsequently killing the organisms. However, *M. tuberculosis* bacilli escape the immune system and have the ability to persist within macrophages, thereby averting the attack by these host cells.[24,25] The cytokine Interferon gamma (IFN-γ) plays an important role in the elimination of *M. tuberculosis* by activating the production of reactive oxygen and nitrogen intermediates in the macrophages, which cause destruction of bacterial pathogens. CD4 T cells recognizing *M. tuberculosis* antigens produce IFN-γ causing activation of *M. tuberculosis*-infected macrophages and kill the bacilli and control their growth.[26,27]

Interferon-γ release assays are blood-based tests assessing the presence of effector and memory immune responses directed against the *M. tuberculosis* antigens. They predominantly measure the presence of *M. tuberculosis*-specific effector memory T cells, the presence of which is considered indicative of previous in vivo exposure to the bacilli. These tests measure the presence of an adaptive immune response to *M. tuberculosis* antigens, and are thus an indirect measure of *M. tuberculosis* exposure.[28,29]

Types of interferon-γ release assays: Two types of IGRAs that have been approved by the US FDA **(Table 2)**.
1. QuantiFERON®-TB Gold In-Tube test (QFT-GIT)
2. T-SPOT®.TB test (T-Spot)

QuantiFERON®-TB Gold In-Tube test: IFN-γ release assays are performed on fresh blood specimens. The QFT-GIT is performed by drawing 1 mL of blood into one of each of the three manufacturer precoated, heparinized tubes. The tubes are then incubated for 16–24 hours at 37°C within 16 hours of blood collection. The plasma is harvested after centrifugation and used to assess the concentration of IFN-α by enzyme-linked immunosorbent assay (ELISA) test. Results are interpreted according to the manufacturer's recommendations.[30]

T-SPOT®.TB test: 8 mL of blood is required and the assay is performed within 8 hours of blood collection (using heparinized tubes). Alternatively, the manufacturer also provides a reagent (T-Cell Xtend) which extends processing time to 32 hours after blood collection. The T cell containing peripheral blood mononuclear cell (PBMC) fraction is separated from

TABLE 2: Comparison between QuantiFERON®-TB Gold In-Tube test (QFT-GIT) AND T-SPOT®.TB test.

	QFT-GIT	T-SPOT
Initial process	Process whole blood within 16 hours	Process peripheral blood mononuclear cells (PBMCs) within 8 hours, or if T-Cell Xtend® is used, within 30 hours
Mycobacterium tuberculosis antigen	Single mixture of synthetic peptides representing ESAT-6, CFP-10, and TB7.7	Separate mixtures of synthetic peptides representing ESAT-6 and CFP-10
Measurement	IFN-γ concentration	Number of IFN-γ producing cells (spots)
Possible results	Positive, negative, and indeterminate	Positive, negative, indeterminate, and borderline

(IFN-γ: interferon gamma)

whole blood and distributed to the microtiter plate wells (250,000 cells/well) provided in the T-SPOT®.TB assay kit. Following 16–20 hours (at 37°C with 5% CO_2) incubation, the number of IFN-γ-secreting T cells (represented as spot-forming units) can be detected by enzyme-linked immunospot (ELISPOT) assay. Results are interpreted according to the manufacturer's recommendations.[31]

Benefits of IFN-γ release assays: The benefits are listed below:
- Single visit
- Not affected by prior BCG vaccination status
- Not dependent on observer (erythema or induration unlike TST)
- It can be used for follow-up as it does not result in boosted reaction unlike TST.

Disadvantages of interferon-γ release assays: The disadvantages are listed below:
- *Cost*: It is an expensive test, as compared to TST. Hence, WHO guidelines suggest that IGRA should not replace TST in low- and middle-income countries for detection of LTBI.
- False positive and poor positive predictive value in low prevalence region.
- Blood samples must be processed within 8–30 hours after collection while white blood cells are still viable.
- Errors in collecting or transporting blood specimens or in running and interpreting the assay can decrease the accuracy of IGRAs.

WHICH TEST TO USE AND HOW TO USE?

It is imperative to screen patients for LTBI before patients are considered for anti-TNF-α agents, as it significantly increases risk of reactivation of TB. First step in screening for LTBI is to rule out active TB by history, clinical examination, and if required necessary investigation (chest radiograph and sputum examination for acid-fast bacilli). All potential candidates should be asked about symptoms of active pulmonary TB (cough, hemoptysis, fever, night sweats, weight loss, chest pain, and shortness of breath).

Test for LTBI should be administered only when active TB is reasonably ruled out because if patient with active TB is treated as LTBI with monotherapy, the treatment will be inadequate and may lead to the development of resistance. Diagnosis of active TB disease needs culture studies, nucleic acid-based tests, and detection of acid-fast bacilli from appropriate clinical material. All psoriasis patients should be enquired for significant exposure to a source of TB (pulmonary or laryngeal) in the family and close contacts.

World Health Organization guidelines suggest use of either TST or IGRA (not both) for detection of LTBI. We propose following steps for detection of LTBI based on relevant literature and cost-effectiveness in our scenario. IGRAs should not replace TST in resource poor settings.

- TST should be used as first test for detection of LTBI.
- IGRA should be done:
  - When results from TST are indeterminate
  - When TST is positive and there is need to increase the acceptability of treatment
  - To follow-up patient who are on biological therapy, when TST is of limited value.
- In case, a patient is positive for TST or IGRA, chest X-ray should be done and any abnormality should prompt evaluation for treatment of active TB. A computed tomography scan can be ordered if chest X-ray reveals any tuberculous foci.

TREATMENT OF LATENT TUBERCULOUS INFECTION

Treatment options available for treatment of LTBI as per National Tuberculosis Controllers Association and CDC, 2020 are as follows:
- 6 months of isoniazid (INH) monotherapy
- 9 months of INH monotherapy[32]
- 3 months regimen of weekly rifapentine and isoniazid
- 3 months isoniazid and rifampicin
- 4 months of rifampicin monotherapy

Pyrazinamide-containing regimens are not used for treatment of LTBI because of unacceptable hepatotoxicity.

There are not enough studies to support or refute superiority of one regimen over another for treatment of LTBI. However, longer treatment has higher risk of hepatotoxicity and compliance issues. Although 9 months of isoniazid was a preferred regimen in the guidelines published in 2000, current guidelines, strongly recommend 6 months of isoniazid as an alternative for those persons unable to take a shorter preferred regimen (e.g., due to drug intolerability or drug-drug interactions), particularly in HIV-negative persons. The longer duration of isoniazid could increase the risk for hepatotoxicity and although increased effectiveness is plausible, the two treatment durations have not been directly compared. For patients without drug intolerability or drug-drug interactions, short-course (3-4 months) rifamycin-based treatment regimens are preferred over the longer-course (6-9 months) isoniazid monotherapy for treatment of LTBI.

American Thoracic Society (ATS) and CDC guidelines suggest use of INH daily for 9 months for treatment of LTBI as first-line therapy.[21]

The WHO and National Institute of Health, United Kingdom recommend 6 months of INH as acceptable treatment for LTBI.

ADVERSE EVENT MONITORING

Patients having LTBI are not sick and are usually in good condition. Hence, it should be kept in mind to minimize the adverse effects due to treatment.

The adverse effects are usually drug specific and include elevation of liver enzymes, peripheral neuropathy, and hepatotoxicity due to isoniazid. Rifamycin group of drugs usually cause cutaneous reactions, flu-like illness, gastrointestinal intolerance, and hepatotoxicity. Out of this adverse reaction, hepatotoxicity is alarming and should always be paid attention to.

In a systematic review of national guidelines, it was concluded that individuals receiving treatment for LTBI should be monitored clinically on a regular monthly basis to identify any adverse effects. The patients should be explained regarding the disease process, rationale of treatment and importance of treatment completion. If the patient is unable to consult the healthcare provider at the time of onset of symptoms, treatment should be stopped immediately.[33,34]

CONCLUSION

Anti-TNF-α therapy has already surpassed the conventional line of treatment for moderate-to-severe psoriasis in most of the developed countries of the world and soon will be an affordable therapeutic option in the Indian subcontinent. TB being an endemic health concern in the Indian subcontinent and further reactivation by use of anti-TNF-α agents warrants existence of region-specific guidelines for screening psoriatic patients, which are potential candidates for receiving anti-TNF-α agents. We hope that this chapter will guide the Indian dermatologist in starting anti-TNF-α therapy with certitude.

REFERENCES

1. World Health Organization. Global tuberculosis report 2021. Geneva: World Health Organization; 2021. p. 15.
2. Stern DK, Tripp JM, Ho VC, Lebwohi M. The use of systemic immune moderators in dermatology. Dermatol Clin. 2005;23(2):259-300.
3. Tzu J, Krulig E, Cardenas V, Kerdel FA. Biological agents in the treatment of psoriasis. G Ital Dermatol Venereol. 2008;143:315-27.
4. Zachariae C, Mørk NJ, Reunala T, Lorentzen H, Falk E, Karvonen SL, et al. The combination of etanercept and methotrexate increases the effectiveness of treatment in active psoriasis despite inadequate effect of methotrexate therapy. Acta Derm Venereol. 2008;88(5):495-501.
5. Gottlieb AB, Casale TB, Frankel E, Goffe B, Lowe N, Ochs HD, et al. CD4+T-cell-directed antibody responses are maintained in patients with psoriasis receiving alefacept: Results of a randomized study. J Am Acad Dermatol. 2003;49(5):816-25.
6. National Psoriasis Foundation. Psoriasis Statistics. [online] Available from https://www.psoriasis.org/psoriasis-statistics/#:~:text=Prevalence&text=125%20million%20people%20worldwide%20—% [Last accessed January, 2024].
7. Mitra A, Fallen RS, Lima HC. Cytokine-based therapy in psoriasis. Clin Rev Allergy Immunol. 2013;44(3):173-82.
8. Raychaudhuri SP. Role of IL-17 in psoriasis and psoriatic arthritis. Clin Rev Allergy Immunol. 2013;44(2):183-93.

9. Brownstone ND, Hong J, Mosca M, Hadeler E, Liao W, Bhutani T, et al. Biologic Treatments of Psoriasis: An Update for the Clinician. Biologics. 2021;15:39-51.
10. Askling J, Fored CM, Brandt L, Baecklund E, Bertilsson L, Cöster L, et al. Risk and case characteristics of tuberculosis in rheumatoid arthritis associated with tumor necrosis factor antagonists in Sweden. Arthritis Rheum. 2005;52:1986-92.
11. Wolfe F, Michaud K, Anderson J, Urbansky K. Tuberculosis infection in patients with rheumatoid arthritis and the effect of infliximab therapy. Arthritis Rheum. 2004;50:372-9.
12. Deodhar A, Mease PJ, McInnes IB, Baraliakos X, Reich K, Blauvelt A, et al. Long-term safety of secukinumab in patients with moderate-to-severe plaque psoriasis, psoriatic arthritis, and ankylosing spondylitis: integrated pooled clinical trial and post-marketing surveillance data. Arthritis Res Ther. 2019;21(1):111.
13. Alkadi A, Alduaiji N, Alrehaily A. Risk of tuberculosis reactivation with rituximab therapy. Int J Health Sci (Qassim). 2017;11(2):41-4.
14. Comstock GW, Livesay VT, Woolpert SF. The prognosis of a positive tuberculin reaction in childhood and adolescence. Am J Epidemiol. 1974;99:131-8.
15. Pai M, Rodrigues C. Management of latent tuberculosis infection: An evidence-based approach. Lung India. 2015;32:205-7.
16. Ponce de León D, Acevedo-Vásquez E, Sánchez-Torres A, Cucho M, Alfaro J, Perich R, et al. Attenuated response to purified protein derivative in patients with rheumatoid arthritis: study in a population with a high prevalence of tuberculosis. Ann Rheum Dis. 2005;64:1360-1.
17. Pai M, Riley LW, Colford JM Jr. Interferon-gamma assays in the immunodiagnosis of tuberculosis: A systematic review. Lancet Infect Dis. 2004;4:761-76.
18. Pai M, Zwerling A, Menzies D. Systematic review: T-cell-based assays for the diagnosis of latent tuberculosis infection: an update. Ann Intern Med. 2008;149:177-84.
19. Jiang W, Shao L, Zhang Y, Zhang S, Meng C, Xu Y, et al. High-sensitive and rapid detection of Mycobacterium tuberculosis infection by IFN-gamma release assay among HIV-infected individuals in BCG-vaccinated area. BMC Immunol. 2009;10:31.
20. American Thoracic Society. The tuberculin skin test, 1981. Am Rev Respir Dis. 1981;124:346-51.
21. Targeted tuberculin testing and treatment of latent tuberculosis infection. American Thoracic Society MMWR Recomm Rep. 2000;49(RR-6):1-51.
22. Nayak S, Acharjya B. Mantoux test and its interpretation. Indian Dermatol Online J. 2012;3:2-6.
23. Tufariello JM, Chan J, Flynn JL. Latent tuberculosis: mechanisms of host and bacillus that contribute to persistent infection. Lancet Infect Dis. 2003;3:578-90.
24. Russell DG. Mycobacterium tuberculosis: here today, and here tomorrow. Nat Rev Mol Cell Biol. 2001;2:569-77.
25. Vergne I, Chua J, Singh SB, Deretic V. Cell biology of Mycobacterium tuberculosis phagosome. Annu Rev Cell Dev Biol. 2004;20:367-94.
26. Caruso AM, Serbina N, Klein E, Triebold K, Bloom BR, Flynn JL. Mice deficient in CD4 T-cells have only transiently diminished levels of IFN-gamma, yet succumb to tuberculosis. J Immunol. 1999;162:5407-16.
27. Nathan CF, Murray HW, Wiebe ME, Rubin BY. Identification of interferon-gamma as the lymphokine that activates human macrophage oxidative metabolism and antimicrobial activity. J Exp Med. 1983;158:670-89.
28. Mack U, Migliori GB, Sester M, Rieder HL, Ehlers S, Goletti D, et al. Latent tuberculosis infection or lasting immune responses to M. tuberculosis? A TBNET consensus statement. Eur Respir J. 2009;33:956-73.
29. Lange C, Pai M, Drobniewski F, Migliori GB. Interferon-gamma release assays in the diagnosis of active tuberculosis: sensible or silly? Eur Respir J. 2009;33:1250-3.

30. Cellestis.com. (2007). QuantiFERON-TB Gold In-Tube Results Interpretation Guide. [online] Available from http://www.cellestis.com/IRM/Company/ShowPage.aspx?CPID=1215 [Last accessed January, 2024].
31. Oxford Immunotec. (2009). T-SPOT.TB technical handbook. [online] Available from http://www.oxfordimmunotec.com/UK%20Technical%20Handbooks [Last accessed January, 2024].
32. Sterling TR, Njie G, Zenner D, Cohn DL, Reves R, Ahmed A, et al. Guidelines for the Treatment of Latent Tuberculosis Infection: Recommendations from the National Tuberculosis Controllers Association and CDC, 2020. MMWR Recomm Rep. 2020;69(1):1-11.
33. Public Health Agency of Canada. Canadian Tuberculosis Standards, 7th edition. Ontario: Canadian Thoracic Society and the Public Health Agency of Canada; 2014.
34. Schaberg T, Bauer T, Castell S, Dalhoff K, Detjen A, Diel R, et al. Recommendations for therapy, chemoprevention and chemoprophylaxis of tuberculosis in adults and children. German Central Committee against Tuberculosis (DZK), German Respiratory Society (DGP). Pneumologie. 2012;66(3):133-71.

CHAPTER 24

Biologics in Presence of Hepatitis B and C Infection

Shekhar Neema, Manish Manrai

INTRODUCTION

Hepatitis B and C infections are common in the Indian population. Hepatitis B virus (HBV) accounts for 15–30% of acute hepatitis in India, while acute infection by hepatitis C virus (HCV) is usually asymptomatic. The transmission of these hepatotropic viruses is by blood transfusion, sexual route, perinatal transmission, intravenous drug abuse, and occupational exposure. The asymptomatic nature of infection mandates screening for these infections prior to administration of immunosuppressive medications, as immunosuppression can result in reactivation of virus and can result in acute liver damage.

HEPATITIS B VIRUS

Hepatitis B virus infection is one of the most common infections in the world. Approximately 2 billion people have been infected and 350 million are chronic carriers. India is an intermediate endemicity country where 4% of population is chronic hepatitis B carrier. Acute infection by HBV presents as hepatitis, but the outcome of infection depends on the age of the patient. Approximately 95% neonate, 20–30% of children aged 1–5 years, and <5% of adults develop chronic carrier state. Immunization has resulted in a decrease in the prevalence of infection where immunization coverage is good.

Diagnosis of Hepatitis B Virus Infection

Diagnosis of HBV infection is based on serological markers, and it is important for dermatologists to understand the variety of serological markers available and their significance. Serological markers available are hepatitis B surface antigen (HBsAg), hepatitis B surface antibody (anti-HBs), hepatitis B envelope antigen (HBeAg), hepatitis B envelope antibody (anti-HBe), anti-HBc immunoglobulin M (IgM) and IgG (core antigen) **(Table 1)**.

TABLE 1: Serological markers available for diagnosis of hepatitis B virus infection.

HBsAg	Anti-HBs	Anti-HBc IgM	Anti-HBc IgG	HBeAg	Anti-HBe	Remarks
−	+	−	−	−	−	• Vaccination • Recovery from infection
+	−	+	−	+	−	Acute infection
+	−	−	+	+	+/−	Chronic carrier state
−	−	−	+	−	+/−	• Isolated HBc • Can result in reactivation on immunosuppression
−	+	−	+	−	+	Recovery from acute infection

(anti-HBs: hepatitis B surface antibody; anti-HBe: hepatitis B envelope antibody; anti-HBc: hepatitis B core antibody; HBeAg: hepatitis B envelope antigen; HBsAg: hepatitis B surface antigen; IgG: immunoglobulin G; IgM: immunoglobulin M)

Hepatitis B surface antigen is considered a hallmark of HBV infection, and persistence of HBsAg 6 months after acute infection defines chronicity. Anti-HBs result from immunity to HBV infection and are the only serological marker present in those who have acquired immunity by vaccination. HBeAg and anti-HBe represent infectivity and viral replication. Anti-HBc IgM and IgG represent serological response to clinical infection. IgM corresponds to symptomatic phase and IgG persists during chronic infection.

Hepatitis B virus deoxyribonucleic acid (DNA) can be measured in blood by polymerase chain reaction (PCR) and is a direct measurement of viral load. The availability of this test has made HBeAg redundant as it is the most reliable marker of viral replication. Quantitative measurement of HBsAg is also available and can predict response to interferon therapy.[1,2] The guidelines suggest HBsAg and HBcAb before starting biologic treatment. HBV DNA should be measured if there is evidence of chronic infection. Alanine aminotransferase (ALT) and serum bilirubin should be done in addition. Patients who have no evidence of infection should complete the vaccination before starting biologics.[3]

Pathogenesis and Clinical Features

Hepatitis B virus is a partially double-stranded DNA virus and belongs to *Hepadnaviridae* family. Liver damage caused by this virus is immune mediated and depends on the host's immune response. Acute exacerbation of chronic hepatitis, fulminant hepatitis, glomerulonephritis, and vasculitis is an immune-mediated phenomenon.

We have already discussed that symptoms and outcome depend on the age at which infection was acquired. Infection acquired in infancy and childhood is asymptomatic but has higher chances of being chronic, while adults are mostly symptomatic but the risk of development of chronic carrier state is <5%. Less than 1% of patients with acute HBV infection develop fulminant hepatic failure.

Patients who become chronic carrier develop the initial phase of immune tolerance for years when they are HBsAg or HBeAg positive and have high HBV DNA levels but normal aminotransferases. The second phase is characterized by a loss of immune tolerance and is known as immune-clearance phase. This is characterized by a decrease in HBsAg and HBV DNA concentration but a rise in aminotransferases. 10–20% of patients become HBeAg negative and develop anti-HBe. These seroconverted patients have low HBV DNA levels and normal aminotransferases; this phase is called inactive phase and has good clinical outcomes. A recurrent increase in aminotransferases and failure to achieve immune clearance increase the risk of development of cirrhosis. 20–30% of the patients who are HBeAg negative develop active disease with an increase in aminotransferases and have a high risk of development of cirrhosis.[1,2]

Reactivation of hepatitis B infection can occur either spontaneously or after immunosuppressive therapy. It is divided into three phases. Host immunity is impaired resulting in viral replication, but ALT remains within normal limits in phase 1 and the patient is asymptomatic. Phase 2 occurs after dose reduction or treatment cessation; the immune system tries to clear the infection, which results in a rise in ALT, malaise, fatigue, and jaundice clinically. Phase 3 results in clearance of HBV, fulminant hepatitis, or cirrhosis.[4]

Treatment of Hepatitis B Virus Infection

Treatment includes general measures and specific pharmacologic therapy. General measures include regular monitoring and preventing the use of hepatotoxic drugs and alcohol. The preferred treatment for chronic hepatitis B infection is pegylated interferon alpha-2a (adults: 180 µg weekly/alpha 2b; children: 6 million IU/m^2 thrice weekly), entecavir (adults: 0.5 mg daily), and tenofovir disoproxil fumarate 300 mg/day. The nonpreferred treatment options are adefovir, lamivudine, and telbivudine. Tenofovir or entecavir is considered first-line anti-viral therapy. These drugs should be prescribed by a hepatologist and are outside of scope of this book.

Hepatitis B Infection and Biologics

In this chapter, we discuss the use of available biologics in the presence of concurrent chronic HBV infection and the monitoring of these patients while on biologics. Every patient in whom biologic therapy is planned should undergo appropriate screening for HBV infection. One should also be aware of the window period of 2–10 weeks before appearance of HBsAg and the development of symptoms after acquiring infection. It is also important to remember that HBsAg negative and anti-HBc IgG positive infection can also occur and it can result in reactivation of infection. If we take into account poor quality control of test kits, false-negative results from test, and risk of acquiring an infection during therapy, this situation becomes more complex and mandates monitoring for liver function in patients who were found negative for infection at baseline.

Tumor Necrosis Factor-alpha Inhibitors

Tumor necrosis factor-alpha (TNF-α) inhibitors are contraindicated in patients with chronic hepatitis B infection for fear of reactivation. There are published reports where TNF-α blockers have been used successfully for the management of psoriasis in the presence of HBV infection. Zingarelli et al.[5] reported that 27 HBV-infected patients were treated with anti-TNF agents, and HBV reactivation was documented in 73% patients without HBV prophylaxis and 14% of patients who were given anti-HBV therapy.[6] A prospective study conducted by Vassilopoulos et al. on the safety of anti-TNF-α agents in the presence of HBV infection included patients who were vaccinated for HBV, resolved HBV infection, and chronic HBV infection. In 19 patients with resolved HBV infection, none developed reactivation of HBV infection or an increase in transaminases. In 19 patients, who had postvaccination status, there was a decrease in anti-HB levels after therapy, but there was no evidence of reactivation. Fourteen patients with chronic HBV infection were included in study; eight patients were classified as inactive hepatitis [negative HBeAg, normal ALT/aspartate aminotransferase (AST), and HBV DNA < 2,000 IU/mL] and six as chronic hepatitis B (HBV DNA > 2,000 IU/mL, persistently elevated ALT/AST). These patients were treated with etanercept (n = 6), adalimumab (n = 4), and infliximab (n = 4). All patients were treated with antiviral therapy along with anti-TNF therapy. One patient developed viral reactivation due to the development of lamivudine-resistant strain, while four patients developed a transient increase in transaminases without any increase in HBV DNA level.[5] A study by Sayar et al. looked at the risk of hepatitis B reactivation during anti-TNF therapy in patients with past HBV infection (anti-HBs and HBc IgG positive) and concluded no risk of hepatitis B reactivation even without prophylactic antiviral treatment after 26 ± 16 weeks follow-up.[7]

The American Gastroenterology Association guidelines define patients on TNF inhibitors as moderate-risk group. They recommend prophylactic antiviral treatment in patients who are HBsAg positive/HBsAg negative and anti-HBc positive.[8]

IL-17 Inhibitor (Secukinumab and Ixekizumab)

Prescribing information suggests that patients should be screened for hepatitis B infection prior to administration of secukinumab. IL-17 has been linked with the development of fibrosis in patients of chronic hepatitis B.[9] A multicentric prospective cohort study included 49 patients with chronic HBV infection on secukinumab. Out of these 45 patients, 25 were HBsAg positive and were included in the first group, the second group had 11 patients (HBsAg negative, HbcAb positive, and HBsAb negative), and the third group had 13 patients (HBsAg negative, anti-HBc positive, and HbsAb positive). There was no viral reactivation in three patients in the first group (HbsAg positive) with antiviral treatment. Viral reactivation was seen in 6 out of 22 patients in whom antiviral prophylaxis was not given. In second and third groups, no antiviral prophylaxis was given and HBV reactivation was seen in one patient in the second group (HbcAb positive and HBsAb negative) and none in the third group (anti-HBc positive and HbsAb positive).[10] In another retrospective study including 37 patients with chronic HBV infection, 6 patients developed reactivation of hepatitis B after 9 ± 5.7 months of secukinumab treatment.[11]

Patients with chronic HBV infection planned for secukinumab treatment should undergo an evaluation to rule out chronic hepatitis B infection. The prophylactic antiviral treatment should be initiated 2-4 weeks before initiation of secukinumab.

Ixekizumab is a relatively new drug and the data regarding its use in patients with chronic HBV infection is limited. There is a case report of the successful use of ixekizumab in a liver transplant patient with chronic HBV infection.[12] It is the same class of drug as ixekizumab and the same precaution should be followed when it is planned to be used in patients with chronic hepatitis B infection.

Rituximab

Chronic HBV infection is a contraindication for the use of rituximab as it can lead to viral reactivation. Acute HBV reactivation can lead to acute liver failure in up to 25% of cases. Patients who are HBsAg positive are at the highest risk, but those who are HBsAg negative and anti-HBc positive can also develop viral reactivation. The risk of reactivation in HBsAg positive patients can be up to 50%, while in HBsAg negative/anti-HBc positive subset, it can be up to 20%. Ideally, patients in whom rituximab is planned should be screened for HBsAg and anti-HBc as the risk of reactivation in patients who are HBsAg negative/anti-HBc positive is quite high **(Flowchart 1)**. The risk of reactivation in patients who are treated with prophylactic antiviral therapy decreases substantially.[13] Antiviral therapy should be started within 1 week of administration of rituximab.[14] American Gastroenterology Association guidelines consider patients on B-cell depleting therapy to be at high risk of reactivation of hepatitis B (>10%). HbsAg positive/anti-HBc positive or HbsAg negative/anti-HbC positive patients should be treated with antivirals before starting rituximab and should be continued for 6-12 months after the last dose of rituximab.[8]

Most of this data is from patients with lymphoproliferative malignancy which is quite different from dermatology patients of autoimmune blistering disorders. Patients with malignancy are administered rituximab for a longer period of time (six cycles or more) and it is used in association with other

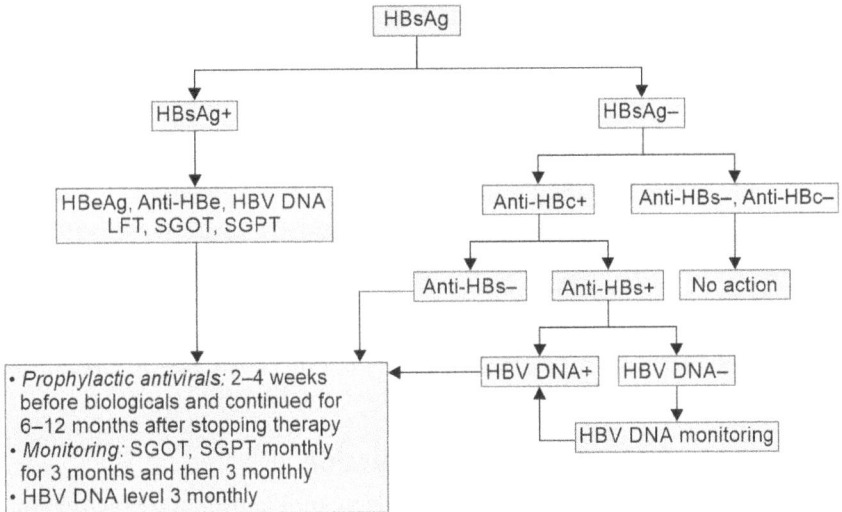

FLOWCHART 1: Practical approach to patient in whom biological therapy is contemplated.[10,11]
(Anti-HBs: hepatitis B surface antibody; Anti-HBe: hepatitis B envelope antibody; Anti-HBc: hepatitis B core antibody; DNA: deoxyribonucleic acid; HBsAg: hepatitis B surface antigen; HBeAg: hepatitis B envelope antigen; HBV: hepatitis B virus; LFT: liver function test; SGOT: serum glutamic oxaloacetic transaminase; SGPT: serum glutamic pyruvic transaminase)

chemotherapeutic agents. The extrapolation of this data to dermatology patients is not entirely correct. However, patients should be screened and those who are positive should be treated with appropriate antivirals before starting rituximab. These patients should be followed up for risk of reactivation of HBV. The data on viral reactivation in dermatology patients is lacking; however, it appears that the risk of reactivation is lower as compared to malignancy patients, and use of antiviral prophylaxis when appropriate can further reduce this risk.[14]

HEPATITIS C VIRUS

Hepatitis C virus is a single-stranded ribonucleic acid (RNA) virus of the *Flavivirus* family. The prevalence of HCV infection is approximately 2%. Modes of transmission of HCV virus are through intravenous drug abuse, infected blood, and perinatal and sexual transmission. Intravenous drug abuse and infected blood are the most efficient modes of transmission. A majority of patients are asymptomatic and show no signs of acute infection. Chronic hepatitis C occurs in 60–85% of the infected population. It is responsible for cirrhosis in 20% of the infected patients, and hepatocellular carcinoma (HCC) develops at the rate of 1–4% per year in patients with cirrhosis.[15] Chronic HCV infection is also responsible for 90% of essential mixed cryoglobulinemia.

Diagnosis of Hepatitis C Virus Infection

Diagnosis of HCV infection is based on either serology or direct detection of the virus. Serology is most commonly utilized for the diagnosis of HCV infection. There are various methods for detection of antibodies like enzyme immunoassay and immunoblot assay. Enzyme immunoassay is the most commonly utilized method and can detect antibodies within 4-10 weeks after infection. The serological test is very sensitive and diagnosis is missed in only 0.5-1% of patients in low-risk settings. False-negative tests can occur in immunocompromised patients and in patients with essential mixed cryoglobulinemia. Viral RNA can be detected using PCR and is utilized for assessing treatment response. Genotyping of virus helps in predicting outcomes of therapy and influences the choice of therapy.[16]

Treatment of Hepatitis C Virus Infection

Every patient with chronic HCV infection is a candidate for antiviral therapy. However, patients with normal aminotransferases and no histologic evidence of necroinflammatory changes have excellent prognoses even without treatment. Patients with raised aminotransferase levels and mild histological changes can be followed up by liver biopsy every 3-5 years and regular aminotransferases measurement. Patients with persistently elevated aminotransferases and moderate-to-severe changes in liver biopsy are candidates for interferon therapy.

Availability of direct-acting antivirals (DAAs) has changed the treatment of HCV infection. These drugs can lead to sustained viral clearance after 12 weeks of therapy. These drugs are sofosbuvir, daclatasvir, simeprevir, ledipasvir, paritaprevir, ombitasvir, and dasabuvir. Many other drugs of the same class are available and are being developed. Interferon-free regimens are now available and have made treatment of HCV infection safe and effective.[17]

Hepatitis C Virus Infection and Biologics

Hepatitis C virus infection is listed as a relative contraindication for use of biologics. We will discuss the available data on the use of biologics in patients with concomitant HCV infection. Treatment options like methotrexate and other hepatotoxic drugs cannot be used. Cyclosporine can be used safely as it inhibits viral replication, but it has certain other problems associated with long-term use **(Flowchart 2)**.

Tumor Necrosis Factor-alpha Inhibitors

The prescribing information on the available TNF inhibitors states chronic HCV infection as one of the contraindications, and prior testing for HCV is advised in all cases in whom biologics are planned. Hepatitis mediated by HCV is autoimmune in nature and TNF-α plays an important role in liver

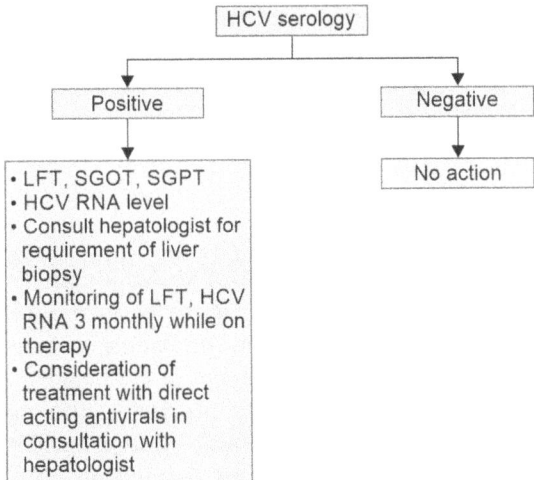

FLOWCHART 2: Practical approach on management of a patient with chronic HCV infection on whom biological therapy is planned.[10,11]
(HCV: hepatitis C virus; LFT: liver function test; RNA: ribonucleic acid; SGOT: serum glutamic oxaloacetic transaminase; SGPT: serum glutamic pyruvic transaminase)

damage caused by the virus. However, it is also known that TNF-α is essential for the host's defense against pathogen. There is a concern that the use of these drugs can lead to reactivation of infection or can result in rapid end-organ damage. In a systemic review, Caso et al. reported the safe use of etanercept and adalimumab in patients of psoriatic arthritis with concomitant HCV infection. Most of these patients were not on any concomitant antiviral therapy. TNF-α inhibitors were found to be effective and there was no deterioration of liver function test (LFT) after therapy.[18] Another study conducted by Costa et al. on 15 patients with psoriatic arthritis reported that TNF-α inhibitors can be safely used in patients with concomitant HCV infection for up to 1 year.[19] Nuzzo et al. described two cases of psoriasis with advanced liver disease due to HCV infection treated with etanercept. These patients developed HCC on long-term use of etanercept despite being on a regular follow-up with a fetoprotein and transaminases. However, whether TNF-α inhibitors played any role in the development of HCC is not known, as these patients had a high risk of development of HCC.[20]

From the currently available literature, it is reasonable to assume that TNF-α inhibitors can be used as second-line therapy in patients with psoriasis with concomitant HCV infection. Etanercept is the drug with maximum data and should be a drug of choice, if biologic therapy is being considered. Caution should be exercised and the patient should be on regular follow-up with LFT, viral load and ultrasound examination of liver being performed at a regular interval, especially in patients with advanced disease.

The availability of DAA for the treatment of HCV infection can change this scenario and antiviral drugs can be combined with biologics and possibly then biologics can be safely administered even for long term in advanced disease. However, TNF inhibitors can be used before, after, or concomitantly with TNF inhibitors, and the timing of antivirals in relation to biologics is not clear.[21]

Secukinumab and Ixekizumab

The data on the availability of the use of secukinumab in patients with hepatitis C infection is scarce. There is a case report where secukinumab has been used in conjunction with DAA and the patient underwent remission at 12 weeks for psoriasis and had undetectable viral load.[22] A multicentric prospective study included 14 patients of psoriasis with concomitant HCV infection treated with secukinumab, and 1 patient developed enhanced viral replication. Unlike chronic hepatitis B infection, the guidelines on management of patients with chronic HCV infection on secukinumab are unclear. European Association for the Study of Liver Diseases 2016 does not recommend antiviral prophylaxis in the setting of biologic therapy.

Due to the paucity of available data, one should be cautious about using secukinumab in patients with HCV infection and hepatologist consultation should be sought along with frequent monitoring of liver functions and viral load while the patient is on therapy. The data on the use of ixekizumab in a patient with chronic HCV infection is scarce and the same precautions are advised as with secukinumab treatment.

Rituximab

Rituximab is an anti-CD20 monoclonal antibody. It is used for the management of HCV-associated cryoglobulinemia. The study done by Quartuccio et al. reported that rituximab is safe for the management of HCV-associated cryoglobulinemia. It does not lead to flare of HCV infection even without the use of concomitant antivirals. It can be safely used for long-term therapy.[23] Rituximab-associated HCV flares have been reported in oncology literature and have resulted in death or liver failure in some cases. However, these patients were on other immunosuppressive and hepatotoxic medications and not only on rituximab monotherapy. The risk of reactivation of HCV infection in rheumatology literature is scant. It has been successfully used in the management of pemphigus with HCV infection without any deterioration of liver function or reactivation of HCV infection.[24]

The existing literature suggests that rituximab can be safely used for the management of pemphigus in the presence of HCV infection. However, one should always be aware of concomitant immunosuppressive medications like corticosteroid or azathioprine, which can increase the risk of viral reactivation and hepatic damage. It is best to administer rituximab in this scenario in consultation with an experienced hepatologist. It is also important to discuss the use of DAA and regular monitoring of liver function and viral load.

CONCLUSION

The presence of chronic hepatitis B and C infection are considered contraindications for the use of biologic therapy. However, biologics are one of the most effective therapies for the management of these diseases and the lack of this therapeutic option makes management unsatisfactory. The available data suggest that biologics can be safely used for the management of these diseases; however, the treating physician should be aware of the diagnosis and management algorithm for chronic hepatitis B and C infection, need for regular follow-up in these patients, and frequent consultation with a hepatologist.

REFERENCES

1. Dienstag JL. Hepatitis B virus infection. N Engl J Med. 2008;359(14):1486-500.
2. Trépo C, Chan HL, Lok A. Hepatitis B virus infection. Lancet. 2014;384(9959):2053-63.
3. European Association for the Study of the Liver; EASL 2017 Clinical Practice Guidelines on the management of hepatitis B virus infection. J Hepatol. 2017;67(2):370-98.
4. Chen YM, Yang SS, Chen DY. Risk-stratified management strategies for HBV reactivation in RA patients receiving biological and targeted therapy: A narrative review. J Microbiol Immunol Infect. 2019;52(1):1-8.
5. Zingarelli S, Frassi M, Bazzani C, Scarsi M, Puoti M, Airò P. Use of tumor necrosis factor-alpha-blocking agents in hepatitis B virus-positive patients: Reports of 3 cases and review of the literature. J Rheumatol. 2009;36(6):1188-94.
6. Papatheodoridis GV, Dimou E, Dimakopoulos K, Manolakopoulos S, Rapti I, Kitis G, et al. Outcome of hepatitis B e antigen-negative chronic hepatitis B on long-term nucleos(t)ide analog therapy starting with lamivudine. Hepatology. 2005;42(1):121-9.
7. Sayar S, Kürbüz K, Kahraman R, Öztürk O, Çalışkan Z, Doğanay HL, et al. Risk of hepatitis B reactivation during anti-TNF therapy; evaluation of patients with past hepatitis B infection. Turk J Gastroenterol. 2020;31(7):522-8.
8. Reddy KR, Beavers KL, Hammond SP, Lim JK, Falck-Ytter YT; American Gastroenterological Association Institute. American Gastroenterological Association Institute guideline on the prevention and treatment of hepatitis B virus reactivation during immunosuppressive drug therapy. Gastroenterology. 2015;148(1):215-9. quiz e16-7.
9. Vassilopoulos D, Apostolopoulou A, Hadziyannis E, Papatheodoridis GV, Manolakopoulos S, Koskinas J, et al. Long-term safety of anti-TNF treatment in patients with rheumatic diseases and chronic or resolved hepatitis B virus infection. Ann Rheum Diss. 2010;69(7):1352-5.
10. Chiu HY, Hui RC, Huang YH, Huang RY, Chen KL, Tsai YC, et al. Safety profile of secukinumab in treatment of patients with psoriasis and concurrent hepatitis B or C: A multicentric prospective cohort study. Acta Derm Venereol. 2018;98(9):829-34.
11. Liu S, He Z, Wu W, Jin H, Cui Y. Safety of secukinumab in the treatment of patients with axial spondyloarthritis and concurrent hepatitis B virus infection or latent tuberculosis infection. Clin Rheumatol. 2023;42(9):2369-76.
12. Lora V, Graceffa D, De Felice C, Morrone A, Bonifati C. Treatment of severe psoriasis with ixekizumab in a liver transplant recipient with concomitant hepatitis B virus infection. Dermatol Ther. 2019;32(3):e12909.
13. Seto WK, Chan TS, Hwang YY, Wong DK, Fung J, Liu KS, et al. Hepatitis B reactivation in patients with previous hepatitis B virus exposure undergoing rituximab-containing chemotherapy for lymphoma: A prospective study. J Clin Oncol. 2014;32(33):3736-43.

14. Huang YH, Hsiao LT, Hong YC, Chiou TJ, Yu YB, Gau JP, et al. Randomized controlled trial of entecavir prophylaxis for rituximab-associated hepatitis B virus reactivation in patients with lymphoma and resolved hepatitis B. J Clin Oncol. 2013;31(22):2765-72.
15. Shepard CW, Finelli L, Alter MJ. Global epidemiology of hepatitis C virus infection. Lancet Infect Dis. 2005;5(9):558-67.
16. Lauer GM, Walker BD. Hepatitis C virus infection. N Eng J Med. 2001;345(1):41-52.
17. Asselah T, Boyer N, Saadoun D, Martinot-Peignoux M, Marcellin P. Direct-acting antivirals for the treatment of hepatitis C virus infection: Optimizing current IFN-free treatment and future perspectives. Liver Int. 2016;36(Suppl 1):47-57.
18. Caso F, Cantarini L, Morisco F, Del Puente A, Ramonda R, Fiocco U, et al. Current evidence in the field of the management with TNF-a inhibitors in psoriatic arthritis and concomitant hepatitis C virus infection. Expert Opin Biol Ther. 2015;15(5):641-50.
19. Costa L, Caso F, Atteno M, Giannitti C, Spadaro A, Ramonda R, et al. Long-term safety of anti-TNF-α in PsA patients with concomitant HCV infection: A retrospective observational multicenter study on 15 patients. Clin Rheumatol. 2014;33(2):273-6.
20. Di Nuzzo S, Boccaletti V, Fantini C, Cortelazzi C, Missale G, Fabrizi G, et al. Are anti-TNF-α agents safe for treating psoriasis in hepatitis C virus patients with advanced liver disease? Case reports and review of the literature. Dermatology. 2016;232(1):102-6.
21. Imperatore N, Castiglione F, Rispo A, Sessa A, Caporaso N, Morisco F. Timing strategies of direct-acting antivirals and biologics administration in HCV-Infected subjects with inflammatory bowel diseases. Front Pharmacol. 2017;8:867.
22. Martinez-Santana V, Rodriguez-Murphy E, Smithson A, Miserachs-Aranda N, Del Río-Gil R, Torre-Lloverás I. Efficacy and safety of direct-acting antiviral agents when combined with secukinumab. Eur J Hosp Pharm. 2017;25(1):53-6.
23. Quartuccio L, Zuliani F, Corazza L, Scaini P, Zani R, Lenzi M, et al. Retreatment regimen of rituximab monotherapy given at the relapse of severe HCV-related cryoglobulinemic vasculitis: Long-term follow up data of a randomized controlled multicentre study. J Autoimmun. 2015;63:88-93.
24. Amber KT, Kodiyan J, Bloom R, Hertl M. The controversy of hepatitis C and rituximab: A multidisciplinary dilemma with implications for patients with pemphigus. Indian J Dermatol Venereol Leprol. 2016;82(2):182-3.

SECTION 8

Biologics in Special Situation

CHAPTER 25

Biologics in Children: Which, When, Why?

Khushboo Minni, Resham Vasani

INTRODUCTION

The management of conditions such as psoriasis (Ps), atopic dermatitis (AD), chronic spontaneous urticaria (CSU), periodic fever syndromes, autoimmune bullous disorders, juvenile collagen vascular diseases, and extensive and refractory alopecia areata (pAA) is challenging among pediatric population as there is limited data regarding efficacy and safety of treatment options. Many conventional immunosuppressive therapies (CISTs) are not appropriate for long-term use in the pediatric population due to the risk of side effects.

Biologics provide important targeted therapeutic options because of higher specificity in their mechanism of action as compared to CIST. Moreover, the use of biologics in general has reported the following advantages over conventional systemic agents:

- Fewer toxicity/serious adverse effects (SAEs) because of higher specificity in their mechanism of action as compared to CIST
- Fixed dosing plan
- Less frequent follow-up schedules

Several factors including the indication, approval for pediatric use, dosing schedule, and safety profile must be considered while choosing the appropriate biologic therapy for the pediatric population. We will dwell on biologics for various dermatological indications and their efficacy and safety in children based on available literature till date. **Table 1** mentions biologics in pediatric dermatology, their mechanism of action, and approval status.

TABLE 1: Biologics in pediatric dermatology with mechanism of action and approval status.

Biologic	Mechanism of action	Approval	Year	Disease
Secukinumab	Human IgG1 mAb that selectively binds to IL-17A cytokine and inhibits its interaction with the IL-17 receptor	*EMA and FDA:* Age ≥ 6 years	• EMA 2020 • FDA 2021	Psoriasis
Ustekinumab	Fully human mAb targeting the p40 subunit of IL-12 and IL-23	*FDA, EMA:* Age ≥6 years	2020	Psoriasis
Ixekizumab	Humanized IgG subclass 4 (IgG4) mAb against IL-17A and prevents it from interacting with the IL-17A receptor	• *FDA:* Age ≥6 years • *EMA:* Not approved for weight <25 kg	2020	Psoriasis
Etanercept	Soluble fusion protein of TNF-α receptor and Fc portion of human IgG	*FDA:* Age ≥4 years	2016	Psoriasis
Adalimumab	Fully humanized monoclonal IgG antibody targeting TNF-α	*EMA:* age ≥4 years	2015	Psoriasis
		FDA and EMA: Age ≥12 years	2015	Moderate-severe hidradenitis suppurativa
Infliximab	Chimeric monoclonal IgG antibody targeting TNF-α	Not approved/off-label		Psoriasis
Brodalumab	IL-17 receptor A inhibitor that blocks the response induced by several IL-17 isoforms	Not approved/off-label		Psoriasis
Omalizumab	Binds to IgE and decreases free IgE levels. Subsequently, IgE receptors (FcεRI) on cells are downregulated	*FDA:* Age ≥12 years	2014	Chronic spontaneous urticaria

Continued

Continued

Biologic	Mechanism of action	Approval	Year	Disease
Dupilumab	Inhibits α subunit of IL-4 and IL-13 receptor	FDA: Age 6 months to 5 years	2022	Atopic dermatitis
		FDA: Age 6–11 years	2020	Atopic dermatitis
		EMA: Age ≥12 years	2019	Atopic dermatitis
		FDA: Age ≥12 years	2017	Atopic dermatitis
Lebrikizumab	IL-13 blocker	EMA: Age ≥12 years with a body weight of at least 40 kg	2023	
Rituximab	CD20-directed cytolytic antibody	FDA: Age ≥2 years	2019	Granulomatosis with polyangiitis (GPA) (Wegener granulomatosis) and microscopic polyangiitis (MPA) in combination with glucocorticoids
Nivolumab	Programmed death receptor-1 (PD-1) blocking antibody	FDA: Age ≥12 years	2023	Completely resected stage IIB or stage IIC melanoma
Ipilimumab	Human cytotoxic T-lymphocyte antigen 4 (CTLA-4)-blocking antibody	FDA: Age ≥12 years	2017	Unresectable or metastatic melanoma
Pembrolizumab	PD-1 inhibitor	FDA: Age ≥12 years	2021	Completely resected stage IIB or stage IIC melanoma
Belimumab	Fully-humanized IgG1 γ mAb directed against soluble B-lymphocyte stimulator	FDA and EMA: Age ≥5 years	2019	Systemic lupus erythematosus as add-on therapy

(EMA: European Medicines Agency; FDA: Food and Drug Administration; IL: interleukin; mAb: monoclonal antibody; TNF-α: tumor necrosis factor-alpha)

PSORIASIS

Psoriasis accounts for approximately 4% of pediatric dermatoses, with up to 33% of cases starting in childhood.[1] Pediatric psoriasis (pPs) is reported to have double the incidence of several cardiovascular, metabolic, gastrointestinal, and psychological comorbidities than their peers.[1,2] Currently, a wide range of biological agents are available for the treatment of pPs, including tumor necrosis factor (TNF)-α inhibitors (TNFi), interleukin (IL)-12/23 inhibitors (IL12/23i), and recently approved IL-17 inhibitors and small molecules.[2] By mid-2020, >14 biologics (TNFi, IL-12/23, and IL-17 inhibitors) have been approved by the Food and Drug administration (FDA) for adult Ps.[3] On the contrary, only secukinumab, etanercept, adalimumab, ustekinumab, and ixekizumab have been approved in pPs **(Table 1)**.[4] Biologics are recommended when first- or second-line therapies fail to control disease in severe plaque pPs.[3]

Indications for the use of biologicals in pPs as per the Joint American Academy of Dermatology-National Psoriasis Foundation (AAD-NPF) 2020 guidelines include:[3]

- Severity of Ps
- Failure of other traditional treatments (topical and other systemic medications and phototherapy)
- Compromised psychosocial quality of life (QoL)
- Comorbidities mainly arthritis
- Ps type—generalized plaque type unresponsive to topical therapy or phototherapy, pustular and erythrodermic forms
- Ps site—scalp, palms, soles, and genital

After informing parents and patients, biologics may be considered in pPs with severe disease—defined as a psoriasis area and severity index (PASI) of ≥10 [or a body surface area (BSA) of ≥10%] and dermatology life quality index (DLQI) >10.[5]

The failure of one biologic therapy does not preclude a successful response to another biologic, even of the same class. Although there is little formal evidence in the pediatric population regarding the use of biologic therapies for severe palmoplantar, nail, or scalp disease or inverse or guttate Ps, these treatments have been used off-label for these indications and anecdotally have been effective. Treatment choices should be individualized to the clinical situation **(Table 2)**.[6,7]

Etanercept

Etanercept is the first biologic to be approved by the FDA and European Medicines Agency (EMA) for management of moderate-to-severe pPs in patients aged ≥4 years.[1] Pharmacokinetic data studying the etanercept dosing regimen in pediatric population revealed a similar exposure to that of the approved dose in adult patients with plaque Ps.[2]

CHAPTER 25: Biologics in Children: Which, When, Why?

TABLE 2: Other biologics with dose, route of administration, and monitoring.

Drugs	Dose	Route	Baseline tests	Follow-up tests
Secukinumab	• *<50 kg*: 75 mg • *>50 kg*: 150 mg as a starting dose (may be increased to 300 mg if needed) at weeks 0, 1, 2, 3, and 4 and every 4 weeks thereafter	SC	CBC, ESR, LFT, RFT, and urinalysis; screening for hepatitis and HIV infection; chest X-ray; tuberculin skin testing or Quantiferon Gold test; pregnancy test in adolescents of childbearing age; serology for varicella-zoster and measles (if clinically indicated)	CBC—3 monthly LFTs, RFTs—3 monthly
Etanercept	0.8 mg/kg weekly; maximum dose: 50 mg/week	SC	• Mantoux test below 5 years; IGRA above 5 years • Chest X-ray • CBC • LFT • HIV, if at risk • HBsAg, HCV, if at risk	• Annual Mantoux test/IGRA • LFT every 4–6 months (may require more frequent with infliximab) • CBC • Other monitoring will depend on situation
Infliximab	3–5 mg/kg at weeks 0, 2, 6, then every 8 weeks	IV		
Adalimumab	• *15 to <30 kg*: Initial dose of 20 mg, followed by 20 mg at week 1 and every 2 weeks thereafter • *≥30 kg*: Initial dose of 40 mg, followed by 40 mg at week 1 and every 2 weeks thereafter • *Maximum dose*: 40 mg	SC		
Ustekinumab	0.75 mg subcutaneous for weight <60 kg; 45 mg for weight ≥60 to ≤100 kg; 90 mg for weight >100 kg; at weeks 0 and 4 and every 12 weeks thereafter	SC		

(CBC: complete blood count; ESR: erythrocyte sedimentation rate; HBsAg: hepatitis B surface antigen; HCV: hepatitis C virus; HIV: human immunodeficiency virus; IGRA: interferon gamma release assay; IV: intravenous; LFT: liver function test; SC: subcutaneous; RFT: renal function test)

An open labeled trial conducted by Paller et al.[8] found etanercept in the dosage of 0.8 mg/kg (maximum dose of 50 mg) to be safe and effective till 264 weeks (5 years). Multiple case series have reported its efficacy in young children up to 22 months of age when used as a monotherapy or as an adjuvant therapy with other conventional regimens in moderate-to-severe plaque Ps, palmoplantar Ps, pustular Ps, and erythrodermic Ps.[3]

Etanercept is associated with fewer AEs than traditional systemic agents such as methotrexate or acitretin.[9] There have been no cases of opportunistic infections or malignancy reported in children or adolescents. Although TNFi carry black-box warnings for increased risk of lymphoma and other malignancies in pediatric populations, a clear relationship between the drug and malignancy has not been established.[9]

Given the quality and quantity of data, etanercept could be used as a first-line agent for systemic treatment of moderate-to-severe pPs in patients ≥4 years.

Adalimumab

Adalimumab has been approved by the EMA for the management of moderate-to-severe Ps in children >4 years in 2015. It is not US-FDA approved yet for use in pPs; however, the FDA approved it for management of juvenile idiopathic arthritis (JIA), ulcerative colitis (UC), and Crohn disease (CD) in this age group.[10]

In a study by Di Lernia et al., 54 patients received standard adalimumab doses according to their body weight. Among the 54 patients, 30 (55.5%) achieved PASI 75 at week 16, 40 (74%) achieved PASI 75 at week 24, and only 33 (61.1%) achieved PASI 75 at week 52. Moreover, among the 54 patients, only 16 (29.6%) achieved PASI 90 at week 16, 30 (55.5%) achieved PASI 90 at week 24, and 30 (55.5%) achieved PASI 90 at week 52. Additionally, no difference was observed in PASI response rates between biologic-naïve and non-naïve patients with pPs. During the study, among 12 patients, treatment was discontinued because of lack of efficacy.[11]

Du et al. in 2022 reported the efficacy of use of adalimumab in pediatric patients with refractory generalized pustular psoriasis (GPP). A total of seven patients had marked clearance and reduction in Physician's Global Assessment (PGA) and systemic/laboratory score within the first week of first subcutaneous injection and achieved almost complete clearance of skin lesions by 1 month follow-up.[12] There is lack of safety data from controlled trials.[9]

Adalimumab has been found to be more effective than methotrexate while having a similar safety profile.[13] In a randomized, double-blind, phase 3 trial of 114 children aged between 4 and 17 years with severe plaque Ps by Papp et al., 58% and 44% patients in adalimumab 0.8 mg/kg and 0.4 mg/kg group achieved PASI 75 in comparison with 32% in methotrexate group (0.1–0.4 mg/kg). But in this trial, average dose of methotrexate was

0.15 mg/kg, which is lower than the standard pediatric dosing of 0.3–0.4 mg/kg.[14] Real-world data on the treatment of pediatric plaque Ps with etanercept and adalimumab seems to corroborate clinical trial findings, with similar results regarding clinical efficacy and safety.[2]

Secukinumab

Secukinumab, a recombinant, fully human, immunoglobulin (Ig) G1κ monoclonal antibody (mAb) targeted against IL-17A is also FDA and EMU approved for the treatment of moderate-to-severe plaque Ps in pediatric patients aged ≥6 years. In pivotal phase III trials in pediatric patients aged 6 to <18 years, both low (75–150 mg) and high (75–300 mg) doses of secukinumab were significantly better than placebo and numerically better than etanercept at week 12 in terms of the proportion of patients achieving ≥75% improvement from baseline in PASI and significantly better than placebo and etanercept in terms of the proportion of patients achieving an Investigator's Global Assessment (IGA) score of 0 or 1.[14,15] The clinical efficacy of secukinumab observed during the first 12 weeks of treatment was maintained long term. Treatment with secukinumab improved health-related QoL and was generally well tolerated.[15]

Mangolo et al. in a phase III, open label, randomized trial without a control arm also evaluated the efficacy and safety of two secukinumab dosage regimens (low dose: 75/75/150 mg; high dose: 75/150/300 mg) stratified and randomized by weight (<25 kg, 25 to <50 kg, ≥50 kg) and disease severity (moderate and severe) in pediatric patients aged 6 to <18 years with moderate-to-severe plaque Ps. They observed that both secukinumab doses were superior to historical placebo with respect to PASI 75/90 and IGA 0/1 responses at week 12. The estimated probability of a positive treatment effect (i.e., log odds ratio >0) for low- or high-dose secukinumab compared with historical placebo is 1 (i.e., 100%). For the low and high doses at week 12, the IGA 0/1 response rates were 78.6% and 83.3%, respectively, and the PASI-90 response rates were 69% and 76.2%, respectively. The PASI-75 response rate was 92.9% for both the doses.[16]

Ustekinumab

Ustekinumab is IL-12/23 blocker approved for the treatment of moderate-to-severe Ps in the pediatric population aged ≥6 years.[7]

The CADMUS study is a phase 3 multicenter, randomized, double-blind, placebo-controlled study evaluating the efficacy and safety of ustekinumab in the treatment of adolescent subjects (12–17 years) with moderate-to-severe plaque-type Ps. In this study, the patients ($n = 110$) were randomly assigned to ustekinumab standard dosing [SD; 0.75 mg/kg (≤60 kg), 45 mg (>60 to ≤100 kg), and 90 mg (>100 kg)] or half-standard dosing [HSD; 0.375 mg/kg (≤60 kg), 22.5 mg (>60 to ≤100 kg), and 45 mg (>100 kg)] at weeks 0 and 4 and every 12 weeks or placebo at weeks 0 and 4 with crossover to ustekinumab

SD or HSD at week 12. At week 12, 67.6% and 69.4% of the patients receiving ustekinumab HSD and SD, respectively, achieved PGA 0/1 versus 5.4% for placebo ($p < 0.001$). Significantly greater proportions receiving ustekinumab achieved PASI 75 (HSD, 78.4%; SD, 80.6%; placebo, 10.8%) or PASI 90 (HSD, 54.1%; SD, 61.1%; placebo, 5.4%) at week 12 ($p < 0.001$). Through week 12, 56.8% of the placebo patients, 51.4% of the HSD patients, and 44.4% of the SD patients reported at least one AE; through week 60, 81.8% reported AEs. SD provided treatment responses comparable to those reported in adults.[17]

A retrospective observational study involving 134 patients compared etanercept ($n = 63$), adalimumab ($n = 44$), and ustekinumab ($n = 27$). The drug survival rate was highest for ustekinumab compared with etanercept and adalimumab ($p < 0.0001$). Severe AEs of infections and weight gain were reported with adalimumab (six) and etanercept (one).[7]

The efficacy of ustekinumab in pediatric palmoplantar pustulosis (PPP) has been highlighted in only a handful of case reports. Thereby, a case report showed that ustekinumab was effective in GPP at 0.9 mg/kg every 9 weeks, with sustained remissions lasting up to 48 months after the initiation of biologic therapy. Likewise, another case in a preschooler female with a de novo mutation in caspase recruitment domain-containing protein 14 showed notable improvement after ustekinumab treatment.[18]

Noticeably, in comparison to other biological agents, ustekinumab requires fewer injections, resulting in easy follow-up for patients.[9] Given the efficacy, safety data, and convenient dosing schedule, ustekinumab can be considered as the first-line treatment for adolescent patients with moderate-to-severe Ps.[7,9]

Ixekizumab

Ixekizumab is the first IL-17A–targeting biologic approved for children.[4] Ixekizumab is an alternative agent for pPs, with a favorable dosing schedule of every 4 weeks and can be considered as a second-line treatment.[7]

In a randomized, double-blind, placebo-controlled, phase III study (IXORA-PEDS) for children aged between 6 and 18 years with moderate-to-severe Ps were given weight-based dosing of ixekizumab. Ixekizumab was superior in terms of PASI 75 and static PGA score at week 4 and 12. The effects were sustained till week 108. Most patients achieved completely clear skin and nails. No new cases of inflammatory bowel disease were observed in the IXORA-PEDS trial, and there were no reported cases of Candida infection.[19]

A 6-month retrospective cohort study demonstrated a comparison between biologics and methotrexate therapies in moderate-to-severe pPs population to evaluate the most potent therapeutic option. Under this study, 163 patients were treated with methotrexate, while 47 patients received biological therapy (etanercept, adalimumab, ustekinumab, and infliximab). Both groups showed significant improvement, but biologics were superior to methotrexate in terms of efficacy and safety. Most of the methotrexate patients left the study due to drug-related adverse effects (nausea, infection, and liver function dysregulation). At the same time, very fewer patients on biologics discontinued their treatment due to mild adverse effects.[20]

Infliximab

Infliximab appears to be effective for management of pPs, but it is not FDA approved. However, it has been used in a few patients not responding to conventional biologic therapy and etanercept. However, its safety is not established and should be used only if the patient is not responding to other TNF-α blockers.[4]

Case reports of pediatric patients with plaque Ps treated with infliximab are scarce, and the vast majority of published data is related to pustular Ps.[2,21-23] Infliximab is recommended for the management of rapidly progressive or unstable, and/or life-threatening pustular Ps that is unresponsive to other systemic medications either as monotherapy or in combination with methotrexate.[20] When used for GPP in children, the average duration for a response to infliximab is reported to be <1 week with no SAE.[21] In refractory chronic plaque Ps, it has been observed to be uniformly effective at doses of 3.3–5 mg/kg administered at weeks 0, 2, 6, and every 7–8 weeks thereafter.[21]

Paradoxically, the development of new-onset Ps or worsening of existing Ps in 10.5% of the children with Crohn disease treated with infliximab has been documented. Hence, its precise role in treating Ps other than pustular Ps, and as maintenance therapy in children is yet to be determined.[5]

Therefore, the use of infliximab in pediatric populations is limited to case reports and anecdotal experience, most often in patients with severe pustular Ps. It is a useful rescue treatment owing to its efficacy and quick onset of action, but patients should avoid sporadic use as this can induce neutralizing antibodies, which decrease efficacy and increase risk of transfusion reactions. In pediatric patients treated with infliximab, higher rates of malignancies have been reported. However, firm conclusions cannot be made due to confounding factors such as concomitant immunosuppressive medications and underlying disease cancer risk.[9]

Other Biologics

Pediatric trials of guselkumab, risankizumab, and tildrakizumab, all targeting the IL-23 receptor-specific p19 subunit, are completed or currently recruiting (NCT03451851, NCT03997786, and NCT04435600) **(Table 3)**.[24]

Brodalumab

Brodalumab is currently being evaluated in the pediatric population with two distinct ongoing clinical trials (one phase II NCT03240809 and one phase III NCT04305327).[24]

TABLE 3: Clinical trials in progress with targeted therapies in pediatric patients with plaque psoriasis.

Drug	Route of administration	Clinical trial	Age group (years)	Phase	Estimated enrollment (number of participants)	Status	Estimated study completion date
Certolizumab pegol	Subcutaneous	NCT04123795	≥6 to <18	III	150	Recruiting	November 2025
Ustekinumab	Subcutaneous	NCT03218488	≥12 to <18	Observational (postauthorization)	75	Recruiting	September 2026
Secukinumab	Subcutaneous	NCT02471144	≥6 to <18	III	162	Active, not recruiting	July 2023
		NCT03668613	≥6 to <18	III	84	Active, not recruiting	September 2023
Ixekizumab	Subcutaneous	NCT03073200	≥6 to <18	III	201	Active, not recruiting	June 2021
Brodalumab	Subcutaneous	NCT03240809	≥6 to <18	II	16	Recruiting	March 2021
		NCT04305327	≥12 to <18	III	120	Not yet recruiting	May 2024
Guselkumab	Subcutaneous	NCT03451851	≥6 to <18	III	125	Recruiting	June 2025
Tildrakizumab	Subcutaneous	NCT03997786	≥6 to <18	II–III	120	Recruiting	November 2023
Risankizumab	Subcutaneous	NCT04435600	≥6 to <18	III	132	Recruiting	August 2025

Certolizumab Pegol

Certolizumab pegol, FDA-approved for Ps and psoriatic arthritis (PsA) in adults is neither FDA- nor EMA-approved for pPs. However, it effectively treats pediatric patients with JIA with a safety profile similar to other TNFi. The plasma concentrations of certolizumab pegol in pediatric patients fall largely within the range seen in adults.[9]

Hence, it is being tested in a phase III placebo-controlled clinical trial (NCT04123795), which is now recruiting patients aged ≥6 to <18 years with an estimated study completion date of November 2025. This study might provide important data and a possible new therapeutic solution for the treatment of pediatric plaque Ps.[2]

Safety Data on Biologics in Pediatric Psoriasis (Table 4)

Refractory skin disease can profoundly affect QoL during childhood and adolescence, a critical time for psychosocial development. In Ps, improvement in QoL is proportional to clearance and is greater when PASI 90 is achieved versus PASI 75. The high efficacy of IL-23 and IL-17A pathway inhibitors now makes achieving at least PASI 90 the new standard in pPs.[24]

In 2015, a case series (age range 5–18 years) demonstrated that clearance rates following etanercept and adalimumab treatments were 67%, whereas the clearance rate following ustekinumab treatment was 33%.[25] A real-life comparative study of 134 children (70 with etanercept, 68 with adalimumab, and 46 with ustekinumab) in 2019 found that ustekinumab had the best drug survival outcome and the side effect profile in children was comparable to that in adults.[26] The authors also reported that age at treatment initiation, age at onset of Ps, and disease severity (baseline PASI and PGA) are factors that affect the choice of the first-line biologic agent for pPs.[26]

Three biologic agents (etanercept, adalimumab, and infliximab) have long-term safety data with no SAE when used up to 1 year.[4] In a recent retrospective review on safety of systemic therapy in pPs, 38.7% patients reported ≥1 AE with use of biologics. Injection site reactions were the most commonly reported AE, seen in 18.9%, followed by infections (primarily of airway) in 11.3%. Infection rate was higher for adalimumab (15.8%) than etanercept (8.8%). Only 2.8% patients reported AE requiring discontinuation of therapy.[5]

There is a safety concern of increased risk of malignancies including lymphoproliferative disorders in children as they may continue to receive biologics through their adolescence into adulthood. But the lack of longitudinal and large studies to assess these risks makes it difficult to ascertain the safety profile of biologic therapy. Although there is lack of pediatric data, data from adult Ps favorably supports the safety profile of biologics in patients with Ps in terms of the risk of developing malignancy with no significantly increased risk of recurrence in those treated with biologics compared with nonbiologic therapy.[5]

TABLE 4: Biologics and reported side effects in children.[16,25,29]

Biologic[16,29]	Contra-indications	Infections	Respiratory	Gastro-intestinal	Metabolic	Rheumatologic	Others	Overall
Etanercept	Active infections, history of heart failure, multiple sclerosis, demyelinating disease	Severe cellulitis	Upper respiratory tract infection (URTI) (37.6%), nasopharyngitis (26.0%)	–	–	–	Purpura fulminans, headache, injection site reactions	No cases of opportunistic infections or malignancy reported, but an increased risk of lymphoma and other malignancies in pediatric populations have been expected
Adalimumab	Active infections, history of heart failure, multiple sclerosis, demyelinating disease	Severe cellulitis	URTI, nasopharyngitis	–	–	–	Headache	*Severe:* Hyperlipidemia
Infliximab		Mild infections					Headache, infusion-related reactions, cytopenias, hepatotoxicity, and malignancies	Higher rates of malignancies have been reported in children treated with infliximab, but the association remains unconfirmed
Secukinumab			Nasopharyngitis, pharyngitis				Headache, arthralgia, hypertension, diarrhea, back pain, pruritus, and cough	One reported death due to hemorrhagic stroke
Repetition			Nasopharyngitis, pharyngitis				Headache, arthralgia, hypertension, diarrhea, back pain, pruritus, and cough	One reported death due to hemorrhagic stroke

Continued

Continued

Biologic[16,29]	Contra-indications	Infections	Respiratory	Gastro-intestinal	Metabolic	Rheumato-logic	Others	Overall
Ustekinumab	Active infections, history of recurrent infections		Common: URTI, nasopharyngitis, pharyngitis				Common: Headache, injection site reaction, headache	Severe: Skin carcinoma
Ixekizumab		Most common					Overdose[2] 4 cases of probable CD	
Omalizumab[3]			Sinusitis, nasopharyngitis, URTI, cough, pneumonia, bronchitis	Appendicitis			Headache, erythema, urticaria	Mild-to-moderate
Dupilumab[3,29]	Hypersensitivity	Skin infections	URTI			Injection site reactions	Most common: Conjunctivitis, blepharitis, Severe: Inflammation of blood vessels, injection site reactions	
Belimumab	Hypersensitivity	Infections		Nausea			Infusion reaction, headache, fatigue, psychiatric events including insomnia, anxiety, depression, and suicidal ideation	Progressive multifocal leukoencephalopathy, most common malignancies—skin cancers (squamous cell carcinoma and basal cell carcinomas)

Summary

The biologics available to treat pPs efficaciously include anti-TNF-α (etanercept and adalimumab), anti-IL-12/23 (ustekinumab), and anti-IL-17A (secukinumab and ixekizumab). Although the efficacy of adalimumab and etanercept is similar to those observed in randomized controlled trials (RCTs), anti-IL-12/23 and anti-IL-17A might have a better efficacy than anti-TNF-α, but more data on the comparison of efficacy profiles among different biologics are needed.[27] As per the recent British Association of Dermatologists (BAD) guidelines, biologic agents can be used in severe childhood Ps, if they fulfill the criteria for biologic therapy.[5]

Biologics appear to be quite efficacious in treating severe plaque, pustular and erythrodermic Ps among children, and are not associated with a significant increase in SAE in the short term. This efficacy data is primarily available for TNFi and to some extent for ustekinumab, but is lacking for several other biologics including the newer ones such as secukinumab. Similarly, the safety data analysis as mentioned in the various trial results is limited by its short-term approach (as expected from trials) and relatively few numbers of AEs. Even among the TNFi, data on efficacy and safety of infliximab is based on small case series rather than the more stringent RCTs.

Furthermore, the AEs of biologics need attention. The most common AE is infection, such as upper respiratory tract infection and nasopharyngitis. The reasons for biologic therapy discontinuation are usually primary and secondary inefficacy. Although several biologics are approved for treating pPs, head-to-head comparisons between different biologics remain limited.[26] This will enable a clearer perspective on first-, second-, and third-line agents for moderate-to-severe disease. Moreover, the patient registries need to follow up with those recruited in the previous trials to increase our knowledge about their long-term safety.[5]

As in adults, there is increasing data that childhood Ps may be associated with obesity, metabolic syndrome, and perhaps related complications. Hence, it will be interesting to see if early treatment with biologics in moderate-to-severe Ps leads to significantly reduced systemic inflammation and has a therapeutic effect on the metabolic syndrome in children.

Another important issue that needs great focus is the accurate assessment of lymphoma/malignancy risk with biologics in children. As at present there is no cure for Ps, children with Ps if exposed to biologics at an early age may require them for a lengthy period (intermittently or continuously or even lifelong therapy as advocated by few pharmaceutical companies). So even if the risk of developing malignancies secondary to biologics use may be small in the short term, it could be cumulative and significant in the long term though speculative at present. As such, the need for long-term safety data and registries cannot be over emphasized.[5]

CHRONIC SPONTANEOUS URTICARIA

Chronic spontaneous urticaria is a common skin disorder, affecting 1–14.5% children.[28]

Omalizumab

Omalizumab, a humanized anti-IgE antibody, is approved by Health Canada, the FDA, and other jurisdictions for the treatment of antihistamine-resistant CSU in patients aged ≥12 years. It is recommended as a third-line option in patients aged ≥12 years in spite being approved for children >6 years suffering with asthma.[29]

Several authors had earlier recommended the baseline value of IgE as a biomarker of response to treatment, suggesting that nonresponders to omalizumab are those with low baseline IgE levels.[28-30] However, recent guidelines suggest omalizumab to be administered subcutaneously at the recommended doses of 150 or 300 mg every 4 weeks, regardless of serum IgE levels. Moreover, in patients experiencing symptoms before 4 weeks, implementation of 150 mg of omalizumab at 2-week intervals might provide better symptom control.[28] It is rapidly acting, sometimes within 24 hours, being highly effective and safe.[30,31]

It has been used for the treatment of CSU not responding to antihistamines in children as young as 4 years of age. The European Academy of Allergy and Clinical Immunology (EAACI) CSU guidelines on Biologics 2022 recommend strongly for 300 mg omalizumab versus 150 mg in adolescents above 12 years irrespective of IgE levels **(Table 5)**.[32]

To date, current guidelines suggest an "until the disease is gone" approach to adopt as criteria to continue treatment.[29]

Overall, 10 RCTs including 1,620 subjects aged 12–75 years treated with omalizumab for 16–40 weeks were evaluated. Omalizumab 150 mg does not result in clinically meaningful improvement (high certainty) of the urticaria activity score (UAS) 7 [mean difference (MD) 5; 95% confidence interval (CI) 7.75 to –2.25], and the itch severity score (ISS) 7 (MD –2.15; 95% CI –3.2 to –1.1) does not increase (moderate certainty) QoL [Dermatology Life Quality Index (DLQI); MD –2.01; 95% CI –3.22 to –0.81] and decreases (moderate certainty) rescue medication use (MD –1.68; 95% CI –2.95 to –0.4). Omalizumab 300 mg results in clinically meaningful improvements (moderate certainty) of the UAS 7 (MD –11.05; 95% CI –12.87 to –9.24), the ISS 7 (MD –4.45; 95%

TABLE 5: Categories of responders to omalizumab in CSU.[29]	
Fast responder	Individuals who improve their symptoms in up to 6 weeks
Slow responders	Require more than three doses of omalizumab
Nonresponder	No response is reported after six months of treatment

CI −5.39 to −3.51), and QoL (high certainty; DLQI; MD −4.03; 95% CI −5.56 to −2.5) and decreases (moderate certainty) rescue medication use (MD −2.04; 95% CI −3.19 to −0.88) and drug-related SAEs [relative risk (RR) 0.77; 95% CI 0.20-2.91].[33]

Other case series, case reports, and pediatric registry assessing treatment with omalizumab (300 mg subcutaneous injections every 4 weeks) included a total of 76 antihistamine-resistant CSU pediatric patients (75 CSU patients and 1 otherwise nonspecified CU patient) aged 4–17 years. Significant improvement of symptoms was reported in 66 out of 76 patients, whereas complete remission (CR) was seen in 44 patients. Clinical improvement was usually seen within 2 months. No unexpected AEs were reported.[31]

Omalizumab use in children aged <12 years remains off-label for CSU despite emerging data suggesting safety and efficacy in this population.[31]

Ligelizumab

Given the promising efficacy and safety profile of ligelizumab, two phase III clinical trials (PEARL 1 and 2, NCT03580369 and NCT03580356) are in the recruitment phase to assess the efficacy and safety of ligelizumab for the treatment of CSU in adolescents and adults not adequately controlled by H1 antihistamines (H1AH).[34]

Another randomized double blind placebo control trial (RDBPCT; NCT03437278) was conducted on 49 adolescents (aged 12-17 years) with treatment-refractory CSU investigated ligelizumab (24 mg, 120 mg, 8-weeks placebo followed by 120 mg ligelizumab), as an add-on treatment to H1AH for 24 weeks. The preliminary results showed that all three groups reported a reduction from the baseline in UAS7, ISS7, HSS7, and DLQI at different endpoints (week 12, 24, and 40).[35]

Summary

Due to scarce data available to support the efficacy and safety of biologics in pCSU, only omalizumab 300 mg showed an improvement in pCSU with moderate certainty with a significant improvement in QoL, with high certainty of evidence.[32,33,35]

ATOPIC DERMATITIS

Treatment selection for AD in pediatric populations depends on patient age/weight, BSA affected, medical comorbidities, QoL, and response to other treatments as well as cost and availability/approval of pharmacologic agents in the locality of the patient. Several novel agents are under clinical investigation as treatments for AD **(Table 3)**.[36,37]

Newly FDA-approved agents for pediatric AD include topical crisaborole [Phosphodiesterase-4 (PDE4) inhibitor], topical ruxolitinib [Janus Kinase (JAK) 1/2 inhibitor], oral upadacitinib (JAK 1 selective inhibitor), and injectable dupilumab (anti-IL-4/13 mAb), though phase 2 and 3 trials support the use of additional topical PDE4 inhibitors and an aryl hydrocarbon receptor agonist (tapinarof), topical and oral JAK inhibitors, and the injectable biologic treatments anti-IL-13 tralokinumab/anti-IL-13Rα lebrikizumab, anti-IL-31Rα nemolizumab, omalizumab, baricitinib (JAK1/2 antagonist), abrocitinib (JAK1 antagonist), upadacitinib (JAK1 antagonist), and tradipitant (neurokinin-1 receptor antagonist).[25,36-40] Many of these medications are not universally available and high cost may prohibit their use.

Dupilumab

Dupilumab is the first biologic that is FDA approved as first-line treatment for moderate-to-severe AD in patients >6 months.[37,40]

In a multicentric trial 55 patients of pAD (6–11 years), dupilumab was administered in the dosage of 300 mg on day 1, followed by 300 mg on day 15 and 300 mg every 4 weeks. Disease severity was assessed at baseline and after week 2, 4, and 16 of dupilumab therapy using Eczema Area Severity Index (EASI), Pruritus Numerical Rating Scale (P-NRS) and Sleep NRS (S-NRS), and Children's DLQI (c-DLQI) score. A significant improvement in EASI, P-NRS, S-NRS, and c-DLQI scores was observed from baseline to week 16 of treatment with dupilumab. In particular, at week 16, the proportion of patients achieving EASI 75 was 74.54%.[41]

Dupilumab in pAD does not increase infection risk overall and is associated with lower rates of skin infections compared with placebo.[42]

Lebrikizumab

Lebrikizumab, a high affinity humanized immunoglobulin G4 mAb was recently EMA approved for moderate-to-severe AD in adult and adolescent patients (12–18 years and >40 kg), making it the second biologic agent approved for AD in adolescents.[42] In a randomized clinical trial (ADhere), where effects of lebrikizumab were studied in AD, a total of 211 patients were enrolled; 46 of which were adolescents. Lebrikizumab was associated with improved physician-reported signs of AD and patient-reported outcomes of pruritus and QoL compared with topical corticosteroid alone, over 16 weeks of treatment.[43]

IL-13RA inhibitors may be as effective as IL-13 inhibitors. Several phase 3 trials that included adolescents met primary endpoints for improvement in pAD. Like IL-13 inhibitors, it remains unclear if there is a unique role for IL-13Rα inhibitors compared with dupimulab.[37]

Nemolizumab

Nemolizumab (previously CIM331) is a humanized IL-31 receptor A (IL-31RA) mAb, which was specifically developed for the treatment of AD-related pruritus and inhibits the IL-31 signaling.[40,44,45]

Nemolizumab is currently not licensed for any indication worldwide.[36] Two recent phase 3 long-term studies in Japanese adolescents demonstrated improved itch with a durable response. Improved EASI, sleep, and life quality was noted by week 16 and persisted through end of treatment. IL-31 expression is increased in children, and nemolizumab may have greater efficacy in this population. Ongoing phase 2/3 trials in adolescents and children are forthcoming (NCT03921411, NCT04921345, NCT03985943, NCT03989349, and NCT03989206).[24,36] In addition, nemolizumab could have a synergistic effect in the treatment of AD and AD-related pruritus.[40]

Tralokinumab

Tralokinumab is a fully human, high-affinity IgG4 mAb, which neutralizes IL-13. Not yet broadly available for pediatric patients, tralokinumab is FDA and EMA approved for adults with AD. The recent ECZTRA 6 trial may lead to FDA approval for adolescents soon. IL-13 inhibitor safety/efficacy appears similar to dupilumab. It is unclear if there will be a unique role for IL-13 inhibitors compared with dupilumab.[37,40]

Omalizumab

Omalizumab is an off-label indication for management of AD.[46,47]

It has been found to be variably effective in various studies. Although two previous RCTs did not demonstrate treatment response with omalizumab,[47] a more recent study showed that omalizumab significantly reduced AD severity and improved QoL in a pediatric population with atopy and severe eczema, despite highly elevated total IgE levels at baseline (NCT02300701). These results were associated with a potent topical corticosteroid (TCS) sparing effect and may suggest that omalizumab is a suitable treatment option for difficult-to-manage severe eczema in children with atopy. The reasons for the discrepancies between the earlier RCTs and the more recent study might include the different treatment responses of children and adults, as well as the maximum doses of omalizumab used.[48]

Future trials with a larger sample size, a longer duration, and perhaps higher affinity anti-IgE antibodies would clarify the precise role of anti-IgE therapy and its ideal AD target population.

There have been various case series involving management of refractory AD in pediatric age group using omalizumab. A case series published by Lane et al. involving three patients in age group of 10–13 years found omalizumab to be effective. The dose used was 150–450 mg twice weekly in this case series.[49] Another case series involving pediatric patients found that omalizumab is effective for management of severe AD. In this case series, patients' age varied from 6 years to 19 years and omalizumab dose was based on IgE and body weight (same as asthma), maximum being 375 mg subcutaneous every 2 weeks.[37]

The available literature suggests that omalizumab is effective for management of pAD, however dose required is more than required for CSU and should be based on weight and serum IgE level. The subset of patients with absence of filaggrin mutation have better control of disease with omalizumab.

Summary

Dupilumab is the first biologic approved for pediatric AD patients as young as 6 months old, while lebrikizumab received fast track designation for moderate-to-severe AD in adult and adolescent patients (12–18 years and >40 kg), making it the second biologic agent approved for AD in adolescents.

PEMPHIGUS

Treating autoimmune bullous diseases in the pediatric population has unique challenges compared with the adult population. More common concerns in pediatric patients are the deleterious effects of pemphigus and its therapy on physical growth, psychosocial development, education, and overall QoL.

Rituximab

Rituximab (RTX) is an anti-CD20 mAb approved by the FDA for the treatment of adult pemphigus vulgaris (PV) in 2018. Despite the robust adult literature, only limited pediatric cases of pemphigus treated with RTX have been reported.[50-52] A review of 12 pediatric PV patients reported that 71.7% had CR when treated with RTX.[51] Another review identified a total of 37 pediatric pemphigus patients [31 with PV, 6 with pemphigus foliaceus (PF)] treated with RTX [rheumatoid arthritis (RA) protocols: 375 mg/m² BSA 15 days apart or lymphoma (LP) protocol: 500 to 1,000 mg 15 days apart as either first-, second-, or third-line therapy]. Of these 37 patients, 26 achieved CR after their first RTX treatment and all patients showed marked clinical improvement.[53]

Another case series described 12 pediatric patients with pemphigus treated with RTX, including six patients who received it as a first-line steroid-sparing agent; this study reported favorable outcomes for individuals treated with RTX first line, including lower mean monthly steroid dosage, shorter time to remission, and longer duration of remission compared with those who received RTX second line. RTX appears to be well-tolerated in children with PV.[54]

A recent systematic review of 1,085 PV patients (adult and pediatric) treated with RTX found that the most common AE were increased bacterial and viral infections. Interestingly, the five pediatric cases included in this review did not experience any AE except for mild infusion reactions in seven patients (52%) and septicemia in one patient (8.3%), with no AE in the remaining four patients (33%).[55]

In a review of 33 pPF cases, 14 (42.4%) patients were treated with RTX, who had previously received CIST. Biologics were utilized largely following the failure of CIST, although five patients were treated with RTX as first-line therapy. All patients in the RTX group had clinical improvement. A total of 12 (85.7%) patients had CR, and two (14.3%) of them had partial remission (PR). Moreover, 10 (71.4%) relapses were reported during a mean follow-up duration of 20.5 months (range = 6–67 months) in the RTX group. One (7.1%) patient had a serious bacterial infection, requiring hospitalization and intravenous antibiotics. Both relapses and AEs occurred only in the patients treated with the LP protocol.[56]

While there are concerns for SAE with RTX, including complications of B-cell depletion and hypogammaglobulinemia, this may be rare in the pediatric PV population, and RTX may possibly be better tolerated than alternative immunosuppressive regimens.[53]

A systematic review found RTX safe and effective for management of pediatric systemic lupus erythematosus (SLE),[57] while in 2019, RTX was FDA approved for management of pediatric granulomatosis with polyangiitis (GPA) and microscopic polyangiitis (MPA) in combination with glucocorticoids.[58]

MALIGNANT MELANOMA

Melanoma accounts for about 4% of all cancers in children aged 15–19 years.[59]

Immune Checkpoint Inhibitors

Four phase I/II studies published between 2020 and 2022 provide the most data; nivolumab (ADVL1412; NCT0230445848), pembrolizumab (KEYNOTE-051; NCT0233266849), atezolizumab (iMATRIX; NCT0254160450), and avelumab (NCT0345182551) were tested as monotherapies against recurrent and refractory pediatric tumors including melanomas. Across all four studies, these immune checkpoint inhibitors (ICIs) were well tolerated in children at weight-based dosing that provided equivalent pharmacokinetics to the approved adult doses: 3 mg/kg of nivolumab every 2 weeks, 2 mg/kg of pembrolizumab every 3 weeks, 15 mg/kg of atezolizumab every 3 weeks, and 20 mg/kg of avelumab every 2 weeks. AEs were similar to those seen in adults, with the exception of more frequent cytopenia (including grade 3–4), possibly reflecting a higher level of pretreatment in these patients than in their adult counterparts. Otherwise, the most common AEs were constitutional (fatigue and fever, grades 1 and 2), and the most common immune-related AE (IRAE) was hepatic toxicity (elevated transaminases, grades 1 and 2). Less common IRAEs included pancreatitis/elevated lipase, thyroiditis, pleural and pericardial effusions, and colitis. Of the 350 pediatric patients treated in these studies, two had grade 5 toxicities that were potentially treatment related (pneumonitis and pleural edema with pembrolizumab treatment in the setting of a chest sarcoma and sepsis, respectively).[60]

Nivolumab

The approved dose of nivolumab for the adjuvant treatment of adult and pediatric patients at least 12 years of age with completely resected stage IIB/C melanoma and who weigh at least 40 kg is 240 mg administered once every 2 weeks or 480 mg administered once every 4 weeks for up to a year, or until disease recurrence or unacceptable toxicity. In those at least 12 years of age who weigh <40 kg, the approved dose is 3 mg/kg once every 2 weeks or 6 mg/kg once every 4 weeks for up to 1 year, or until disease recurrence or unacceptable toxicity.[61,62]

Ipilimumab

The EMA and FDA approved ipilimumab for adolescents aged ≥12 years with recommended induction regimen of 3 mg/kg administered intravenously over a 30-minute period every 3 weeks for a total of 4 doses as monotherapy or in combination with nivolumab is indicated for the treatment of advanced (unresectable or metastatic) melanoma. Relative to nivolumab monotherapy, an increase in progression-free survival (PFS) and overall survival (OS) for the combination of nivolumab with ipilimumab is established only in patients with low tumor PD-L1 expression.[63]

Pembrolizumab

In 2021, the FDA approved pembrolizumab for the adjuvant treatment of adult and pediatric patients aged ≥12 years with stage IIb or IIc melanoma following complete resection by evaluating efficacy in KEYNOTE-716, a multicenter, randomized 1:1, double-blind, placebo-controlled trial in patients. The recommended pembrolizumab dose and schedule for the adjuvant treatment of melanoma is 200 mg administered as an IV infusion over 30 minutes every 3 weeks until disease recurrence or unacceptable toxicity, for a maximum of 1 year.[64]

ALOPECIA AREATA

Ustekinumab

Only one case series of three pediatric patients has documented hair regrowth with ustekinumab use,[65] in contrast with several reports showing that new-onset AA occurred after this drug administration.[66]

Biologics (quality of evidence IIb) although TNF-α has been found to be significantly elevated in the sera of AA patients, anti-TNF-α therapies have been found to be ineffective in AA. As such, biologics cannot be recommended for treatment of pediatric AA at this juncture.

SYSTEMIC LUPUS ERYTHEMATOSUS

Belimumab

Intravenous belimumab is the first biologic approved by the FDA and EMA to treat SLE in children aged ≥5 years as an add-on therapy.[67] It is effective in moderately active, autoantibody-positive LE with predominantly mucocutaneous and/or musculoskeletal manifestations.[68] A RCT-PLUTO study (pediatric lupus trial of belimumab and background standard therapy) that evaluated the efficacy, safety, and pharmacokinetics of intravenous belimumab in 93 patients aged 5–17 years with active LE concluded that the drug was safe, efficacious, and well tolerated in children. Belimumab reduced the overall disease activity and the incidence and severity of flares.[69]

BIOLOGICS AND OTHER DERMATOLOGICAL DISORDERS

There are case reports in literature citing the efficacy of various biologicals in different dermatology disorders **(Table 6)**.[18,67]

BIOLOGICS AND HYPERSENSITIVITY REACTIONS

Hypersensitivity reactions (HSRs) have been observed with the use of biologics in children. The management of HSRs in children is mainly based on experiences from the adult population. With regard to HSRs to biologics in children, few data are available. Compared with the adult population, there is a lack of knowledge in the endophenotypes, management, and the standardization of protocols including premedication regimens in children. An international consensus is needed to provide clinicians with new

TABLE 6: Off-label indications for biologicals in pediatric dermatology.[67]

Biologic	Reported off-label use
Etanercept	Pityriasis rubra pilaris (PRP), hidradenitis suppurativa (HS), atopic dermatitis (AD), pyoderma gangrenosum (PG), SJS/TEN, Kawasaki disease, Juvenile PRP
Infliximab	pAD, TEN, HS
Ustekinumab	AD, PRP, HS, Ichthyosis
Omalizumab	Moderate-to-severe AD
Rituximab	• AD • *Autoimmune disorders*: Pemphigus vulgaris, pemphigus foliaceus, bullous pemphigoid, mucous membrane pemphigoid, and epidermolysis bullosa acquisita • Neoplastic disorders • *Connective tissue disorders*: Juvenile dermatomyositis, antiphospholipid antibody syndrome with cutaneous necrosis, systemic lupus erythematosus (SLE) • *Vasculitis disorders*: Cutaneous polyarteritis nodosa

insight on how to apply personalized management and to perform tailored desensitization protocols in pediatric populations.[70]

MONITORING AND VACCINATIONS

Absolute contraindications to the use of biologicals include hypersensitivity and active infections including active tuberculosis and hepatitis.[3] Recent guidelines have proposed there is no need for regular bloodwork in children receiving biologic treatment unless they are predisposed to certain risks (such as infectious exposure, comorbidities, etc.), further lowering the burden for families compared to nonbiologic therapies.[8]

Infants exposed in utero to anti-TNF drugs, vedolizumab or ustekinumab, mount adequate serological responses to vaccines. No relevant adverse events for non-live inactivated vaccines have been reported in newborns exposed in utero to biologics. Studies assessing the safety of live-attenuated vaccines administered to infants exposed to biologics in utero have not observed, in general, SAEs. However, although no severe complications have been reported with rotavirus live vaccination, several fatal disseminated tuberculosis infections after administration of the BCG live vaccine in infants exposed to anti-TNFs in utero have been reported. To summarize, vaccines appear to be effective in infants exposed to biologics in utero. Inactivated vaccines are probably safe, whereas live-attenuated vaccines should be avoided while the children have detectable levels of biological drugs.[71]

Recent publications revealed that immunogenicity of vaccines in children treated with biologics was lower than in the healthy population, especially on long-term follow-up. Children treated with biologic therapy are at greater danger of infections, compared to the healthy population. Therefore, they should be vaccinated according to national guidelines. Regardless of the therapy, non-live vaccines are recommended. However, it is common practice to advise postponing vaccination with live-attenuated vaccines in children while they are on immunosuppressive therapy. Newly published data suggest that booster dose MMR/V is safe for children treated with biologic therapy.[72] Monitoring and vaccinations of drugs used in Ps are given in **Table 2**.

Following principles should be adhered to while vaccinating a child with Ps:[72]
- Update vaccinations
- Avoid live and live attenuated vaccines (e.g., varicella, MMR, oral typhoid, yellow fever, intranasal influenza, herpes zoster, BCG)
- Vaccinate household contacts prior to treatment initiation

Although there are no guidelines or studies on the use of vaccines in pediatric patients receiving biologics for dermatological disorders from India, international data and guidelines for use of vaccines in rheumatological diseases suggest safe use of seasonal influenza vaccines, MMR booster, but each case should be reviewed for risk-benefit ratio.[72] Also, these data cannot be directly extrapolated to Indian settings.

To summarize, the vaccination schedule of the children should be considered before administering biologics. It is better to finish the vaccination schedule before starting biologics. Live vaccines should be given 4 weeks before and inactivated vaccines 2 weeks before starting biologics. Live vaccines should generally be avoided during therapy, but if they need to be given then the biologics should be discontinued for at least 3 half-lives of that particular biologic. Inactivated vaccines are safe to administer concurrently with biologics, but the response may be inadequate.

CONCLUSION

There is a growing body of evidence that biologics are safe to use in the pediatric age group and should be used, if necessary, keeping vaccination protocols in mind.

Biologics are targeted molecules that theoretically lack many of the toxicities of traditional agents, are convenient to use, and require less frequent dosing and laboratory monitoring. Still, concerns remain regarding their long-term safety. Hence, despite the obvious advantages, these are often indicated as second- or third-line agents in children. Also, biologics are costly, require repeated injections (which can be difficult in pediatric patients), and are not curative. If treatment is discontinued or patients have poor adherence, disease relapse or rebound can occur. There is an increased need for patient monitoring and post-market registries are necessary to evaluate long-term adverse effects in pediatric patients who may be on biologics for decades. It may thus be concluded that the clear advantages of using biologic agents must be balanced with a measure of caution.

REFERENCES

1. Eichenfield LF, Paller AS, Tom WL, Sugarman J, Hebert AA, Friedlander SF, et al. Pediatric psoriasis: evolving perspectives. Pediatr Dermatol. 2018;35(2):170-81.
2. Nogueira M, Paller AS, Torres T. Targeted therapy for pediatric psoriasis. Paediatr Drugs. 2021;23(3):203-12.
3. Aslam N, Saleem H, Murtazaliev S, Quazi SJ, Khan S. FDA Approved Biologics: Can etanercept and ustekinumab be considered a first-line systemic therapy for pediatric/adolescents in moderate to severe psoriasis? A Systematic Review. Cureus. 2020;12(8):e9812.
4. Katakam BK, Munisamy M, Rao TN, Chiramel MJ, Panda M, Gupta S, et al. Recommendations for management of childhood psoriasis. Indian Dermatol Online J. 2021;12(Suppl 1):S71-S85.
5. Dogra S, Mahajan R. Biologics in pediatric psoriasis—efficacy and safety. Expert Opin Drug Saf. 2018;17(1):9-16.
6. Menter A, Cordoro KM, Davis DMR, Kroshinsky D, Paller AS, Armstrong AW, et al. Joint American Academy of Dermatology-National Psoriasis Foundation guidelines of care for the management and treatment of psoriasis in pediatric patients. J Am Acad Dermatol. 2020;82(1):161-201.
7. Thatiparthi A, Martin A, Liu J, Egeberg A, Wu JJ. Biologic treatment algorithms for moderate-to-severe psoriasis with comorbid conditions and special populations: A Review. Am J Clin Dermatol. 2021;22(4):425-42.

8. Paller AS, Siegfried EC, Pariser DM, Rice KC, Trivedi M, Iles J, et al. Long-term safety and efficacy of etanercept in children and adolescents with plaque psoriasis. J Am Acad Dermatol. 2016;74(2):280-7.e1-3.
9. Zangrilli A, Bavetta M, Bianchi L. Adalimumab in children and adolescents with severe plaque psoriasis: a safety evaluation. Expert Opin Drug Saf. 2020;19(4):433-8.
10. Traczewski P, Rudnicka L. Adalimumab in dermatology. Br J Clin Pharmacol. 2008;66(5):618-25.
11. Di Lernia V, Bianchi L, Guerriero C, Stingeni L, Gisondi P, Filoni A, et al. Adalimumab in severe plaque psoriasis of childhood: a multi-center, retrospective real-life study up to 52 weeks observation. Dermatol Ther. 2019;32:e13091.
12. Du Y, Yan Q, Chen M, Dong Z, Wang F. Efficacy of adalimumab in pediatric generalized pustular psoriasis: case series and literature review. J Dermatolog Treat. 2022;33(6):2862-8.
13. Cline A, Bartos GJ, Strowd LC, Feldman SR. Biologic treatment options for pediatric psoriasis and atopic dermatitis. Children (Basel). 2019;6(9):103.
14. Papp K, Thaci D, Marcoux D, Weibel L, Philipp S, Ghislain PD, et al. Efficacy and safety of adalimumab every other week versus methotrexate once weekly in children and adolescents with severe chronic plaque psoriasis: A randomised, double-blind, phase 3 trial. Lancet. 2017;390(10089):40-9.
15. Blair HA. Secukinumab: A review in moderate to severe pediatric plaque psoriasis. Paediatr Drugs. 2021;23(6):601-8.
16. Magnolo N, Kingo K, Laquer V, Browning J, Reich A, Szepietowski JC, et al. A phase 3 open-label, randomized multicenter study to evaluate efficacy and safety of secukinumab in pediatric patients with moderate to severe plaque psoriasis: 24-week results. J Am Acad Dermatol. 2022;86(1):122-30.
17. Landells I, Marano C, Hsu MC, Li S, Zhu Y, Eichenfield LF, et al. Ustekinumab in adolescent patients age 12 to 17 years with moderate-to-severe plaque psoriasis: results of the randomized phase 3 CADMUS study. J Am Acad Dermatol. 2015;73(4):594-603.
18. Chehad AS, Boutrid N, Rahmoune H. Ustekinumab in pediatric dermatology: An updated review. J Explor Res Pharmacol. 2023;8(1):66-73.
19. Paller AS, Seyger MMB, Magariños GA, Pinter A, Cather JC, Rodriguez-Capriles C, et al; IXORA-PEDS Investigators. Long-term efficacy and safety of up to 108 weeks of ixekizumab in pediatric patients with moderate to severe plaque psoriasis: The IXORA-PEDS Randomized Clinical Trial. JAMA Dermatol. 2022;158(5):533-41.
20. Bronckers IMGJ, Paller AS, West DP, Lara-Corrales I, Tollefson MM, Tom WL, et al; Psoriasis Investigator Group, the Pediatric Dermatology Research Alliance, and the European Working Group on Pediatric Psoriasis. A Comparison of Psoriasis Severity in Pediatric Patients Treated with Methotrexate vs Biologic Agents. JAMA Dermatol. 2020;156(4):384-92.
21. Menter MA, Cush J. Successful treatment of pediatric psoriasis with infliximab. Pediatr Dermatol. 2004;21(1):87-8.
22. Tsang V, Dvorakova V, Enright F, Murphy M, Gleeson C. Successful use of infliximab as first line treatment for severe childhood generalized pustular psoriasis. J Eur Acad Dermatol Venereol. 2016;30(11):e117-e119.
23. Skrabl-Baumgartner A, Weger W, Salmhofer W, Jahnel J. Childhood generalized pustular psoriasis: longtime remission with combined infliximab and methotrexate treatment. Pediatr Dermatol. 2015;32(1):e13-4.
24. Scott JB, Paller AS. Biologics in pediatric psoriasis and atopic dermatitis: revolutionizing the treatment landscape. Cutis. 2020;106(5):224-6.
25. Garber C, Creighton-Smith M, Sorensen EP, Dumont N, Gottlieb AB. Systemic treatment of recalcitrant pediatric psoriasis: a case series and literature review. J Drugs Dermatol. 2015;14(8):881-6.

26. Phan C, Beauchet A, Burztejn AC, Severino-Freire M, Barbarot S, Girard C, et al. Biological treatments for paediatric psoriasis: a retrospective observational study on biological drug survival in daily practice in childhood psoriasis. J Eur Acad Dermatol Venereol. 2019;33(10):1984-92.
27. Wang W-M, Jin H-Z. Biologics in pediatric psoriasis. J Dermatol. 2023;50(4):415-21.
28. Zuberbier T, Aberer W, Asero R, Abdul Latiff AH, Baker D, Ballmer-Weber B, et al. The EAACI/GA^{2}LEN/EDF/WAO guideline for the definition, classification, diagnosis and management of urticaria. Allergy. 2018;73(7):1393-414.
29. Castagnoli R, De Filippo M, Votto M, Marseglia A, Montagna L, Marseglia GL, et al. An update on biological therapies for pediatric allergic diseases. Minerva Pediatr. 2020;72(5):364-71.
30. Licari A, Manti S, Marseglia A, De Filippo M, De Sando E, Foiadelli T, et al. Biologics in Children with Allergic Diseases. Curr Pediatr Rev. 2020;16(2):140-7.
31. Netchiporouk E, Nguyen CH, Thuraisingham T, Jafarian F, Maurer M, Ben-Shoshan M. Management of pediatric chronic spontaneous and physical urticaria patients with omalizumab: case series. Pediatr Allergy Immunol. 2015;26(6):585-8.
32. Agache I, Akdis CA, Akdis M, Brockow K, Chivato T, Del Giacco S, et al. EAACI Biologicals Guidelines-Omalizumab for the treatment of chronic spontaneous urticaria in adults and in the paediatric population 12-17 years old. Allergy. 2022;77(1):17-38.
33. Chang J, Cattelan L, Ben-Shoshan M, Le M, Netchiporouk E. Management of pediatric chronic spontaneous urticaria: A review of current evidence and guidelines. J Asthma Allergy. 2021;14:187-99.
34. Muntyanu A, Ouchene L, Ben-Shoshan M, Netchiporouk E. Ligelizumab is superior to omalizumab for chronic spontaneous urticaria. J Cutan Med Surg. 2020;24(2):201-2.
35. Manti S, Giallongo A, Papale M, Parisi GF, Leonardi S. Monoclonal antibodies in treating chronic spontaneous urticaria: New drugs for an old disease. J Clin Med. 2022;11(15):4453.
36. Chu CY. Treatments for childhood atopic dermatitis: An update on emerging therapies. Clin Rev Allergy Immunol. 2021;61(2):114-27.
37. Kondratuk K, Netravali IA, Castelo-Soccio L. Modern interventions for pediatric atopic dermatitis: An updated pharmacologic approach. Dermatol Ther (Heidelb). 2023;13(2):367-89.
38. Blauvelt A, Teixeira HD, Simpson EL, Costanzo A, De Bruin-Weller M, Barbarot S, et al. Efficacy and safety of upadacitinib vs dupilumab in adults with moderate-to-severe atopic dermatitis: A randomized clinical trial. JAMA Dermatol. 2021;157(9):1047-55.
39. Wollenberg A, Christen-Zäch S, Taieb A, Paul C, Thyssen JP, de Bruin-Weller M, et al.; European Task Force on Atopic Dermatitis/EADV Eczema Task Force. ETFAD/EADV Eczema task force 2020 position paper on diagnosis and treatment of atopic dermatitis in adults and children. J Eur Acad Dermatol Venereol. 2020;34(12):2717-44.
40. Wollenberg A, Kinberger M, Arents B, Aszodi N, Avila Valle G, Barbarot S, et al. European guideline (EuroGuiDerm) on atopic eczema: part I—systemic therapy. J Eur Acad Dermatol Venereol. 2022;36(9):1409-31.
41. Napolitano M, Fabbrocini G, Neri I, Stingeni L, Boccaletti V, Piccolo V, et al. Dupilumab treatment in children aged 6–11 years with atopic dermatitis: a multicentre, real-life study. Pediatric Drugs. 2022;24(6):671-8.
42. Moreno A, Renert-Yuval Y, Guttman-Yassky E. Shedding light on key pharmacological knowledge and strategies for pediatric atopic dermatitis. Expert Rev Clin Pharmacol. 2023;16(2):119-31.
43. Simpson EL, Gooderham M, Wollenberg A, Weidinger S, Armstrong A, Soung J, et al. Efficacy and safety of lebrikizumab in combination with topical corticosteroids in adolescents and adults with moderate-to-severe atopic dermatitis: a randomized clinical trial (ADhere). JAMA dermatology. 2023;159(2):182-91.

44. Paller AS, Beck LA, Blauvelt A, Siegfried EC, Cork MJ, Wollenberg A, et al. Infections in children and adolescents treated with dupilumab in pediatric clinical trials for atopic dermatitis-A pooled analysis of trial data. Pediatr Dermatol. 2022;39(2):187-96.
45. Szegedi K, Lutter R, Res PC, Bos JD, Luiten RM, Kezic S, et al. Cytokine profiles in interstitial fluid from chronic atopic dermatitis skin. J Eur Acad Dermatol Venereol. 2015;29(11):2136-44.
46. Zhou S, Qi F, Gong Y, Zhang J, Zhu B. Biological therapies for atopic dermatitis: A systematic review. Dermatology. 2021;237(4):542-52.
47. Hotze M, Baurecht H, Rodríguez E, Chapman-Rothe N, Ollert M, Fölster-Holst R, et al. Increased efficacy of omalizumab in atopic dermatitis patients with wild-type filaggrin status and higher serum levels of phosphatidylcholines. Allergy. 2014;69(1):132-5.
48. Heil PM, Maurer D, Klein B, Hultsch T, Stingl G. Omalizumab therapy in atopic dermatitis: depletion of IgE does not improve the clinical course—a randomized, placebo-controlled and double blind pilot study. J Dtsch Dermatol Ges. 2010;8(12):990-8.
49. Lane JE, Cheyney JM, Lane TN, Kent DE, Cohen DJ. Treatment of recalcitrant atopic dermatitis with omalizumab. J Am Acad Dermatol. 2006;54(1):68-72.
50. Connelly EA, Aber C, Kleiner G, Nousari C, Charles C, Schachner LA. Generalized erythrodermic pemphigus foliaceus in a child and its successful response to rituximab treatment. Pediatr Dermatol. 2007;24(2):172-6.
51. de Sena Nogueira Maehara L, Huizinga J, Jonkman MF. Rituximab therapy in pemphigus foliaceus: report of 12 cases and review of recent literature. Br J Dermatol. 2015;172(5):1420-3.
52. Kincaid L, Weinstein M. Rituximab Therapy for Childhood Pemphigus Vulgaris. Pediatr Dermatol. 2016;33(2):e61-4.
53. Mistry BD, Leis M, Lee DM, Levy R. Management of pediatric pemphigus vulgaris with rituximab: A case report and review of the literature. Pediatr Dermatol. 2022;39(6):960-6.
54. Kianfar N, Dasdar S, Mahmoudi H, Tavakolpour S, Balighi K, Daneshpazhooh M. Rituximab in childhood and juvenile autoimmune bullous diseases as first-line and second-line treatment: a case series of 13 patients. J Dermatol Treat. 2022;33(2):869-74.
55. Tavakolpour S, Mahmoudi H, Balighi K, Abedini R, Daneshpazhooh M. Sixteen-year history of rituximab therapy for 1085 pemphigus vulgaris patients: A systematic review. Int Immunopharmacol. 2018;54:131-8.
56. Carver C, Kalesinskas M, Dheden N, Ahmed AR. Treatment of pediatric pemphigus foliaceus. Cureus. 2023;15(9):e45373.
57. Sawhney S, Agarwal M. Rituximab use in pediatric systemic lupus erythematosus: Indications, efficacy and safety in an Indian cohort. Lupus. 2021;30(11):1829-36.
58. Jamois C, Gibiansky L, Chavanne C, Cheu M, Lehane PB, Pordeli P, et al. Rituximab pediatric drug development: Pharmacokinetic and pharmacodynamic modeling to inform regulatory approval for rituximab treatment in patients with granulomatosis with polyangiitis or microscopic polyangiitis. Clin Transl Sci. 2022;15(9):2172-83.
59. Bleyer A, O'Leary M, Barr R, Ries LAG (Eds). Cancer Epidemiology in Older Adolescents and Young Adults 15 to 29 Years of Age, Including SEER Incidence and Survival: 1975-2000. Bethesda: National Cancer Institute; 2006.
60. Long AH, Morgenstern DA, Leruste A, Bourdeaut F, Davis KL. Checkpoint immunotherapy in pediatrics: Here, gone, and back again. Am Soc Clin Oncol Educ Book. 2002;42:781-94.
61. Bristol Myers Squibb. (2023). U.S. Food and Drug Administration approves Opdivo (nivolumab) as adjuvant treatment for eligible patients with completely resected stage IIB or stage IIC melanoma. [online] Available from https://news.bms.com/news/details/2023/U.S.-Food-and-Drug-Administration-Approves-Opdivonivolumab-as-Adjuvant-Treatment-for-Eligible-Patients-with-Completely-Resected-Stage-IIB-or-Stage-IIC-Melanoma1/default.aspx [Last accessed January, 2024].

62. ClinicalTrials.gov. (2023). Effectiveness study of nivolumab compared to placebo in prevention of recurrent melanoma after complete resection of stage IIB/C melanoma (CheckMate76K). [online] Available from https://classic.clinicaltrials.gov/ct2/show/NCT04099251 [Last accessed January, 2024].
63. Geoerger B, Bergeron C, Gore L, Sender L, Dunkel IJ, Herzog C, et al. Phase II study of ipilimumab in adolescents with unresectable stage III or IV malignant melanoma. Eur J Cancer. 2017;86:358-63.
64. Rutkowski P, Czarnecka AM. Pembrolizumab for the adjuvant treatment of IIB or IIC melanoma. Expert Rev Anticancer Ther. 2023;23(9):897-902.
65. Aleisa A, Lim Y, Gordon S, Her MJ, Zancanaro P, Abudu M, et al. Response to ustekinumab in three pediatric patients with alopecia areata. Pediatr Dermatol. 2019;36(1):e44-e45
66. Ortolan LS, Kim SR, Crotts S, Liu LY, Craiglow BG, Wambier C, et al. IL-12/IL-23 neutralization is ineffective for alopecia areata in mice and humans. J Allergy Clin Immunol. 2019;144(6):1731-4.
67. Gautam M, Shukla R. Biologics in pediatric dermatology. Indian J Paediatr Dermatol. 2021;22(2):107-17.
68. Dubey AK, Handu SS, Dubey S, Sharma P, Sharma KK, Ahmed QM. Belimumab: First targeted biological treatment for systemic lupus erythematosus J Pharmacol Pharmacother. 2011;2:317-9.
69. ClinicalTrials.gov. (2020). Study of subcutaneous (SC) belimumab in pediatric participants with systemic lupus erythematosus (SLE). [online] Available from https://www.medthority.com/clinical-trials/benlysta/study-of-subcutaneous-sc-belimumab-in-pediatric-participants-with-systemic-lupus-erythematosus-sle/ [Last accessed January, 2024].
70. de Las Vecillas L, Caimmi D, Isabwe GAC, Madrigal-Burgaleta R, Soyer O, Tanno L, et al. Hypersensitivity reactions to biologics in children. Expert Opin Biol Ther. 2023;23(1):61-72.
71. Gisbert JP, Chaparro M. Vaccines in children exposed to biological agents in utero and/or during breastfeeding: Are they effective and safe? J Crohns Colitis. 2023;17(6):995-1009.
72. Jansen MH, Rondaan C, Legger G, Minden K, Uziel Y, Toplak N, et al. Efficacy, immunogenicity and safety of vaccination in Pediatric Patients with Autoimmune Inflammatory Rheumatic Diseases (pedAIIRD): A systematic literature review for the 2021 Update of the EULAR/PRES Recommendations. Front Pediatr. 2022;10:910026.

CHAPTER 26

Biologics in Pregnancy, Lactation, and Other Situations

Shekhar Neema, Vikas Pathania

INTRODUCTION

Biologics are a newer group of drugs, and like all new drugs, trials are conducted and approval obtained in the most physiologically robust population—adults (18-60 years). The pediatric and geriatric population and pregnant and lactating mothers are vulnerable population and generally not included in drug trials. Inclusion of this population in trials is fraught with ethical issues and is generally avoided. This noninclusion results in inability to use drugs freely in this population even when indications exist. With continuous use and anecdotal reports, evidence in this population builds up slowly and physicians develop more confidence in using new drugs (which are no longer new) in vulnerable populations. Etanercept was approved for the management of chronic plaque psoriasis in adults in 2004, while approval for pediatric psoriasis was given in November 2016. This reflects fear of regulatory authorities in the mind of physicians about using newer drugs in special population and situations. Biologics in the pediatric age group has already been discussed in a separate chapter and in this chapter, we will discuss other special situations and populations.

BIOLOGICS IN PREGNANCY

Pregnancy is a complex physiological state, where the maternal immune system undergoes changes and shifts from T helper 1 (Th1) to Th2 response. This shift is required for immune tolerance toward a developing fetus. Psoriasis is a Th1-mediated disease and approximately half of the patients improve while the other half either report no change or worsening of disease. Severity of psoriasis has been linked with poor pregnancy outcomes due to immune dysregulation; other factors like drug intake and concomitant metabolic syndrome also add to poor pregnancy outcomes in patients with psoriasis.[1]

Pregnancy is a state in which any decision taken for the patient has potential effect on two lives, one of them is unborn and is in a developmental stage. The decision to administer any drug during pregnancy is difficult because of the potential risk to fetus. The decision to give any drug to pregnant women is a fine balance between benefit to mother and risk of potential adverse effects in fetus; this algorithm gets further complicated by the effect of an untreated disease in the mother on fetus, risk of progression of disease in the mother causing severe morbidity or mortality, and general reluctance on part of the mother to take any drug to safeguard her unborn child.

Drugs used for the management of psoriasis like cyclosporine and apremilast are pregnancy category C drugs and methotrexate and acitretin are category X drugs, while most of the biologics in use are pregnancy category B drugs and are considered reasonably safe. The teratogenic risk is highest during the first trimester, but immunoglobulin G (IgG) transport across the placenta is limited. The fetal immunoglobulin level is lower than the maternal level till the 22nd week of period of gestation after which it increases rapidly facilitated by neonatal Fc receptor on syncytiotrophoblast. Hence, exposure to biologic agents during the third trimester is associated with elevated cord blood levels. Various monoclonal antibodies have different affinity for Fc receptors. IgG1 monoclonal antibodies (adalimumab, infliximab, secukinumab, ustekinumab, guselkumab, tildrakizumab, risankizumab, and bimekizumab) followed by IgG4 (ixekizumab) and IgG3 and IgG2 (brodalumab) antibodies are most easily transmissible. Etanercept has low affinity being fusion protein and certolizumab pegol has no to minimum transfer due to the absence of an Fc receptor. Most exposures to biologics occur during the first trimester and data in patients with late pregnancy exposure is limited.[2]

The issues that need to be discussed are:
- Inadvertent administration of biologics in an unplanned pregnancy
- Decision to give biologics to a pregnant mother for treatment

Effect on fetus and/or neonate: The question that one commonly comes across when a patient in the reproductive age group on biologics becomes pregnant is teratogenicity. Should one continue pregnancy or terminate it because of the risk of congenital malformations? The data which is available is mostly from use in rheumatology and gastroenterology patients and registry data is about pregnancy outcome and congenital malformation.

Antitumor Necrosis Factor-alpha Therapy
Risk of Adverse Fetal Outcome
There are various case series when pregnant women were exposed to infliximab. In infliximab safety database 2004, the outcome of 96 infliximab-exposed pregnancy was reported. Rate of miscarriage was the same as general population.[3] In Crohn's treatment registry, 117 patients had infliximab

exposure during conception and first-trimester period. The rate of miscarriage and neonatal complications were the same as general population.[4] Another series of 42 patients who were exposed to infliximab ($n = 35$) and adalimumab ($n = 7$) reported six low-birth-weight babies and seven preterm deliveries. These outcomes were not statistically significant as compared to controls.[5] A systematic review and meta-analysis discussed use of tumor necrosis factor (TNF) inhibitors in pregnancy in immune-mediated diseases and noted an increased risk of preterm birth and low birth weight. This risk was seen in inflammatory bowel disease patients but not in patients with psoriasis and rheumatoid arthritis (RA).[6] Another systematic review published in 2023 included psoriasis patients on biologics and included 740 pregnant patients on various biologics. The study concluded that prevalence of miscarriage and congenital malformation was the same as general population; however, the rates of preterm birth are higher.[2] It is prudent to be careful about infusion reaction and anaphylaxis, as it can precipitate labor in advanced pregnancy.

Teratogenicity

A systematic review has been published by the European League Against Rheumatism (EULAR) on use of disease-modifying antirheumatic drugs in pregnancy. The registry data and systematic literature review support the use of anti-TNF-α treatment in the first half of pregnancy. Carter et al. have reported association of anti-TNF-α drugs with vertebral, anal, cardiac, tracheoesophageal, renal, and limb (VACTERL) group of anomalies; however, this paper was criticized because of poor methodology. The current evidence suggests that there is no increased risk of congenital malformations in babies whose mothers were exposed to anti-TNF therapy during conception and the first half of pregnancy.[7,8]

Effect on Fetus or Neonate

As we have already discussed, the use of anti-TNF drugs in the first half of pregnancy appears to be safe. Use of these drugs in second and third trimesters can result in transplacental transfer. Since IgG is actively transported from maternal to fetal circulation, fetal serum concentration can exceed that of maternal drug levels. Affinity of neonatal Fc receptor on the trophoblast cell is highest for monoclonal antibodies (infliximab) and low for fusion protein (etanercept). Infliximab administered during the third trimester can persist for 6–12 months in infant circulation.[9] To prevent neonatal exposure to these drugs, infliximab should be discontinued by 21–22 weeks, gestation, adalimumab by 26–28 weeks, and etanercept by 30–32 weeks.

All neonates who are exposed to anti-TNF therapy after 22 weeks, gestation should undergo complete immunization except live vaccines [bacillus Calmette-Guérin (BCG) vaccine, oral polio-virus vaccine, and rotavirus vaccine].[10]

Interleukin-17 Blockers
Secukinumab and Ixekizumab
Animal studies suggested no adverse fetal outcome. The human data is limited; however, secukinumab and ixekizumab are likely to have a low risk of adverse maternal and fetal outcome. A systematic review which included 44 pregnant patients exposed to ixekizumab and 11 patients exposed to secukinumab found a low risk of adverse fetal outcome.[2] In unplanned pregnancy, where pregnant women are exposed to secukinumab, expert advice is recommended. The patient should be reassured that the available data do not suggest any adverse fetal outcome. She should be counseled about limited availability of human data and managed in consultation with a fetomaternal medicine specialist.[11]

Rituximab
Pemphigus is an uncommon disease in pregnancy. Severe pemphigus requiring biologic therapy for management is rare. Prednisolone and intravenous immunoglobulin (IVIg) are traditionally considered safe in pregnancy. Rituximab is a pregnancy category C drug. Its prescribing information states that contraception should be advised during and after 12 months of rituximab use in women in the reproductive age group. British Society of Rheumatology (BSR) guidelines recommend that rituximab be stopped 6 months prior to conception. BSR registry data of 32 pregnant patients who were exposed to rituximab prior to conception reported that the rate of live births and absence of congenital malformation were reassuring.[12] Rituximab global drug safety database identified 231 pregnancies with maternal rituximab exposure. Pregnancy outcome was known in 153 pregnancies (90 live births, 22 premature, 1 neonatal death at 6 weeks, 4 neonatal infections, and 2 congenital malformations).[13] Patients of child-bearing age should be advised not to become pregnant for 12 months after rituximab administration. Patients who become pregnant inadvertently should be counseled about the risks and comanaged with a fetomaternal medicine specialist. Rituximab can cause neonatal cytopenia or B-cell depletion and can increase the risk of infections in neonates. Neonate should also remain under the care of an expert.

Omalizumab
Omalizumab is a pregnancy category B drug. Prescribing information by manufacturer states that data on use in pregnancy is insufficient. There are various case reports of use of omalizumab in pregnancy for urticaria with successful treatment as well as favorable outcomes of pregnancy.[14] Omalizumab pregnancy registry [Xolair pregnancy registry (EXPECT)] has been collecting data on the safety of omalizumab in pregnancy. Pregnancy outcome was consistent with baseline outcome seen in asthma patients. No pattern of anomalies has been reported.[15] A real-life study on 29 pregnant

CHAPTER 26: Biologics in Pregnancy, Lactation, and Other Situations

TABLE 1: Biologics use during pregnancy.

Drug	Pregnancy category	Preconception	During pregnancy	Unplanned pregnancy	Neonate
Etanercept	B	• Limited data • Appears to be safe	• Safe in first and second trimesters • Increased risk of maternal infection	• Can be continued • Increased maternal infection risk • No increased risk of congenital malformation	• Neonatal immunosuppression, if used in third trimester • Should be stopped by 30–32 weeks • Avoid live vaccine for 6 months
Adalimumab	B	• Limited data • Appears to be safe	• Safe in first and second trimesters • Risk of maternal infection	• Can be continued • No increased risk of congenital malformation	• Neonatal infection • Stop by 26–28 weeks • Avoid live vaccine for 6 months
Infliximab	B	• Limited data • Appears to be safe	• Safe in first and early second trimesters • Risk of maternal infection	• Can be continued • No increased risk of congenital malformation	• Neonatal infection • Stop by 20–22 weeks • Avoid live vaccine for 6–12 months
Secukinumab	B	Limited data	• No data • Should not be used	• Stop the drug • Specialist consultation • Can continue pregnancy	• Risk of neonatal immunosuppression • Avoid live vaccines for 6 months
Ixekizumab	B	Limited data	• No data • Should not be used	• Stop the drug • Specialist consultation • Can continue pregnancy	• Risk of neonatal immunosuppression • Avoid live vaccines for 6 months
Rituximab	C	Should be stopped 6 months prior to conception	Should not be used during pregnancy	Specialist consultation with fetomaternal medicine expert required	• Neonatal infection • B-cell depletion and lymphocytopenia • Avoid live vaccine for 12 months after exposure
Omalizumab	B	• Limited data • Appears to be safe	Appears to be safe and can be used	• Can be continued • No increased risk of congenital malformation	Appears to be safe

patients receiving omalizumab for chronic urticaria did not find any adverse event, pregnancy complications, or congenital anomalies.[16] It should also be noted that second-generation antihistamines like cetirizine, loratadine, and levocetirizine are pregnancy category B drugs, while fexofenadine and desloratadine are pregnancy category C drugs. Prednisolone and cyclosporine are pregnancy category C drugs. This leaves us with a little choice for urticaria in pregnancy **(Table 1)**.

BIOLOGICS DURING LACTATION

Most of the drugs administered to mothers get secreted in breast milk. The quantity of drugs that gets secreted varies and they may or may not be harmful to baby. Biologics are IgG molecules, while predominantly IgA is secreted in breast milk. These drugs are protein and likely to be metabolized in the gastrointestinal system of infants. The available studies suggest that anti-TNF drug concentration in breast milk is minimal and unlikely to be of any clinical significance. In absence of large data, guidelines suggest that mothers on anti-TNF therapy should be encouraged to breastfeed.[6] There is insufficient data to comment on the safety of interleukin-17 (IL-17) inhibitors, secukinumab and ixekizumab, in lactation.

There is no data on rituximab use in breastfeeding and should be avoided. Omalizumab is compatible with breastfeeding and breastfeeding should be encouraged in patients who are already doing so.[17]

BIOLOGICS IN GERIATRIC POPULATION

Elderly patients have special concerns. They are more prone to infections and are often on multiple drugs. Most of the trials which are conducted are on patients between 18 and 65 years; therefore, safety and efficacy data in elderly population is scant. Most of the data on elderly patients are based on postmarketing case series and studies.

Antitumor Necrosis Factor-alpha and Interleukin-17 Blockers

A retrospective study conducted by Momose et al. in Japan reported that biologics are effective in patients >75 years. Biologics used in this study were infliximab, adalimumab, secukinumab, and ustekinumab. There was increased frequency of adverse events, which requires observation.[18] Another retrospective study conducted by Ikari et al. in elderly patients with RA reported that the rate of discontinuation of biologics in elderly patients (>75 years) was significantly high.[19] The study conducted by Garber et al. compared safety and efficacy of biologics and conventional systemic agents for treatment of moderate-to-severe psoriasis in elderly (>65 years) and adults. They reported that there was no statistically significant difference in safety and efficacy of biologic agents in adults and elderly; however, in elderly population, the risk of adverse events with conventional therapy was found to be higher as compared to biologic therapy.[20] A systematic review conducted in 2020 found similar efficacy of TNF inhibitors (etanercept, adalimumab, and infliximab) and IL-17 inhibitors (secukinumab and ixekizumab) in young and elderly patients (>65 years). The rate of adverse events and discontinuation was higher among elderly population.[21]

Rituximab
The French rituximab registry with 2 years of follow-up had patients in different age groups. This registry data is mainly based on RA data and does not include the pemphigus group of disorders. They reported that drug is less effective in patients > 75 years, and elderly were more prone to infections.[22] Available literature in dermatology suggests that rituximab is effective in the treatment of elderly pemphigus patients. There is no data to suggest that it is less effective for management of pemphigus in elderly patients. However, caution should be exercised while administering rituximab in elderly patients as they are more prone to infections, cardiovascular events, and hematologic adverse effects. Vaccination should be completed to prevent infections.

Omalizumab
Omalizumab is approved for management of asthma in children > 6 years and chronic spontaneous urticaria for children >12 years. There is no upper limit of age for administration of omalizumab; however, prescribing information states that data on elderly patients is scant. It has been used for management of uncontrolled asthma and chronic spontaneous urticaria in elderly patients effectively in various case series. The available data supports use of omalizumab for management of chronic spontaneous urticaria. However, higher-than-expected arterial thrombotic events have been reported in asthma patients on omalizumab.[23,24]

BIOLOGICS IN PRESENCE OF OTHER COMORBIDITIES

Chronic Renal Failure
Psoriasis is associated with metabolic syndrome in 30–40% patients. These patients are at a high risk of development of chronic renal failure. Psoriasis per se can increase the risk of renal dysfunction; however, the exact mechanism of this is not known. Drugs like cyclosporine are nephrotoxic and can lead to renal dysfunction. Drugs and their active and inactive metabolites get excreted by kidneys, thereby complicating treatment algorithms in the presence of organ dysfunction. It is important to be aware of this risk while managing psoriasis and a patient at risk should be followed up for the development of renal dysfunction, especially when the patient is on cyclosporine and nonsteroidal anti-inflammatory drug (NSAID). The physician should also be able to manage psoriasis in the presence of established chronic kidney disease.

Management of psoriasis in the presence of renal dysfunction remains challenging as conventional systemic therapy like cyclosporine is nephrotoxic and kidney is the primary route of elimination for methotrexate precluding their use. Phototherapy may not be feasible because of frequent hospital visits that it requires. Biologics are protein molecules that are metabolized by proteolysis and fragments are excreted in bile and urine. Pharmacokinetic data of biologics in the presence of renal dysfunction is not available as this group of population has not been studied. Studies conducted by Gisondi and Girolomoni reported that the glomerular filtration rate in patients on etanercept does not change.[25] There are various case reports of successful use of anti-TNF therapy for management of psoriasis in the presence of end-stage renal disease (ESRD) on hemodialysis.[26,27] Infliximab should be used with caution as it can lead to fluid overload in these patients. There is a case series involving three psoriasis patients on hemodialysis treated successfully with secukinumab without any adverse events.[28] Biologics are large molecules and are not removed in hemodialysis. Patients with kidney dysfunction do not need any dose adjustments. There is a report suggesting improvement in renal function in psoriasis after ixekizumab administration.[29] Patients with ESRD have impaired host defenses, and careful monitoring for infections is required in these patients.

Rituximab is used in management of kidney diseases of autoimmune etiology [antineutrophil cytoplasmic antibodies (ANCAs) associated renal vasculitis, antiglomerular basement membrane (anti-GBM) disease, and lupus nephritis]. Rituximab can be used for management of autoimmune blistering diseases in the presence of impaired renal function; however, it should be used in consultation with a nephrologist. High risk of infection and fluid overload should be addressed in these patients.

The guidelines for management of chronic spontaneous urticaria suggest use of second-generation antihistamines as first-line therapy and omalizumab in cases in which the patient is not responding to a fourfold increase in dose of antihistamines. Commonly used antihistamines like levocetirizine, desloratadine, and fexofenadine require dose adjustment in the presence of renal failure. The availability of literature on use of omalizumab in chronic urticaria in the presence of renal dysfunction is scant. However, omalizumab is an IgG molecule and is metabolized by proteolysis. There is no evidence of renal toxicity of omalizumab in pharmacokinetic studies. As per available literature, omalizumab can be used if indicated.

Chronic Liver Disease

Psoriasis is associated with an increased risk of metabolic dysfunction-associated liver disease, and use of hepatotoxic drugs like methotrexate, acitretin, and azathioprine for longer duration further increases the risk of development of chronic liver disease. As psoriasis is a common disease, it can also coexist with chronic liver disease of various etiologies. Treatment of psoriasis in the presence of chronic liver failure can be challenging as hepatotoxic drugs and drugs which are primarily metabolized in the liver have to be used with caution. Pharmacokinetic data of biologics in the presence of chronic liver failure is not available. This is further complicated by fact that TNF-α blockers have been linked to drug-induced liver injury (DILI). The median latency period before development of DILI was 13 weeks.[30] The etiological evaluation of chronic liver disease should be done prior to starting any biologic therapy as hepatitis B- and C-induced chronic liver disease requires specialist consultation before treatment with biologics is contemplated.

There are various case series and individual case reports of successful use of TNF inhibitors for management of psoriasis with chronic liver disease resulting from various etiologies. Data on secukinumab use in the presence of cirrhosis of liver is scant and no recommendation is available; the author has used secukinumab in two patients with cirrhosis of liver and found it to be safe and effective (unpublished observation). Large safety data of biologic use in this setting is not available. Etanercept is a biologic with maximum available literature in this setting; the risk of development of autoimmune hepatitis with its use is minimal unlike monoclonal antibodies (infliximab and adalimumab) and is safe in the presence of hepatitis C virus (HCV) infection. The available literature suggests that etanercept is a preferable drug in this setting. Biologics in the presence of hepatitis B and C have been discussed in a separate chapter.

Autoimmune blistering diseases are rare diseases and coexistent chronic liver disease with this group of disorders is quite rare. Screening of concomitant hepatitis B and C infection should be done prior to initiation of rituximab as reactivation of hepatitis B and C can occur, and thus rituximab is contraindicated. However, it can be used with careful consideration in consultation with a hepatologist.

Rituximab is used for management of HCV-associated cryoglobulinemia. Since hepatitis C-induced liver damage is immune mediated in nature and liver function also tends to improve in these patients. There are case reports of successful treatment of pemphigus with concomitant HCV infection; however, reactivation of HCV infection can occur and treatment should be done in consultation with a hepatologist.[31]

Chronic hepatitis B infection has a significant risk of worsening or reactivation on administration of rituximab. Complete serological evaluation and hepatitis B virus (HBV) DNA level should be done. Antiviral therapy (lamivudine, entecavir, and tenofovir) should be started in consultation with a hepatologist. Rituximab should be used after adequate viral suppression has been achieved and antiviral should be continued for 6-12 months after the last dose of rituximab to prevent late reactivation.[32]

Cardiac Disease

Psoriasis is associated with risk factors for coronary artery disease (diabetes, hypertension, obesity, and metabolic syndrome) and increased risk of ischemic heart disease. The risk of cardiovascular events is significantly reduced with anti-TNF-α therapy or methotrexate. Anti-TNF therapy significantly reduces the risk of myocardial infarction and major adverse cardiac events but not heart failure.[33] The circulating TNF may induce or exacerbate the development of cardiac failure, and therefore, blocking TNF should improve heart failure but various trials have suggested otherwise. Anti-TNF therapy is contraindicated in patients with advanced congestive heart failure (CHF) [New York Heart Association III or IV (NYHA III or IV)]; however, it can be used in mild-to-moderate CHF (NYHA I or II).[34]

A randomized double-blind placebo-controlled trial to evaluate cardiovascular risk factors found significant improvement in endothelial dysfunction demonstrated by increase in flow-mediated dilation.[35] Another randomized controlled trial did not find any improvement in aortic vascular inflammation after 52 weeks of secukinumab.[36] The data on the effect of ixekizumab on cardiovascular biomarkers is scant.

Various case reports of myocardial infarction, coronary spasm, and ventricular tachycardia have been reported with rituximab. These events generally occur after first infusion but can occur in subsequent infusions also. Ischemic events generally occur in patients with underlying cardiovascular risk factors, but may occur in patients without any risk factors.[37] In a patient with underlying risk factors, cardiologist consultation should be obtained prior to starting rituximab. Infusion should be done where facilities for cardiopulmonary resuscitation are available, especially in patients with underlying heart disease.

Cancer

There are two issues which need to be discussed under this heading. The first issue is the increased risk of malignancy associated with use of biologicals, which has been discussed in detail in adverse effect chapter. The second issue which needs to be discussed is the use of biologics in patients with current or treated malignancy. Patients with current or treated cancer can have associated moderate-to-severe psoriasis requiring systemic therapy. The decision to treat such patients can be quite challenging as one has to choose between conventional systemic therapy or biological agents. There is an unknown risk of cancer recurrence in patients on immunosuppressive medications, and definite guidelines for treatment in such situations are scarce.

There are various systematic reviews, which suggest that there is an increased risk of nonmelanoma skin cancer and lymphoma in patients treated with anti-TNF therapy; however, there has been no significant increase in risk of solid organ malignancy.[38] There are studies that have compared the relative risk of development of malignancy in patients treated with disease-modifying antirheumatic drugs (DMARDs) or biologics in cancer survivors. A systematic review found a slightly increased risk of cancer in psoriasis, but there was no increase in cancer risk in patients treated with biologics.[39] The available data suggests that there is no increase in the risk of cancer recurrence in patients treated with biologics as compared to conventional systemic therapy; however, the available data is limited and is confounded by various other factors.[40] Experts recommend that for cancer survivors, the malignancy should be in remission for 5 years before treatment initiation with biologic. Till the time more robust evidence emerges in this group of population, it is recommended that patients should be informed about a possible increase in the risk of recurrence of cancer in patients being treated with biologic therapy.[41]

CONCLUSION

Biologics are relatively new drugs, and their use in special situations is not yet clear. Despite being an effective therapy, there is some hesitation on part of the treating physician in such situations. This hesitation stems from the fact that data in these scenarios is scant. We have tried to provide current data available, but it leaves a lot to be discussed and their usage will attain clarity as more and more data becomes available.

REFERENCES

1. Bobotsis R, Gulliver WP, Monaghan K, Lynde C, Fleming P. Psoriasis and adverse pregnancy outcomes: A systematic review of observational studies. Br J Dermatol. 2016;175(3):464-72.
2. Sánchez-García V, Hernández-Quiles R, de-Miguel-Balsa E, Giménez-Richarte Á, Ramos-Rincón JM, Belinchón-Romero I. Exposure to biologic therapy before and during pregnancy in patients with psoriasis: Systematic review and meta-analysis. J Eur Acad Dermatol Venereol. 2023;37(10):1971-90.
3. Antoni CE, Furst D, Manger B, Lichtenstein GR, Keenan GF, Healy DE, et al. Outcome of pregnancy in women receiving Remicade® (infliximab) for the treatment of Crohn's disease or rheumatoid arthritis. Arthritis Rheum. 2001;44(9):S152.
4. Lichtenstein GR, Feagan BG, Cohen RD, Salzberg BA, Diamond RH, Price S, et al. Serious infection and mortality in patients with Crohn's disease: More than 5 years of follow-up in the TREATTM registry. Am J Gastroenterol. 2012;107(9):1409-22.
5. Schnitzler F, Fidder H, Ferrante M, Ballet V, Noman M, Van Assche G, et al. Outcome of pregnancy in women with inflammatory bowel disease treated with antitumor necrosis factor therapy. Inflamm Bowel Dis. 2011;17(9):1846-54.
6. Barenbrug L, Groen MT, Hoentjen F, van Drongelen J, Reek JMPAVD, Joosten I, et al. Pregnancy and neonatal outcomes in women with immune mediated inflammatory diseases exposed to anti-tumor necrosis factor-α during pregnancy: A systemic review and meta-analysis. J Autoimmun. 2021;122:102676.
7. Götestam Skorpen C, Hoeltzenbein M, Tincani A, Fischer-Betz R, Elefant E, Chambers C, et al. The EULAR points to consider for use of antirheumatic drugs before pregnancy, and during pregnancy and lactation. Ann Rheum Dis. 2016;75(5):795-810.

8. Carter JD, Ladhani A, Ricca LR, Valeriano J, Vasey FB. A safety assessment of tumor necrosis factor antagonists during pregnancy: A review of the Food and Drug Administration database. J Rheumatol. 2009;36(3):635-41.
9. Förger F. Treatment with biologics during pregnancy in patients with rheumatic diseases. Reumatologia. 2017;55(2):57-8.
10. Soh MC, MacKillop L. Biologics in pregnancy—for the obstetrician. Obstet Gynaecol. 2016;18(1):25-32.
11. Rademaker M, Agnew K, Andrews M, Armour K, Baker C, Foley P, et al. Psoriasis in those planning a family, pregnant or breast-feeding. The Australasian Psoriasis Collaboration. Australas J Dermatol. 2018;59(2):86-100.
12. De Cock D, Birmingham L, Watson KD, Kearsley-Fleet L; BSRBR Control Centre Consortium; Symmons DP, Hyrich KL. Pregnancy outcomes in women with rheumatoid arthritis ever treated with rituximab. Rheumatology (Oxford). 2017;56(4):661-3.
13. Chakravarty EF, Murray ER, Kelman A, Farmer P. Pregnancy outcomes after maternal exposure to rituximab. Blood. 2011;117(5):1499-506.
14. Pardo LBC, Blanch MAB, Radojicic C. Use of omalizumab for treatment of antihistamine and steroid resistant chronic idiopathic urticaria during pregnancy. J Allergy Clin Immunol. 2015;135(2):AB129.
15. Namazy JA, Blais L, Andrews EB, Scheuerle AE, Cabana MD, Thorp JM, et al Pregnancy outcomes in the omalizumab pregnancy registry and a disease-matched comparator cohort. J Allergy Clin Immunol. 2020;145(2):528-36.e1.
16. Patruno C, Guarneri F, Nettis E, Bonzano L, Filippi F, Ribero S, et al. Safety of omalizumab for chronic urticaria during pregnancy: A real-life study. Clin Exp Dermatol. 202313:llad386.
17. Saito J, Yakuwa N, Sandaiji N, Uno C, Yagishita S, Suzuki T, et al. Omalizumab concentrations in pregnancy and lactation: A case study. J Allergy Clin Immunol Pract. 2020;8(10):3603-4.
18. Momose M, Asahina A, Hayashi M, Yanaba K, Umezawa Y, Nakagawa H. Biologic treatments for elderly patients with psoriasis. J Dermatol. 2017;44(9)1020-3.
19. Ikari Y, Miwa Y, Yajima N. The association between elderly rheumatoid arthritis patients using biologics and adverse events: Retrospective cohort study. Ann Rheum Dis. 2017;76(Suppl 2):801.
20. Garber C, Plotnikova N, Au SC, Sorensen EP, Gottlieb A. Biologic and conventional systemic therapies show similar safety and efficacy in elderly and adult patients with moderate to severe psoriasis. J Drugs Dermatol. 2015;14(8):846-52.
21. Sandhu VK, Ighani A, Fleming P, Lynde CW. Biologic treatment in elderly patients with psoriasis: A systematic review. J Cutan Med Surg. 2020;24(2):174-86.
22. Payet S, Soubrier M, Perrodeau E, Bardin T, Cantagrel A, Combe B. Efficacy and safety of rituximab in elderly patients with rheumatoid arthritis enrolled in a French Society of Rheumatology registry. Arthritis Care Res (Hoboken). 2014;66(9):1289-95.
23. Sussman G, Gonçalo M, Sánchez-Borges M. Treatment dilemmas in chronic urticaria. J Euro Acad Dermatol Venereol. 2015;29(Suppl 3):33-7.
24. Presa IJ, Rodríguez BN, Bareño BR, Setien PG, Etxebarria IU, Ercoreca IA. Chronic urticaria in special populations: Children, pregnancy, lactation and elderly people. Curr Treat Options Allergy. 2016;3(4):423-38.
25. Gisondi P, Girolomoni G. Glomerular filtration rate in patients with psoriasis treated with etanercept. J Int Med Res. 2016;44(1 suppl):106-8.
26. Cassano N, Vena GA. Etanercept treatment in a hemodialysis patient with severe cyclosporine-resistant psoriasis and hepatitis C virus infection. Int J Dermatol. 2008;47(9):980-1.

27. Saougou I, Papagoras C, Markatseli TE, Voulgari PV, Drosos AA. A case report of a psoriatic arthritis patient on hemodialysis treated with tumor necrosis factor blocking agent and a literature review. Clin Rheumatol. 2010;29(12):1455-9.
28. Mukai M, Kurihara Y, Ito Y, Shintani Y, Takahashi H, Kubo A, et al. Successful treatment with secukinumab of three psoriatic patients undergoing dialysis. J Dermatol. 2020;47(1):e26-8.
29. Amoruso GF, Nisticò SP, Iannone L, Russo E, Rago G, Patruno C, et al. Ixekizumab may improve renal function in psoriasis. Healthcare (Basel). 2021;9(5):543.
30. Ghabril M, Bonkovsky HL, Kum C, Davern T, Hayashi PH, Kleiner DE. Liver injury from tumor necrosis factor-α antagonists: Analysis of thirty-four cases. Clin Gastroenterol Hepatol. 2013;11(5):558-64.e3.
31. Amber KT, Kodiyan J, Bloom R, Hertl M. The controversy of hepatitis C and rituximab: A multidisciplinary dilemma with implications for patients with pemphigus. Indian J Dermatol Venereol Leprol. 2016;82(2):182-3.
32. de Sena Nogueira Maehara L, Huizinga J, Jonkman MF. Rituximab therapy in pemphigus foliaceus: report of 12 cases and review of recent literature. Br J Dermatol. 2015;172(5):1420-3.
33. Roubille C, Richer V, Starnino T, McCourt C, McFarlane A, Fleming P, et al. Evidence-based recommendations for the management of comorbidities in rheumatoid arthritis, psoriasis, and psoriatic arthritis: Expert opinion of the Canadian Dermatology-Rheumatology Comorbidity Initiative. J Rheumatol. 2015;42(10):1767-80.
34. Heslinga SC, Sijl AM, De Boer K, Van Halm VP, Nurmohamed MT. Tumor necrosis factor blocking therapy and congestive heart failure in patients with inflammatory rheumatic disorders: A systematic review. Curr Med Chem. 2015;22(16):1892-902.
35. von Stebut E, Reich K, Thaçi D, Koenig W, Pinter A, Körber A, et al. Impact of secukinumab on endothelial dysfunction and other cardiovascular disease parameters in psoriasis patients over 52 weeks. J Invest Dermatol. 2019;139(5):1054-62.
36. Gelfand JM, Shin DB, Duffin KC, Armstrong AW, Blauvelt A, Tyring SK, et al. A randomized placebo-controlled trial of secukinumab on aortic vascular inflammation in moderate-to-severe plaque psoriasis (VIP-S). J Invest Dermatol. 2020;140(9):1784-93.e2.
37. Armitage JD, Montero C, Benner A, Armitage JO, Bociek G. Acute coronary syndromes complicating the first infusion of rituximab. Clin Lymphoma Myeloma. 2008;8(4):253-5.
38. Jung JM, Kim YJ, Chang SE, Lee MW, Won CH, Lee WJ. Cancer risks in patients with psoriasis administered biologics therapy: A nationwide population-based study. J Cancer Res Clin Oncol. 2023;149(19):17093-102.
39. Vaengebjerg S, Skov L, Egeberg A, Loft ND. Prevalence, incidence, and risk of cancer in patients with psoriasis and psoriatic arthritis: a systematic review and meta-analysis. JAMA Dermatol. 2020;156(4):421-9.
40. Mastorino L, Dapavo P, Avallone G, Merli M, Cariti C, Rubatto M, et al. Biologic treatment for psoriasis in cancer patients: Should they still be considered forbidden? J Dermatolog Treat. 2022;33(5):2495-502.
41. Majewksi S, Kheterpal M, Nardone B, Sable K, West DP, Lacouture ME. First line biologic agent therapy for moderate-to-severe psoriasis in cancer survivors. J Am Acad Dermatol. 2016;74(5):AB250.

SECTION 9

Miscellaneous Issues with Biologics

CHAPTER 27

Miscellaneous Uses of Biologics

Manas Chatterjee, Dipali Rathod

INTRODUCTION

In 2003, alefacept was the first biological agent to be used in the treatment of psoriasis. Following this, many biological agents have been tried and approved for their use in various dermatological and nondermatological diseases. Over the last few decades, there has been an exponential growth in the direction of the development of newer biologics with receptor specific actions, better pharmacological properties, and in a nutshell, newer biologics with a better safety profile. With the advent of technological developments in this area, the concept of treatment directed to patient-specific target has emerged recently. In this chapter, we have dealt about the various newer biologicals and their off-label uses within dermatology.

DERMATOLOGICAL CONDITIONS

Inflammatory and Granulomatous Dermatoses

In the field of dermatology, the off-label use of biologics has emerged as a groundbreaking frontier in the management of inflammatory dermatoses. While initially developed to target specific immune pathways in conditions such as rheumatoid arthritis and psoriasis, biologics have demonstrated remarkable efficacy beyond their approved indications. This upcoming modality explores the untapped potential of these biological agents in treating a spectrum of inflammatory skin disorders caused by both Th1 and Th2 pathway dysregulation. The intricate interplay between immune dysregulation and dermatologic manifestations has spurred innovative approaches to repurpose biologics, addressing unmet needs in patient care.

Sarcoidosis

There are numerous reports of successful treatment with infliximab infusions in sarcoidosis patients with cutaneous involvement.[1-3] A recent double-blind, randomized, placebo-controlled trial with adalimumab showed modest results, whereas there is lack of evidence to suggest benefits with etanercept in patients with sarcoidosis. Ustekinumab and golimumab have also been tried in a single randomized, double-blind, placebo-controlled trial comprising 173 patients of cutaneous sarcoidosis with no statistically significant improvement.[4] However, it should be borne in mind that few case reports have documented triggering or exacerbation of sarcoid with all of the tumor necrosis factor-alpha (TNF-α) inhibitors.[5,6]

Pityriasis Rubra Pilaris[7-9]

The off-label utilization of biologics has undergone extensive exploration in pityriasis rubra pilaris (PRP), leveraging its pronounced clinical and pathogenic parallels with psoriasis. The efficacy spectrum of anti-TNF-α, anti-interleukin (IL)-17, and anti-IL-12/23 treatments reveals notable to complete responses spanning the spectrum of 50–78%. Infliximab, adalimumab, ustekinumab, secukinumab, and ixekizumab has been tried in PRP with variable efficacy.

Alopecia Areata[10,11]

The TNF-α inhibitors, IL-12/23, and IL-17 inhibitors have been used in alopecia areata (AA) with variable success. Recently, dupilumab that acts on Th2 cytokines (IL-4/13) has also been tried in AA and patients with high IgE or background atopy showed better response to the drug. However, paradoxical AA has also been described with dupilumab possibly due to Th2 inhibition induced by dupilumab amplifying alternative immune pathways, such as Th1 or Th17, implicated in AA adverse outcomes.

Granuloma Annulare

Tumor necrosis factor-alpha plays an important role in the pathogenesis of granuloma annulare (GA), as well in any granulomatous process as a critical regulator of inflammatory granuloma formation.[12] Many case reports have successfully shown good results with TNF-α inhibitors in treating refractory or challenging cases of these conditions but they have not been treated in a randomized controlled trial (RCT). There are case reports of mixed results, improvement,[13] and failure[14] with etanercept while both infliximab[15,16] and adalimumab[17-19] have shown to improve GA (mostly the disseminated form). However, paradoxical appearance of GA lesions postinitiation of biologic (anti-TNF, anti-IL-17, anti-IL-6, and anti-IL-12/23) is also known.[20]

Necrobiosis Lipoidica

In the literature, there are some case reports showing successful treatment of necrobiosis lipoidica with the TNF-α inhibitors.[21-23] The best and most strong data in context to the granulomatous disorders exist for infliximab, followed by adalimumab and etanercept, respectively.

Sweet Syndrome
There exists direct evidence that TNF-α levels are increased in patients with Sweet syndrome. Two case reports have shown good efficacy of etanercept in the treatment of Sweet syndrome with presumed inflammatory arthritis.[24,25] Neutrophilic dermatosis due to various biologics in the form of Sweet syndrome and pyoderma gangrenosum (PG) have also been reported. These biologics include adalimumab, tocilizumab, rituximab, infliximab, etanercept, golimumab, secukinumab, and certolizumab. However, due to association of neutrophilic dermatosis (ND) with underlying disease, the causal relationship between biologic and ND is difficult to establish.[26]

Pyoderma Gangrenosum
Although there is a relative paucity of RCTs to confirm the evidence of biologic use for the treatment of PG, there exists successful case reports[21-26] of treatment with infliximab and also a RCT of 30 patients which showed significant ($p = 0.025$) improvement compared to the control.[27] Mixed results showing treatment failure[28] and treatment successes[29-31] have been observed with the use of both etanercept and adalimumab, whereas a paradoxical case eventually responded to adalimumab, which showed treatment failure with both infliximab and etanercept earlier.[32] A recalcitrant case of PG recently showed elevated expression of IL-23, which after treatment with ustekinumab showed complete healing.[33]

Autoimmune Bullous Dermatoses
The newer biologics in autoimmune bullous dermatoses (AIBDs) have been dealt in detail in previous chapter (newer biologics in autoimmune bullous disorder). A summary of various biologics used in AIBDs is mentioned in **Table 1**.

Connective Tissue Diseases
Various therapeutic options exist for connective tissue diseases such as systemic lupus erythematosus (SLE), scleroderma/morphea, and dermatomyositis (DM) for managing the cutaneous and systemic manifestations of these conditions. However, to treat the recalcitrant cases, newer treatment options are crucial. The data regarding biologic treatment of scleroderma/morphea or DM are relatively sparse.

Systemic Lupus Erythematosus
The TNF-α inhibitors have been used successfully in the treatment of SLE patients, along with rituximab and tocilizumab, a monoclonal antibody to the IL-6 receptor.[34] The efficacy of rituximab in SLE and other systemic autoimmune disorder patients was demonstrated in a large study ($n = 107$).[35]

Belimumab, a human monoclonal antibody to the soluble B-lymphocyte stimulator was given in a study of 867 patients, which according to the SLE

TABLE 1: Various biologics in autoimmune bullous dermatoses.

Biological agents	Target of action
• *First generation*: Rituximab, ofatumumab, veltuzumab, and ocrelizumab • *Second generation*: Tositumomab and obinutuzumab	Anti-CD20 (inhibit stimulatory signals provided by CD20 to memory B-cells, causes depletion of memory B-cells)
Blinatumomab and inebilizumab	Anti-CD19 (inhibit stimulatory signals provided by CD19 to B-cells and plasma cells)
Epratuzumab	CD22 modulators (augments inhibitory signals provided by CD-22 to B-cells)
• Belimumab • VAY736	• Anti-BAFF • Anti-BAFF receptor monoclonal antibody
Atacicept	Anti-APRIL
Omalizumab	Anti-immunoglobulin E monoclonal antibodies
Sutimlimab	Anti-complement C1s monoclonal antibody
Bertilimumab	Anti-eotaxin-1 monoclonal antibody
Mepolizumab	Anti-IL-5 monoclonal antibody
Dupilumab	IL-4 receptor antagonist
Ixekizumab	IL-17 inhibitor
• Efgartigimod, rozanolixizumab, SYNT001 • Intravenous immunoglobulins	FcRn antagonists
Live T-cells possessing chimeric autoantibody receptors are composed of the autoantigen (desmoglein 3 for pemphigus) fused to the signaling domain CD137	CAAR T-cells (CAAR T-cells recognize autoantigen-specific autoreactive B-cells)

(APRIL: A proliferation-inducing ligand; BAFF: B-cell activating factor; CAAR: chimeric autoantibody receptor; CD: cluster of differentiation; FcRn: neonatal Fc receptor; IL: interleukin)

Responder Index [defined as a ≥4-point improvement on a validated scale of SLE, the SELENA-SLEDAI (safety of estrogen in lupus erythematosus national assessment–SLE disease activity index)] showed significant improvement versus the control ($p < 0.02$ in both treatment groups of 1 mg/kg and 10 mg/kg).[35] In the treatment of active SLE, the United States Food and Drug Administration (US FDA) approval has been granted, which may prove valuable.

Many possible targets for which biologics are at various stages of trials are mentioned in **Figure 1**.

Morphea

Few case reports of generalized morphea showed promising results with infliximab,[36] while another study of 16 patients failed to demonstrate

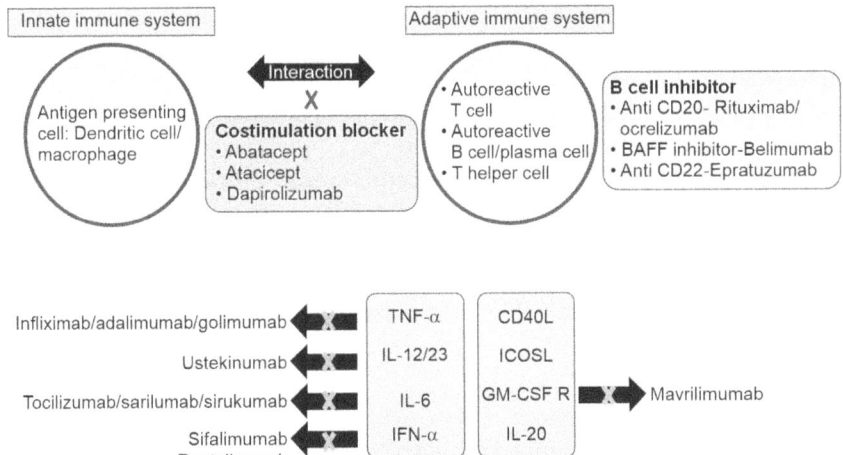

FIG. 1: Schematic representation of different biologics and their therapeutic targets.
(BAFF: B-cell activating factor; GM-CSF: granulocyte-macrophage colony stimulating factor; ICOSL: inducible costimulator ligand; IFN: interferon; IL: interleukin)

significant clinical improvement at 26 weeks, wherein 50% of the patients dropped out likely due to the drug related adverse events.[37]

Dermatomyositis

Similar to morphea, there have been dermatomyositis case reports demonstrating successful treatment with infliximab,[38] whereas infliximab seemed to be a therapeutic failure in a patient who developed sepsis and then thereafter lymphoma a few months after the infliximab infusion.[39] Tocilizumab, an IL6 inhibitor has also been tried successfully in morphea in both pediatric and adult population.[40]

DISORDERS OF FOLLICULAR OCCLUSION

Hidradenitis Suppurativa

Hidradenitis suppurativa (HS) is an extremely morbid condition, a disorder of follicular occlusion, is both distressing and painful, and is often difficult to manage.[41] One study showed elevated levels of TNF-α in patients with HS,[42] and further the successful treatment of HS patients with TNF-α inhibitors illustrates a relationship between pathophysiologic mechanisms of the disease and effective treatment. A phase 2 trial of 154 patients with moderate-to-severe HS (no improvement with oral antibiotics) showed a significantly improved clinical response in those treated weekly with adalimumab versus the control ($p = 0.025$).[43]

Infliximab was one of the earliest used TNF-α inhibitor in the treatment of HS patients.[44] As of May 2014, a PubMed search of MEDLINE indexed articles using the search terms hidradenitis suppurativa and infliximab yielded >80 results. A small RCT of 38 participants demonstrated statistically significant improvement with infliximab (5 mg/kg at 0, 2, and 6 weeks) in the severity index scores of HS at 8 weeks ($p < 0.005$) compared with the control.[45] A meta-analysis of five RCTs suggested that both adalimumab and infliximab are effective therapeutic option in treating HS patients, however infliximab showed a better early response.[46]

Two open-label studies of etanercept showed efficacy in treating HS patients, however both studies only recruited 10 patients each.[47,48]

Table 2 shows the list of biologics proven effective/that have shown efficacy in HS with evidence. These include bermekimab, guselkumab, brodalumab, bimekizumab, IFX-1, risankizumab, CSL324, and adalimumab.

Acne Conglobata[65]

Acne conglobata, in instances of systemic retinoid failure, can manifest as a disfiguring ailment with limited therapeutic alternatives. Notably, Sand and Thomsen documented a favorable response to TNF-α inhibitors in 64% (7 out of 11) of patients grappling with severe and refractory acne conglobata.

The pathophysiological link becomes apparent as *Propionibacterium acnes* incites keratinocytes to unleash IL-1α and TNF-α. Moreover, the stimulation of peripheral blood mononuclear cells (PBMCs) in acne patients by *P. acnes* induces heightened production of TNF-α and IL-8, underscoring the pivotal role of TNF-α in this dermatological condition.

Others

Toxic Epidermal Necrolysis[66,67]

Given its status as one of the most perilous dermatological conditions, the management of toxic epidermal necrolysis (TEN) assumes paramount importance. The presence of TNF-α has been discerned in both blister fluid and serum among TEN patients. The bulk of available evidence stems from case series and individual case reports. Nevertheless, a prevailing trend emerges wherein a substantial majority of cases exhibit marked responsiveness, yielding outcomes that surpass anticipated mortality rates.

An intriguing case series featuring 10 patients, all achieving exemplary outcomes through the utilization of etanercept, has been documented. An RCT pitting etanercept ($n = 48$) against corticosteroids ($n = 43$) revealed a lower mortality rate associated with etanercept (8.3%), in stark contrast to the predicted outcome (17.7%). Although the disparity with the corticosteroid cohort (16.3%) did not achieve statistical significance, it is noteworthy that the time required for complete skin healing was notably abbreviated.

However, a notable paradox persists, with >50 documented cases wherein individuals developed TEN despite concurrent treatment with TNF-α blockers.

Mastocytosis

Given its remarkable effectiveness in treating urticaria, the application of omalizumab in other mast cell–mediated conditions, such as mastocytosis,

CHAPTER 27: Miscellaneous Uses of Biologics

TABLE 2: Biologics for hidradenitis suppurativa (HS).

Biologicals	Target	Status of study/efficacy

• Bermekimab
• Dosed at 7.5 mg/kg every 14 days up to 7 infusions
	IL-1α	• Low (one double-blind RCT of 20 patients)[49]
		• Two clinical trials updated on clinicaltrials.gov as active but not yet recruiting:
		   ○ NCT03512275[50]
		   ○ NCT04019041[51]

Guselkumab	IL-23	• One open-label trial of 3 patients,[52] one retrospective chart review of 8 patients,[53] and one case study[54] • A phase II clinical trial registered on clinicaltrials.gov (NCT03628924)[55] • A pilot open-label study is active but not recruiting (NCT04084665)[56]
Brodalumab	IL-17	• A phase 0 clinical trial to assess for safety on clinicaltrials.gov is recruiting (NCT03960268)[57] • A phase II clinical trial is currently listed but not yet recruiting (NCT03910803)[58]
Bimekizumab	IL-17A and IL-17F	Completed phase II study on clinicaltrials.gov, no results available yet (NCT03248531)[59]
IFX-1	C5a	A phase II clinical trial has been completed but results have not been published (NCT03001622);[60] another phase II clinical trial is active but not recruiting (NCT03487276)[61]
Risankizumab	IL-23/17, JAK2	Phase II recruiting (NCT03926169)[62]
CSL324	G-CSF stimulating mAb	A phase I clinical trial on clinicaltrials.gov is listed but not recruiting (NCT03972280)[63]
MSB11022 (adalimumab biosimilar)	TNF-α	A phase I clinical trial listed on clinicaltrials.gov is currently recruiting (NCT04018599)[64]

(G-CSF: granulocyte colony stimulating factor; IL: interleukin; JAK: Janus Kinase; mAb: monoclonal antibody; RCT: randomized controlled trial; TNF-α: tumor necrosis factor alpha)

holds considerable promise. Published cases consistently highlight the notable efficacy of omalizumab in alleviating systemic symptoms, ranging from gastrointestinal issues to pruritus. Intriguingly, there have been instances where patients experienced a resolution of cutaneous lesions.

A multicenter RCT involved seven patients administered omalizumab and nine receiving a placebo.[68] At the 6-month mark, the omalizumab group demonstrated a superior improvement in the French Association for the Initiatives of Research on Mastocyte and Mastocytosis (AFIRMM) score (52-26 vs. 104-102), although statistical significance was not achieved. The findings suggest a potential positive impact, although further investigation is warranted.

Recurrent Aphthous Stomatitis and Behçet Syndrome[69-71]

In challenging cases of recurrent aphthous stomatitis, the utility of anti-TNF-α inhibitors has proven significant. Adalimumab, etanercept, and infliximab all exhibit commendable efficacy. Adalimumab, in particular, has demonstrated complete responses in approximately two-thirds of treated patients. Notably, its effectiveness extends to mitigating other manifestations of *Behçet* syndrome, including the resolution of venous thrombosis.

Secukinumab has exhibited favorable outcomes in five patients with *Behçet* syndrome, concurrently presenting with ankylosing spondylitis or psoriatic arthritis and refractory to conventional treatments and anti-TNF-α therapy. Improvement in active mucocutaneous manifestations was evident, with the rapid resolution of oral ulcerations standing out as particularly remarkable. Various studies have corroborated the involvement of IL-17 in the pathogenesis. Ustekinumab also demonstrated efficacy in a small prospective study involving 14 patients. After 12 weeks, a complete response was observed in 64%, a partial response in 21%, with 14% showing no response.

IL-1 antagonism (Anakinra) has predominantly been explored for its impact on uveitis in *Behçet* syndrome, although a limited pilot study has delved into its effects on mucocutaneous complaints. In five out of six patients, there was an improvement in the severity and number of ulcers, with two cases achieving a complete response.

CONCLUSION

The use of biological agents has completely revolutionized the dermatological practice in today's era. Various biological agents have been tried with good response in several other dermatologic diseases, however the continuing research and development efforts have shed light on the benefit-risk profiles of these agents.

Although these agents seem effective, the cost should be borne in mind while ascertaining the various management options in comparison to the traditional agents.

Nonetheless, the cost of a biological agent may be counterbalanced due to their effectiveness leading to significant reductions in the use of other systemic therapies, number of hospital stays, and thereby increased satisfaction by the patients.[72] Therefore, understanding the mechanisms of action of these agents, their on-label and off-label indications in various dermatological diseases along with the commonly encountered adverse effects may aid in appropriate decision making, thus improving the end results.

REFERENCES

1. Tu J, Chan J. Cutaneous sarcoidosis and infliximab: evidence for efficacy in refractory disease. Australas J Dermatol. 2014;55(4):279-81.
2. Tuchinda P, Bremmer M, Gaspari AA. A case series of refractory cutaneous sarcoidosis successfully treated with infliximab. Dermatol Ther (Heidelb). 2012;2(1):11.
3. Sené T, Juillard C, Rybojad M, Cordoliani F, Lebbé C, Morel P, et al. Infliximab as a steroid-sparing agent in refractory cutaneous sarcoidosis: single-center retrospective study of 9 patients. J Am Acad Dermatol. 2012;66(2):328-32.
4. Judson MA, Baughman RP, Costabel U, Drent M, Gibson KF, Raghu G, et al. Safety and efficacy of ustekinumab or golimumab in patients with chronic sarcoidosis. Eur Respir J. 2014;44(5):1296-307.
5. Clementine RR, Lyman J, Zakem J, Mallepalli J, Lindsey S, Quinet R. Tumor necrosis factor-alpha antagonist-induced sarcoidosis. J Clin Rheumatol. 2010;16(6):274-9.
6. Santos G, Sousa LE, João AM. Exacerbation of recalcitrant cutaneous sarcoidosis with adalimumab—a paradoxical effect? a case report. An Bras Dermatol. 2013;88(6 Suppl 1):26-8.
7. Bonomo L, Levitt JO. Secukinumab emerges as a rapidly effective therapy for pityriasis rubra pilaris. Cutis. 2018;101(5):367-9.
8. Heibel MD, Heibel HD. Successful treatment of type I pityriasis rubra pilaris with ixekizumab. JAAD Case Rep. 2018;4(8):774-6.
9. Wain T, Choy B, Satchell AC, Woods JA, Frew JW. Secukinumab in pityriasis rubra pilaris: a case series demonstrating variable response and the need for minimal clinical datasets. JAAD Case Rep. 2018;4(5):500-5.
10. Guttman-Yassky E, Renert-Yuval Y, Bares J, Chima M, Hawkes JE, Gilleaudeau P, et al. Phase 2a randomized clinical trial of dupilumab (anti-IL-4Rα) for alopecia areata patients. Allergy. 2022;77(3):897-906.
11. Sachdeva M, Witol A, Mufti A, Maliyar K, Yeung J. Alopecia areata related paradoxical reactions in patients on dupilumab therapy: a systematic review. J Cutan Med Surg. 2021;25(4):451-2.
12. Fayyazi A, Schweyer S, Eichmeyer B, Herms J, Hemmerlein B, Radzun HJ, et al. Expression of IFNgamma, coexpression of TNFalpha and matrix metalloproteinases and apoptosis of T lymphocytes and macrophages in granuloma annulare. Arch Dermatol Res. 2000;292(8):384-90.
13. Shupack J, Siu K. Resolving granuloma annulare with etanercept. Arch Dermatol. 2006;142(3):394-5.
14. Kreuter A, Altmeyer P, Gambichler T. Failure of etanercept therapy in disseminated granuloma annulare. Arch Dermatol. 2006;142(9):1236-7.
15. Murdaca G, Colombo BM, Barabino G, Caiti M, Cagnati P, Puppo F. Anti-tumor necrosis factor-α treatment with infliximab for disseminated granuloma annulare. Am J Clin Dermatol. 2010;11(6):437-9.
16. Hertl MS, Haendle I, Schuler G, Hertl M. Rapid improvement of recalcitrant disseminated granuloma annulare upon treatment with the tumour necrosis factor-α inhibitor, infliximab. Br J Dermatol. 2005;152(3):552-5.
17. Kozic H, Webster GF. Treatment of widespread granuloma annulare with adalimumab: a case report. J Clin Aesthet Dermatol. 2011;4(11):42-3.
18. Werchau S, Enk A, Hartmann M. Generalized interstitial granuloma annulare—response to adalimumab. Int J Dermatol. 2010;49(4):457-60.

19. Rosmarin D, LaRaia A, Schlauder S, Gottlieb AB. Successful treatment of disseminated granuloma annulare with adalimumab. J Drugs Dermatol. 2009;8(2):169-71.
20. Lytvyn Y, Mufti A, Sachdeva M, Maliyar K, Yeung J. Development of granuloma annulare in patients on biologic therapies: A systematic review. J Am Acad Dermatol. 2021;85(6):1594-7.
21. Zhang KS, Quan LT, Hsu S. Treatment of necrobiosis lipoidica with etanercept and adalimumab. Dermatol Online J. 2009;15(12):12.
22. Suárez-Amor O, Pérez-Bustillo A, Ruiz-González I, Rodríguez-Prieto MA. Necrobiosis lipoidica therapy with biologicals: an ulcerated case responding to etanercept and a review of the literature. Dermatology. 2010;221(2):117-21.
23. Hu SW, Bevona C, Winterfield L, Qureshi AA, Li VW. Treatment of refractory ulcerative necrobiosis lipoidica diabeticorum with infliximab: report of a case. Arch Dermatol. 2009;145(4):437-9.
24. Ambrose NL, Tobin AM, Howard D. Etanercept treatment in Sweet's syndrome with inflammatory arthritis. J Rheumatol. 2009;36(6):1348-9.
25. Yamauchi PS, Turner L, Lowe NJ, Gindi V, Jackson JM. Treatment of recurrent Sweet's syndrome with coexisting rheumatoid arthritis with the tumor necrosis factor antagonist etanercept. J Am Acad Dermatol. 2006;54(suppl 2):S122-S126.
26. Haber R, Dib N, El Gemayel M, Makhlouf M. Paradoxical neutrophilic dermatosis induced by biologics and immunosuppressive drugs: A systematic review. J Am Acad Dermatol. 2021;85(4):1048-9.
27. Campos-Muñoz L, Conde-Taboada A, Aleo E, Toledano E, López-Bran E. Refractory pyoderma gangrenosum treated with infliximab in an infant. Clin Exp Dermatol. 2014;39(3):336-9.
28. Bhatti H, Khalid N, Rao B. Superficial pyoderma gangrenosum treated with infliximab: a case report. Cutis. 2012;90(6):297-9.
29. Hayashi H, Kuwabara C, Tarumi K, Makino E, Fujimoto W. Successful treatment with infliximab for refractory pyoderma gangrenosum associated with inflammatory bowel disease. J Dermatol. 2012;39(6):576-8.
30. Fernández A, Velasco A, Prieto V, Canueto J, Alvarez A, Rodríguez A. Response to infliximab in atypical pyoderma gangrenosum associated with ulcerative colitis. Am J Gastroenterol. 2008;103(11):2951-2.
31. Cocco A, Angelucci E, Viscido A, Caprilli R. Successful treatment with infliximab of refractory pyoderma gangrenosum in 2 patients with inflammatory bowel diseases. Inflamm Bowel Dis. 2007;13(10):1317-9.
32. Stichweh DS, Punaro M, Pascual V. Dramatic improvement of pyoderma gangrenosum with infliximab in a patient with PAPA syndrome. Pediatr Dermatol. 2005;22(3):262-5.
33. Brooklyn TN, Dunnill MG, Shetty A, Bowden JJ, Williams JD, Griffiths CE, et al. Infliximab for the treatment of pyoderma gangrenosum: a randomised, double blind, placebo controlled trial. Gut. 2006;55(4):505-9.
34. Aringer M, Burkhardt H, Burmester GR, Fischer-Betz R, Fleck M, Graninger W, et al. Current state of evidence on 'off-label' therapeutic options for systemic lupus erythematosus, including biological immunosuppressive agents, in Germany, Austria and Switzerland—a consensus report. Lupus. 2012;21(4):386-401.
35. Ramos-Casals M, García-Hernández FJ, de Ramón E, Callejas JL, Martínez-Berriotxoa A, Pallarés L, et al; BIOGEAS Study Group. Off-label use of rituximab in 196 patients with severe, refractory systemic autoimmune diseases. Clin Exp Rheumatol. 2010;28(4):468-76.
36. Diab M, Coloe JR, Magro C, Bechtel MA. Treatment of recalcitrant generalized morphea with infliximab. Arch Dermatol. 2010;146(6):601-4.
37. Denton CP, Engelhart M, Tvede N, Wilson H, Khan K, Shiwen X, et al. An open-label pilot study of infliximab therapy in diffuse cutaneous systemic sclerosis. Ann Rheum Dis. 2009;68(9):1433-9.

38. Hengstman GJ, van den Hoogen FH, Barrera P, Netea MG, Pieterse A, van de Putte LB, et al. Successful treatment of dermatomyositis and polymyositis with anti-tumor-necrosis-factor-alpha: preliminary observations. Eur Neurol. 2003;50(1):10-5.
39. Roddy E, Courtney PA, Morris A. Non-Hodgkin's lymphoma in a patient with refractory dermatomyositis which had been treated with infliximab. Rheumatology (Oxford). 2002;41(10):1194-5.
40. Lonowski S, Goldman N, Kassamali B, Shahriari N, LaChance A, Vleugels RA. Tocilizumab for refractory morphea in adults: A case series. JAAD Case Reports. 2022;30:27-9.
41. von der Werth JM, Jemec GB. Morbidity in patients with hidradenitis suppurativa. Br J Dermatol. 2001;144(4):809-13.
42. Matusiak L, Bieniek A, Szepietowski JC. Increased serum tumour necrosis factor-alpha in hidradenitis suppurativa patients: is there a basis for treatment with anti-tumour necrosis factor-alpha agents? Acta Derm Venereol. 2009;89(6):601-3.
43. Kimball AB, Kerdel F, Adams D, Mrowietz U, Gelfand JM, Gniadecki R, et al. Adalimumab for the treatment of moderate to severe hidradenitis suppurativa: a parallel randomized trial. Ann Intern Med. 2012;157(12):846-55.
44. Martínez F, Nos P, Benlloch S, Ponce J. Hidradenitis suppurativa and Crohn's disease: response to treatment with infliximab. Inflamm Bowel Dis. 2001;7(4):323-6.
45. Grant A, Gonzalez T, Montgomery MO, Cardenas V, Kerdel FA. Infliximab therapy for patients with moderate to severe hidradenitis suppurativa: a randomized, double-blind, placebo-controlled crossover trial. J Am Acad Dermatol. 2010;62(2):205-17.
46. Thorlund K, Druyts E, Mills EJ, Fedorak RN, Marshall JK. Adalimumab versus infliximab for the treatment of moderate to severe ulcerative colitis in adult patients naïve to anti-TNF therapy: an indirect treatment comparison meta-analysis. J Crohns Colitis. 2014;8(7):571-81.
47. Pelekanou A, Kanni T, Savva A, Mouktaroudi M, Raftogiannis M, Kotsaki A, et al. Long-term efficacy of etanercept in hidradenitis suppurativa: results from an open-label phase-II prospective trial. Exp Dermatol. 2010;19(6):538-40.
48. Giamarellos-Bourboulis EJ, Pelekanou E, Antonopoulou A, Petropoulou H, Baziaka F, Karagianni V, et al. An open-label phase-II study of the safety and efficacy of etanercept for the therapy of hidradenitis suppurativa. Br J Dermatol. 2008;158(3): 567-72.
49. Kanni T, Argyropoulou M, Spyridopoulos T, Pistiki A, Stecher M, Dinarello CA, et al. MABp1 Targeting IL-1α for moderate to severe hidradenitis suppurativa not eligible for adalimumab: A randomized study. J Invest Dermatol. 2018;138(4):795-801.
50. ClinicalTrials.gov. (2022). A study of bermekimab in patients with hidradenitis suppurativa. [online] Available from https://clinicaltrials.gov/ct2/show/NCT03512275 [Last accessed January, 2024].
51. ClinicalTrials.gov. (2023). A study to evaluate the efficacy, safety and tolerability of bermekimab in patients with hidradenitis suppurativa. [online] Available from https://clinicaltrials.gov/ct2/show/NCT04019041 [Last accessed January, 2024].
52. Kovacs M, Podda M. Guselkumab in the treatment of severe hidradenitis suppurativa. J Eur Acad Dermatol Venereol. 2019;33(3):e140-e141.
53. Berman H, Villa NM, Shi VY, Hsiao JL. Guselkumab in the treatment of concomitant hidradenitis suppurativa, psoriasis, and Crohn's disease. J Dermatolog Treat. 2021;32(2):261-3.
54. Casseres RG, Kahn JS, Her MJ, Rosmarin D. Guselkumab in the treatment of hidradenitis suppurativa: A retrospective chart review. J Am Acad Dermatol. 2019;81(1): 265-7.
55. ClinicalTrials.gov. (2021). A study to evaluate the efficacy, safety and tolerability of guselkumab for the treatment of participants with moderate to severe hidradenitis suppurativa (HS) (NOVA). [online] Available from https://clinicaltrials.gov/ct2/show/NCT03628924?cond=hidradenitis+suppurativa &rank=13 [Last accessed January, 2024].

56. ClinicalTrials.gov. (2020). Biomarkers in participants with hidradenitis suppurativa receiving guselkumab. [online] Available from https://clinicaltrials.gov/ct2/show/NCT04084665 [Last accessed January, 2024].
57. ClinicalTrials.gov. (2020). Biomarkers in hidradenitis suppurativa participants receiving brodalumab. [online] Available from https://clinicaltrials.gov/ct2/show/NCT03960268 [Last accessed January, 2024].
58. ClinicalTrials.gov. (2019). Treatment of moderate hidradenitis suppurativa. [online] Available from https://clinicaltrials.gov/ct2/show/NCT03910803 [Last accessed January, 2024].
59. ClinicalTrials.gov. (2020). A study to test the efficacy, safety and pharmacokinetics of bimekizumab in subjects with moderate to severe hidradenitis suppurativa. [online] Available from https://classic.clinicaltrials.gov/ct2/show/NCT04242498 [Last accessed January, 2024].
60. GlobeNewswire. (2019). InflaRx announces top-line SHINE phase IIb results for IFX-1 in hidradenitis suppurativa. [online] Available from http://www.globenewswire.com/news-release/2019/06/05/1864534/0/en/InflaRx-Announces-Top-Line-SHINE-Phase-IIb-Results-for-IFX-1-in-Hidradenitis-Suppurativa.html [Last accessed January, 2024].
61. ClinicalTrials.gov. (2021). Efficacy and safety study of IFX-1 in patients with moderate to severe hidradenitis suppurativa (HS) (SHINE). [online] Available from https://clinicaltrials.gov/study/NCT03487276 [Last accessed January, 2024].
62. ClinicalTrials.gov. (2022). A global study comparing risankizumab to placebo in adult participants with moderate to severe hidradenitis suppurativa. [online] Available from https://clinicaltrials.gov/ct2/show/NCT03926169 [Last accessed January, 2024].
63. ClinicalTrials.gov. (2023). Safety and pharmacokinetics of repeat doses of CSL324 in subjects with hidradenitis suppurativa and palmoplantar pustulosis. [online] Available from https://clinicaltrials.gov/ct2/show/NCT03972280 [Last accessed January, 2024].
64. ClinicalTrials.gov. (2020) Comparison of PK and tolerability of MSB11022 administered by AI or PFS. [online] Available from https://clinicaltrials.gov/ct2/show/NCT04018599 [Last accessed January, 2024].
65. Yiu ZZN, Madan V, Griffiths CEM. Acne conglobata and adalimumab: use of tumour necrosis factor-α antagonists in treatment-resistant acne conglobata, and review of the literature. Clin Exp Dermatol. 2015;40(4):383-6.
66. Woolridge KF, Boler PL, Lee BD. Tumor necrosis factor alpha inhibitors in the treatment of toxic epidermal necrolysis. Cutis. 2018;101(1):E15-21.
67. Paradisi A, Abeni D, Bergamo F, Ricci F, Didona D, Didona B. Etanercept therapy for toxic epidermal necrolysis. J Am Acad Dermatol. 2014;71(2):278-83.
68. Jendoubi F, Gaudenzio N, Gallini A, Negretto M, Paul C, Bulai Livideanu C. Omalizumab in the treatment of adult patients with mastocytosis: A systematic review. Clin Exp Allergy. 2020;50(6):654-61.
69. Emmi G, Bettiol A. Adalimumab-based treatment versus disease-modifying antirheumatic drugs for venous thrombosis in Behçet's syndrome: a retrospective study of seventy patients with vascular involvement. Arthritis Rheumatol. 2018;70(9):1500-7.
70. Di Scala G, Bettiol A, Cojan RD, Finocchi M, Silvestri E, Emmi G. Efficacy of the anti-IL 17 secukinumab in refractory Behçet's syndrome: a preliminary study. J Autoimmun. 2019;97:108-13.
71. Mirouse A, Barete S, Monfort J-B, Resche-Rigon M, Bouyer A-S, Comarmond C, et al. Ustekinumab for Behçet's disease. J Autoimmun. 2017;82:41-6.
72. Cheng J, Feldman SR. The cost of biologics for psoriasis is increasing. Drugs Context. 2014;3:212266.

CHAPTER 28

Adverse Effects of Biologics: Feared or Real?

Sunil Dogra, Narayanan B

INTRODUCTION

Biological products are large complex molecules that target specific proteins implicated in immune-mediated disease. They are defined by the United States Food and Drug Administration as "products produced through biotechnology in a living system, such as a microorganism, plant cell or animal cell, and are often more difficult to characterize than small molecule drugs." There has been a paradigm shift in the treatment of dermatological conditions from conventional immunomodulatory and immunosuppressive therapy to more targeted biological agents in the past two decades. The use of biological therapies in the treatment of chronic skin diseases has led to improved therapeutic response, prognosis, control of symptoms, and better quality of life. Biologic therapies owing to their targeted action are claimed to have reduced risk of cumulative adverse effects when compared with older drugs. With the widespread use of these agents, there is more literature available on their associated adverse effects. This chapter summarizes the side effects seen with biologic therapy commonly used in various dermatological disorders.

DEFINITION

An adverse drug reaction is defined as "an appreciably harmful or unpleasant reaction, resulting from an intervention related to the use of a medicinal product, which predicts hazard from future administration and warrants prevention or specific treatment, or alteration of dosage regimen, or withdrawal of the product."[1] In 1972, the World Health Organization (WHO) also defined it as "a response to a drug which is noxious and unintended, and which occurs at doses normally used in man for the prophylaxis, diagnosis, or therapy of disease, or for the modifications of physiological function."

TABLE 1: Differences between traditional drugs and biologic agents.[2]	
Traditional drugs	**Biologic agents**
Small molecules (MW<1 kDa)	Larger and complex molecules (MW>1 kDa)
Synthetic compounds	Structurally similar to autologous proteins
Stable	Heat-sensitive
Pharmacological effect	Biological effect
Undergoes metabolism to active and inactive products	Catabolized to amino acids, not metabolized
Cytochrome P450 involvement and possible drug interactions	No cytochrome P450 involvement and drug interactions
Less chance of antigenicity and antibody formation	More chance of antigenicity and antibody formation

(MW: molecular weight)

DIFFERENCE BETWEEN BIOLOGICS AND TRADITIONAL DRUGS

For a better understanding of the adverse effects of biologics, some key differences between small molecule drugs and biologics should be known, which are summarized in **Table 1**. Although the adverse effects of traditional drugs are related to their pharmacological effects, the adverse effects of biologics are often target related and linked to the biological consequences of their mechanism. The toxicity of biologics is also related to their manufacturing quality, including the cell type choice, culture medium, and the purification process. In addition, because of the larger molecular size and foreign non-self-protein nature, biologics can be intrinsically immunogenic and may induce antidrug antibodies, which may lead to both adverse effects and reduced efficacy.[2,3]

CLASSIFICATION OF ADVERSE DRUG REACTIONS

The original classification of adverse effects of biologics was proposed by Pichler,[3] which was subsequently modified by Hausmann et al.[4] The classification is based on the pathomechanism of these effects, which might help in guiding future courses of action including re-exposure, premedication, and switching to another biologic. **Table 2** summarizes the mechanisms and examples of different types of adverse effects of biologics.

ADVERSE DRUG REACTIONS OF BIOLOGICS USED IN DERMATOLOGY

Biologics that are commonly used in various disorders in dermatology are mentioned in **Table 3**.

TABLE 2: Classification of adverse effects of biologics.[4]

Type	Mechanism	Relation to dose	Relation to function	Clinical features	Examples
α	• Overstimulation • Cytokine storm (increased IL-1β, IL-6, IL-8, TNFα, IFN)	Yes	Yes	• Acute infusion reaction (fever, headache, arthralgia, myalgia) • Flu-like symptoms • Gastrointestinal symptoms (nausea, vomiting, diarrhea)	Muromonab, IFN-α, GM-CSF, TGN1412
β	Hypersensitivity IgE/non-IgE mediated	No	No	• Immediate reaction • Cutaneous reaction (urticaria, angioedema and recall phenomenon) • Systemic reaction (anaphylaxis)	Rituximab, omalizumab
	Immunogenicity IgG-mediated	Yes	No	Delayed reaction	Infliximab, adalimumab
γ	Immunosuppression	Yes	Yes	Risk of tuberculosis	Infliximab, adalimumab
				Risk of PML	Rituximab, infliximab
	Autoimmunity (immune/cytokine imbalance)	Unknown	Unknown	Lupus-like syndrome, paradoxical psoriasis, atopic dermatitis	• Infliximab • Adalimumab
δ	Cross-reactivity	Yes	Yes	Acneiform eruption	Cetuximab
ε	Nonimmunological	Unknown	Possible	• Neuropsychiatric effects • Aggravation of heart failure (major adverse cardiovascular events)	• IFN-α • Infliximab, adalimumab

(GM-CSF: granulocyte monocyte–colony stimulating factor; IFN: interferon; IL: interleukin; PML: progressive multifocal leukoencephalopathy; TNF: tumor necrosis factor)

TABLE 3: Commonly used biologics in dermatology.

Disease group	Category of biologic used	Examples
• Autoimmune bullous dermatoses • Connective tissue disorders	Anti-CD20 monoclonal antibody	Rituximab
Psoriasis	TNF-α antagonists	Infliximab, adalimumab, etanercept, golimumab, certolizumab pegol
	IL-12/23 antibodies	Ustekinumab
	Anti-IL-23 inhibitors	Tildrakizumab, guselkumab, risankizumab, mirikizumab
	IL-17/IL-17R inhibitors	Secukinumab, ixekizumab, brodalumab, bimekizumab
	Anti-CD6 antibody	Itolizumab
Pustular psoriasis	IL-36 receptor antagonist	Spesolimab
Hidradenitis suppurativa	TNF-α antibody	Adalimumab
Atopic dermatitis	IL-4/IL-13 inhibitor	Dupilumab
	IL-13 inhibitor	Tralokinumab, lebrikizumab
	IL-5 inhibitor	Mepolizumab
	IL-31 Rα inhibitor	Nemolizumab
	IL-22	Fezakinumab
	TSLP	Tezepelumab
Urticaria	Anti-IgE antibody	Omalizumab, ligelizumab

(IgE: immunoglobulin E; IL: interleukin, TNF-α: tumor necrosis factor alpha)

SIDE EFFECTS OF INDIVIDUAL DRUGS

Anti-CD20 Monoclonal Antibodies

Rituximab

Rituximab is a chimeric monoclonal antibody that targets the B-cell-specific CD20 transmembrane glycoprotein to deplete the normal and pathogenic B cells. Although approved for pemphigus vulgaris, it has gained importance in the treatment of other autoimmune blistering disorders and connective tissue disorders.

Early Adverse Effects

Hypersensitivity reactions: There are several types of hypersensitivity reactions reported due to rituximab, which vary in their pathomechanism.[5]
- *Infusion-related reactions*: They are the most common adverse effect of rituximab and occur most commonly during the initial 30 minutes to 2 hours of infusion. Rituximab has the highest rate of infusion reactions

among biologicals, with the risk being maximum during the first infusion (up to 77%).[6] The common symptoms include thoracic oppression, chills, nausea, vomiting, skin rash, and respiratory problems. They are generally mild in severity and subside with subsequent infusions, however, fatal reactions have also been reported.[5] The risk factors for infusion reactions include the first or second exposure to the drug, the rate of infusion of the drug, and a higher baseline CD20 cell level.[7] Predictive models based on parameters including CD20 positive cells, CD16 positive natural killer cells, levels of CD16 and CD20 expressions, and FCGR3A polymorphisms have been proposed for identifying occurrence and severity of infusion reaction rates with rituximab.[8] The incidence of infusion reactions is higher when rituximab is used for treatment of lymphoma when compared with autoimmune disorders such as pemphigus and rheumatoid arthritis, the reasons proposed being the tumor burden and cytokine disarray in lymphoma and protective role of concomitant corticosteroid use in pemphigus. Premedication with antihistamines, acetaminophen, and corticosteroids significantly lower the risk of infusion reactions, the incidence reducing from 41 to 8% as shown in a study of 389 patients treated with rituximab.[9] Mild-to-moderate infusion reactions (grade 1 or 2) can be managed by slowing the rate of infusion or stopping the infusion until the symptoms improve, thereafter the infusion can be restarted at half the previous infusion rate. Grade 3 or 4 reactions require stopping of infusion and emergency rescue management **(Table 4)**.[10]

- *Cytokine-release reactions*: Cytokine-release syndrome is rare in patients with pemphigus treated with rituximab and is common in patients with lymphoproliferative disorders, during the initial 90 minutes of infusion. The mechanism behind this syndrome is increased levels of proinflammatory cytokines such as interleukin 8 (IL-8), interferon-gamma (IFN-γ), and tumor necrosis factor-alpha (TNF-α) due to rapid infusion of the drug. In severe cytokine-release syndrome, the elevation of liver enzymes, D-dimer levels, and prolonged prothrombin time can occur. This is clinically characterized by dyspnea, fever, chills, urticaria, and pulmonary insufficiency and is associated with considerable mortality. These patients may be treated with aggressive hydration and anti-inflammatory drugs and lesser doses/slower infusion of subsequent therapy.[11]
- *Type 1 reactions*: They are generally immunoglobulin-E (IgE) mediated and include flushing, pruritus, urticaria, shortness of breath, wheezing, hypotension, and life-threatening anaphylaxis. They differ from infusion-related reactions by their mechanism, they are caused by mast cell degranulation leading to release of histamine, prostaglandins, and leukotrienes.[5] They usually recur with subsequent infusions and can be predicted by skin intradermal tests and measuring IgE specific to rituximab. These reactions are less common than infusion-related

TABLE 4: Common terminology criteria for adverse events (CTCAE): Common for all biologicals including rituximab and infliximab.[18]		
Grades	Definition	Management
1	Mild-transient reaction; infusion interruption not indicated; intervention not indicated	Slow the rate of infusion
2	Therapy or infusion interruption indicated but responds promptly to symptomatic treatment; prophylactic medications indicated for ≤24 hours after the current infusion	Slow rate/short-term cessation of infusion; IV diphenhydramine 50 mg + IV ranitidine 50 mg. If needed IV corticosteroids (methylprednisolone). Restart infusion at 50% rate and titrate to tolerance
3	Prolonged (not rapidly responsive to symptomatic medication and/or brief interruption of infusion); recurrence of symptoms following initial improvement; hospitalization indicated for clinical sequelae	• Stop infusion • Epinephrine 0.2–0.5 mg (1 mg/mL) IM; repeat after 5–15 minutes • Normal saline 1–2 L IV infusion at rate of 5–10 mL/kg first 5 minutes. Crystalloids or colloids in boluses of 20 mL/kg followed by slow infusion; IV diphenhydramine 50 mg + IV ranitidine 50 mg • IV corticosteroids (methylprednisolone) 1–2 mg/kg every 6 hours • If bradycardia—atropine; if hypotension—dopamine or vasopressin
4	*Life-threatening consequences*: Urgent intervention indicated	
5	Death	

reactions and respond to antihistamines and corticosteroids.[12] Desensitization has also been found successful in preventing further episodes in IgE-mediated reactions.[13]

- *Mixed reactions*: They represent an overlap between cytokine release syndrome and IgE-mediated reaction. They are characterized clinically by flushing, urticaria, and pruritus, associated with fever/chills, wheezing, nausea, pain, headache, and rigor.[5]
- *Type 3 reactions*: Rituximab-associated serum sickness is rare, reported in patients majorly with underlying rheumatological disorders. The complement-fixing IgM and IgG antibodies targeted at an immunological part of the drug are implicated and corticosteroids are helpful in treatment.[14]
- *Type 4 reactions*: Rare cases of Stevens–Johnson syndrome (SJS) and toxic epidermal necrolysis (TEN) have been reported with rituximab.[15-17]

Late Adverse Events
- *Infections*: The incidence of serious infections is 5.3/100 patient-years and most of them occur within the first year of infusion.[19] The infection rate

with rituximab is comparable with conventional immunosuppressants including methotrexate. Serious infections and sepsis are the major cause of death post-rituximab treatment.
Upper respiratory tract infections including nasopharyngitis are the most common, followed by urinary tract infections, bronchitis, sinusitis, and diarrhea. Most infections are bacterial in etiology, followed by viral and fungal infections.[20] The most common serious infection is pneumonia, seen in about 2% of cases.[6] A review by Aksoy et al., on viral infections post rituximab, showed that the median time to diagnosis of infection was 5 months.[21] The most common viral infection noted was hepatitis B, followed by cytomegalovirus infection, influenza, and herpes zoster. The risk of tuberculosis reactivation/flare is minimal. The rare serious infections reported include *Candida* septicemia, *Pneumocystis jirovecii* pneumonia, bacterial arthritis, *Listeria monocytogenes* sepsis, and progressive multifocal leukoencephalopathy (PML). PML, a JC virus infection of the brain, has been reported in patients treated for rheumatoid arthritis and lymphomas, but not for pemphigus.[22,23] The risk factors for infections in patients receiving rituximab include older age, concomitant steroid, or immunosuppressant use, other metabolic or endocrine comorbidities, and severe pemphigus.[24] There is also a lack of correlation between the infection risk and the levels of immunoglobulins.

- *Cardiac side effects*: Sinus tachycardia, dysrhythmia, and myocardial ischemia can occur in patients receiving rituximab. They have been reported in about 8% of patients receiving treatment for lymphoma, all having at least one conventional risk factor for the same.[25] These are more common in patients with pre-existing cardiac disorders. Cardiac monitoring is essential during and post rituximab infusion in patients with cardiac disease or risk factors.[26] Rare reports of new-onset cardiogenic shock, fatal myocarditis, and nonischemic cardiomyopathy have been reported during and after rituximab therapy.[27-29] Pre-existing cardiovascular disease is however not an absolute contraindication to rituximab use.
- *Immune/autoimmune adverse events*: Uveitis, optic neuritis, systemic vasculitis, pleuritis, lupus-like syndrome, serum sickness, polyarticular arthritis, and vasculitis with rash are the immune-mediated adverse reactions seen with rituximab.[30]
- *Hypogammaglobulinemia*: Hypogammaglobulinemia can occur in patients receiving rituximab. This is common in patients who receive maintenance doses of rituximab. In a study, the mean interval to document this was after 1.2 years of rituximab infusion.[31] Prophylactic antibiotics are not indicated for the prevention of infections. Rituximab-induced hypogammaglobulinemia may persist for years but usually is not symptomatic. Patients with infections may be considered for intravenous immunoglobulin (IVIg) treatment.[32]

- *Neoplasia*: Most studies have shown that there is no increased risk of malignancies after rituximab when compared to age- and sex-matched standardized incidence rates for malignancy in the general population.[33] Second primary malignancy rates for lymphoma patients treated with rituximab have also been similar to those treated without rituximab. Malignancies noted post rituximab include skin tumors such as squamous cell carcinoma and Merkel cell carcinoma, breast carcinoma, and lymphomas.[34] Disease progression of Kaposi sarcoma in human immunodeficiency virus (HIV) patients has occurred with rituximab.[35]
- *Gastrointestinal side effects*: In patients receiving rituximab in combination with chemotherapy, rituximab-induced colitis leading to bowel obstruction and perforation can occur. The incidence of rituximab-induced colitis confirmed by colonoscopy and histology in a large study was 4%. The symptoms, most common being diarrhea, begin generally >8 months after rituximab infusion. The proposed mechanisms of colitis include the depletion of the protective CD20 lymphocytes in the colon and T-cell regulatory dysfunction leading to colon inflammation. Colon perforation is very rare, seen in only one patient in the above study.[36] Rituximab-induced transaminitis has been reported in a patient treated for pemphigus foliaceus.[37]
- *Pulmonary side effects*: Pulmonary adverse effects have been noted in around 5% of patients treated with rituximab, most of them being infections.[38] Other rare pulmonary adverse effects noted include interstitial lung disease, bronchiolitis obliterans, hypersensitivity pneumonitis, status asthmaticus, and diffuse alveolar hemorrhage.[39-41] There are also reports of deep vein thrombosis and pulmonary embolism after infusion.[42,43] The proposed pathogenesis is platelet aggregation following rituximab therapy, leading to thrombosis. However, it is difficult to assert rituximab as the only factor leading to thrombosis in such cases, as pemphigus vulgaris itself is a risk factor and all reported cases were also on concomitant corticosteroids and immunosuppressants including azathioprine.[42] The possible risk factors include severe pemphigus leading to immobilization, high cumulative dose of steroids, and thrombocytopenia post the rituximab infusion. Patients who develop deep vein thrombosis need to be treated with anticoagulants. Early ambulation, pneumatic compression pumps, and prophylactic low-molecular weight heparin can be considered for high-risk patients.
- *Hematological side effects*:
  - Late-onset neutropenia (LON): It is defined as unexplained neutropenia in the absence of an alternative explanation, usually of grade 3 or 4 starting at least 28 days after the last dose of rituximab.[32] The incidence of LON is generally reported to be in the range of 3–27%.[44] An increased risk of LON is seen in patients with stem cell transplant, and lymphoma, with multiple doses and rarely in patients

with autoimmune diseases. However, the risk factors in patients with pemphigus is not well-studied, possible factors being severity of disease and multiple infusions of rituximab. Also, there are reports of LON in pemphigus patients occurring after 19 weeks of exposure.[45] A multifactorial etiology is likely to underlie the blood dyscrasia. This may occur 1 month to 1 year post rituximab with a prevalence of around 8% in lymphoma patients.[46] Complete blood count with differential count should be conducted at regular intervals (after 1 month, thereafter every 2-3 months) to detect neutropenia. Several mechanisms have been suggested for LON, which include the direct toxic effect of rituximab on the bone marrow,[44] immune-mediated neutropenia,[47] and apoptosis of neutrophils by Fas-Fas ligand secretion by infiltrated granular lymphocytes in the bone marrow,[48] but none of them has been proven. In some patients, treatment with granulocyte colony-stimulating factor has been required.
  ○ Prolonged neutropenia: It is defined as neutropenia that has not resolved between 24 and 42 days after the last dose of rituximab treatment.
- *Neurological side effects*: Neurological adverse effects are rare with rituximab and include cerebrovascular infarcts and seizures.[49]
- *Cutaneous side effects*:
  ○ Urticaria: It is commonly seen in patients treated with rituximab with the incidence ranging from 3 to 14% in nonrandomized trials.[50]
  ○ Severe mucocutaneous reactions: The onset of these reactions has varied from 1 to 13 weeks following rituximab exposure and there are rare reports of occurrence. These reactions include Stevens–Johnson syndrome,[15-17] lichenoid dermatitis, vesiculobullous dermatitis, and paraneoplastic pemphigus.[51]
  ○ Vasculitis flare: Rituximab has been shown to cause a flare of type 2 cryoglobulinemic vasculitis in 3.4% of treated cases. Cutaneous vasculitis has also been reported in patients treated with rituximab.[52]

Tumor Necrosis Factor-alpha Inhibitors
Infliximab
Infliximab is an IgG1 murine-human monoclonal antibody that binds to the soluble and transmembrane forms of TNF-α. It is approved for use in psoriasis and psoriatic arthritis.
- *Infusion-related reactions*: Infusion reactions occur in 3–22% of patients with psoriasis treated with infliximab. Reactions are generally mild to moderate, usually within the initial 3 hours of infusion.[53] Infusion reactions are common in patients with neutralizing antibodies to infliximab. Common manifestations include urticaria, pruritus, rash, headache, flushing, fever, chills, nausea, tachycardia, or dyspnea. Severe reactions such as anaphylaxis and hypotension occur in <1% of patients

receiving infliximab. Delayed reactions also do occur, presenting with fever, myalgia, arthralgia, urticarial rash, and malaise between 24 hours to 14 days after infusion.[54] Management of delayed reactions includes antihistamines and nonsteroidal anti-inflammatory drugs for symptom control and a short course of oral corticosteroids for severe cases. Studies have shown that concomitant administration of immunosuppressants such as methotrexate would reduce the formation of antibodies and thereby reduce the incidence of infusion reactions.[55]

- *Paradoxical reactions*: Paradoxical reactions are defined as de novo or worsening immune-mediated reactions that would normally respond to the same biologic that is causing it.[56]
  - Paradoxical psoriasis: It may occur in 2-5% of patients receiving infliximab treatment for psoriasis and inflammatory bowel disease (IBD).[57] The mean reported latency is about 14 months but can be variable, and the clinical presentations include palmoplantar pustulosis, plaque psoriasis, guttate psoriasis, and nail and scalp psoriasis. Genetic factors and immune alteration leading to excess IFN-α and T-lymphocyte activation are proposed in pathogenesis. TNF-α signaling inhibition is thought to relieve TNF-α dependent negative feedback to plasmacytoid dendritic cells (pDCs), resulting in overproduction of type I IFNs. T-cell polarization skewing with inhibition of one arm leading to hyperstimulation of other is also a factor. Apart from this, antidrug antibodies may interact with host immune cells to trigger innate immune activation. Many patients show antinuclear antibody (ANA) and anti-dsDNA positivity after being treated with TNF-α inhibitors. However, despite all these postulations we are yet to figure out why only few patients develop such paradoxical reaction, the long and variable latency and different manifestation of paradoxical reaction in different patients. Generally, the reactions are mild and can be treated with topical agents. Complete resolution or partial improvement is still common despite continuing the drug, and severe reactions may require drug discontinuation and biologic class switching. Paradoxical psoriasis can occur with other TNF-α inhibitors including etanercept and adalimumab. Switching to another TNF-α inhibitor can lead to recurrence of this problem as it is a class effect, thereby, switching to IL-12/23 inhibitors or IL-17 inhibitors is advised for severe reactions. Future doses of the same drug can be given for mild-to-moderate reactions, as 33% have total resolution and 57% have partial improvement of paradoxical reaction despite maintaining the same drug.[58]
  - Cutaneous vasculitis: Infliximab has been associated with the paradoxical development of leukocytoclastic vasculitis due to increased inflammatory activity. Among targeted therapies, TNF-α

inhibitors such as infliximab are reported to be the most common agents causing cutaneous vasculitis (59.5%).[59]
  o Others: The other debatable paradoxical reactions reported include alopecia areata, vitiligo, acneiform eruptions, lichen planus and lichenoid eruptions, sarcoidosis, dermatomyositis,[60] bullous pemphigoid,[61] pyoderma gangrenosum,[62] granuloma annulare,[63] and interstitial granulomatous dermatitis.[56]
- *Lupus-like syndrome*: Infliximab has been reported to induce lupus-like syndrome, which improves after the discontinuation of the drug. The reason for the development of lupus is proposed to be an increased level of autoantibodies after infliximab. The onset of symptoms ranges from <1 month to >4 years. Clinical features are most commonly cutaneous with reports of malar rash, pruritic rash, photosensitivity, purpura, discoid rash, mucosal ulcers, and alopecia. Other features include constitutional symptoms, arthralgia, pericarditis, pleural or pericardial effusions, deep venous thrombosis, pneumonitis, and neuritis. The mainstay of treatment is the withdrawal of the offending drug. Symptoms generally resolve within 3 weeks to 6 months after withdrawal. However, many patients require traditional therapy for idiopathic systemic lupus erythematosus (SLE), including topical or systemic steroids, antimalarials, and less frequently immunosuppressants.[64,65]
- *Other cutaneous adverse effects*: Other reported cutaneous adverse effects with infliximab include erythema nodosum, Sweet's syndrome, bullous eruptions, necrotizing fasciitis, cutaneous ulcerations, eczematid-like purpura of Doucas and Kapetanakis, atopic dermatitis, nevi, etc.[66]
- *Infections*: Patients receiving infliximab are at a high risk of acquiring infections so cautious use is advised. Patients with mycobacterial and deep fungal infections are a contraindication for its use. There is an increased risk of viral [human herpesvirus (HHV)-8, CMV, herpes zoster, molluscum], bacterial [pneumococcal, *Legionella*, and *Moraxella*) and fungal [histoplasmosis, cryptococcosis, *Pneumocystis pneumonia* (PCP), and aspergillosis] infections in patients receiving infliximab. TNF-α is necessary for granuloma formation, macrophage activation, phagosome formation, and killing of intracellular pathogens. This explains the increased risk of above stated infections with infliximab.[67,68]
- *Tuberculosis*: Tuberculosis has been most closely linked to the use of infliximab. Reviews have shown that 0.57% of patients who received TNF-α antagonists developed tuberculosis with the odds ratio for infliximab being 1.82.[69] Of patients developing tuberculosis, 68.8% developed an extrapulmonary infection and 25% developed disseminated tuberculosis.[70] Infliximab can also lead to the activation of latent tuberculosis infection. Patients need to be screened for tuberculosis before infliximab to prevent the reactivation of latent tuberculosis. If infliximab is required in patients positive for latent tuberculosis infection,

then they should be started on prophylaxis before infliximab, which has been shown to reduce the risk of reactivation significantly. Latent tuberculosis prophylaxis includes isoniazid monotherapy for a period of 6–9 months or a combination of isoniazid and rifampicin for a period of 3 months. Biological therapy can be commenced 2 months after initiation of latent tuberculosis treatment.[71,72]

- *Cardiovascular disease*: TNF exerts negative inotropic effects and can promote fibrosis, hypertrophy, and cardiomyopathy in animal models. The association of cardiac complications with infliximab is controversial, with reviews and meta-analyses showing no statistically significant risk of major adverse cardiac events in psoriasis patients treated with the biologic.[73,74] However, there is also evidence of worsening heart failure with infliximab, thereby caution should be exercised in patients with moderate-to-severe congestive heart failure.[75] Infliximab is contraindicated at doses >5 mg/kg in patients with moderate-to-severe (New York Classification III or IV) congestive cardiac failure. However, as the dosage range for psoriatic arthritis and psoriasis is from 3 to 5 mg/kg, this complication is unlikely in our patients.

- *Demyelinating diseases*: Infliximab infusion has been associated with the rare development of demyelinating disorders such as multiple sclerosis, optic neuritis, and Guillain–Barré syndrome.[76] Infliximab should be avoided in patients with pre-existing demyelinating disorders.

- *Autoantibodies*: It has been seen in various studies that there is the development of ANAs and anti-dsDNA antibodies in patients receiving infliximab, which is a transient phenomenon. ANA positivity is seen in around 60% of patients receiving infliximab.[77,78] These antibodies do not have much clinical significance and are not contraindications for further doses of infliximab. The development of lupus-like syndrome is rare, as mentioned earlier. Anti-drug antibodies (ADAs) are also formed in 60% of patients, which may be implicated in adverse effects and loss of efficacy of infliximab.[79] Concomitant immunotherapy, premedication with corticosteroids, continuing maintenance dose after induction therapy, and decreasing the frequency or increasing the dose might help in reducing the formation of ADA.[80]

- *Malignancy*: Malignancies reported in patients who received infliximab include lymphomas (non-Hodgkin lymphoma and hepatosplenic T-cell lymphoma), skin cancers (melanoma and Merkel cell carcinoma), cervical cancer, and other malignancies. Large trials have shown lymphoma rates of 0.08 and 0.10 cases per 100 patient-years of follow-up in patients of rheumatoid arthritis and all inflammatory disorder patients receiving infliximab, respectively, which is higher than expected in the general population. However, these disorders per se may also contribute to baseline increased risk.[81,82] The British Society for Rheumatology Rheumatoid Arthritis Register (BSRBR-RA) compared the risk of lymphoma in patients with RA who were treated with nonbiologic disease-modifying antirheumatic drug (DMARD) versus those treated with TNF-α inhibitors. Overall, 12,000 patients who were given TNF-α inhibitors were compared with 3,367 biologic naïve and nonbiologic DMARD patients. In 8 years follow-up study, there was no statistical difference in risk of lymphoma in the two groups, after adjusting for baseline differences in patient characteristic.[83] The incidence of nonlymphoma cancers is not increased in patients receiving infliximab as compared with the control population.

- *Hepatotoxicity*: Severe hepatic reactions, including acute liver failure, jaundice, hepatitis, and cholestasis, have been reported in post marketing data in patients receiving infliximab. Autoimmune hepatitis has been diagnosed in some of these cases.[64] These reactions develop 2 weeks to >1 year after initiation of infliximab with no pretreatment elevations in hepatic aminotransferase levels. Patients with symptoms or signs of liver dysfunction should be evaluated for evidence of liver injury. If jaundice and/or marked liver enzyme elevations (e.g., ≥5 times the upper limit of normal) develop, infliximab should be discontinued, and a thorough investigation of the abnormality should be undertaken.
- *Hematological effects*: Cases of leukopenia, neutropenia, thrombocytopenia, and pancytopenia have been reported in patients receiving infliximab.[84]
- *Other systemic complications*: Other rare, reported complications include aseptic meningitis, polymyositis, serum sickness, acute idiopathic pancreatitis, anaphylactic-like reactions, etc.[85]

Adalimumab

Adalimumab is a fully human monoclonal antibody against TNF-α approved for use in psoriasis, psoriatic arthritis, and hidradenitis suppurativa. The adverse effect profile of adalimumab is similar to infliximab.

- *Injection site reactions*: Injection site reactions are the most common side effect of adalimumab. These occur in the form of erythema, itching, pain, and swelling. These are mild to moderate, which do not lead to discontinuation of the drug and usually do not tend to recur.[86]
- *Paradoxical reactions*: Paradoxical reactions such as psoriasis have been reported with adalimumab, however, the risk is lesser than with infliximab.[56,57]
- *Infections*: Adalimumab increases the risk of nonserious infections marginally:[86]
  - Upper respiratory tract infection
  - Sinusitis
  - Flu-like symptoms
  - Urinary tract infections

  It also increases the risk of serious infections such as the follows:
  - Tuberculosis: The odds ratio of adalimumab causing tuberculosis is 2.11. Reactivation of latent tuberculosis is seen with adalimumab.

Miliary, lymphatic, pulmonary, and peritoneal tuberculosis have been seen with adalimumab treatment. Most cases occur in the first 8 months.[87]
   ○ Deep fungal infections: Adalimumab treatment also exposes the patient to the risk of deep fungal infections such as histoplasmosis, coccidioidomycosis, aspergillosis, nocardiosis, etc.[86]
- *Cardiovascular diseases*: It can increase the risk of congestive cardiac failure, which is lesser than infliximab. So, it should be avoided in severe congestive cardiac failure.
- *Demyelinating disorders*: It increases the risk of demyelinating disorders. So, it should not be used in cases of multiple sclerosis and other demyelinating disorders and should be discontinued if these develop.
- *Lupus-like syndrome*: Lupus-like syndrome can occur with adalimumab, which remits after discontinuation of the drug.
- *Immunogenicity*: Neutralizing antibodies are seen in patients receiving adalimumab and have a decreased efficacy in those with positive neutralizing antibodies.
- *Lymphoma and other neoplasms*: The observed rate of lymphoma in patients treated with adalimumab for various inflammatory disorders is 0.11 per 100 patient years, which is higher than expected for the general population. There is no increased risk of other malignancies when compared to the general population.[88]
- *Cutaneous side effects*: Infectious skin complications such as cellulitis, herpes zoster, and erysipelas can be seen. Other skin complications include anaphylactoid reactions such as urticaria, angioedema, and pruritus.[86]
- *Systemic complications*: Pancytopenia and transaminitis can be seen with adalimumab, which warrants intermittent laboratory monitoring.[86]

Etanercept

Etanercept is a TNF inhibitor; the drug acts as a soluble TNF receptor and binds TNF-α and TNF-β. It is approved for use in plaque psoriasis and psoriatic arthritis.
- *Injection site reactions*: Injection site bleeding and bruising have been seen commonly with etanercept. These occur in around 37% of cases and last an average of 3–5 days and eventually, tolerance develops to these reactions. The mechanism of these reactions is suggested to be a delayed-type hypersensitivity reaction that is T-cell mediated, which wanes over time due to the induction of tolerance.[89]
- *Paradoxical reactions*: Paradoxical psoriasis, and more importantly new-onset psoriatic arthritis, has been reported in patients treated with etanercept for psoriasis.[56,57]
- *Infections*: Upper respiratory tract infections are commonly associated with etanercept treatment. Reports of multifocal septic arthritis and

osteomyelitis are also there. Other rare reports of orbital myositis, viral pneumonia, histoplasmosis, toxoplasmosis, and aspergillosis are documented with etanercept. Reactivation of latent tuberculosis is seen with etanercept treatment. The chances of reactivation are however lesser than infliximab. Tubercular tonsillitis and peritonitis have also been reported.[62,90]

- *Lymphoma and other malignancies*: Among 4,410 adult patients of psoriatic arthritis treated with etanercept, the observed rate of lymphoma was 0.05 cases per 100 patient years, which is comparable with the general population. Nonlymphoma cancers are not associated with etanercept.[91]
- *Cardiovascular complications*: It should be avoided in patients with severe congestive cardiac failure as worsening of heart failure may occur.
- *Demyelinating disorders*: There are rare reports of the development of demyelinating disorders after treatment with etanercept.[92]
- *Lupus-like syndrome*: Drug-induced lupus is seen with etanercept treatment.[93] Subacute cutaneous lupus-like lesions can be commonly seen.[94] Cases of autoimmune hepatitis have also been reported.[95]
- *Immunogenicity*: Around 5% of patients receiving etanercept develop antibodies, but these are not related to the efficacy or adverse effects.[96]
- *Cutaneous side effects*: Cutaneous vasculitis can occur with etanercept.[59] Other reported cutaneous adverse effect is erythema multiforme.[97]
- *Other systemic complications*: Aplastic anemia, lung injury, and silent thyroiditis have also been reported rarely.[66]

Other newer drugs in this class including golimumab and certolizumab also have similar adverse effect profiles; however, long-term safety in psoriasis is yet to be established.

Interleukin-17 Inhibitors

Secukinumab

Secukinumab is a human monoclonal IgG1 antibody that blocks the action of IL-17A. It is approved for use in psoriasis and psoriatic arthritis.

In the ERASURE study, during the 12-week induction period, 55.1% of patients had at least one adverse event in the 300 mg secukinumab group and the most common were upper respiratory tract infection, nasopharyngitis, and headache. In the FIXTURE study, nasopharyngitis, headache, and diarrhea were commonly seen, which were common in induction as well as the entire treatment period.[98-100]

Various side effects seen with secukinumab are as follows:
- *Infections*: IL-17 is involved in host defense against extracellular bacteria and fungi, which explains the risk of such infections in patients treated with secukinumab. Commonly reported are upper respiratory tract infections, including nasopharyngitis, seen in 7% of patients. Other minor infections include diarrhea, urinary tract infections, orolabial herpes, herpes zoster, tinea pedis, and otitis externa.[98-100] The risk of tuberculosis

in patients treated with secukinumab is minimal, and pooled cohort study has shown that no active cases of tuberculosis or latent tuberculosis reactivation were seen in patients treated with secukinumab for psoriasis and psoriatic arthritis.[101] However, all patients need to be screened for tuberculosis and prophylaxis is required for latent tuberculosis before giving secukinumab. Other rare serious infections noted include herpes keratitis, necrotizing fasciitis, invasive *Hemophilus influenzae* infection, and ocular *Histoplasma* infection.

- *Mucocutaneous candidiasis*: There is a strong association between secukinumab and candidiasis, including cutaneous, oropharyngeal, vulvovaginal, esophageal candidiasis, and candida onychomycosis. IL-17 is involved defense against *Candida* infections. It has been proposed IL-17 plays a major role in recruitment of neutrophils to site of *Candida* infection, and thereby there is an increased risk of skin and mucosal candidiasis when this process is impaired. However, systemic candidiasis is not seen as circulating neutrophils are not affected. The risk of candida infection increases 2–16-fold after secukinumab. Most cases are mild to moderate, do not require discontinuation of therapy, and are treated with oral fluconazole for 7–14 days.[102]
- Minor adverse effects include dizziness, headache, pruritus, and fatigue.
- Injection site reactions such as erythema, pruritus, and hemorrhage can occur.
- *Neutropenia*: IL-17A stimulates neutrophil trafficking and granulopoiesis. So, neutropenia is an important adverse event and must be considered in patients for secukinumab. Rich et al., have reported neutropenia in 19 patients in the 12-week induction phase and 30 patients in the maintenance phase (weeks 12–32). Dosing was not interrupted or withheld as no clinically significant adverse events were associated with the development of neutropenia. The neutropenia resolved during the study in all cases.[99]
- *Inflammatory bowel disease*: Exacerbation of IBD has been seen in patients with psoriasis and arthritis treated with secukinumab. In a review by Onac et al., gastrointestinal adverse effects were seen in 7.8% of patients after starting secukinumab. The risk was higher in patients who had pre-existing IBD, however, the absolute rate of new IBD in treated patients was low.[103] Secukinumab should thereby be avoided in patients with inflammatory bowel disease.
- *Treatment-emergent anti-secukinumab antibodies—very uncommonly formed*: In the FIXTURE study, 0.4% of patients developed these antibodies but had no relation with loss of efficacy or adverse events. These are generally non-neutralizing antibodies and do not have any clinical significance.[100]
- *Cutaneous adverse effects*: Rare cutaneous manifestations reported include urticaria, eczema, cutaneous vasculitis, sarcoidosis, and drug-

induced lupus erythematosus. Rare paradoxical flare of arthritis has also been reported.[98-100] Eczema like paradoxical reaction has been reported with secukinumab and ixekizumab. This includes classic generalized atopic dermatitis-like eruptions,[104] facial dermatitis, and/or dyshidrotic eczema,[105,106] among others. They usually occur within 6 months of starting therapy. Rarely worsening of psoriasis and change in morphology of psoriasis have also been reported.[107]
- Ophthalmological adverse effects—rare episode of conjunctivitis and endophthalmitis have been reported.[108]

Ixekizumab

Ixekizumab is a humanized monoclonal IgG antibody that selectively binds to and inhibits IL-17A. The adverse effects are as follows:
- In the UNCOVER 2 and 3 trials that compared ixekizumab with etanercept or placebo, the adverse effects profile was similar for ixekizumab and etanercept. The most common adverse effects included nasopharyngitis and upper respiratory tract infections. The other minor common adverse effects include injection site erythema, pain and reaction, pruritus, headache, and arthralgia.[109]
- *Infections:* In the above trials, most infections with ixekizumab were mild and severe infections were seen in <1% of cases. The most frequent infections were nasopharyngitis and upper respiratory tract infections. Mucocutaneous candidiasis were reported in <1% of cases. No cases of tuberculosis reactivation were seen.[109]
- Hypersensitivity reactions can occur in about 4% of cases, and are usually mild. A case of leukocytoclastic vasculitis has also been reported. Exacerbation of inflammatory bowel disease can occur, however, the incidence of new onset IBD is very low.[109,110]
- No increased risk of depression or suicidal ideation has been reported with ixekizumab.

Other IL-17 inhibitors such as brodalumab also have comparable and similar adverse effect profiles. Suicidal ideation and behavior have been reported with brodalumab, and thereby it is contraindicated in patients with depression or suicidal ideation.[111,101]

Interleukin 12/23 Inhibitors

Ustekinumab

Ustekinumab is a fully human monoclonal IgG1 antibody targeting the interleukin 12/23 shared p40 subunit. It is approved for use in psoriasis and psoriatic arthritis.

It is generally a well-tolerated drug with minimal adverse effects. The adverse effects are as follows:
- *Infusion reactions*: Acute infusion reactions can be seen in 1-4.5% of patients treated with ustekinumab. The symptoms include shortness of

breath, flushing, cough, diaphoresis, stomach pain, and palpitations. Hypersensitivity reactions such as urticaria and angioedema can also occur.[112]
- *Infections*: Ustekinumab is associated with a lower risk of infections when compared with other classes of biologics used for psoriasis. The most common include nasopharyngitis and sinusitis. The risk of tuberculosis and reactivation of latent tuberculosis infection is minimal.[113] Serious infections such as pneumonia, gastroenteritis, osteomyelitis, diverticulitis, cholecystitis, and sepsis are rare.
- *Paradoxical reactions*: Paradoxical pustular psoriasis, new-onset psoriatic arthritis, vitiligo, eczematous reaction, lichenoid reaction, and sarcoidosis have been reported in patients treated with ustekinumab.[56]
- *Reversible posterior leukoencephalopathy syndrome (RPLS)*: It is a rarely reported adverse effect of ustekinumab, presenting with headache, seizures, confusion, and visual disturbances.[114]
- Multiple studies have shown no increased risk of malignancy in patients treated with ustekinumab as compared with controls.[115]
- *Major adverse cardiovascular event (MACE)*: During the initial years of use of ustekinumab, there was an increased concern of MACE among the users of this biologic. However, a recent meta-analysis of randomized clinical trials was conducted to evaluate the risk of MACE in patients with plaque psoriasis that are exposed to biologic therapies including anti-TNF-α agents (adalimumab, etanercept, and infliximab), anti-IL 12/23 agent (ustekinumab), and anti-IL-17A agents (secukinumab and ixekizumab) and no statistically significant difference in the risk of MACE between patients on biologic therapies and patients on placebo was found. Similarly, no significant difference of MACE was present between different class of biologic users. The risk of MACE appears to be primarily caused by the disease status (e.g., severe inflammatory condition) and/or the patient population (e.g., associated comorbidities predisposing to cardiovascular events).[73]

Interleukin-23 Inhibitors

Interleukin-23 inhibitors include tildrakizumab, risankizumab, and guselkumab. They are approved for use in psoriasis.

These drugs are well-tolerated with common adverse effects including upper respiratory tract infections, nasopharyngitis, urinary tract infections, injection site reactions, diarrhea, headache, back pain, and eczema.[116] Long-term safety is yet to be established.

Omalizumab

Omalizumab is a recombinant, humanized, monoclonal antibody against human immunoglobulin E. It is approved for use in chronic urticaria.

Serious adverse effects are very uncommon with omalizumab. Various side effects seen with omalizumab are as follows:[117]
- Injection site reactions are the most common adverse reaction. Reactions often manifest within 1 hour of administration and resolved within 8 days.
- Other adverse effects include upper respiratory tract infection, headache, pharyngitis fatigue, arthralgia, dizziness, pruritus, dermatitis, and ear ache.
- *Anaphylaxis*: The mechanism of anaphylaxis with omalizumab is poorly understood. The suggested mechanism is because omalizumab is composed of 5% mouse polypeptide, it is possible that IgE-mediated reactions may occur against the murine sequences. It has a very low incidence and occurs during the first 2 hours of infusion. In a postmarketing trial during the first three injections, these reactions occur after 1 hour of injection and during further injections within 30 minutes. So recommended time for monitoring during initial injections is 2 hours and subsequent injections are 30 minutes. However, it is important to note that rarely these reactions can occur up to 4 days after administration of the drug. Another recommendation is to educate patients about signs and symptoms and prescribe them epinephrine autoinjectors. No premedication is recommended prior to omalizumab administration to prevent anaphylaxis.[118]
- *Helminthic infections*: Due to the role of IgE in protection against helminthic infections, there is a theoretical possibility of such infections in patients treated with omalizumab. In a one-year clinical trial conducted in Brazil in adult and adolescent patients at high risk for helminthic infections (roundworm, hookworm, whipworm, and threadworm), 53% (36/68) of Xolair-treated patients experienced an infection, as diagnosed by standard stool examination, compared with 42% (29/69) of placebo controls.[119] Patients at high risk may require monitoring for helminthic infections.
- Serum sickness-like reaction and delayed anaphylactoid reaction have also been reported with the use of omalizumab.
- *Cardiovascular and cerebrovascular event*: A post marketing cohort observational study (EXCELS) has reported increased cardiovascular and cerebrovascular events with omalizumab.[120]
- No significant laboratory abnormalities are seen with omalizumab, so no routine monitoring is recommended.

Dupilumab

Dupilumab is a fully human monoclonal IgG4 antibody that inhibits IL-4 and IL-13. It is approved for use in moderate to severe atopic dermatitis.

The adverse effects of dupilumab are as follows:
- *Conjunctivitis*: It is seen in 8–22% of patients treated with dupilumab. The risk factors include a more severe atopic dermatitis at baseline, and

increased baseline serum biomarkers such as thymus and activation-regulated chemokine (TARC), IgE, and serum eosinophils. The pathogenic theories postulated include a reduction in ocular cytokines providing a favorable environment for *Demodex* mites to grow, causing IL-17-mediated inflammation; eosinophilia after dupilumab administration; increased downstream activity of the OX40 ligand in the eye; and systemic IL-13 inhibition indirectly leading to a reduction in conjunctival goblet cells and mucin production. Most cases are mild, treated conservatively, and do not require discontinuation of therapy.[110,121] Though less common than conjunctivitis, keratitis has also been reported with the use of dupilumab.[122]

- Nasopharyngitis and upper respiratory tract infections
- Headache
- *Hypersensitivity reactions*: Hypersensitivity reactions, including generalized urticaria and serum sickness or serum sickness-like reactions, were reported in <1% of subjects who received dupilumab. Injection site reactions can also occur.[123]

ADVERSE EFFECTS IN PREGNANCY AND FERTILITY STATUS

Rituximab is not recommended for use in pregnancy or lactation (pregnancy category C). All female patients receiving rituximab should be advised 1 year of contraception. A review of pregnancy outcomes with maternal rituximab exposure from the rituximab global drug safety database assessed 231 such cases of pregnancy. Of the 153 pregnancies with outcomes known, 90 resulted in live births, 33 resulted in spontaneous abortion, one stillbirth at 20 weeks' gestation, and 28 elective terminations. Moreover, 22 of the live births had abnormalities at birth; 4 neonatal infections and 2 congenital malformations were reported.[124] Another study assessing pregnancy outcomes in 19 women with pemphigus exposed to rituximab before or during pregnancy concluded that no relevant serious adverse pregnancy outcome occurred except for a case of neonatal sepsis.[125] Rituximab has also been used for the treatment of pemphigoid gestationis during and after pregnancy. Rituximab has no effect on the fertility status.[126,127] Human IgG passes into breast milk, so lactating women should refrain from nursing, until circulating rituximab levels are undetectable. Practically, it is advised to wait 6 months after rituximab administration.

Tumor necrosis factor alpha inhibitors come under pregnancy category B. Most TNF-α inhibitors have data regarding pregnancy and neonatal outcomes in patients with IBD and rheumatoid arthritis. A meta-analysis of IBD patients treated with TNF-α inhibitors showed that the rate of elective terminations was 17% in exposed group versus 0.02% in the background population.[128] There are conflicting studies regarding the risk of adverse neonatal outcomes among pregnant women exposed to TNF-α inhibitors.[129-131]

Secukinumab has also been shown in global safety database that exposure during pregnancy is not associated with an increased risk of spontaneous abortions or neonatal malformations, however, data is limited.[119,132]

The British Association of Dermatologists states in their guideline that decision making on treatment during pregnancy should be made on a case-by-case basis, with no defined gestational cutoff for drug discontinuation. It also states that live vaccines should be avoided for first 6 months of life of infants born to mothers taking biologic therapy beyond 16 weeks' gestation.[67] Certolizumab pegol differs structurally from other drugs in this class as it is a humanized pegylated antibody Fab fragment that lacks the IgG1 Fc fragment, and thereby the transfer across the placenta is low/negligible.

Omalizumab also comes under pregnancy category B. There has been no increase in major congenital defects in the pregnant asthma patients exposed to omalizumab.[133]

Biologics have gained a very popular role in the treatment of dermatological disorders. Biologics targeting a particular cytokine, leading to an efficient control of the disease with minimal side effects have become a boon to the treatment of several skin diseases. Hence, it is of utmost importance for all dermatologists to be well versed with the use of biologics and their potential safety concerns.

CONCLUSION

The use of biologics in dermatology is increasing day by day. Common dermatological diseases such as psoriasis, urticaria, atopic dermatitis and pemphigus are being treated using biologics routinely. It is important to be aware of common and uncommon adverse effect of these biologics which we use routinely.

REFERENCES

1. Edwards IR, Aronson JK. Adverse drug reactions: definitions, diagnosis and management. Lancet. 2000;356(9237):1255-9.
2. Aubin F, Carbonnel F, Wendling D. The complexity of adverse side-effects to biological agents. J Crohn's Colitis. 2013;7(4):257-62.
3. Pichler WJ. Adverse side-effects to biological agents. Allergy Eur J Allergy Clin Immunol. 2006;61(8):912-20.
4. Hausmann OV, Seitz M, Villiger PM, Pichler WJ. The complex clinical picture of side effects to biologicals. Med Clin North Am. 2010;94(4):791-804.
5. Fouda GE, Bavbek S. Rituximab hypersensitivity: From clinical presentation to management. Front Pharmacol. 2020;11:572863.
6. Van Vollenhoven RF, Emery P, Bingham CO 3rd, Keystone EC, Fleischmann RM, Furst DE, et al. Long-term safety of rituximab in rheumatoid arthritis: 9.5-year follow-up of the global clinical trial programme with a focus on adverse events of interest in RA patients. Ann Rheum Dis. 2013;72(9):1496-502.

7. Courville J, Nastoupil L, Kaila N, Kelton J, Zhang J, Alcasid A, Nava-Parada P. Factors Influencing Infusion-Related Reactions Following Dosing of Reference Rituximab and PF-05280586, a Rituximab Biosimilar. BioDrugs. 2021;35(4):459-68.
8. Paul F, Cartron G. Infusion-related reactions to rituximab: frequency, mechanisms and predictors. Expert Rev Clin Immunol. 2019;15(4):383-9.
9. Jung JW, Kang HR, Lee SH, Cho SH. The incidence and risk factors of infusion-related reactions to rituximab for treating B cell malignancies in a single tertiary hospital. Oncology. 2014;86(3):127-34.
10. Rombouts MD, Swart EL, VAN DEN Eertwegh AJM, Crul M. Systematic review on infusion reactions to and infusion rate of monoclonal antibodies used in cancer treatment. Anticancer Res. 2020;40(3):1201-18.
11. Kulkarni HS, Kasi PM. Rituximab and cytokine release syndrome. Case Rep Oncol. 2012;5(1):134-41.
12. Patel SV, Khan DA. Adverse reactions to biologic therapy. Immunol Allergy Clin North Am. 2017;37(2):397-412.
13. Wong JT, Long A. Rituximab hypersensitivity: Evaluation, desensitization, and potential mechanisms. J Allergy Clin Immunol Pract. 2017;5(6):1564-71.
14. Karmacharya P, Poudel DR, Pathak R, Donato AA, Ghimire S, Giri S, et al. Rituximab-induced serum sickness: A systematic review. Semin Arthritis Rheum. 2015;45(3): 334-40.
15. Chen CB, Wu MY, Ng CY, Lu CW, Wu J, Kao PH, et al. Severe cutaneous adverse reactions induced by targeted anticancer therapies and immunotherapies. Cancer Manag Res. 2018;10:1259-73.
16. Fallon MJ, Heck JN. Fatal Stevens-Johnson syndrome/toxic epidermal necrolysis induced by allopurinol-rituximab-bendamustine therapy. J Oncol Pharm Pract. 2015;21(5):388-92.
17. Lowndes S, Darby A, Mead G, Lister A. Stevens-Johnson syndrome after treatment with rituximab. Ann Oncol. 2002;13(12):1948-50.
18. Roselló S, Blasco I, García Fabregat L, Cervantes A, Jordan K; ESMO Guidelines Committee. Management of infusion reactions to systemic anticancer therapy: ESMO Clinical Practice Guidelines. Ann Oncol. 2017;28(suppl_4):iv100-iv118.
19. Tony HP, Burmester G, Schulze-Koops H, Grunke M, Henes J, Kötter I, et al. Safety and clinical outcomes of rituximab therapy in patients with different autoimmune diseases: experience from a national registry (GRAID). Arthritis Res Ther. 2011;13(3):R75.
20. Kasi PM, Tawbi HA, Oddis CV, Kulkarni HS. Clinical review: Serious adverse events associated with the use of rituximab: a critical care perspective. Crit Care. 2012;16(4):231.
21. Aksoy S, Harputluoglu H, Kilickap S, Dede DS, Dizdar O, Altundag K, et al. Rituximab-related viral infections in lymphoma patients. Leuk Lymphoma. 2007;48(7):1307-12.
22. Berger JR, Malik V, Lacey S, Brunetta P, Lehane PB. Progressive multifocal leukoencephalopathy in rituximab-treated rheumatic diseases: a rare event. J Neurovirol. 2018;24(3):323-31.
23. D'Alò F, Malafronte R, Piludu F, Bellesi S, Cuccaro A, Maiolo E, et al. Progressive multifocal leukoencephalopathy in patients with follicular lymphoma treated with bendamustine plus rituximab followed by rituximab maintenance. Br J Haematol. 2020;189(4):e140-e144.
24. Gottenberg JE, Ravaud P, Bardin T, Cacoub P, Cantagrel A, Combe B, et al; Autoimmunity and Rituximab registry and French Society of Rheumatology. Risk factors for severe infections in patients with rheumatoid arthritis treated with rituximab in the autoimmunity and rituximab registry. Arthritis Rheum. 2010;62(9):2625-32.
25. Coiffier B, Lepage E, Briere J, Herbrecht R, Tilly H, Bouabdallah R, et al. CHOP chemotherapy plus rituximab compared with CHOP alone in elderly patients with diffuse large-B-cell lymphoma. N Engl J Med. 2002;346(4):235-42.

26. Patil VB, Lunge SB, Doshi BR. Cardiac side effect of rituximab. Indian J Drugs Dermatol. 2020:6(1):49-52.
27. Millward PM, Bandarenko N, Chang PP, Stagg KF, Afenyi-Annan A, Hay SN, et al. Cardiogenic shock complicates successful treatment of refractory thrombotic thrombocytopenia purpura with rituximab. Transfusion. 2005;45(9):1481-6.
28. Diarra A, Gantois G, Lazrek M, Verdier B, Elsermans V, Zephir H, et al. Fatal enterovirus-related myocarditis in a patient with Devic's syndrome treated with rituximab. Card Fail Rev. 2021;7:e09.
29. Cheungpasitporn W, Kopecky SL, Specks U, Bharucha K, Fervenza FC. Non-ischemic cardiomyopathy after rituximab treatment for membranous nephropathy. J Renal Inj Prev. 2016;6(1):18-25.
30. Hočevar A, Alibegović A, Jurčić V, Tomšič M, Rotar Ž. An immune-mediated adverse event potentially related to rituximab. J Clin Rheumatol. 2021;27(8S):S743-S744.
31. Casulo C, Maragulia J, Zelenetz AD. Incidence of hypogammaglobulinemia in patients receiving rituximab and the use of intravenous immunoglobulin for recurrent infections. Clin Lymphoma Myeloma Leuk. 2013;13(2):106-11.
32. Hincks I, Woodcock BE, Thachil J. Is rituximab-induced late-onset neutropenia a good prognostic indicator in lymphoproliferative disorders? Br J Haematol. 2011;153(3):411-3.
33. Emery P, Furst DE, Kirchner P, Melega S, Lacey S, Lehane PB. Risk of malignancies in patients with rheumatoid arthritis treated with rituximab: Analyses of Global Postmarketing Safety Data and Long-term Clinical Trial Data. Rheumatol Ther. 2020;7(1):121-31.
34. Aksoy S, Arslan C, Harputluoglu H, Dizdar O, Altundag K. Malignancies after rituximab treatment: just coincidence or more? J BUON. 2011;16(1):112-5.
35. Alkan A, Yaşar A, Toprak S. Kaposi sarcoma associated with rituximab-based cytotoxic therapy. J Oncol Pharm Pract. 2020;26(1):220-3.
36. Mallepally N, Abu-Sbeih H, Ahmed O, Chen E, Shafi MA, Neelapu SS, et al. Clinical features of rituximab-associated gastrointestinal toxicities. Am J Clin Oncol. 2019;42(6):539-45.
37. Joy N, Sobhanakumari K, Celine MI, Mathew R, Athir S. Rituximab induced transaminitis in pemphigus foliaceus. J Skin Sex Transm Dis. 2019;1:45-7.
38. Kang HJ, Park JS, Kim DW, Lee J, Jeong YJ, Choi SM, et al. Adverse pulmonary reactions associated with the use of monoclonal antibodies in cancer patients. Respir Med. 2012;106(3):443-50.
39. Biehn SE, Kirk D, Rivera MP, Martinez AE, Khandani AH, Orlowski RZ. Bronchiolitis obliterans with organizing pneumonia after rituximab therapy for non-Hodgkin's lymphoma. Hematol Oncol. 2006;24(4):234-7.
40. Tonelli AR, Lottenberg R, Allan RW, Sriram PS. Rituximab-induced hypersensitivity pneumonitis. Respiration. 2009;78(2):225-9.
41. Heresi GA, Farver CF, Stoller JK. Interstitial pneumonitis and alveolar hemorrhage complicating use of rituximab: case report and review of the literature. Respiration. 2008;76(4):449-53.
42. Wu KJ, Wei KC. Venous thromboembolism in a case with pemphigus vulgaris after infusion of rituximab plus systemic glucocorticoids and azathioprine: A possible adverse effect of rituximab?. Dermatol Sin. 2021;39:103-4.
43. Londhe PJ, Kalyanpad Y, Khopkar US. Intermediate doses of rituximab used as adjuvant therapy in refractory pemphigus. Indian J Dermatol Venereol Leprol. 2014;80(4):300-5.
44. Wolach O, Bairey O, Lahav M. Late-onset neutropenia after rituximab treatment: case series and comprehensive review of the literature. Medicine (Baltimore). 2010;89(5):308-18.

45. Goh MS, McCormack C, Dinh HV, et al. Rituximab in the adjuvant treatment of pemphigus vulgaris: a prospective open-label pilot study in five patients. Br J Dermatol. 2007;156(5):990-6.
46. Salmon JH, Cacoub P, Combe B, Sibilia J, Pallot-Prades B, Fain O, et al. Late-onset neutropenia after treatment with rituximab for rheumatoid arthritis and other autoimmune diseases: data from the Autoimmunity and Rituximab registry. RMD Open. 2015;1(1):e000034.
47. Voog E, Morschhauser F, Solal-Céligny P. Neutropenia in patients treated with rituximab. N Engl J Med. 2003;348(26):2691-4; discussion 2691-4.
48. Papadaki T, Stamatopoulos K, Stavroyianni N, Paterakis G, Phisphis M, Stefanoudaki-Sofianatou K. Evidence for T-large granular lymphocyte-mediated neutropenia in rituximab-treated lymphoma patients: report of two cases. Leuk Res. 2002;26(6): 597-600.
49. Siddiqi AI. Rituximab as a possible cause of posterior reversible encephalopathy syndrome. Australas Med J. 2011;4(9):513-5.
50. Bremmer M, Deng A, Gaspari A. A mechanism-based classification of dermatologic reactions to biologic agents used in the treatment of cutaneous disease: Part 2. Dermatitis. 2009;20(5):243-56.
51. Bhandari PR, Pai VV. Novel applications of Rituximab in dermatological disorders. Indian Dermatol Online J. 2014;5(3):250-9.
52. Desbois AC, Biard L, Sène D, Brocheriou I, Rouvier P, Lioger B, et al. Rituximab-associated Vasculitis Flare: Incidence, Predictors, and Outcome. J Rheumatol. 2020;47:896-902.
53. Lichtenstein L, Ron Y, Kivity S, Ben-Horin S, Israeli E, Fraser GM, et al. Infliximab-related infusion reactions: Systematic review. J Crohns Colitis. 2015;9(9):806-15.
54. Steenholdt C, Svenson M, Bendtzen K, Thomsen OØ, Brynskov J, Ainsworth MA. Severe infusion reactions to infliximab: aetiology, immunogenicity and risk factors in patients with inflammatory bowel disease. Aliment Pharmacol Ther. 2011;34(1):51-8.
55. Vermeire S, Noman M, Van Assche G, Baert F, D'Haens G, Rutgeerts P. Effectiveness of concomitant immunosuppressive therapy in suppressing the formation of antibodies to infliximab in Crohn's disease. Gut. 2007;56(9):1226-31.
56. Munera-Campos M, Ballesca F, Carrascosa JM. Paradoxical reactions to biologic therapy in psoriasis: A review of the literature. Actas Dermosifiliogr (Engl Ed). 2018;109(9): 791-800.
57. Bucalo A, Rega F, Zangrilli A, Silvestri V, Valentini V, Scafetta G, et al. Paradoxical psoriasis induced by anti-TNFα treatment: Evaluation of disease-specific clinical and genetic markers. Int J Mol Sci. 2020;21(21):7873.
58. Brown G, Wang E, Leon A, Huynh M, Wehner M, Matro R, et al. Tumor necrosis factor-α inhibitor-induced psoriasis: Systematic review of clinical features, histopathological findings, and management experience. J Am Acad Dermatol. 2017;76(2):334-41.
59. da Silva Cendon Duran C, da Paz AS, Barreto Santiago M. Vasculitis induced by biological agents used in rheumatology practice: A systematic review. Arch Rheumatol. 2021;37(2):300-10.
60. Klein R, Rosenbach M, Kim EJ, Kim B, Werth VP, Dunham J. Tumor necrosis factor inhibitor-associated dermatomyositis. Arch Dermatol. 2010;146(7):780-4.
61. Zhang J, Wang SH, Zuo YG. Paradoxical phenomena of bullous pemphigoid induced and treated by identical biologics. Front Immunol. 2023;13:1050373.
62. Romagnuolo M, Moltrasio C, Iannone C, Gattinara M, Cambiaghi S, Marzano AV. Pyoderma gangrenosum following anti-TNF therapy in chronic recurrent multifocal osteomyelitis: drug reaction or cutaneous manifestation of the disease? A critical review on the topic with an emblematic case report. Front Med (Lausanne). 2023;10: 1197273.
63. Ratnarathorn M, Raychaudhuri SP, Naguwa S. Disseminated granuloma annulare: a cutaneous adverse effect of anti-TNF agents. Indian J Dermatol. 2011;56(6):752-4.

64. Dang LJ, Lubel JS, Gunatheesan S, Hosking P, Su J. Drug-induced lupus and autoimmune hepatitis secondary to infliximab for psoriasis. Australas J Dermatol. 2014;55(1):75-9.
65. Poulin Y, Thérien G. Drug-induced hepatitis and lupus during infliximab treatment for psoriasis: case report and literature review. J Cutan Med Surg. 2010;14(2):100-4.
66. Scheinfeld N. A comprehensive review and evaluation of the side effects of the tumor necrosis factor alpha blockers etanercept, infliximab and adalimumab. J Dermatolog Treat. 2004;15(5):280-94.
67. Ali T, Kaitha S, Mahmood S, Ftesi A, Stone J, Bronze MS. Clinical use of anti-TNF therapy and increased risk of infections. Drug Healthc Patient Saf. 2013;5:79-99.
68. Wallis RS. Biologics and infections: lessons from tumor necrosis factor blocking agents. Infect Dis Clin North Am. 2011;25(4):895-910.
69. Souto A, Maneiro JR, Salgado E, Carmona L, Gomez-Reino JJ. Risk of tuberculosis in patients with chronic immune-mediated inflammatory diseases treated with biologics and tofacitinib: a systematic review and meta-analysis of randomized controlled trials and long-term extension studies. Rheumatology (Oxford). 2014;53(10):1872-85.
70. Borekci S, Atahan E, Demir Yilmaz D, Mazıcan N, Duman B, Ozguler Y, et al. Factors affecting the tuberculosis risk in patients receiving anti-tumor necrosis factor-α treatment. Respiration. 2015;90(3):191-8.
71. Smith CH, Yiu ZZN, Bale T, Burden AD, Coates LC, Edwards W, et al; British Association of Dermatologists' Clinical Standards Unit. British Association of Dermatologists guidelines for biologic therapy for psoriasis 2020: a rapid update. Br J Dermatol. 2020;183(4):628-37.
72. Doherty SD, Van Voorhees A, Lebwohl MG, Korman NJ, Young MS, Hsu S; National Psoriasis Foundation. National Psoriasis Foundation consensus statement on screening for latent tuberculosis infection in patients with psoriasis treated with systemic and biologic agents. J Am Acad Dermatol. 2008;59(2):209-17.
73. Rungapiromnan W, Yiu ZZN, Warren RB, Griffiths CEM, Ashcroft DM. Impact of biologic therapies on risk of major adverse cardiovascular events in patients with psoriasis: systematic review and meta-analysis of randomized controlled trials. Br J Dermatol. 2017;176(4):890-901.
74. Bissonnette R, Kerdel F, Naldi L, Papp K, Galindo C, Langholff W, et al. Evaluation of risk of major adverse cardiovascular events with biologic therapy in patients with psoriasis. J Drugs Dermatol. 2017;16(10):1002-13.
75. Danila MI, Patkar NM, Curtis JR, Saag KG, Teng GG. Biologics and heart failure in rheumatoid arthritis: are we any wiser? Curr Opin Rheumatol. 2008;20(3):327-33.
76. Tristano AG. Neurological adverse events associated with anti-tumor necrosis factor α treatment. J Neurol. 2010;257(9):1421-31.
77. Poulalhon N, Begon E, Lebbé C, Lioté F, Lahfa M, Bengoufa D, et al. A follow-up study in 28 patients treated with infliximab for severe recalcitrant psoriasis: evidence for efficacy and high incidence of biological autoimmunity. Br J Dermatol. 2007;156(2):329-36.
78. Bobbio-Pallavicini F, Alpini C, Caporali R, Avalle S, Bugatti S, Montecucco C. Autoantibody profile in rheumatoid arthritis during long-term infliximab treatment. Arthritis Res Ther. 2004;6(3):R264-72.
79. Valenzuela F, Flores R. Immunogenicity to biological drugs in psoriasis and psoriatic arthritis. Clinics (Sao Paulo). 2021;76:e3015.
80. Cheifetz A, Mayer L. Monoclonal antibodies, immunogenicity, and associated infusion reactions. Mt Sinai J Med. 2005;72(4):250-6.
81. Ferraro S, Leonardi L, Convertino I, Blandizzi C, Tuccori M. Is there a risk of lymphoma associated with anti-tumor necrosis factor drugs in patients with inflammatory bowel disease? A systematic review of observational studies. Front Pharmacol. 2019;10:247.
82. Dahmus J, Rosario M, Clarke K. Risk of lymphoma associated with anti-TNF therapy in patients with inflammatory bowel disease: Implications for therapy. Clin Exp Gastroenterol. 2020;13:339-50.

83. Mercer LK, Galloway JB, Lunt M, Davies R, Low AL, Dixon WG, et al. Risk of lymphoma in patients exposed to antitumour necrosis factor therapy: results from the British Society for Rheumatology Biologics Register for Rheumatoid Arthritis. Ann Rheum Dis. 2017;76(3):497-503.
84. Reich K, Wozel G, Zheng H, van Hoogstraten HJ, Flint L, Barker J. Efficacy and safety of infliximab as continuous or intermittent therapy in patients with moderate-to-severe plaque psoriasis: results of a randomized, long-term extension trial (RESTORE2). Br J Dermatol. 2013;168(6):1325-34.
85. Subedi S, Gong Y, Chen Y, Shi Y. Infliximab and biosimilar infliximab in psoriasis: efficacy, loss of efficacy, and adverse events. Drug Des Devel Ther. 2019;13:2491-502.
86. Scheinfeld N. Adalimumab: a review of side effects. Expert Opin Drug Saf. 2005;4(4):637-41.
87. Zhang Z, Fan W, Yang G, Xu Z, Wang J, Cheng Q, et al. Risk of tuberculosis in patients treated with TNF-α antagonists: a systematic review and meta-analysis of randomised controlled trials. BMJ Open. 2017;7(3):e012567.
88. Mariette X, Tubach F, Bagheri H, Bardet M, Berthelot JM, Gaudin P, et al. Lymphoma in patients treated with anti-TNF: results of the 3-year prospective French RATIO registry. Ann Rheum Dis. 2010;69(2):400-8.
89. Murphy FT, Enzenauer RJ, Battafarano DF, David-Bajar K. Etanercept-associated injection-site reactions. Arch Dermatol. 2000;136(4):556-7.
90. Chiang YC, Kuo LN, Yen YH, Tang CH, Chen HY. Infection risk in patients with rheumatoid arthritis treated with etanercept or adalimumab. Comput Methods Programs Biomed. 2014;116(3):319-27.
91. Campanati A, Diotallevi F, Martina E, Paolinelli M, Radi G, Offidani A. Safety update of etanercept treatment for moderate to severe plaque psoriasis. Expert Opin Drug Saf. 2020;19(4):439-48.
92. Ibrahim WH, Hammoudah M, Akhtar N, Al-Hail H, Deleu D. Central nervous system demyelination associated with etanercept in a 51 years old woman. Libyan J Med. 2007;2(2):99-102.
93. Kang MJ, Lee YH, Lee J. Etanercept-induced systemic lupus erythematosus in a patient with rheumatoid arthritis. J Korean Med Sci. 2006;21(5):946-9.
94. Bleumink GS, ter Borg EJ, Ramselaar CG, Stricker BH. Etanercept-induced subacute cutaneous lupus erythematosus. Rheumatology (Oxford). 2001;40(11):1317-9.
95. Fathalla BM, Goldsmith DP, Pascasio JM, Baldridge A. Development of autoimmune hepatitis in a child with systemic-onset juvenile idiopathic arthritis during therapy with etanercept. J Clin Rheumatol. 2008;14(5):297-8.
96. Hsu L, Armstrong AW. Anti-drug antibodies in psoriasis: a critical evaluation of clinical significance and impact on treatment response. Expert Rev Clin Immunol. 2013;9(10):949-58.
97. Ahdout J, Haley JC, Chiu MW. Erythema multiforme during anti-tumor necrosis factor treatment for plaque psoriasis. J Am Acad Dermatol. 2010;62(5):874-9.
98. Papp KA, Langley RG, Sigurgeirsson B, Abe M, Baker DR, Konno P, et al. Efficacy and safety of secukinumab in the treatment of moderate-to-severe plaque psoriasis: a randomized, double-blind, placebo-controlled phase II dose-ranging study. Br J Dermatol. 2013;168(2):412-21.
99. Rich P, Sigurgeirsson B, Thaci D, Ortonne JP, Paul C, Schopf RE, et al. Secukinumab induction and maintenance therapy in moderate-to-severe plaque psoriasis: a randomized, double-blind, placebo-controlled, phase II regimen-finding study. Br J Dermatol. 2013;168(2):402-11.
100. Langley RG, Elewski BE, Lebwohl M, Reich K, Griffiths CE, Papp K, et al; ERASURE Study Group; FIXTURE Study Group. Secukinumab in plaque psoriasis—results of two phase 3 trials. N Engl J Med. 2014;371(4):326-38.

101. Elewski BE, Baddley JW, Deodhar AA, Magrey M, Rich PA, Soriano ER, et al. Association of Secukinumab Treatment with Tuberculosis Reactivation in Patients with Psoriasis, Psoriatic Arthritis, or Ankylosing Spondylitis. JAMA Dermatol. 2021;157:43-51.
102. Davidson L, van den Reek JMPA, Bruno M, van Hunsel F, Herings RMC, Matzaraki V, et al. Risk of candidiasis associated with interleukin-17 inhibitors: A real-world observational study of multiple independent sources. Lancet Reg Health Eur. 2021;13:100266.
103. Onac IA, Clarke BD, Tacu C, Lloyd M, Hajela V, Batty T, et al. Secukinumab as a potential trigger of inflammatory bowel disease in ankylosing spondylitis or psoriatic arthritis patients. Rheumatology (Oxford). 2021;60(11):5233-8.
104. Burlando M, Cozzani E, Russo R, Parodi A. Atopic-like dermatitis after secukinumab injection: A case report. Dermatol Ther. 2019;32(1):e12751.
105. Eichhoff G. Secukinumab-induced pompholyx in a psoriasis patient. Dermatol Online J. 2020;26:13030/qt3669k149.
106. Bose R, Beecker J. Dyshidrotic eczema in two patients on secukinumab for plaque psoriasis: A case report. SAGE Open Med Case Rep. 2020;8:2050313X20904561.
107. Dogra S, Bishnoi A, Narang T, Handa S. Secukinumab-induced paradoxical pustular psoriasis. Clin Exp Dermatol. 2019;44(1):72-3.
108. M Castillejo Becerra C, Ding Y, Kenol B, Hendershot A, Meara AS. Ocular side effects of antirheumatic medications: a qualitative review. BMJ Open Ophthalmol. 2020;5(1):e000331.
109. Griffiths CE, Reich K, Lebwohl M, van de Kerkhof P, Paul C, Menter A, et al; UNCOVER-2 and UNCOVER-3 investigators. Comparison of ixekizumab with etanercept or placebo in moderate-to-severe psoriasis (UNCOVER-2 and UNCOVER-3): results from two phase 3 randomised trials. Lancet. 2015;386(9993):541-51.
110. Blegvad C, Skov L, Zachariae C. Ixekizumab for the treatment of psoriasis: an update on new data since first approval. Expert Rev Clin Immunol. 2019;15(2):111-21.
111. Lebwohl MG, Papp KA, Marangell LB, Koo J, Blauvelt A, Gooderham M, et al. Psychiatric adverse events during treatment with brodalumab: Analysis of psoriasis clinical trials. J Am Acad Dermatol. 2018;78(1):81-89.e5.
112. Spencer EA, Kinnucan J, Wang J, Dubinsky MC. Real-world experience with acute infusion reactions to ustekinumab at 2 large tertiary care centers. Crohns Colitis. 2020;2(2):otaa022.
113. Cho SI, Kang S, Kim YE, Lee JY, Jo SJ. Ustekinumab does not increase tuberculosis risk: Results from a national database in South Korea. J Am Acad Dermatol. 2020;82(5):1243-5.
114. Gratton D, Szapary P, Goyal K, Fakharzadeh S, Germain V, Saltiel P. Reversible posterior leukoencephalopathy syndrome in a patient treated with ustekinumab: case report and review of the literature. Arch Dermatol. 2011;147(10):1197-202.
115. Hasan B, Tandon KS, Miret R, Khan S, Riaz A, Gonzalez A, et al. Ustekinumab does not increase risk of new or recurrent cancer in inflammatory bowel disease patients with prior malignancy. J Gastroenterol Hepatol. 2022;37(6):1016-21.
116. Naik PP. Adverse effects of anti-interleukin-23 agents employed in patients with psoriasis: A systematic review. Dermatology. 2022;238(5):886-96.
117. Chia J, Mydlarski PR. Omalizumab in dermatology: a review of the literature. J Am Acad Dermatol. 2015;72:AB210.
118. Kim HL, Leigh R, Becker A. Omalizumab: Practical considerations regarding the risk of anaphylaxis. Allergy Asthma Clin Immunol. 2010;6(1):32.
119. Cooper PJ, Ayre G, Martin C, Rizzo JA, Ponte EV, Cruz AA. Geohelminth infections: a review of the role of IgE and assessment of potential risks of anti-IgE treatment. Allergy. 2008;63(4):409-17.
120. Iribarren C, Rahmaoui A, Long AA, Szefler SJ, Bradley MS, Carrigan G et al. Cardiovascular and cerebrovascular events among patients receiving omalizumab: Results from

EXCELS, a prospective cohort study in moderate to severe asthma. J Allergy Clin Immunol. 2017;139(5):1489-95.
121. Agnihotri G, Shi K, Lio PA. A clinician's guide to the recognition and management of dupilumab-associated conjunctivitis. Drugs RD. 2019;19(4):311-8.
122. Wilson MM, Roberts PK, Daniell M. Dupilumab-associated ulcerative keratitis. Int J Ophthalmol. 2022;15(6):1020-2.
123. Halling AS, Loft N, Silverberg JI, Guttman-Yassky E, Thyssen JP. Real-world evidence of dupilumab efficacy and risk of adverse events: A systematic review and meta-analysis. J Am Acad Dermatol. 2021;84(1):139-47.
124. Chakravarty EF, Murray ER, Kelman A, Farmer P. Pregnancy outcomes after maternal exposure to rituximab. Blood. 2011;117(5):1499-506.
125. Dehghanimahmoudabadi A, Kianfar N, Akhdar M, Dasdar S, Balighi K, Mahmoudi H, Daneshpazhooh M. Pregnancy outcomes in women with pemphigus exposed to rituximab before or during pregnancy. Int J Womens Dermatol. 2022;8(3):e038.
126. Tourte M, Brunet-Possenti F, Mignot S, Gavard L, Descamps V. Pemphigoid gestationis: a successful preventive treatment by rituximab. J Eur Acad Dermatol Venereol. 2017;31(4):e206-e207.
127. Narayanan A, Pangti R, Agarwal S, Bhari N. Pemphigoid gestationis: a rare pregnancy dermatosis treated with a combination of IVIg and rituximab. BMJ Case Rep. 2021;14(3):e241496.
128. Cornish J, Tan E, Teare J, Teoh TG, Rai R, Clark SK, et al. A meta-analysis on the influence of inflammatory bowel disease on pregnancy. Gut. 2007;56(6):830-7.
129. Pottinger E, Woolf RT, Exton LS, Burden AD, Nelson-Piercy C, Smith CH. Exposure to biological therapies during conception and pregnancy: a systematic review. Br J Dermatol. 2018;178(1):95-102.
130. Bröms G, Granath F, Ekbom A, Hellgren K, Pedersen L, Sørensen HT, et al. Low risk of birth defects for infants whose mothers are treated with anti-tumor necrosis factor agents during pregnancy. Clin Gastroenterol Hepatol. 2016;14(2):234-41.e1-5.
131. Shihab Z, Yeomans ND, De Cruz P. Anti-tumour necrosis factor α therapies and inflammatory bowel disease pregnancy outcomes: A meta-analysis. J Crohns Colitis. 2016;10(8):979-88.
132. Warren RB, Reich K, Langley RG, Strober B, Gladman D, Deodhar A, et al. Secukinumab in pregnancy: outcomes in psoriasis, psoriatic arthritis and ankylosing spondylitis from the global safety database. Br J Dermatol. 2018;179(5):1205-7.
133. Levi-Schaffer F, Mankuta D. Omalizumab safety in pregnancy. J Allergy Clin Immunol. 2020;145(2):481-3.

CHAPTER 29

Adult Immunization Prior to Initiation of Biologic Therapy

Ankan Gupta, Himadri

INTRODUCTION

Immunization is the process through which a person is made immune to an infectious agent, typically by the administration of a vaccine which stimulates body's own immune system to protect against subsequent exposure to that particular agent.[1] The concept is based on immunological memory where exposing the foreign molecules which are "non-self", orchestrate an immune response, which develops the ability to quickly respond to a subsequent encounter. Immunization is a proven tool for controlling and eliminating life-threatening infectious diseases and is estimated to avert between 2 and 3 million deaths each year.[1,2] Immunization in pediatric age group has been quite successful in our country, but adult "at risk" population is still vulnerable.[3] Patients with autoimmune diseases (AIDs) are arguably the most neglected group surprisingly in this respect knowing the fact that immunizing them helps in a long term in a multifactorial way.

- Vaccination prevents these patients from acquiring infections which would otherwise worsen the morbidity and mortality due to the immunosuppressive nature of the disease [most noticeable in atopic dermatitis, complement deficiency in systemic lupus erythematosus (SLE), etc.], and the drug therapy used for its management.[4-8]
- There is an increased risk not only of acquiring an infection but also of infections being more severe.[5,7]
- *Malignancies*: These patients are also "at risk" of developing infection-induced malignancies, e.g., human papillomavirus (HPV) causing squamous cell carcinoma and hepatitis B virus (HBV) causing liver cancer.
- Infection itself is one of the most consistent factors in etiopathogenesis of AID. Making them immunosuppressed would initiate a vicious cycle of infection-relapse-drugs-immunosuppression-infection.[8]

With obvious benefits of immunizing such a patient, convincing them or their relatives is still a difficult task with reports of serious adverse events, such as paralysis, encephalomyelitis, and demyelinating disorders making rounds in social media and with internet doctors. Vaccination in itself can trigger the disease theoretically, making the entire exercise controversial, but the present evidence does not indicate that it increases the clinical or laboratory parameters of disease activity in AID.[9,10]

USE OF BIOLOGICS IN DERMATOLOGY

Psoriasis, autoimmune vesiculobullous disorders, hidradenitis suppurativa, alopecia areata, vitiligo, SLE, dermatomyositis, scleroderma, and chronic urticaria are some of the well-established indications for the use of immunosuppressives and biologics in dermatology. All these share a common set of cytokine dysregulation and therefore a similar approach to management, which is using the traditional immunosuppressants or the biologics.[11]

IMMUNOSUPPRESSION

Immunosuppressants commonly used in dermatology are corticosteroids, azathioprine, mycophenolate mofetil, cyclosporine, methotrexate, cyclophosphamide, and biologics, such as rituximab, interleukin-17A (IL-17A) blockers, and tumor necrosis factor-alpha (TNF-α) inhibitors. There are several other newer smaller molecules that are getting launched each day to add to their ever-increasing number. Most of these are being interchangeably used as an off-label indication for a disease, which has its own approved biologic. The inherent immunosuppressive properties of these diseases, various molecules having a different length and depth of immunosuppression and different doses and duration of the same molecule make it arduous for the experts to make protocols for immunization. What constitutes immunosuppression is also debated with common agreement presently dictating that drugs like biologics, cyclophosphamide, cyclosporine, leflunomide, and mycophenolate mofetil cause immune suppression at any dose while corticosteroids, methotrexate, and azathioprine increase the risk of infection in dose-dependent manner.[12,13] A concept of "low-dose immunosuppression" has been put forward which is defined as:
- Low-dose corticosteroid (< 20 mg/day of prednisone or equivalent)
- Glucocorticoid replacement therapy in adrenal insufficiency
- Topical steroids or intra-articular, intrabursa, or intratendon steroid injection
- Low-dose methotrexate (< 0.4 mg/kg/week or < 20 mg/week)
- Low-dose azathioprine (< 3 mg/kg/day)
- Low-dose 6-mercaptopurine (< 1.5 mg/kg/day)[14]

Old age in itself is considered a state of immunosuppression with the concept of immune senescence defining it as "changes that reduce the protection of the vaccines as a result of aging and the effects of aging on natural and acquired immunities".[15] In the present text, we have not limited ourselves to the role of vaccines with biologics, but expanded to include vaccination with traditional immunosuppressants and vaccination in old age.

VACCINES

The available vaccines can be categorized into live vaccines and inert or the killed or inactivated vaccines as shown in **Table 1**.

General Principles of Vaccination in Autoimmune Diseases[14,16,17]

- Vaccination status of patients must ideally be assessed at the time of diagnosis of an AID.
- Vaccination should ideally be completed before starting any immunosuppressant. A catch-up vaccination may be considered for missed vaccinations that are recommended for the general population. If the therapy has already been initiated, vaccines should be administered in the period of the lowest level of disease activity and the lowest dose of immunosuppressive therapy.
- Live vaccines are contraindicated in immunosuppressed individuals and pregnancy, but recombinant and inactivated vaccines can safely be given.
  - Live vaccines should be administered ideally at least 4 weeks before starting any immunosuppressant.

TABLE 1: Live vaccines and killed/inactivated or recombinant vaccines.	
Live vaccines	**Inactivated/Recombinant vaccines**
• Oral polio* • BCG*,† • MMR*,† • Human papillomavirus† • Yellow fever • Herpes zoster†	• Pneumococcal*,† • Influenza† • Diphtheria* • Pertussis* • Tetanus* • Injectable polio* • Hepatitis B*,† • Hepatitis A • COVID-19† • Herpes zoster (recombinant)† • Japanese encephalitis* • Meningococcal • Tick-borne encephalitis

*Routinely given as per the National Program.
†Increased risk in the individuals with autoimmune diseases.
(BCG: bacillus Calmette–Guérin; COVID-19: coronavirus disease 2019; MMR: measles, mumps, and rubella)

- Nonlive vaccines can be safely administered during immunosuppressant treatment; however, 2 weeks are required for the development of an immune response to inactivated vaccines. Therefore, if possible, inactivated vaccines should be administered at least 2 weeks before the commencement of immunosuppressive therapy without delaying the treatment.
- The safe time intervals for the administration of live vaccines after cessation of immunosuppressive therapy is:
  - At least 6 months after B-cell depleting therapy. Biologics targeting cytokines and T-cells may have less suppressive effect on vaccine response.
  - 4 weeks after high-dose corticosteroid therapy (≥20 mg/day prednisone or equivalent, for longer than 2 weeks)
  - 4 weeks after etanercept and 3 months after other TNF inhibitor (infliximab and adalimumab)
  - 4–12 weeks after the doses of ≥0.4 mg/kg/week or ≥20 mg/week of methotrexate
  - 2 years after leflunomide
  - For 6 months for other immunosuppressants not mentioned above
  - *Vaccination with intravenous immunoglobulin (IVIg)*: Inactivated vaccines and IVIg products may be administered simultaneously or within any time interval. An exception to this is the hepatitis A vaccine, which like other live vaccines should be administered either 2 weeks before the IVIg therapy or should be delayed for 3–11 months after the therapy. If a need for IVIg therapy arises within 14 days after the vaccination, the vaccine should be readministered 3–11 months after the IVIg therapy in patients without serological evidence of an antibody response.
- Live vaccines can be administered during sulfasalazine and hydroxychloroquine therapies.
- Vaccination of close contacts should be strongly considered in certain situations. Few live vaccines should not be given to immunocompromised hosts or their household contacts, (e.g., oral polio); though measles, mumps, and rubella (MMR), herpes zoster, and bacillus Calmette-Guérin (BCG) are safe for household contacts. Highly immunocompromised patients should avoid handling diapers of infants vaccinated against rotavirus for at least 4 weeks following the administration of the vaccine. Conversely, if a patient cannot be vaccinated because of certain reasons, people who are in close contact with the patient can be vaccinated to reduce the risk of infection.
- Live-attenuated vaccines should be avoided during the first 6 months of life in newborns of mothers exposed to anti-TNF biologics during the second half of pregnancy. Children exposed to biologics only before a gestational age of 22 weeks, can receive vaccinations according to standard protocols including live vaccines.

- Severe allergic reaction to the previously administered same vaccine is a contraindication for further vaccination.
- Increased interval between doses of a multidose vaccine does not diminish vaccine effectiveness; therefore, it is not necessary to restart the vaccine series or add doses to the series because of an extended interval between doses.
- If not administered on the same day, separate live vaccines should be given by at least 28 days.

Efficacy of a Vaccine

It should ideally be demonstrated through clinical endpoints, e.g., incidence of infection, hospitalization, and death; however, most research is based on demonstration of B-cell generated antibodies as a surrogate marker for vaccination-induced protection, antibody titers, as well as the quality of the antibody response in terms of binding avidity and bactericidal or neutralizing activity of antibodies.

Essential Vaccines

Pneumococcal Vaccine[18]

This is probably the most controversial and researched vaccination in individuals with immunosuppression or with acquired immune deficiency syndrome (AIDS).[19] There are various vaccines available in the market for pneumococcus.
- The 23-valent pneumococcal polysaccharide vaccine (PPSV23) which contains antigens of the 23 most common pneumococcal strains. It is effective against approximately 90% of all pneumococcal infections.
- 13-valent pneumococcal conjugate vaccine (PCV13)
- 20-valent (PCV20) and 15-valent (PCV15) pneumococcal vaccines have been licensed by US FDA recently.
  - PCV15 contains pneumococcal polysaccharide serotype 22F and 33F in addition to those in PCV13
  - PCV20 contains pneumococcal polysaccharide serotypes 8, 10A, 11A, 12F, 15B, 22F, and 33F, in addition to PCV13 serotypes

Though the Advisory Committee on Immunization Practices (ACIP) recommendations are succinct to guide us in different clinical scenarios, the few points not to be forgotten including:
- Only a single dose of PCV (PCV13, 15, or 20) is recommended currently for any age group due to lack of data showing waning of protection after PCV administration.
- There should be a gap of at least 8 weeks between the administrations of PCV and PPSV23.

Preferred dosing schedule is to vaccinate with PCV20 alone, or PCV15 followed by PPSV23 at least 8 weeks later.

In India, PCV15 and PCV20 are not available. As per the older schedule, start vaccination with PCV13, administer PPSV23 at least 8 weeks after PCV13 and repeat PPSV23 at least 5 years after the previous PPSV23 dose. All adults who already received PPSV23 should receive a dose of PCV13 ≥1 year after receipt of PPSV23. Revaccinations with PPSV23 should occur 5 years after the last dose. A caution is warranted when planning pneumococcal vaccine in patients with Behçet's disease because of a theoretical risk of flaring up of the disease and those with cryopyrin-associated periodic syndromes (CAPS), who may develop severe local and systemic reactions to PPSV23.[14]

Lower efficacy with or without shorter seroprotection period has been reported in SLE patients, in other AID being treated with methotrexate and rituximab, but not with TNF inhibitor.[20,21]

Influenza Vaccine

The risk of hospital admission for influenza is higher in elderly patients (≥65 years) with AID or vasculitis, compared with the ones with no underlying medical condition.[22]

- *Preferred dosing schedule*: Yearly injectable anti-influenza vaccination should be given to all patients regardless of current therapy including pregnant women. It is not contraindicated in those with allergies to eggs. The live attenuated nasal spray vaccination is contraindicated in immunosuppressed and pregnant patients.

The efficacy of concurrent immunosuppressants has been contradictory with reports of lower immunogenicity with steroids above 20 mg, azathioprine, mycophenolate, rituximab, and methotrexate but in most studies, neither disease-modifying antirheumatic drugs (DMARDs) nor biologics, except rituximab and abatacept, hampered humoral immune responses to influenza vaccination.[23,24] A second booster dose improved immunogenicity.[14,25] A list of currently available influenza vaccines is available at https://www.cdc.gov/flu/prevent/vaccinations.htm.

Herpes Zoster Vaccine[26,27]

Immunosuppressed patients have a higher risk of severe rash, visceral dissemination, or death, and hence, the prevention is desirable. Treatment with immunosuppressive drugs, particularly corticosteroids, increases this risk.[28] Recombinant zoster vaccine (RZV) is preferable to zoster vaccine live (ZVL), when available. The live-attenuated herpes zoster vaccine bears the potential risk of invasive infection in susceptible individuals. Centers for Disease Control and Prevention Advisory Committee on Immunization Practices (CDC-ACIP) Recommendations recommend RZV for adults ≥19 years old, who are or will become immunocompromised. Ideally, the vaccine should be given when patients are on "low-dose immunosuppression."

- *Preferred dosing schedule:* RZV is given as intramuscular injection, two doses 2–6 months apart (at least 1–2 months apart). ZVL should be given

≥4 weeks before initiating immunosuppressants, and it is only approved for those ≥50 years old.

Although the risk–benefit of the ZVL vaccine must be individually assessed, it is best avoided with:
- Treatment with all biologics, cyclosporine, cyclophosphamide, leflunomide, and higher doses of corticosteroids, methotrexate, and azathioprine
- Active leukemia, lymphoma, and malignant neoplasm affecting bone marrow or lymphatics
- Acquired immune deficiency syndrome or human immunodeficiency virus (AIDS or HIV) patients and those with CD4 lymphocyte counts <200/mm^3
- Clinical or laboratory evidence of cellular immunodeficiency
- Pregnancy and severe acute illness

Tetanus and Diphtheria Vaccines[29]
- *Preferred dosing schedule*: Administer a single dose of tetanus toxoid, diphtheria, and acellular pertussis (Tdap) followed by booster dose with tetanus and diphtheria (Td) every 10 years; however, passive immunization with tetanus Ig is required in cases of history of rituximab infusion in the past 24 weeks due to a possible reduction in immunogenicity due to rituximab. Though the literature does not suggest doing it in pemphigus, the authors recommend following this protocol in patients with autoimmune bullous disorders where raw skin is culture media for the microbe.

Adults with an unknown or incomplete history of a three-dose primary series in childhood with Td toxoid-containing vaccines should complete the primary series (0, 4 weeks, and 6–12 months), with at least one Tdap (other two being Tdap or Td) followed by 10-yearly Td or Tdap boosters. Pregnant women should receive one dose of Tdap during each pregnancy, preferably during 27–36 weeks, regardless of prior history of receiving TdaP.

Hepatitis B Vaccine
- It is recommended for all patients <60 years regardless of risk and ≥60 years old at-risk patients with negative serology [hepatitis B surface antigen (HBsAg), anti-HB core antigen (HBc), and anti-HBs negative]. At-risk, patients include HBV-seronegative patients who travel to or are residents in endemic countries, and those at increased risk of exposure to HBV (e.g., healthcare workers, household contacts or sexual partners of known persons with chronic HBV infection, intravenous drug users, and men who have sex with men).
    - *Preferred dosing schedule*: To be given in three doses at 0, 1–2, and 6 months. Postvaccination measurement of the anti-HBs titers 1–2 months after completion of the primary vaccination series is

indicated in immunocompromised patients to assess the response. Seroprotection is defined as a serum titer ≥10 IU/L and if it is not achieved, revaccination should be considered. Treatment with immunosuppressants can be started after the first two doses.
- In case of an exposure to HBV (e.g., percutaneous needle stick, laceration, bite, or per mucosal) in an unvaccinated patient or a patient with an insufficient response to HBV vaccine, a booster or passive immunization with hepatitis B immune globulin is indicated according to the CDC recommendations.

Human Papillomavirus Vaccine

Human papillomavirus infection is of relevance in young girls suffering from SLE as there is a higher incidence, florid presentation, and lower rate of spontaneous clearance of infection in women affected with SLE.[30] Hence, HPV vaccination should be encouraged in patients with AIDs, especially those with SLE until the age of 26 years.
- *Preferred dosing schedule*: Three doses at 0, 1–2, and 6 months.

COVID-19 Vaccines

Current data suggest that neither AID nor concurrent biologic use is a contraindication to coronavirus disease 2019 (COVID-19) vaccination. However, patients receiving biologics, particularly those on B-cell depleting therapy, may produce diminished immune responses. Therefore, vaccination should be completed 2 weeks prior to the start of rituximab treatment whenever possible; otherwise, it is best to wait 4–6 months after the last rituximab infusion.

It is essential to keep these patients under follow-up to determine the safety, efficacy, and duration of the vaccine.[31]

There is no indication for BCG vaccine in adults as most of the tuberculosis cases in adulthood are due to the activation of latent tuberculosis cases. BCG vaccine should not be administered to persons older than 6 years of age even if it has not been administered before.

Vaccines for Travelers

Patients with severe immunosuppression should avoid traveling in yellow fever endemic countries. If it is mandatory to travel in endemic area or when yellow fever vaccination is mandatory, temporary discontinuation of treatment with immunosuppressive drugs is required in combination with rigorous mosquito protection measures. A complete destination-wise list of travel vaccines can be referred to at https://www.cdc.gov/travel/destinations/list.

Safety of Vaccines

Autoimmune diseases are known to coexist. Their etiology is still not clear, but environmental factors are considered to be important triggers which are

not evident unless an environmental factor produces an overt expression. The term autoimmune inflammatory syndrome induced by adjuvants (ASIA) is a clinical condition of autoimmune nature, which is induced by the exposure to an environmental factor which may include vaccines and the adjuvants which are used to increase the immunogenicity.[32,33] Vaccine use has been associated with onset of AID, especially in patients already suffering from an AID, e.g., Guillain-Barré syndrome (GBS) with Td, polio and measles vaccine, autoimmune thrombocytopenia with MMR, development of multiple sclerosis with HBV vaccine, and autism with measles vaccine. However, practically the risk-to-benefit ratio is overwhelmingly in favor of vaccination and any untoward effect, though cannot be ignored still warrants a detailed evaluation to establish the causality.

Individuals who might be susceptible to develop vaccination-induced ASIA include patients with prior postvaccination autoimmune phenomena, patients with a medical history of autoimmunity, or a history of atopy.[34,35]

Vaccination Schedule for Adults[36,37]

The vaccination schedule for adults has been given in **Table 2**.

TABLE 2: Vaccination schedule for adults.			
Vaccine	Schedule	Age group	Contraindications
Pneumococcus: • PCV20 • PCV15/13 followed by PPSV23	• Single dose • PCV15/13 single dose followed by PPSV23 1 year (minimum 8 weeks) later	Adults aged >65 years or aged 19–64 years with immuno-suppression	Previous severe allergic reaction to previous vaccine or vaccine component or diphtheria-toxoid containing vaccine
Influenza	Annually	All age groups	History of GBS within 6 weeks after previous vaccination. Previous severe allergic reaction to any influenza vaccine or its component (except egg)
Herpes zoster: • RZV • ZVL	• Two doses (0, 2–6 months) • Single dose	Adults aged >60 years or aged 19–64 years with immuno-suppression	Severe allergic reaction to vaccine component
Td	Every 10 years booster	All age groups	• GBS within 6 weeks after a previous dose of tetanus toxoid • History of Arthus-type hypersensitivity reaction
Hepatitis B	Three doses (0, 1–2, and 6 months)	All age groups	Previous severe allergic reaction to vaccine or its component, including yeast

Continued

Continued

Vaccine	Schedule	Age group	Contraindications
Human papillomavirus (HPV)	Three doses (0, 1–2, and 6 months)	Between 9 and 26 years and preferably completed before the start of sexual activity	Receipt of acyclovir or congeners 24 hours before vaccination (avoid use of these antiviral drugs for 14 days after vaccination)
COVID-19: • Corbevax • Covovax • Covaxin • Covishield • Sputnik V • ZyCoV-D	• Two doses (0, 4 weeks) • Two doses (0, 3 weeks) • Two doses (0, 4–6 weeks) • Two dose (0, 12–16 weeks) • Two doses (0, 3 weeks) • Two doses (0, 4 weeks) • *Precaution dose*: 6 months after second dose	• All age groups ≥ 12 years • *Children 12–17 years*: Corbevax or Covovax • *Children 15–17 years*: Covaxin	

(COVID-19: coronavirus disease 2019; GBS: Guillain–Barré syndrome; PCV15: 15-valent pneumococcal conjugate vaccine; PCV20: 20-valent pneumococcal conjugate vaccine; PPSV23: 23-valent pneumococcal polysaccharide vaccine; RZV: recombinant zoster vaccine; Td: tetanus and diphtheria; ZVL: zoster vaccine live)

CONCLUSION

Every dermatologist and especially the ones, who wish to dwell in the world of biologics, should understand the importance of vaccination in patients with AID and should use the first visit as an opportunity to inquire about the vaccination status of the individual. The immunization should start prior to the initiation of immunosuppressants. As of now scientific data regarding vaccination efficacy before biologic therapy for dermatological indications is scarce, but extrapolating the evidence from rheumatology literature should be a good first step. In Indian population, influenza, pneumococcal, hepatitis B, and COVID-19 vaccines are safe and generally sufficiently immunogenic, whereas HPV and herpes zoster vaccination might be considered in select subgroups of patients.

REFERENCES

1. World Health Organization. (2023). Vaccines and immunization. [online] Available from https://www.who.int/health-topics/vaccines-and-immunization [Last accessed January, 2024].
2. Plotkin SA. Vaccines: correlates of vaccine-induced immunity. Clin Infect Dis Off Publ Infect Dis Soc Am. 2008;47(3):401-9.

3. Glück T, Müller-Ladner U. Vaccination in patients with chronic rheumatic or autoimmune diseases. Clin Infect Dis Off Publ Infect Dis Soc Am. 2008;46(9):1459-65.
4. Lindegård B. Diseases associated with psoriasis in a general population of 159,200 middle-aged, urban, native Swedes. Dermatologica. 1986;172(6):298-304.
5. Doran MF, Crowson CS, Pond GR, O'Fallon WM, Gabriel SE. Frequency of infection in patients with rheumatoid arthritis compared with controls: a population-based study. Arthritis Rheum. 2002;46(9):2287-93.
6. Conti F, Rezai S, Valesini G. Vaccination and autoimmune rheumatic diseases. Autoimmun Rev. 2008;8(2):124-8.
7. Blumentals WA, Arreglado A, Napalkov P, Toovey S. Rheumatoid arthritis and the incidence of influenza and influenza-related complications: a retrospective cohort study. BMC Musculoskelet Disord. 2012;13:158.
8. Doria A, Zampieri S, Sarzi-Puttini P. Exploring the complex relationships between infections and autoimmunity. Autoimmun Rev. 2008;8(2):89-91.
9. Takayama K, Satoh T, Hayashi M, Yokozeki H. Psoriatic skin lesions induced by BCG vaccination. Acta Derm Venereol. 2008;88(6):621-2.
10. Guimarães LE, Baker B, Perricone C, Shoenfeld Y. Vaccines, adjuvants and autoimmunity. Pharmacol Res. 2015;100:190-209.
11. Kuek A, Hazleman BL, Ostör AJK. Immune-mediated inflammatory diseases (IMIDs) and biologic therapy: a medical revolution. Postgrad Med J. 2007;83(978):251-60.
12. Bernatsky S, Hudson M, Suissa S. Anti-rheumatic drug use and risk of serious infections in rheumatoid arthritis. Rheumatol Oxf Engl. 2007;46(7):1157-60.
13. Schneeweiss S, Korzenik J, Solomon DH, Canning C, Lee J, Bressler B. Infliximab and other immunomodulating drugs in patients with inflammatory bowel disease and the risk of serious bacterial infections. Aliment Pharmacol Ther. 2009;30(3):253-64.
14. Furer V, Rondaan C, Heijstek MW, Agmon-Levin N, van Assen S, Bijl M, et al. 2019 update of EULAR recommendations for vaccination in adult patients with autoimmune inflammatory rheumatic diseases. Ann Rheum Dis. 2020;79(1):39-52.
15. Lang PO, Govind S, Michel JP, Aspinall R, Mitchell WA. Immunosenescence: Implications for vaccination programmes in adults. Maturitas. 2011;68(4):322-30.
16. Tanrıöver MD, Akar S, Türkçapar N, Karadağ Ö, Ertenli İ, Kiraz S. Vaccination recommendations for adult patients with rheumatic diseases. Eur J Rheumatol. 2016;3(1):29-35.
17. Centers for Disease Control and Prevention. (2023). Vaccine Recommendations and Guidelines of the ACIP. Timing and Spacing of Immunobiologics. [online] Available from https://www.cdc.gov/vaccines/hcp/acip-recs/general-recs/timing.html [Last accessed January, 2024].
18. Kobayashi M, Farrar JL, Gierke R, Britton A, Childs L, Leidner AJ, et al. Use of 15-Valent Pneumococcal Conjugate Vaccine and 20-Valent Pneumococcal Conjugate Vaccine Among U.S. Adults: Updated Recommendations of the Advisory Committee on Immunization Practices—United States, 2022. MMWR Morb Mortal Wkly Rep. 2022;71(4):109-17.
19. Coulson E, Saravanan V, Hamilton J, So KL, Morgan L, Heycock C, et al. Pneumococcal antibody levels after pneumovax in patients with rheumatoid arthritis on methotrexate. Ann Rheum Dis. 2011;70(7):1289-91.
20. Mease PJ, Ritchlin CT, Martin RW, Gottlieb AB, Baumgartner SW, Burge DJ, et al. Pneumococcal vaccine response in psoriatic arthritis patients during treatment with etanercept. J Rheumatol. 2004;31(7):1356-61.
21. Elkayam O, Ablin J, Caspi D. Safety and efficacy of vaccination against streptococcus pneumonia in patients with rheumatic diseases. Autoimmun Rev. 2007;6(5):312-4.
22. Nichol KL, Wuorenma J, von Sternberg T. Benefits of influenza vaccination for low-, intermediate-, and high-risk senior citizens. Arch Intern Med. 1998;158(16):1769-76.

23. Gelinck LBS, van der Bijl AE, Beyer WEP, Visser LG, Huizinga TWJ, van Hogezand RA, et al. The effect of anti-tumour necrosis factor alpha treatment on the antibody response to influenza vaccination. Ann Rheum Dis. 2008;67(5):713-6.
24. Fomin I, Caspi D, Levy V, Varsano N, Shalev Y, Paran D, et al. Vaccination against influenza in rheumatoid arthritis: the effect of disease modifying drugs, including TNF alpha blockers. Ann Rheum Dis. 2006;65(2):191-4.
25. Mathian A, Devilliers H, Krivine A, Costedoat-Chalumeau N, Haroche J, Huong DB, et al. Factors influencing the efficacy of two injections of a pandemic 2009 influenza A (H1N1) nonadjuvanted vaccine in systemic lupus erythematosus. Arthritis Rheum. 2011;63(11):3502-11.
26. Centers for Disease Control and Prevention. (2022). Vaccines and Preventable Diseases: Shingrix Recommendations. [online] Available from https://www.cdc.gov/vaccines/vpd/shingles/hcp/shingrix/recommendations.html [Last accessed January, 2024].
27. Anderson TC, Masters NB, Guo A, Shepersky L, Leidner AJ, Lee GM, et al. Use of Recombinant Zoster Vaccine in Immunocompromised Adults Aged ≥19 Years: Recommendations of the Advisory Committee on Immunization Practices—United States, 2022. MMWR Morb Mortal Wkly Rep. 2022;71(3):80-4.
28. Veetil BMA, Myasoedova E, Matteson EL, Gabriel SE, Green AB, Crowson CS. Incidence and time trends of herpes zoster in rheumatoid arthritis: a population-based cohort study. Arthritis Care Res. 2013;65(6):854-61.
29. Liang JL, Tiwari T, Moro P, Messonnier NE, Reingold A, Sawyer M, et al. Prevention of Pertussis, Tetanus, and Diphtheria with Vaccines in the United States: Recommendations of the Advisory Committee on Immunization Practices (ACIP). MMWR Recomm Rep Morb Mortal Wkly Rep Recomm Rep. 2018;67(2):1-44.
30. Chen Y, Wu X, Liu L. Association between systemic lupus erythematosus and risk of cervical atypia: A meta-analysis. Lupus. 2021;30(13):2075-88.
31. Wack S, Patton T, Ferris LK. COVID-19 vaccine safety and efficacy in patients with immune-mediated inflammatory disease: Review of available evidence. J Am Acad Dermatol. 2021;85(5):1274-84.
32. Shoenfeld Y, Agmon-Levin N. "ASIA"—autoimmune/inflammatory syndrome induced by adjuvants. J Autoimmun. 2011;36(1):4-8.
33. Perricone C, Colafrancesco S, Mazor RD, Soriano A, Agmon-Levin N, Shoenfeld Y. Autoimmune/inflammatory syndrome induced by adjuvants (ASIA) 2013: Unveiling the pathogenic, clinical and diagnostic aspects. J Autoimmun. 2013;47:1-16.
34. Lee SH. Detection of human papillomavirus L1 gene DNA fragments in postmortem blood and spleen after Gardasil® vaccination—A case report. Adv Biosci Biotechnol. 2012;3(8):1214-24.
35. Soriano A, Nesher G, Shoenfeld Y. Predicting post-vaccination autoimmunity: who might be at risk? Pharmacol Res. 2015;92:18-22.
36. Ministry of Health and Family Welfare, Government of India. (2023). Information Regarding COVID-19 Vaccine. [online] Available from https://www.mohfw.gov.in/covid_vaccination/vaccination/index.html [Last accessed January, 2024].
37. US Department of Health and Human Services. (2023). Recommended Adult Immunization Schedule for Ages 19 Years or Older, United States, 2024. [online] Available from https://www.cdc.gov/vaccines/schedules/downloads/adult/adult-combined-schedule.pdf [Last accessed January, 2024].

CHAPTER 30

Cost Effectiveness and Quality of Life with Biologic Therapy

Ankan Gupta, Jaya Krishna, Shekhar Neema

INTRODUCTION

Chronic skin diseases result in a significant economic burden to patients and society. It can limit daily activities, require frequent hospital visits and admissions, and result in a loss of productivity. The cost of illness can be divided into direct medical costs, which often include physician consultations, cost of the medicine, investigations, and need for hospitalizations, which can be quantified roughly, and indirect medical costs due to absence from work, early mortality, and time contributed by caregivers, which leads to loss of productivity and the costs of pain and suffering that cannot be quantified generally in monetary aspects as it varies from person to person.[1]

Biologics are rapidly evolving novel groups of drugs that provide better quality of life and superior clinical outcomes in terms of faster and sustained improvement and prevention of long-term morbidity compared with traditional immunosuppressives. Though biologics are one of the top-selling drugs worldwide, the main limitations of using it in developing countries such as India are the exorbitant cost of the drug, poor insurance coverage, and less awareness among health care professionals.[2] Whether the superior clinical outcome or improvement in quality of life is worth the cost difference is debatable and a subjective determinant. Still, the authors feel that every patient should be given a choice of the available therapeutic options and their expected outcomes. The following chapter is an effort to compare the cost-effectiveness with available therapeutics in dermatology. Indirect cost is difficult to calculate, varies from person to person, and is not considered for summation. We have also not included the cost of hospitalizations as it is difficult to predict its duration and frequency. The therapeutics' dosage, schedule, and monitoring protocols are based on standard guidelines. We recognize the heterogeneity in monitoring protocols and follow-up visit schedules with immunosuppressants at various centers. Consultation charges and daycare costs are chosen arbitrarily, and investigation costs are based on a popular private laboratory available in most cities in the country.

In countries where the treatment is neither funded by the government nor covered by the insurance companies consistently, pharmacoeconomic studies are needed to assess the cost-effectiveness of various therapeutic options from time to time. Till there is a conclusive answer, the option of using biologics should be a personal preference for the patient and the treating physician. This chapter attempts to assess the cost-effectiveness of various therapeutics in psoriasis, pemphigus, hidradenitis suppurativa, and chronic urticaria.

PSORIASIS

Psoriasis is a common, chronic, immune-mediated skin disorder affecting 2–3% of the general population.[3] Almost 20–30% of those affected have moderate-to-severe disease requiring systemic therapy. Psoriasis severely impairs the quality of life and results in an economic burden to those affected and society.[4] Systemic treatment options for psoriasis include photochemotherapy, methotrexate, cyclosporine, acitretin, hydroxyurea, and fumaric acid esters. Biologics give better clinical outcomes regarding faster and sustained reduction in psoriasis area severity index (PASI) and health-related quality of life (HRQoL) indices.[5]

Cost Analysis for Systemic Therapy in Psoriasis

For the purpose of this chapter, we have attempted to calculate only the direct costs of available treatment options for one year cycle. The cost of treatment for 2nd year and afterward is expected to be much lesser than the 1st year with the biologics because of their infrequent dosing in maintenance regimens **(Tables 1 and 2)**.

Comparison of Cost and Efficacy of Systemic and Biologic Therapy for Psoriasis (Tables 3 and 4)

Psoriasis area severity index-75 (PASI-75) is the meaningful endpoint for managing psoriasis, defined as a 75% improvement in PASI score from baseline that leads to an improvement in quality of life.[6] However, with the introduction of biologics with high efficacy, PASI 90/100 has also been established as a measure of effectiveness.[7]

Out of available systemic therapy for psoriasis, apremilast is the most cost-effective followed by narrowband ultraviolet B (NBUVB) as almost similar PASI-75 is achieved in 58% and 65% of patients respectively,[8,9] and therapy is relatively free of adverse effects. If available, NBUVB is a reasonable first-line therapy for managing chronic plaque psoriasis. Methotrexate is very efficacious for managing psoriasis and is cost-effective, though it requires

CHAPTER 30: Cost Effectiveness and Quality of Life with Biologic Therapy

TABLE 1: Cost analysis for systemic therapy in psoriasis for 1 year of therapy.

Drug	Cost of medicine	Schedule of treatment	Total cost for 1 year	Consultation	Investi-gations	Total cost
Metho-trexate Folic acid	₹43/- (15 mg) ₹2/- (5 mg)	15 mg/week 10 mg/week	₹2,064/- ₹208/-	Initial, after 15 days in the 1st month and monthly for 3 months, 3 monthly thereafter—total cost = 8 × 700 = ₹5,600/-	Initial: ₹8,000/- Monitoring: ₹5,280/- Cost of baseline FibroScan: ₹5,000/-	₹26,152/-

- Initial investigations include complete blood count (CBC), blood urea, serum creatinine, liver function test (LFT), blood sugar fasting and postprandial, chest X-ray, Mantoux or interferon-gamma release assays (IGRA), bloodborne virus screening
- Monitoring includes CBC, aspartate aminotransferase (SGOT), and alanine aminotransferase (SGPT)—after 7 days, 15 days, monthly for 3 months, and 3 monthly thereafter.
- A baseline FibroScan is ideal for all patients planned for long-term methotrexate. This is followed in authors' practice also

| Cyclo-sporine | ₹95/- (100 mg) | 300 mg/day—1 month 250 mg/day—1 month 200 mg/day—10 months | ₹72,390/- | Initial, after 15 days and monthly Total cost = 14 × 700 = ₹9,800/- | Initial: ₹3530/- Monitoring: ₹39,390/- | ₹1,25,110/- |

- Initial investigations include CBC, blood urea nitrogen, serum creatinine (twice in gap of 1 day), urinalysis, lipid profile, LFTs, serum potassium, magnesium, and uric acid level
- Monitoring test to be done every 15 days for 1 month and monthly thereafter. It includes CBC, LFT, urea, creatinine, triglycerides, cholesterol, uric acid, magnesium, and potassium
- Dose has been calculated as a stepdown approach for a 60 kg individual with normal renal function: 5 mg/kg for one month, 4 mg/kg for 1 month, and 3 mg/kg for rest of the duration. Cyclosporine is generally continued as a single drug for not >3–6 months and is rotated with some other drug such as acitretin. However, for ease of understanding and simplify the calculation, it has been shown to be used as monotherapy for 12 months

| Acitretin | ₹70/- (25 mg) | 50 mg once a day | ₹51,100/- | Initial and monthly—total cost 12 × 700 = ₹8,400/- | Initial: ₹2600/- Monitoring: ₹10,400/- Cost of X-ray wrist joint: ₹300/- | ₹72,800/- |

Continued

Continued

Drug	Cost of medicine	Schedule of treatment	Total cost for 1 year	Consultation	Investigations	Total cost
<td colspan="7">• Initial investigations include CBC, LFT, lipid profile, renal function test, and pregnancy test in women of childbearing potential • Monitoring—monthly for 3 months and 3 monthly thereafter. Includes CBC, LFT, lipid profile, renal function test, pregnancy test • Yearly X-ray of wrist or symptomatic joints in patient in long-term retinoid therapy • Dose can be used as 25, 50, or 75 mg once a day. Psoriasis area severity index (PASI) 75 is reached in 75% of patients on higher doses of retinoids than those who are on 25 mg (46%). 50 mg once a day has been used in calculation as it is effective in majority of cases on monotherapy with acitretin</td>
Narrow-band ultraviolet B (NBUVB) therapy	₹400/-	Start with 300 mg and increase as per guidelines	400 × 54 = ₹21,600/-	Initial and monthly— total cost 12 × 700 = ₹8,400/-	–	₹30,000/-
<td colspan="7">• Initial induction thrice weekly for 12 weeks, maintenance dose—twice a month. Total sessions 54 in a year. Psoralen and ultraviolet-A (PUVA) is more effective than NBUVB for management of psoriasis, however, it is more cumbersome to use. The cost of therapy will also increase, if we use psoralen</td>
Apremilast	₹295 (starter pack) ₹266 (30 mg BD for 10 tablets)	Starter pack for 1 week Maintenance pack of 30 mg BD for rest of the year	₹295/- ₹9,522/-	Initial, 3 monthly once 5 × 700 = ₹3,500/-	Initial = ₹150/- Monitoring = ₹600/-	₹14,067/-
<td colspan="7">• Initial investigations include serum creatinine • Monitoring includes serum creatinine</td>

frequent monitoring for adverse effects. Acitretin monotherapy can also be used to manage psoriasis; however, it may result in dose-limiting adverse effects when used at a dose of 50 mg/day. Cyclosporine is extremely effective for the management of psoriasis and results in PASI-75 and PASI-90 in almost 90% and 40% of patients, respectively;[10,11] however, it is more expensive as compared with other first-line treatments and cannot be used for longer periods. Cyclosporine is used intermittently as a crisis-buster drug to manage exacerbations.

Among biological therapy, adalimumab appears to be the most cost-effective as it leads to PASI-75 response in 75% of patients and PASI-90 response in 51% of patients at week 16.[12]

CHAPTER 30: Cost Effectiveness and Quality of Life with Biologic Therapy

TABLE 2: Cost analysis for biologics and biosimilar drugs in psoriasis for 1 year of therapy.

Drug	Cost of medicine	Schedule of treatment	Total cost	Consultation	Investigations	Total cost
Etanercept	₹17,170/- (MRP) Patient support programme (PSP)—first 6 pen—₹60,000/-, then every pen ₹6,000/- (50 mg)	• 50 mg twice weekly for 3 months • 50 mg once a week for 9 months = 60 injections	₹3,84,000/-	Initial, after 15 days, month and then 3 monthly 700 × 7 = ₹4,900/-	Initial: 5,400 Monitoring: ₹400 × 3 = ₹1,200/-	₹3,95,500/-
Biosimilar Intacept (Intas)	₹10,000/- (MRP) ₹5,833/- (PSP)	Same as above	₹3,49,980/-	Same	Same	₹3,60,080/-
Biosimilar Etacept (Cipla)	₹6700/- (MRP) for 25 mg injection ₹3000/- (reduced price)	Same	₹3,60,000/-	Same	Same	₹3,70,100/-

- Dose used is 50 mg twice weekly for 3 months and 50 mg/week thereafter. With this dose psoriasis area and severity index (PASI)-75 reached in 50% patients at the end of 12 weeks
- Maintenance dose can be reduced to 50 mg once a week or even 50 mg once every 2 weeks, thereby reducing the cost
- Initial investigations to be done are same as before initiating methotrexate, monitoring investigations are complete blood count (CBC) and liver function test (LFT) every 3 months. With tumor necrosis factor inhibitor (TNFi), we perform both QuantiFERON Tb assay and Mantoux test
- PASI-75, immunogenicity, and remission data for etanercept biosimilars are not available
- Median time to relapse after achieving remission with originator molecule is 84 days and drug can be discontinued for 3 months in a year, which will further reduce the cost of therapy

Infliximab

Remicade (original molecule)	₹20,500/- (MRP) for 100 mg vial PSP—₹16,400/- (100 mg vial)	5 mg/kg (3 vials) 0, 2, and 6 weeks and 8 weekly thereafter 27 vials	₹4,42,800/-	Initial, after 15 days for first infusion, after 2 weeks	Initial: ₹5,400/- Monitoring: ₹3,200/-	₹4,65,400/-

Continued

Continued

Drug	Cost of medicine	Schedule of treatment	Total cost	Consultation	Investigations	Total cost
		3 mg/kg 18 vials	₹2,95,200/-	For second infusion, after 4 weeks and 8 weekly Total 8 × 1,750 = ₹14,000/-		₹317,800/-
Biosimilar Infimab (Sun Pharma)	₹32,000 (MRP) for 100 mg vial ₹12,000/- (PSP)	Same	₹3,24,000/- (3 mg/kg ₹2,16,000/-)	Same	Same	₹3,46,600/- ₹2,38,600/-

- Dose has been calculated for a 60 kg patient at the rate of 5 mg/kg. PASI-75 response is seen in 80% patients with this dose
- 3 mg/kg dose can also be used, which results in PASI-75 response in almost 70% patients and results in significant reduction in cost
- Cost of consultation is higher as patient is required to be admitted in a daycare center for infusion
- Initial investigations are same as which are done for methotrexate except baseline antinuclear antibodies (ANA) needs to be done, monitoring requires CBC and LFT before every infusion

Adalimumab

| Biosimilar Exemptia (Zydus) Biosimilars Adfrar P (Torrent) Adalirel (Reliance) | ₹26,000/- (MRP) PSP—₹11,000/- | 80 mg loading dose. 40 mg week 1 and 40 g once every 2 weeks | 25 × 11,000 = ₹2,75,000/- | Initial, after 15 days, after 1 month and the 3 monthly 6 × 700 = ₹4,200/- | Initial: ₹5,400/- Monitoring: 400 × 3 = ₹1,200/- | ₹2,84,600/- |

- Initial investigations are same as other TNF alpha blockers, monitoring requires CBC and LFT every 3 months
- Scheduled dose results in PASI-75 improvement in almost 80% patients
- Originator molecule of adalimumab (Humira) is not available in India. Exemptia is most well-studied biosimilar, whereas other two molecules are intended copies (biosimilar) while cost almost remains same for all three

Continued

CHAPTER 30: Cost Effectiveness and Quality of Life with Biologic Therapy

Continued

Drug	Cost of medicine	Schedule of treatment	Total cost	Consultation	Investigations	Total cost
Secukinumab originator molecule, no biosimilar	₹16,000/- (150 mg vial) PSP—₹12,800/-	300 mg on week 0, 1, 2, 3, and 4 and monthly thereafter	₹4,09,600/- (32 × 12,800)	Initial, after 15 days, 1 month, and 3 monthly 7 × 700 = ₹4,900/-	Initial: ₹5,400/- Monitoring: 400 × 3 = ₹1,200/-	₹4,21,140/-
Itolizumab	₹7,950 (25 mg vial) (MRP) PSP—₹5,300/	1.6 mg/kg every 2 weeks for 12 week and once in 4 weeks till 24 weeks (for 70 kg—5 vial)	30 vials in induction and 15 vials in maintenance 45 × 5,300 = ₹2,38,500/-	Initial, every 2 weeks for 12 weeks and once in 4 weeks for 3 months and 3 monthly = 9 × 2,000 = ₹18,000/- (infusion) 2 × 700 = ₹1,400/- (follow-up)	Initial: ₹5,400/- Monitoring: 400 × 3 = ₹1,200/-	₹2,64,500/-
Ixekizumab	₹20,870/- per 80 mg pen	160 mg once, followed by 80 mg at every 2 weeks till 12 weeks, thereafter 80 mg every 4 weeks = 17 injections	₹3,54,790/-	Initial, after 15 days, 1 month, and then 3 monthly 700 ×7 = ₹4,900/-	Initial: ₹5,400/- Monitoring: ₹400 × 3 = ₹1,200/-	₹3,66,290/-

- Dose is administered for 6 months and patient to be observed without therapy, assuming that patient will maintain remission for next 6 months else cost of therapy could increase
- Initial and monitoring investigations are same as TNF alpha blockers
- Cost of consultation is high as it requires infusion
- PASI-75 response was seen in almost 45% patients

- Dose used is 160 mg once, followed by 80 mg at every 2 weeks till 12 weeks, thereafter 80 mg every 4 weeks
- With this dose PASI-75 reached in 89% patients at the end of 12 weeks
- Initial investigations and monitoring investigations to be done are same as like before initiating secukinumab

TABLE 3: Comparison of cost and efficacy of systemic and biologic therapy for psoriasis.

Drug	Efficacy		Studies	Cost in ₹ (For one year therapy)	Approximate cost of the therapy, 2nd year onwards
	Psoriasis area severity index (PASI)-75	PASI-90/100			
Methotrexate	35%	40%	CHAMPION (2008) Heydendael VM (2003)	₹ 26,152/-	₹ 13,152/-
	60%				
Cyclosporine (5 mg/kg)	97%	–	IMSGCP (1993) Laburte (1994)	₹ 1,25,110/-	–
	88.6%				
Acitretin	53%	–	Dogra (2013)	₹ 72,800/-	₹ 46,200/-
Apremilast	58%	29%	Shah (2020)	₹ 14,067/-	₹ 13,109/-
Phototherapy	65%	–	Dawe RS (2003)	₹ 30,000/-	₹ 30,000/-
Enbrel	49%	–	Leonardi CL (2003)	₹ 3,94,100/-	₹ 3,12,000/-
Intacept	–	–	No data available	₹ 3,60,080/-	₹ 3,03,316/-
Remicade (5 mg/kg)	80%	57%	Reich K (2005)	₹ 4,65,400/-	₹ 3,19,800/-
Remicade (3 mg/kg)	70%	37%	Menter A (2007)	₹ 2,95,200/-	₹ 2,13,200/-
Infimab	–	–	No data available	₹ 3,24,000/-	₹ 2,05,700/-
Adalimumab	75%	51%	CHAMPION (2008) Study done on originator molecule No studies in psoriasis available for biosimilar	₹ 2,84,600/-	₹ 2,62,600/-
Itolizumab	46%	–	Krupashankar DS (2014)	₹ 2,64,500/-	–
Secukinumab	86%	55%	Ohtsuki (2014)	₹ 4,21,440/-	₹ 3,48,000/- (300 mg) ₹ 1,74,000/- (150 mg)
Ixekizumab	89%	70%	Gordan (2016)	₹ 3,66,290/-	₹ 2,56,000/- (80 mg every 4 weeks)

- Reduction in cost of therapy in second year for most biologics is because of not using induction therapy in these patients

CHAPTER 30: Cost Effectiveness and Quality of Life with Biologic Therapy

TABLE 4: Comparison of cost per PASI and efficacy of systemic and biologic therapy for psoriasis.

Drug	Efficacy			Cost in ₹ (For one year therapy)	Cost per PASI reduction (Based on PASI 75 response)
	Psoriasis area severity index (PASI)-75	PASI-90/100	Studies		
Methotrexate	35% 60%	40%	CHAMPION (2008) Heydendael VM (2003)	₹ 26,152/-	₹ 871/- (PASI 75—40%)
Cyclosporine (5 mg/kg)	97% 88.6%	–	IMSGCP (1993) Laburte (1994)	₹ 1,25,110/-	₹ 1,853/- (PASI 75—90%)
Acitretin	53%	–	Dogra (2013)	₹ 72,800/-	₹ 1,941/-
Apremilast	58%	29%	Shah (2020)	₹ 14,067/-	₹ 323/-
Phototherapy	65%	–	Dawe RS (2003)	₹ 30,000/-	₹ 615/-
Enbrel	49%	–	Leonardi CL (2003)	₹ 3,94,100/-	₹ 10,761/-
Intacept	–	–	No data available	₹ 3,60,080/-	–
Remicade (5 mg/kg)	80%	57%	Reich K (2005)	₹ 4,65,400/-	₹ 7,756/-
Remicade (3 mg/kg)	70%	37%	Menter A (2007)	₹ 2,95,200/-	₹ 5,622/-
Infimab	–	–	No data available	₹ 3,24,000/-	–
Adalimumab	75%	51%	CHAMPION (2008) Study done on originator molecule No studies in psoriasis available for biosimilar	₹ 2,84,600/-	₹ 5,059/-
Itolizumab	46%	–	Krupashankar DS (2014)	₹ 2,64,500/-	₹ 7,666/-
Secukinumab	86%	55%	Ohtsuki (2014)	₹ 4,21,140/-	₹ 6,529/-
Ixekizumab	89%	70%	Gordan (2016)	₹ 3,66,290/-	₹ 5,487/-

- Cost per PASI was calculated as mentioned below
- For example, 80% of the patient achieved PASI-75. The total cost is let's say ₹ 10,000/-. So, we multiply 10,000 × 100/80 = 12,500/75 = ₹ 166/-. The cost to achieve per PASI would be 166

Adalimumab is followed by ixekizumab, secukinumab, infliximab (3 mg/kg), and infliximab (5 mg/kg).[13-16] However, infliximab is given as an infusion and requires repeated visits to a healthcare establishment. Etanercept appears to be the least cost-effective among biologicals, as it leads to PASI-75 response in 49% of patients and is more expensive than adalimumab and infliximab (5 mg/kg), with a much smaller number of patients achieving PASI-75.[17]

The National Institute of Clinical Excellence (NICE), UK guidelines (2012) suggest that biologics should be used when first-line conventional therapy cannot control the disease. The 2017 NICE guidelines for using biologics in psoriasis suggest that adalimumab should be the first line of biological treatment, especially when psoriatic arthritis is present. Secukinumab and ixekizumab are approved as first-line therapy and can be used as first-line biological therapy, irrespective of arthropathy. Infliximab should be reserved for patients with severe disease or when other biologics have failed.[18]

Various studies have been conducted to understand the cost-effectiveness of biologicals. A study was conducted on the economic impact of high-need psoriasis in the Netherlands before and after the introduction of biologics in 2010. The study concluded that patients during biological treatment resulted in a decrease in direct costs despite high treatment costs, this reduction in direct costs results from the decrease in medical consultation and hospitalization.[19] A study conducted by Fonia et al. in London had similar findings that while the cost of treatment increases significantly after the introduction of biologics, this cost reduces due to changes in the pattern of healthcare delivery in patients using biologics.[20] Nelson et al. conducted a cost-effectiveness study of biologics based on a literature review. In this study, the considered outcomes were PASI-75 and dermatology life quality index (DLQI) minimally important difference (MID). PASI-75 is a 75% improvement in the PASI score from baseline, while the five-point change in DLQI from baseline represents DLQI MID. As per this study, the most cost-effective medication for cost per patient achieving DLQI MID was etanercept 25 mg subcutaneously weekly, followed by infliximab 3 mg/kg for three infusions. The most cost-effective medication in terms of cost per patient achieving PASI-75 scores was infliximab 3 mg/kg, three infusions followed by adalimumab 40 mg subcutaneously every other week.[21] This study did not include drugs such as ustekinumab and secukinumab, as these drugs were unavailable when the study was conducted. Wu et al. in the United States and Riveros et al. in Brazil concluded that adalimumab 40 mg subcutaneously every other week was the most cost-effective drug to achieve PASI-75 scores.[22,23] Introducing new biologics in those patients who have failed or responded poorly to one biologic is a cost-effective alternative. It improves the quality of life in patients with severe psoriasis.[24] **Table 4** shows cost required to achieve per unit improvement in PASI. Apremilast appears to be most cost-effective drug as it does not require regular monitoring. NBUVB follows apremilast in cost effectiveness, however, indirect cost (travel and absence of work) is quite high with this form of treatment. Adalimumab is the most cost-effective biologic followed by ixekizumab and secukinumab.

PEMPHIGUS

Pemphigus is a group of immune blistering disorders characterized by acantholysis resulting in intraepithelial blisters in the skin and mucosa.[25] The different forms of pemphigus are distinguished by their clinical features and associated autoantigens, and pemphigus vulgaris represents the most common form. The incidence rate in an Indian study has been postulated to be 0.09–1.8%.[26,27]

Pemphigus usually occurs in adults, with an average age of onset at 40–60 years,[28] making it a high socioeconomic burden for the patient and the family, both in terms of direct and indirect costs. The initial treatment for the pemphigus group of diseases involves initiation of systemic steroids at 1–2 mg/kg body weight/day, which is universally accepted; however, the choice of the steroid-sparing agent for the treatment of the refractory cases and maintenance of remission is still an area of argument. The use of intravenous immunoglobulin (IVIg) as an emergency measure in nonresponsive cases, a norm in the West, is seldom practiced in India because of the high cost. Steroid-sparing immunosuppressants, such as azathioprine (Aza), mycophenolate mofetil (MMF), methotrexate, and cyclophosphamide (Cyc) are popularly used to minimize the risk of adverse effects of long-term steroids. They are prescribed either at the onset or subsequently in the treatment course.[29] Rituximab (Rtx), which was traditionally reserved for refractory pemphigus, is now routinely prescribed in nonrefractory cases to achieve sustained long-term complete remission.[30,31]

Cost Analysis for Systemic Therapy in Pemphigus (Tables 5 and 6)

Widespread loss of the skin barrier leads to hypoproteinemia, blood and fluid loss, electrolyte imbalances, and increased risk for local and systemic infections, which warrant supportive management and add to the cost of the therapy, which cannot be quantified and will not be discussed further in the chapter. Topical steroids and calcineurin inhibitors with daily therapeutic baths and dressings are also mandatory, and their cost depends upon the percentage of body area involved; hence difficult to quantify in monetary aspects.

Management of pemphigus vulgaris will be discussed hereafter to reference the pharmacoeconomic aspect of all vesiculobullous disorders. The scoring system used to measure the severity of pemphigus is the pemphigus disease activity index (PDAI) score, which is seldom used in most studies. Instead, definitions used for disease extent, severity, time to disease control, serum antibody titers, remission, relapses, and mortality are used according to the widely accepted consensus statement.[32] Although published literature does not support one therapeutic modality over another.[33]

TABLE 5: Cost analysis for systemic therapy in pemphigus.

Drug	Cost of medicine	Schedule of treatment	Total cost	Consultation	Investigations	Total cost
Azathioprine (2.5 mg/kg)	50 mg for ₹9.50/-	2.5 mg/kg for 12 weeks followed by tapering by 0.5 mg every 6–8 weeks	₹4,250/-	Every 2 weeks for first 2 months and every 2 months thereafter 14 × 500 = ₹7,000/-	a. ₹2,600/- b. 900 × 14 = ₹12,600/-	₹19,450/-
a. Initial investigations that are not done as a part of presteroid workup include liver function test (LFT) and thiopurine methyltransferase activity						
b. Monitoring includes LFT every 2 weeks for first 2 months and every 2 months thereafter						
Mycophenolate mofetil	500 mg for ₹62/-	1–3 g/day	₹18,350/- to ₹55,000/-	Every 2 weeks during the first 2 months, once monthly thereafter 500 × 18 = ₹9,000/-	a. ₹1,100/- b. ₹1,100 × 18 = ₹19,800/-	₹48,250/- to ₹84,900/-
a. Initial extra investigations include LFT and renal function test (RFT)						
b. Monitoring includes LFT and RFT every 2 weeks during the first 2 months, once monthly within the first year, and every 3 months thereafter						
Cyclophosphamide	50 mg for ₹4/-	1–3 mg/kg/day	₹1,160/- to ₹3,480/-	Every 2 weeks during the first 2 months, once monthly thereafter 500 × 18 = ₹9,000/-	a. ₹1,100/- b. ₹1,100 × 18 = ₹19,800/-	₹31,060/- to ₹33,380/-
a. Initial extra investigations include LFT and RFT						
b. Monitoring includes LFT and RFT every 2 weeks during the first month followed by monthly for as long as on the drug						
Rituximab	500 mg for ₹37,675/-	Schedule A: 1 g on days 1 and 14	₹1,50,700/-	Every month for the first 3 months and quarterly thereafter 500 × 6 = ₹3000/-	₹12,500/-	₹1,66,200/-
		Schedule B: 500 g on days 1 and 14	₹75,350/-	Same as above	Same as above	₹90,850/-

Continued

Continued

Drug	Cost of medicine	Schedule of treatment	Total cost	Consultation	Investigations	Total cost
Rituximab (IPCA) (Biosimilar)	500 mg for 12,000/-	Schedule A: 1 g on days 1 and 14	₹48,000/-	Every month for the first 3 months and quarterly thereafter 500 × 6 = ₹ 3,000/-	₹12,500/-	₹60,500/-
		Schedule B: 500 g on days 1 and 14	₹24,000/-	Same as above	Same as above	₹36,500/-

- Initial extra investigations include blood borne virus screening along with Hepatitis-B core antibody, QuantiFERON Tb assay, echocardiography (ECHO) with echocardiogram (ECG)
- Monitoring includes no investigations, particularly blood counts are monitored as with other immunosuppressives

Drug	Cost of medicine	Schedule of treatment	Total cost	Consultation	Investigations	Total cost
Dexamethasone-cyclophosphamide pulse	Dexamethasone injection for ₹75/- Cyclophosphamide injection for ₹75/- Dextrose for ₹35/- Daily Tab Cyclophosphamide 50 mg for ₹3.79/-	Dexamethasone 100 mg on day 1, 2, and 3 in 5% of 500 mL dextrose Cyclophosphamide 500 mg on day 2 Daily cyclophosphamide at 50 mg/day	₹6,133/-	Every month in a day-care facility for 3 days 3,000 × 12 = ₹36,000/-	2280 × 12 = ₹27,360/-	₹69,493/-

a. Daily ECG and serum electrolytes on all 3 days of pulse and urinalysis prior to and after the 2nd day is practiced in most centers
b. The regimen does not include daily steroids and that cost may be deducted from the other regimens mentioned above, which include continuous use of steroids
c. The cost of consultation is higher as it includes 3 days of daycare admission also

TABLE 6: Cost analysis for adjuvant drugs in pemphigus for one year of therapy.	
The adjuvant drug	Cost in ₹ (for 1 year therapy)
Azathioprine	19,450/-
Mycophenolate mofetil	48,250/-
Cyclophosphamide	31,060/-
Rituximab	90,850/- (Schedule B)
Rituximab (IPCA)—biosimilar	36,500/- (Schedule B)
Dexamethasone-cyclophosphamide (DCP) pulse	69,493/-

In the author's experience, Rtx is a far superior therapy for pemphigus, especially when used early in the disease for early control and sustained remission of the disease process. It was approved by the United States Food and Drug Administration (USFDA) for moderate-to-severe pemphigus vulgaris in 2018. The adjuvants discussed here include Aza, MMF, Cyc, and Rtx **(Tables 5 and 6)**. The general toxicity of Cyc makes it a lesser favorable option. Most literature on the treatment aspect of pemphigus suggests avoidance of Cyc as a steroid-sparing agent as far as possible.[34-36] Another popular therapy conceptualized in India and widely practiced is dexamethasone-cyclophosphamide or plain dexamethasone pulse therapy.[37] The rationale of the duration and dosage of therapy is poorly understood, and outcome data concerning the attainment of early and late endpoints (Murrell et al.,) is unavailable.[32]

The timing of the introduction of the steroid-sparing drug is also controversial. Few dermatologists introduce them at the start of the treatment along with systemic steroids or use them in treatment-resistant cases or when disease flares, and some introduce them later in the course of the illness after decreasing the doses of steroids to maintain remission, reduce the risk of relapse and to avoid profound immunosuppression at once. An increase in doses of steroids rather than adding an adjuvant, all of which are slow-acting drugs, helps more in the disease control process.[38]

For a fair calculation, we assume a 60 kg adult male with no comorbidities who initially started on systemic steroids. The adjuvant is introduced later in the disease when the steroid has been tapered to 40 mg/day (0.66 mg/kg/day). Like psoriasis, the indirect cost of disease and cost of hospitalization is not calculated, and the cost of a 12-month treatment period is chosen for cost-effective analysis purposes as that (8–16 months) is the average period after which a pemphigus patient achieves complete remission on therapy.[39-42]

The calculations are based on the premise that the treatment with the adjuvant was given until the patient achieved complete remission on therapy which hypothetically is 12 months on average, which is not the case in every patient and is created to have a logical comparison.

CHAPTER 30: Cost Effectiveness and Quality of Life with Biologic Therapy

We will fail in our duties if we do not mention that the total amount of steroid needed is much less and the average duration to achieve initial and eventual clinical remission is far lesser with Rtx as compared with the other steroid-sparing adjuvant options, which brings down the indirect costs of the therapy by a huge amount. The studies used to calculate the average duration of treatment also mention failure and relapse cases, which are the least with Rtx. Though the difference between Aza and Rtx with this calculation is a lot, it would be interesting to calculate it in a real-life prospective study, which should be much lesser, according to the author's opinion. The initial one-time expense is a limiting factor in the Indian population that usually deters the clinician and patient from opting for Rtx. Still, the overall treatment cost would not differ much to achieve sustained complete remission. According to most experts, healthcare professionals should encourage using Rtx, which has been a game changer in managing vesiculobullous disorders.

Cost Analysis for Biologics and Biosimilar Drugs of Rituximab

The maximum retail price of Ristova, the biologics, and the biosimilars such as Reditux, Ikgdar, Rituxirel, Ipca, and Mabtas is almost the same. Still, most biosimilars are available at 50% of the cost to most institutes, which brings the cost of Rtx therapy down. Although there are no head-to-head trials between biologics and biosimilars for pemphigus in the literature, the efficacy of biosimilars has been proven beyond doubt based on the author's experience.

HIDRADENITIS SUPPURATIVA

Hidradenitis suppurativa (HS) is a chronic, painful follicular occlusive disorder that affects the pilosebaceous glands, mainly at intertriginous skin, which causes profound psychosocial distress and a significant life impact in many patients.[43] The estimated prevalence of HS ranges from 1 to 4%.[44] It usually occurs in adolescents and adults with an average onset of age between 20 and 40 years,[45] who are the main workforce in the country, making it a high socioeconomic burden for the patient and family in terms of direct and indirect costs. Being simple, most of the clinicians used Hurley staging to assess the disease severity; however, validated scoring systems such as Hidradenitis suppurativa clinical response (HiSCR) and the International Hidradenitis suppurativa severity scoring system (IHS4) were used as clinical trial outcome measures,[46,47] along with DLQI and physician global assessment (PGA).

Cost Analysis of Systemic Therapy in Hidradenitis Suppurativa (Tables 7 and 8)

Management of HS involves systemic medical therapy and surgical therapy, often in Hurley stage 2 or 3. It also involves wound and skin care, including

TABLE 7: Cost analysis for conventional and biologics drugs in hidradenitis suppurativa (HS) for 12 weeks of therapy.

Drug	Cost of medicine	Schedule of treatment	Total cost	Consultation	Investigations	Total cost
Infliximab						
Remicade (original molecule)	₹20,500/- (MRP) for 100 mg vial ₹16,400/- (100 mg vial)—PSP (patient support programme)	5 mg/kg at 0, 2, 6 weeks and 8 weekly thereafter	₹65,600/-	Initial, after 2 weeks for second infusion, after 4 weeks and 8 weekly Total of 4 × 1,750 = ₹7,000/-	Initial: ₹5,400/- Monitoring: ₹3,200/-	₹81,200/-
Biosimilar Infimab (Sun Pharma)	₹32,000/- (MRP) for 100 mg vial ₹12,000/ (PSP—patient support programme)	Same	₹48,000/-	Same	Same	₹63,600/-

- Dose has been calculated for 60 kg patient at the rate of 5 mg/kg. Hidradenitis Suppurativa Severity Index (HSSI) >50% reduction in >30% patients by week 8.[55]
- Cost of consultation is higher as patient is required to be admitted in daycare center for infusion
- Initial investigations are same as which are done for methotrexate except baseline antinuclear antibodies (ANA) need to be done, monitoring requires complete blood count (CBC) and liver function test (LFT) before every infusion

Drug	Cost of medicine	Schedule of treatment	Total cost	Consultation	Investigations	Total cost
Adalimumab						
Biosimilar Exemptia (Zydus)	₹26,000/- (MRP) PSP—₹11,000/- (40 mg)	160 mg subcutaneous (SUBQ) over first 2 days, then 80 mg after 2 weeks, thereafter 40 mg every week	16 × 11,000 = ₹1,76,000/-	Initial, after 15 days, after 1 month and the 3 monthly 4 × 700 = ₹2,800/-	Initial: ₹5,400/- Monitoring: 400 × 2 = ₹800/-	₹1,85,000/-

- Initial investigations are same as other tumor necrosis factor (TNF) alpha blockers, monitoring requires CBC and LFT every 3 months
- Scheduled dose resulted HS clinical response (HiSCR) >50% reduction in >48% patients by week 12 **(Abbvie et al.)**[66]
- Originator molecule of adalimumab (Humira) is not available in India. Exemptia is the most well-studied biosimilar

Continued

Continued

Drug	Cost of medicine	Schedule of treatment	Total cost	Consultation	Investigations	Total cost
Secukinumab Originator molecule, no biosimilar	₹16,000/- (150 mg vial) PSP—₹12,800/-	300 mg on week 0, 1, 2, 3, 4, and monthly thereafter	₹89,600/- (7 × 12,800)	Initial, after 15 days, one month and 3 monthly 6 × 700 = ₹4,200/-	Initial: ₹6,300/- Monitoring: ₹400 × 3 = ₹1,200/-	₹1,01,300/-
• Scheduled dose resulted HiSCR> 50% reduction in >42% patients by week 16[56]						
• Initial investigations include CBC, blood urea, serum creatinine, LFT, blood sugar fasting and postprandial, chest X-ray, Mantoux or interferon-gamma release assay (IGRA), bloodborne virus screening, C-reactive protein (CRP), stool occult blood, and stool calprotectin						
Ertapenem rescue therapy	₹3,100/- (1 g vial)	1 g once daily for 6 weeks intravenous route via peripherally inserted central catheter (PICC) line	3100 × 42 = ₹1,32,000/-	Initial, after 3 weeks for PICC line replacement 2 × 2500 = ₹5,000/-	Initial: ₹2,000/- Monitoring: ₹2,000/-	₹1,41,000/-
• Scheduled dose resulted >50% reduction in sartorius scores and 67% and 26% into remission of Hurley stage 1 and stage 2 respectively at the end of treatment[54]						
• Initial and monitoring investigations include CBC, serum creatinine, and LFT						
Doxycycline	100 mg – ₹8/-	100 mg twice daily for 12 weeks	₹1344 /-	Initial consultation = ₹750/-	Initial: ₹2,000/- Monitoring: ₹2,000/-	₹6,094/-
• Initial and monitoring investigations include CBC, serum creatinine, and LFT						
Rifampicin + clindamycin combination therapy	₹3,100 (1 g vial) Rifampicin 300 mg: ₹5/- Clindamycin 300 mg: ₹23/-	Rifampicin 600 mg once daily and clindamycin 300 mg twice daily for 10–12 weeks	₹4,704/-	Initial consultation = ₹750/-	Initial: ₹2,000/- Monitoring: ₹2,000/-	₹9,454/-
• Scheduled dose resulted clinical response in 73% of patients at week 12[53]						
• Initial and monitoring investigations include CBC, serum creatinine, and LFT						

TABLE 8: Cost analysis for therapeutic option in hidradenitis suppurativa (HS) for 12 weeks.

The drug	Cost in ₹ (for 12 weeks therapy)
Doxycycline	6,094/-
Rifampicin + clindamycin	9,454/-
Adalimumab	1,85,000/-
Infimab (Biosimilar infliximab)	63,600/-
Secukinumab	1,01,300/-
Ertapenem rescue therapy for 6 weeks	1,41,000/-

topical medications and therapeutic baths and pain management, which warrant supportive management and add to the cost of the therapy, which cannot be quantified in general as it varies from person to person depending upon the area of involvement and hence will not be discussed further in the chapter.

The European S1 guideline (2015) for the treatment of HS recommends systemic antibiotics as initial measures such as doxycycline (Doxy), rifampicin + clindamycin (R+C) are indicated when more severe lesions present. Biologics, such as adalimumab or infliximab, are recommended if there is no satisfactory sustained disease control to systemic antibiotic therapy.[48] Biologics of IL-17 blockers such as secukinumab were the next preferred option, which had no sufficient improvement with adalimumab as per the European Commission.

Patients with HS may be at high risk of multiple comorbid conditions,[49,50] which cannot be quantified in general. For a fair calculation, we assume a 60 kg adult male with no comorbidities is started on conventional systemic medical therapy without surgical intervention. Management of HS will be discussed hereafter to reference the pharmacoeconomic aspects.

Like psoriasis, the indirect cost of disease and hospitalization is not calculated. The cost of a 12-week treatment period is chosen for cost-effective analysis purposes as that (10–12 weeks) is the average period after which an HS patient achieves good clinical response with Doxy, R+C, adalimumab.[48,51,52] However long-term benefit of treatment was highly variable. Still, sustained responses were more in patients treated with biologics though not cost-effective. The R+C combination seems more cost-effective in achieving good clinical response in almost 73% of patients at week 12.[53,54] Among biologics, infliximab and secukinumab showed almost similar results.[55,56] However, biosimilar infliximab is less expensive than secukinumab in achieving almost similar HiSCR. Surgical treatment might be a long-term, cost-effective option, based on the body region and disease severity, which is not accounted for in this chapter.

CHRONIC URTICARIA

Chronic spontaneous urticaria (CSU) is defined by the appearance of recurrent wheals, angioedema, or both, for 6 weeks or longer without any identifiable trigger, which is the most common form of chronic urticaria,[57] which significantly affects the patient's quality of life. Its prevalence varies from region to region, but the estimated lifetime prevalence is around 1.4%.[58] CSU exhibits natural remission typically within 1–5 years, though in some cases, the condition may be present for over 20 years.[59,60] Although it affects all age groups, the peak incidence is seen between the 20 and 40 age group,[60] which accounts for the high socioeconomic burden to patients and families regarding direct healthcare costs and indirect costs like loss of working hours. The initial treatment for this group of diseases involves the initiation of second-generation antihistamines, which can go up to a maximum of a fourfold increase in the dose. A short course of glucocorticoids may be considered in cases of acute severe exacerbation; however, it may not be a long-term solution as it poses potential severe side effects.[57] There were no potential biomarkers to predict response to various therapies for refractory CSU.[61] Among all, at least 35% of CSU patients are refractory to antihistamines and require additional second-line therapy such as omalizumab (Omz) or cyclosporine for control of disease as per the European Academy of Allergy and Clinical Immunology (EAACI) 2018 guidelines.[57,62] Omalizumab is the only biologic licensed currently for CSU.[63]

Cost Analysis of Biologics in Chronic Spontaneous Urticaria (Tables 9 to 11)

Management of chronic urticaria will be discussed hereafter regarding the pharmacoeconomic aspect. The scoring systems used to assess the severity and predict the clinical response in CSU were the Urticaria Activity Score (UAS), Urticaria Activity Score over seven days (UAS7), DLQI, and Chronic Urticaria Quality of Life Questionnaire (CU-Q2oL).[57] Acute exacerbation management with a short course of steroids and angioedema with anaphylaxis episodes were not accounted for in this chapter, as these episodes vary from person to person and cannot be quantified. Thus, adding omalizumab to the combination of maximally dosed H1 antihistamines in refractory cases achieved significant satisfactory disease control in approximately 80% of patients by week 12, with sustained effects up to 24 weeks with just an additional 20,000 rupees extra.[64] It was shown that omalizumab therapy for 1 year allows tapering to 150 mg with gradual lengthening between injections at intervals of 8 weeks.[65] On long-term tapering of omalizumab with less dosage and more intervals, we can achieve satisfactory results with sustained outcomes at a lesser cost.

TABLE 9: Cost analysis of drugs in chronic spontaneous urticaria (CSU) before omalizumab for 16 weeks of therapy.

Drug	Cost of medicine	Standard of treatment	Total cost	Consultation	Investigations	Total cost of CSU before omalizumab
Standard of care (nonsedating antihistamines up to four-fold the standard dose) Cetirizine 10 mg	One tablet of 10 mg = ₹3/-	4 weeks × 1 time dosing = 56 units 4 weeks × 2 times dosing = 112 units 4 weeks × 3 times dosing = 168 units 4 weeks × 4 times dosing = 224 units	560 × 3 = ₹1,680/-	Two consultations at initial visit and then after 4 weeks 2 × 700 = ₹1,400/-	Baseline investigations = ₹ 4,650/-	₹ 7,730/-

Note:
- Initial investigations include antinuclear antibody (ANA), thyroid-stimulating hormone (TSH), T4, thyroid antibodies, fasting blood sugar (FBS), postprandial blood sugar (PPBS), complete blood count (CBC), IgE
- As per the European Academy of Allergy and Clinical Immunology (EAACI) 2018 guidelines, treatment with antihistamines OD dose and up dose titrate up to 4 times with interval assessment of 4 weeks[57]

CONCLUSION

Biologics are an important addition to the armamentarium of physicians managing chronic skin diseases. Biologics increase the direct cost of therapy and increase the disease's economic burden during the initial treatment period. Still, the indirect cost comes down significantly with superior clinical outcomes. The use of biologics only for treatment-resistant cases just because of the cost is not justified and every patient should be foretold the treatment options and given a choice to choose the modality he prefers. Soon, as market size increases and people's awareness about insurance increases, biologics could be the most cost-effective option with significant clinical outcomes in most chronic skin diseases.

ADDENDUM

The authors have taken the costs of investigations and drugs from prevailing market rates and verified them to the best of their knowledge. However, India is a huge and heterogeneous market, and rates of drugs may vary from place to place and from time to time. These calculations have only been done to understand the cost-effectiveness of various drugs for these diseases and have no legal or financial implications. Brand names have been used in this chapter liberally for understanding purpose. The authors have no financial conflict of interest.

TABLE 10: Cost analysis of drugs in chronic spontaneous urticaria after adding omalizumab for 12 weeks of therapy in addition to antihistamines care for a total of 28 weeks.

Drug	Cost of medicine	Standard of treatment	Total cost	Consultation	Investigations	Total cost for antihistamines	Total cost for omalizumab	Total cost for antihistamines + omalizumab
Standard of care (nonsedating antihistamines up to fourfold the standard dose) Cetirizine 10 mg	Same as in **Table 9** before adding omalizumab					For standard antihistamines of initial 4 months) + extra 3 months while on omalizumab ₹7,730 + ₹2,772 = ₹10,502/-	₹20,000/-	₹30,502/-
Omalizumab 3 × 700 = ₹2,100/- -NA-	₹8,400/ for 150 mg vial ₹6,000/ (PSP)— patient support programe	300 mg subcutaneous (SUBQ) every 4 weeks once	₹6000/- × 3 = ₹18,000/-	Monthly once consultation for injection				

Note:
- Initial investigations include antinuclear antibody (ANA), thyroid-stimulating hormone (TSH), T4, thyroid antibodies, fasting blood sugar (FBS), postprandial blood sugar (PPBS), complete blood count (CBC), IgE
- As per the European Academy of Allergy and Clinical Immunology (EAACI) 2018 guidelines, omalizumab is considered to be added in addition to standard of care which up to fourfold antihistamines[57]
- No special investigations are required before initiating omalizumab—just to monitor for anaphylaxis episodes
- Omalizumab standard dosing achieves satisfactory control of CSU in terms of Urticaria Activity Score (UAS) in approximately 80% of patients by week 12 along with antihistamines[64]

TABLE 11: Cost analysis for therapeutic option in chronic spontaneous urticaria (CSU) for a period of 28 weeks.

Cost of therapy	Cost in ₹
Before adding omalizumab for 16 weeks	7,730/-
After adding omalizumab along with antihistamines at 17th week till 28th week	30,502/-

REFERENCES

1. Centers for Disease Control and Prevention. (2021). Cost of Illness. POLARIS. Policy, Performance, and Evaluation. [online]. Available from https://www.cdc.gov/policy/polaris/economics/cost-illness/index.html#:~:text=Cost%20of%20illness%20analysis%20may,and%20drugs%20and%20medical%20supplies [Last accessed January, 2024].
2. O'Callaghan J, Bermingham M, Leonard M, Hallinan F, Morris JM, Moore U, et al. Assessing awareness and attitudes of healthcare professionals on the use of biosimilar medicines: A survey of physicians and pharmacists in Ireland. Regul Toxicol Pharmacol. 2017;88:252-61.
3. Rajagopalan M, Mital A. Biologics use in Indian psoriasis patients. Indian Dermatol Online J. 2016;7(6):489-97.
4. Parisi R, Symmons DPM, Griffiths CEM, Ashcroft DM, Identification and Management of Psoriasis and Associated ComorbidiTy (IMPACT) project team. Global epidemiology of psoriasis: a systematic review of incidence and prevalence. J Invest Dermatol. 2013;133(2):377-85.
5. Merola JF, Lockshin B, Mody EA. Switching biologics in the treatment of psoriatic arthritis. Semin Arthritis Rheum. 2017;47(1):29-37.
6. Reich K, Griffiths CEM. The relationship between quality of life and skin clearance in moderate-to-severe psoriasis: lessons learnt from clinical trials with infliximab. Arch Dermatol Res. 2008;300(10):537-44.
7. Puig L. PASI90 response: the new standard in therapeutic efficacy for psoriasis. J Eur Acad Dermatol Venereol JEADV. 2015;29(4):645-8.
8. Shah BJ, Mistry D, Chaudhary N, Shah S. Real-world efficacy and safety of apremilast monotherapy in the management of moderate-to-severe psoriasis. Indian Dermatol Online J. 2020;11(1):51-7.
9. Dawe RS. A quantitative review of studies comparing the efficacy of narrow-band and broad-band ultraviolet B for psoriasis. Br J Dermatol. 2003;149(3):669-72.
10. Marsili F, Travaglini M, Stinco G, Manzoni R, Tiberio R, Prignano F, et al. Effectiveness of cyclosporine A in patients with moderate to severe plaque psoriasis in a real-life clinical setting in Italy: the TRANSITION study. J Dermatol Treat [Internet]. 2022;33(1):401-7.
11. Thaçi D, Bräutigam M, Kaufmann R, Weidinger G, Paul C, Christophers E. Body-weight-independent dosing of cyclosporine micro-emulsion and three times weekly maintenance regimen in severe psoriasis. A randomised study. Dermatol Basel Switz. 2002;205(4):383-8.
12. Saurat JH, Stingl G, Dubertret L, Papp K, Langley RG, Ortonne JP, et al. Efficacy and safety results from the randomized controlled comparative study of adalimumab vs. methotrexate vs. placebo in patients with psoriasis (CHAMPION). Br J Dermatol. 2008;158(3):558-66.
13. Menter A, Feldman SR, Weinstein GD, Papp K, Evans R, Guzzo C, et al. A randomized comparison of continuous vs. intermittent infliximab maintenance regimens over 1

year in the treatment of moderate-to-severe plaque psoriasis. J Am Acad Dermatol. 2007;56(1):31.e1-31.e15.
14. Krupashankar DS, Dogra S, Kura M, Saraswat A, Budamakuntla L, Sumathy TK, et al. Efficacy and safety of itolizumab, a novel anti-CD6 monoclonal antibody, in patients with moderate to severe chronic plaque psoriasis: results of a double-blind, randomized, placebo-controlled, phase-III study. J Am Acad Dermatol. 2014;71(3):484-92.
15. Ohtsuki M, Morita A, Abe M, Takahashi H, Seko N, Karpov A, et al. Secukinumab efficacy and safety in Japanese patients with moderate-to-severe plaque psoriasis: subanalysis from ERASURE, a randomized, placebo-controlled, phase 3 study. J Dermatol. 2014;41(12):1039-46.
16. Gordon KB, Blauvelt A, Papp KA, Langley RG, Luger T, Ohtsuki M; UNCOVER-1 Study Group; UNCOVER-2 Study Group; UNCOVER-3 Study Group. Phase 3 trials of ixekizumab in moderate-to-severe plaque psoriasis. N Engl J Med. 2016;375(4):345-56.
17. Papp KA, Tyring S, Lahfa M, Prinz J, Griffiths CEM, Nakanishi AM, et al. A global phase III randomized controlled trial of etanercept in psoriasis: safety, efficacy, and effect of dose reduction. Br J Dermatol. 2005;152(6):1304-12.
18. Smith CH, Jabbar-Lopez ZK, Yiu ZZ, Bale T, Burden AD, Coates LC, et al. British Association of Dermatologists guidelines for biologic therapy for psoriasis 2017. Br J Dermatol. 2017;177(3):628-36.
19. Driessen RJB, Bisschops LA, Adang EMM, Evers AW, Van De Kerkhof PCM, De Jong EMGJ. The economic impact of high-need psoriasis in daily clinical practice before and after the introduction of biologics. Br J Dermatol. 2010;162(6):1324-9.
20. Fonia A, Jackson K, Lereun C, Grant DM, Barker JNWN, Smith CH. A retrospective cohort study of the impact of biologic therapy initiation on medical resource use and costs in patients with moderate to severe psoriasis. Br J Dermatol. 2010;163(4):807-16.
21. Nelson AA, Pearce DJ, Fleischer AB, Balkrishnan R, Feldman SR. Cost-effectiveness of biologic treatments for psoriasis based on subjective and objective efficacy measures assessed over a 12-week treatment period. J Am Acad Dermatol. 2008;58(1):125-35.
22. Wu JJ, Feldman SR, Rastogi S, Menges B, Lingohr-Smith M, Lin J. Comparison of the cost-effectiveness of biologic drugs used for moderate-to-severe psoriasis treatment in the United States. J Dermatol Treat. 2018;29(8):769-74.
23. Riveros BS, Ziegelmann PK, Correr CJ. Cost-effectiveness of biologic agents in the treatment of moderate-to-severe psoriasis: A Brazilian Public Health Service Perspective. Value Health Reg Issues. 2014;5:65-72.
24. Sawyer LM, Wonderling D, Jackson K, Murphy R, Samarasekera EJ, Smith CH. Biological therapies for the treatment of severe psoriasis in patients with previous exposure to biological therapy: a cost-effectiveness analysis. PharmacoEconomics. 2015;33(2):163-77.
25. Mihai S, Sitaru C. Immunopathology and molecular diagnosis of autoimmune bullous diseases. J Cell Mol Med. 2007;11(3):462-81.
26. Kanwar AJ, Ajith AC, Narang T. Pemphigus in North India. J Cutan Med Surg. 2006;10(1):21-5.
27. Mascarenhas MF, Hede RV, Shukla P, Nadkarni NS, Rege VL. Pemphigus in Goa. J Indian Med Assoc. 1994;92(10):342-3.
28. Joly P, Litrowski N. Pemphigus group (vulgaris, vegetans, foliaceus, herpetiformis, brasiliensis). Clin Dermatol. 2011;29(4):432-6.
29. Bystryn JC, Steinman NM. The adjuvant therapy of pemphigus. An update. Arch Dermatol. 1996;132(2):203-12.
30. Ahmed AR, Spigelman Z, Cavacini LA, Posner MR. Treatment of pemphigus vulgaris with rituximab and intravenous immune globulin. N Engl J Med. 2006;355(17):1772-9.
31. Schmidt E, Goebeler M, Zillikens D. Rituximab in severe pemphigus. Ann N Y Acad Sci. 2009;1173(1):683-91.

32. Murrell DF, Dick S, Ahmed AR, Amagia M, Barnadas MA, Borradori L, et al. Consensus statement on definitions of disease, end points, and therapeutic response for pemphigus. J Am Acad Dermatol. 2008;58(6):1043-6.
33. Martin LK, Werth VP, Villanueva EV, Murrell DF. A systematic review of randomized controlled trials for pemphigus vulgaris and pemphigus foliaceus. J Am Acad Dermatol. 2011;64(5):903-8.
34. Zhao CY, Murrell DF. Pemphigus vulgaris: an evidence-based treatment update. Drugs. 2015;75(3):271-84.
35. Vanstreels L, Alkhateeb A, Megahed M. [Pemphigus vulgaris. Therapy with cyclophosphamide]. Hautarzt Z Dermatol Venerol Verwandte Geb. 2013;64(5):330-2.
36. Ruocco E, Wolf R, Ruocco V, Brunetti G, Romano F, Lo Schiavo A. Pemphigus: associations and management guidelines: facts and controversies. Clin Dermatol. 2013;31(4):382-90.
37. Kanwar AJ, De D. Pemphigus in India. Indian J Dermatol Venereol Leprol. 2011;77(4):439-49.
38. Atzmony L, Hodak E, Leshem YA, Rosenbaum O, Gdalevich M, Anhalt GJ, et al. The role of adjuvant therapy in pemphigus: A systematic review and meta-analysis. J Am Acad Dermatol. 2015;73(2):264-71.
39. Mutalik SD, Rasal Y. Sustained remission of pemphigus in Indian patients with a modified lymphoma rituximab protocol. J Dermatol Res. 2018;3(1):135-8.
40. Iranzo P, Pigem R, Giavedoni P, Alsina-Gibert M. Remission time after rituximab treatment for autoimmune bullous disease: A proposed update definition. Skin Pharmacol Physiol. 2015;28(5):255-6.
41. Almugairen N, Hospital V, Bedane C, Duvert-Lehembre S, Picard D, Tronquoy AF, et al. Assessment of the rate of long-term complete remission off therapy in patients with pemphigus treated with different regimens including medium- and high-dose corticosteroids. J Am Acad Dermatol. 2013;69(4):583-8.
42. Joly P, Maho-Vaillant M, Prost-Squarcioni C, Hebert V, Houivet E, Calbo S, et al. First-line rituximab combined with short-term prednisone versus prednisone alone for the treatment of pemphigus (Ritux 3): a prospective, multicentre, parallel-group, open-label randomised trial. Lancet Lond Engl. 2017;389(10083):2031-40.
43. Kouris A, Platsidaki E, Christodoulou C, Efstathiou V, Dessinioti C, Tzanetakou V, et al. Quality of life and psychosocial implications in patients with hidradenitis suppurativa. Dermatol Basel Switz. 2016;232(6):687-91.
44. Prens LM, Bouwman K, Troelstra LD, Prens EP, Alizadeh BZ, Horváth B. New insights in hidradenitis suppurativa from a population-based Dutch cohort: prevalence, smoking behaviour, socioeconomic status and comorbidities. Br J Dermatol. 2022;186(5):814-22.
45. Garg A, Lavian J, Lin G, Strunk A, Alloo A. Incidence of hidradenitis suppurativa in the United States: A sex- and age-adjusted population analysis. J Am Acad Dermatol. 2017;77(1):118-22.
46. Kimball AB, Jemec GBE, Yang M, Kageleiry A, Signorovitch JE, Okun MM, et al. Assessing the validity, responsiveness and meaningfulness of the Hidradenitis Suppurativa Clinical Response (HiSCR) as the clinical endpoint for hidradenitis suppurativa treatment. Br J Dermatol. 2014;171(6):1434-42.
47. Zouboulis CC, Tzellos T, Kyrgidis A, Jemec GBE, Bechara FG, Giamarellos-Bourboulis EJ, et al. Development and validation of the International Hidradenitis Suppurativa Severity Score System (I4), a novel dynamic scoring system to assess HS severity. Br J Dermatol. 2017;177(5):1401-9.
48. Zouboulis C, Desai N, Emtestam L, Hunger R, Ioannides D, Juhász I, et al. European S1 guideline for the treatment of hidradenitis suppurativa/acne inversa. J Eur Acad Dermatol Venereol. 2015;29(4):619-44.
49. Miller IM, McAndrew RJ, Hamzavi I. Prevalence, risk factors, and comorbidities of hidradenitis suppurativa. Dermatol Clin. 2016;34(1):7-16.

50. Shlyankevich J, Chen AJ, Kim GE, Kimball AB. Hidradenitis suppurativa is a systemic disease with substantial comorbidity burden: a chart-verified case-control analysis. J Am Acad Dermatol. 2014;71(6):1144-50.
51. Zouboulis CC, Okun MM, Prens EP, Gniadecki R, Foley PA, Lynde C, et al. Long-term adalimumab efficacy in patients with moderate-to-severe hidradenitis suppurativa/acne inversa: 3-year results of a phase 3 open-label extension study. J Am Acad Dermatol. 2019;80(1):60-69.e2.
52. van der Zee HH, Boer J, Prens EP, Jemec GBE. The effect of combined treatment with oral clindamycin and oral rifampicin in patients with hidradenitis suppurativa. Dermatol Basel Switz. 2009;219(2):143-7.
53. Dessinioti C, Zisimou C, Tzanetakou V, Stratigos A, Antoniou C. Oral clindamycin and rifampicin combination therapy for hidradenitis suppurativa: a prospective study and 1-year follow-up. Clin Exp Dermatol. 2016;41(8):852-7.
54. Join-Lambert O, Coignard-Biehler H, Jais JP, Delage M, Guet-Revillet H, Poirée S, et al. Efficacy of ertapenem in severe hidradenitis suppurativa: a pilot study in a cohort of 30 consecutive patients. J Antimicrob Chemother. 2016;71(2):513-20.
55. Grant A, Gonzalez T, Montgomery MO, Cardenas V, Kerdel FA. Infliximab therapy for patients with moderate to severe hidradenitis suppurativa: a randomized, double-blind, placebo-controlled crossover trial. J Am Acad Dermatol. 2010;62(2):205-17.
56. Kimball AB, Jemec GBE, Alavi A, Reguiai Z, Gottlieb AB, Bechara FG, et al. Secukinumab in moderate-to-severe hidradenitis suppurativa (SUNSHINE and SUNRISE): week 16 and week 52 results of two identical, multicentre, randomised, placebo-controlled, double-blind phase 3 trials. Lancet Lond Engl. 2023;401(10378):747-61.
57. Zuberbier T, Aberer W, Asero R, Abdul Latiff AH, Baker D, Ballmer-Weber B, et al. The EAACI/GA2LEN/EDF/WAO guideline for the definition, classification, diagnosis and management of urticaria. Allergy. 2018;73(7):1393-414.
58. Fricke J, Ávila G, Keller T, Weller K, Lau S, Maurer M, et al. Prevalence of chronic urticaria in children and adults across the globe: Systematic review with meta-analysis. Allergy. 2020;75(2):423-32.
59. Beltrani VS. An overview of chronic urticaria. Clin Rev Allergy Immunol. 2002;23(2):147-69.
60. Maurer M, Weller K, Bindslev-Jensen C, Giménez-Arnau A, Bousquet PJ, Bousquet J, et al. Unmet clinical needs in chronic spontaneous urticaria. A GA2LEN task force report. Allergy. 2011;66(3):317-30.
61. Sánchez-Borges M, Capriles-Hulett A, Caballero-Fonseca F, González-Aveledo L. Biomarkers of treatment efficacy in patients with chronic spontaneous urticaria. Eur Ann Allergy Clin Immunol. 2018;50(1):5-9.
62. Alen Coutinho I, Regateiro FS, Fernandes RA, Pita JS, Gomes R, Coelho C, et al. Refractory chronic urticaria in adults: clinical characterization and predictors of severity. Allergy Asthma Clin Immunol. 2020;16(1):97.
63. Vestergaard C, Toubi E, Maurer M, Triggiani M, Ballmer-Weber B, Marsland A, et al. Treatment of chronic spontaneous urticaria with an inadequate response to H1-antihistamines: an expert opinion. Eur J Dermatol. 2017;27(1):10-9.
64. Kaplan A, Ledford D, Ashby M, Canvin J, Zazzali JL, Conner E, et al. Omalizumab in patients with symptomatic chronic idiopathic/spontaneous urticaria despite standard combination therapy. J Allergy Clin Immunol. 2013;132(1):101-9.
65. Türk M, Maurer M, Yılmaz İ. How to discontinue omalizumab in chronic spontaneous urticaria? Allergy. 2019;74(4):821-4.
66. AbbVie. A Phase 4, Double-blind, Randomized, Placebo-Controlled, Multicenter Study to Assess the Safety and Efficacy of Adalimumab Used in Conjunction With Surgery in Subjects With Moderate to Severe Hidradenitis Suppurativa [Internet]. clinicaltrials.gov; 2020 May [cited 2023 Jul 19]. Report No.: NCT02808975. Available from: https://clinicaltrials.gov/study/NCT02808975.

SECTION 10

Small Molecules and IVIG

CHAPTER 31

Janus Kinase Inhibitors

Part A: Classification of Janus Kinase Inhibitors

Siddharth Mani, Manish Khandare

INTRODUCTION

Janus kinases (JAKs) are intracytoplasmic nonreceptor tyrosine kinases that bind the cytoplasmic region of transmembrane cytokine receptors and initiate a variety of downstream intracellular effects. In humans, the JAK family comprises four members: JAK1, JAK2, JAK3, and TYK2 (tyrosine kinase).[1] Each member can dimerize in different combinations at the intracytoplasmic end of cytokine receptors and each combination selectively responds to certain extracellular signals. The four JAKs play an essential role in the transduction of the cytokine-mediated signals, which takes place through the JAK-signal transducers and activators of the transcription (STAT) pathway. The targeting of JAK-associated pathways by using JAK inhibitors has rapidly entered the clinical arena for a wide array of disease states, including inflammatory dermatosis, myeloproliferative neoplasms, rheumatoid arthritis and other immune-mediated arthropathies, and inflammatory bowel disease, and has revolutionized the management of many diseases.

JAK–STAT PATHWAY

Irrespective of type, all cytokine receptors are associated with one or more of the JAKs to facilitate signal transduction. Upon binding of specific cytokine to its cellular receptor, there is a confirmation change which in turns leads to recruitment and activation of JAK. Activated JAK phosphorylates specific sites on the intracellular part of the receptor. These act as docking site for

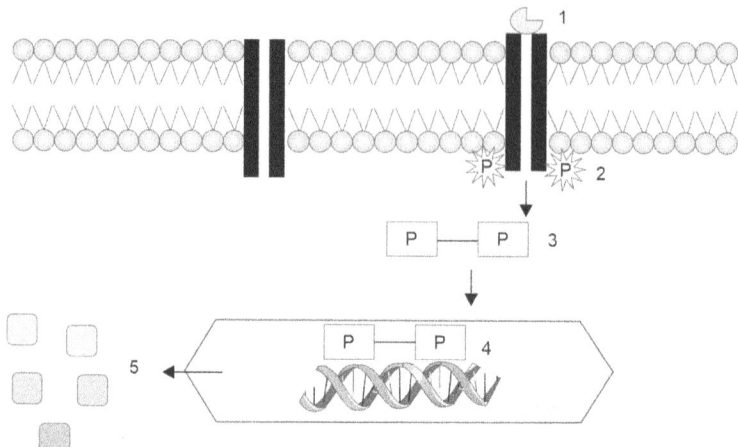

FIG. 1: (1) Binding of cytokine to its receptor; (2) Attachment, activation, and phosphorylation of JAK; (3) Docking and phosphorylation of STAT; (4) Translocation of dimerized and phosphorylated STAT to the nucleus; (5) STAT causes increased transcription and increasing inflammatory cytokines.
(JAK: Janus kinase; STAT: signal transducers and activators of the transcription)

STAT proteins. This is followed by phosphorylation of STAT which then dissociates from the receptor, dimerizes, and translocate to the nucleus. The STAT leads to gene transcription which leads to increase in a number of different cytokines.[2] The mechanism of action of JAK–STAT pathway is explained in **Figure 1**.

Both type 1 and 2 cytokines can cause activation of JAK–STAT pathways. Since there are multiple cytokines, 4 JAKs, and 7 STATs, hence activation and dimerization of different JAK-STAT molecules can occur which in turn will lead to different types of responses as lymphocyte proliferation, homeostasis, T-cell differentiation, myelopoiesis, and erythropoiesis, innate antiviral defense to name a few **(Fig. 2)**.[3,4]

CLASSIFICATION OF JAK INHIBITORS

Based on selectivity:
- *First-generation JAK inhibitors*: These include nonselective inhibitors of JAK. Target multiple JAK isoforms. Examples are tofacitinib, baricitinib, ruxolitinib, peficitinib, and ifidancitinib
- *Second-generation JAK inhibitors*: Selective inhibitory activity against certain JAK.
  Examples are filgotinib and upadacitinib.

Based on mode of binding and type of interaction with amino acid:
- *Reversible inhibitors*: These molecules form reversible or noncovalent bond or interactions with the amino acids in the four JAKs. The reversible inhibitors can be further classified as:

- ATP-competitive inhibitors: The mechanism of action of these inhibitors depends on their competition with ATP for the catalytic ATP-binding site in JAKs.[5,6] These inhibitors are of two types.
    i. Type 1 JAK inhibitors: Bind to the ATP-binding site of the JAKs under the active conformation of the kinase domain.[7,8]
    Example: Filgotinib-selective JAK 1 inhibitor, fedratinib-selective JAK 2 inhibitor, nonselective JAK inhibitors—tofacitinib, peficitinib.[9] The ability of type 1 inhibitors to bind to multiple kinases is due to highly conserved structure of the ATP-binding site in the four JAKs.[10]
    ii. Type 2 JAK inhibitors: Bind to the ATP-binding site of the kinase domain in the inactive conformation of JAKs.
- Allosteric JAK inhibitors: Bind to a site other than the ATP-binding site in JAKs. Example—deucravacitinib[11]
- *Irreversible JAK inhibitors*: This is due to covalent bond formation and is seen mainly with JAK 3.[12] Example—ritlecitinib

A list of JAK inhibitors with target sites and indications has been mentioned in **Table 1**.

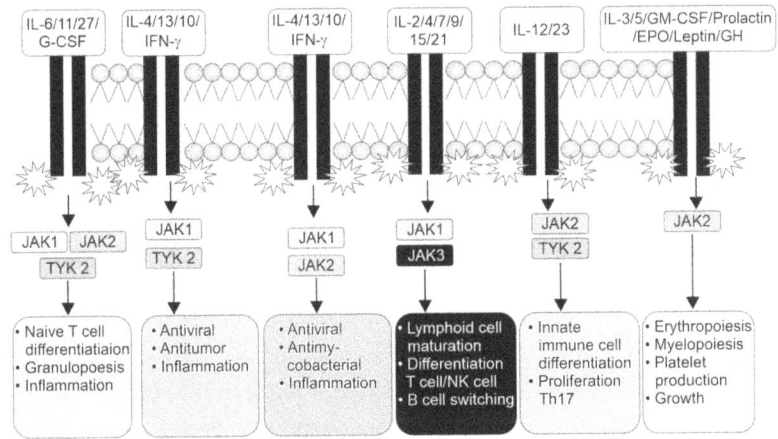

FIG. 2: Different response of body to different cytokines and different JAK molecules.
(EPO: erythropoietin; GH: growth hormone; JAK: Janus kinase; TYK: tyrosine kinase)

TABLE 1: JAK inhibitors with their target sites and US FDA approved indications.			
Drug	**Target JAK**	**Disease**	**US FDA approval**
Abrocitinib	JAK1, JAK2	Atopic dermatitis	2022
Baricitinib	JAK1, JAK2	• Rheumatoid arthritis • Alopecia areata	2018 2022
Delgocitinib	Pan JAK	Atopic dermatitis	2020 (Approved only in Japan—in topical form)

Continued

Continued

Drug	Target JAK	Disease	US-FDA approval
Fedratinib	JAK2, JAK2V617F	Myelofibrosis	2019
Filgotinib	JAK1	Rheumatoid arthritis	Approved by European Union
Pacritinib	JAK2, JAK2V617F	Myelofibrosis	2022
Peficitinib	Pan JAK	Rheumatoid arthritis	Approved in Japan—2019
Ruxolitinib	JAK1, JAK2 JAK2V617F	• Myelofibrosis • Polycythemia vera • Acute and chronic graft-versus-host disease • Vitiligo (in topical form) • Atopic dermatitis	2011 2014 2019, 2021 2022 2021
Tofacitinib	JAK1 and JAK3, >> JAK 2	• Rheumatoid arthritis • Psoriatic arthritis • Ulcerative colitis • Juvenile idiopathic arthritis • Ankylosing spondylitis	2012 2017 2018 2020 2021
Upadacitinib	JAK1	• Rheumatoid arthritis • Psoriatic arthritis • Atopic dermatitis • Ulcerative colitis	2019 2021 2022 2022
Ritlecitinib	JAK3	Alopecia areata	2023

(USFDA United States: Food and Drug Administration; JAK: Janus kinase)

CONCLUSION

The use of JAK inhibitors in dermatology has led to a transformative effect in clinical practice. The class of drug has been accepted by both patients and practitioners alike. The drugs are being used for various inflammatory dermatosis where conventional therapies are not working and giving biologics is not feasible. Their ability to modulate key signaling pathways involved in immune responses and inflammatory cascades underscores their versatility and efficacy in addressing diverse dermatological manifestations. As research continues to elucidate the intricate mechanisms underlying skin pathology, the role of JAK inhibitors is poised to expand further, potentially encompassing a broader spectrum of dermatosis. However, a continuous vigilance is required as long term safety data for many of the newer drugs is not available dermatosis broadertions.

REFERENCES

1. Rawlings JS, Rosler KM, Harrison DA. The JAK/STAT signalling pathway. J Cell Sci. 2004;117:1281-3.
2. Haan C, Kreis S, Margue C, Behrmann I. Jaks and cytokine receptors—an intimate relationship. Biochem Pharmacol. 2006;72:1538-46.
3. Clark JD, Flanagan ME, Telliez JB. Discovery and development of Janus Kinase (JAK) inhibitors for inflammatory diseases: Miniperspective. J Med Chem. 2014;57:5023-38.
4. Danese S, Grisham M, Hodge J, Telliez JB. JAK inhibition using tofacitinib for inflammatory bowel disease treatment: a hub for multiple inflammatory cytokines. Am J Physiol Gastrointest Liver Physiol. 2016;310:G155-62.
5. Leroy E, Constantinescu SN. Rethinking JAK2 inhibition: Towards novel strategies of more specific and versatile Janus kinase inhibition. Leukemia. 2017;31:1023-38.
6. Vainchenker W, Leroy E, Gilles L, Marty C, Plo I, Constantinescu SN. JAK inhibitors for the treatment of myeloproliferative neoplasms and other disorders. F1000Research. 2018;7:82.
7. Schwartz DM, Kanno Y, Villarino A, Ward M, Gadina M, O'Shea JJ. JAK inhibition as a therapeutic strategy for immune and inflammatory diseases. Nat Rev Drug Discov. 2017;16:843-62.
8. Wernig G, Kharas MG, Okabe R, Moore SA, Leeman DS, Cullen DE, et al. Efficacy of TG101348, a selective JAK2 inhibitor, in treatment of a murine model of JAK2V617F-induced polycythemia vera. Cancer Cell. 2008;13:311-20.
9. Singh D, Bogus M, Moskalenko V, Lord R, Moran EJ, Crater GD, et al. A phase 2 multiple ascending dose study of the inhaled pan-JAK inhibitor nezulcitinib (TD-0903) in severe COVID-19. Eur Respir J. 2021;58:2100673.
10. Virtanen AT, Haikarainen T, Raivola J, Silvennoinen O. Selective JAKinibs: Prospects in inflammatory and autoimmune diseases. Bio Drugs. 2019;33:15-32.
11. Burke JR, Cheng L, Gillooly KM, Strnad J, Zupa-Fernandez A, Catlett IM, et al. Autoimmune pathways in mice and humans are blocked by pharmacological stabilization of the TYK2 pseudokinase domain. Sci Transl Med. 2019;11:eaaw1736.
12. Casimiro-Garcia A, Trujillo JI, Vajdos F, Juba B, Banker ME, Aulabaugh A, et al. Identification of cyanamide-based Janus kinase 3 (JAK3) covalent inhibitors. J Med Chem. 2018;61:10665-99.

Part B: Tofacitinib

Siddharth Mani, Manish Khandare

INTRODUCTION

Tofacitinib is a small-molecule Janus kinase (JAK) inhibitor that has been approved for the treatment of a variety of inflammatory diseases, including rheumatoid arthritis (RA), psoriatic arthritis (PsA), ulcerative colitis (UC), and ankylosing spondylitis (AS). JAKs are a family of enzymes that play a critical role in the signaling of cytokines, which are important mediators of inflammation. By blocking the activity of JAKs, tofacitinib can effectively suppress inflammation and improve clinical outcomes in patients with inflammatory diseases. The mechanism of action of tofacitinib is described in the previous chapter of "Classification of JAK inhibitors".

PHARMACOKINETICS AND PHARMACODYNAMICS

The drugs pharmacokinetic and pharmacodynamic properties are mentioned in **Table 1**.

TABLE 1: Pharmacological properties of tofacitinib.[1]

Tofacitinib		Tofacitinib XR	
Absorption and bioavailability	*Peak levels:* 0.5–1 hour	Absorption and bioavailability	*Peak levels:* 4 hours
	Bioavailability: 74%		*Bioavailability:* 74%
	Steady state concentration: 24–48 hours		*Steady state concentration:* 48 hours
Elimination	*Half-life:* 3 hours	Elimination	*Half-life:* 6 hours
	Metabolism and excretion: 70% hepatic metabolism and 30% renal excretion of the parent drug, primarily mediated by CYP3A4 with minor contribution from CYP2C19		*Metabolism and excretion:* 70% hepatic metabolism and 30% renal excretion of the parent drug, primarily mediated by CYP3A4 with minor contribution from CYP2C19
Dose adjustment	• Required in both moderate hepatic and renal impairment • No dose adjustment in mild hepatic and renal impairment		

INDICATIONS

Most of the indications of tofacitinib in the field of dermatology are off label. A comprehensive list of its indications is mentioned in **Table 2**.

STUDIES OF TOFACITINIB PERTAINING TO DERMATOLOGY CONDITIONS

Psoriasis

Numerous studies assessing the efficacy of tofacitinib for psoriasis have been completed, including for both oral and topical routes of administration. Most of the studies have used Physician's Global Assessment (PGA) and Psoriasis Area and Severity Index (PASI) over placebo. Few trials have also looked at Nail Psoriasis Severity Index (NAPSI) score improvements. The major studies are mentioned in **Table 3**.

Three randomized controlled trials (RCTs) have been conducted to evaluate the efficacy of topical tofacitinib (TT) in the treatment of psoriasis. An intra-subject placebo-controlled trial comparing 2%, 0.2%, and 0.02% tofacitinib ointments did not find a statistically significant difference in target plaque severity score (TPSS) between the tofacitinib and placebo groups.[6] However, the study authors noted the presence of tofacitinib in placebo-treated patches, suggesting potential cross-contamination due to unsupervised patient application. Another RCT comparing two tofacitinib

TABLE 2: Various indications of tofacitinib.		
FDA approved	**Off label**	**Topical formulation**
Rheumatoid arthritis	Psoriasis	Alopecia areata
Psoriatic arthritis	Alopecia areata	Vitiligo
Ulcerative colitis	Atopic dermatitis	Psoriasis
Juvenile idiopathic arthritis	Vitiligo	
Ankylosing spondylitis	Lichen planus	
	Morphea	
	Dermatomyositis	
	Nail dystrophy	
	Granuloma Annulare	
	Hypereosinophilic syndrome	
	Pyoderma gangrenosum	
	Lichen planopilaris	
	Contact dermatitis	

TABLE 3: Studies pertaining to use of tofacitinib in psoriasis.

Author and number of patients (n)	Clinical endpoint	Remarks
Bachelez et al.[2] (n = 1,101)	Phase III placebo-controlled RCT Four groups—3:3:3:1 1. Tofacitinib 5 mg BD 2. Tofacitinib 10 mg BD 3. Etanercept twice-a-week (subcutaneous) 4. Placebo PASI 75 and PGA observed	• PASI75 and PGA responses at 12 weeks • Tofacitinib 5 mg BD—39.5 and 47.1% • Tofacitinib 10 mg BD—63.6 and 68.2% • Etanercept twice weekly—58.8% and 66.3% • Placebo—5.6% and 15%
Valenzuela et al.[3] (n = 1,092)	Phase III placebo-controlled RCT Four groups—3:3:3:1 1. Tofacitinib 5 mg BD 2. Tofacitinib 10 mg BD 3. Etanercept twice-a-week (subcutaneous) 4. Placebo Patient-reported outcomes (PROs) including DLQI, Itch Severity Item Score (ISIS), and Patient Global Assessment of Psoriasis (PtGA)	DLQI • Tofacitinib 5 mg BD—30.9% • Tofacitinib 10 mg BD—47.3% • Etanercept twice weekly—43.6% • Placebo—7.8% • Itch was significantly reduced by tofacitinib compared with etanercept and placebo within 1 day of starting treatment
Lloyd–Lavery[4] (n = 2,867)	• Multiple phase II and global phase III trials with open-label long-term extension (LTE) study • Tofacitinib 10 mg BD for 3 months then 5–10 mg BD for a median duration of 35.6 months • PASI 75 and PGA observed	• PGA response and PASI75 • Achieved by 52–62% and 56–74% of patients
Merola et al.[5] (n = 1,196)	Two 52-week, randomized, controlled phase III studies 2:2:1 1. Tofacitinib 5 mg BD 2. Tofacitinib 10 mg BD 3. Placebo Week 16—placebo patients rerandomized to tofacitinib group Observed ≥ 50% reduction in NAPSI from baseline (NAPSI50), NAPSI75, or NAPSI100	• Week 16; Tofacitinib 5 mg vs. 10 mg vs. placebo • *NAPSI 50*: 32.8%, 44.2%, 12.0% • *NAPSI75*: 16.9%, 28.1%, 6.8% • *NAPSI100*: 10.3%, 18.2%, 5.1% • Improvements sustained till week 52

(DLQI: Dermatology Life Quality Index; RCT: randomized controlled trial)

ointment formulations to vehicle control demonstrated significant improvements over vehicle control for one of the two formulations. Minimal adverse effects were observed in all treatment groups.[7]

A RCT comparing the treatment efficacy of 1% and 2% tofacitinib ointment to vehicle control demonstrated statistically significant improvements over vehicle control in Calculated Physician's Global assessment (PGA-C) scores at week 8. However, this improvement was not sustained at study completion (week 12) for the 2% daily (QD) and twice daily (BID) dosing groups.[8]

PSORIATIC ARTHRITIS

This is a US Food and Drug Administration (FDA) approved indication. Mease et al. studied the effects of tofacitinib in patients of PsA not responding to disease-modifying anti-rheumatic drugs (DMARDs) and tumor necrosis factor-alpha (TNF-α) inhibitors. A total of 422 patients were studied and American College of Rheumatology (ACR) 20 along with HAQ-DI (Health Assessment Questionnaire Disability Index) scores was studied. 50% patient in tofacitinib 5 mg BD, 61% patients in tofacitinib 10 mg BD as compared to 52% in adalimumab group showed improvement in ACR 20. The HAQ-DI scores were comparable in all three groups.[9]

The drug also demonstrated efficacy in patients who did not respond to at least one TNF-α inhibitor after 6 months of treatment.[10] While the higher dose of 10 mg twice daily yielded better results, 5 mg twice daily is currently the recommended dose for PsA due to its superior safety profile.[11]

Alopecia Areata

Both the oral and topical forms of this drug have been used in the management of alopecia areata (AA). A summary of various important clinical trials and their effects is mentioned in **Table 4**.

A 24-week, open-label pilot study involving 10 patients with AA treated with TT 2% ointment applied twice daily revealed hair regrowth in 3 patients, with an average decrease of 34.6% in the SALT score. The hair regrowth response was less pronounced than that observed with oral tofacitinib but comparable to that reported with clobetasol 0.05% ointment under occlusion.[15] While the results for AA, alopecia totalis (AT), and alopecia universalis (AU) have been mixed and modest,[16] TT may be a favorable treatment option for inducing hair regrowth in specific areas, such as the eyebrows and eyelashes. In a patient who had previously tried several ineffective treatments, near-complete eyelash regrowth was achieved with TT 2% solution by 4 months.[17]

Vitiligo

Tofacitinib has been tried successfully in vitiligo. Repigmentation has been achieved with oral tofacitinib 5–10 mg administered twice daily.[18]

TABLE 4: Studies pertaining to use of tofacitinib in alopecia areata (AA).

Author and number of patients (n)	Clinical endpoint	Remarks
Liu et al.[12] (n = 90)	• Tofacitinib 5 mg BD (43%) or more (29%) alone or with prednisolone (28%) • *Duration*: 4–18 months • *Desired outcome*: >50% improvement in SALT score	• >50% patient achieved clinical outcome. • Patients with AA experienced a higher percent change in SALT score than did patients with alopecia totalis or alopecia universalis (81.9% vs. 59.0%)
Jabbari et al.[13] (n = 12)	• Tofacitinib 5 mg BD escalated to 10 mg BD in nonresponders • *Duration*: 4–18 months • *Desired outcome*: >50% improvement in SALT score	66% of patients achieved SALT reduction >50%, 25% achieved SALT reduction of 5–50%, and 8% achieved no response. 6 of 7 patients followed were noted to have shedding of hair following cessation of tofacitinib
Shin et al.[14] (n = 74)	• Retrospective comparative study • 18 patients treated with tofacitinib 5–10 mg BD, 26 treated with conventional oral treatment (steroid ± cyclosporine), and 30 treated with DPCP • *Duration*: 6 months • *Desired outcome*: >50% improvement in SALT score	44.4% of patients in tofacitinib group, 37.5% in conventional oral treatment group, and 11.1% in DPCP group

Improvement was more pronounced in sun-exposed areas and when combined with narrowband ultraviolet B (NB-UVB) therapy.[19,20]

Atopic Dermatitis

An RCT comparing 2% tofacitinib ointment to vehicle control demonstrated significantly greater treatment efficacy for mild-to-moderate atopic dermatitis (AD), with Eczema Area and Severity Index (EASI) scores showing a significant improvement at week 4. An initial response was observed by week 1 of treatment.[21] A study involving 6 patients with moderate-to-severe AD treated with oral tofacitinib (5 mg twice daily) demonstrated a 54.8% reduction in Scoring of Atopic Dermatitis (SCORAD) scores within the initial 14 weeks of treatment.[22] An additional 66.6% reduction in SCORAD scores was noted in the following 15 weeks of treatment. Secondary endpoints included subjective improvements in pruritus (itching) and sleep quality over the course of this study. Notably, one patient with a history of AD, alopecia, and vitiligo was treated with tofacitinib and achieved complete remission of AD symptoms within 3 months of treatment.[23]

TABLE 5: Case Series and reports of off-label uses of tofacitinib.

Disease/study	Remarks
Kurtzman et al.[24] Dermatomyositis ($n = 3$)	• Roughly 50% improvement in CDASI (Cutaneous Dermatomyositis Disease Area and Severity Index) score, with improvement in pruritus, strength and fatigue noted • 1 of 3 patient was also on HCQ
Moghadam-Kia et al.[25] Dermatomyositis ($n = 4$)	• Near-complete remission of skin and joint symptoms • Adjunctive treatment—prednisolone all • IVIG-3 out of 4
Yang et al.[26] Lichen planopilaris ($n = 10$)	LPPAI (Lichen Planopilaris Activity Index) score improvement of 30–94% for 8 patients; no improvement for 2 patients
Jaller et al.[27] Nail dystrophy ($n = 2$)	Complete resolution of nail symptoms
Dhayalan and King[28] Nail dystrophy ($n = 3$)	Complete resolution of nail symptoms
Kochar et al.[29] Pyoderma gangrenosum ($n = 3$)	Complete or near-complete clearance

The patient also demonstrated marked improvements in alopecia, with hair regrowth observed on the scalp, beard region, extremities, eyebrows, and eyelashes. Improvements in vitiligo were more modest, with a 15.6% decrease in Vitiligo Area Scoring Index (VASI).

Other Off-label Indications

Case reports have documented the use of tofacitinib for the treatment of a variety of dermatological conditions, including chronic actinic dermatitis, dermatomyositis, pyoderma gangrenosum, and several others. In these case reports, tofacitinib is administered either as a monotherapy or in combination with other medications. The outcomes of these case series and case reports are discussed in detail in **Table 5**.

ADVERSE EFFECTS

Dermatologists should be aware of and vigilant about the major groups of adverse events (AEs) associated with tofacitinib, summarized below. These include:
- *Infections*: Cutaneous or systemic infections, new-onset infections, reactivation of latent infections, nasopharyngitis, severe infections, and opportunistic infections (OIs) are all associated with tofacitinib.[1]

   There is risk of invasive fungal infection including cryptococcosis, histoplasmosis, esophageal candidiasis and pneumocystosis which may present with disseminated, rather than localized disease. Bacterial (listeria), viral, including herpes zoster/HSV/BK/CMV have also been reported in various studies.[1] There is increased risk of reactivation of herpes zoster. In patients that are high risk for herpes zoster infections, including older patients, smokers and those on concomitant oral corticosteroids (CS), pretreatment prophylactic zoster vaccination should be considered.

There is risk of active tuberculosis (TB), both pulmonary and extra-pulmonary variant. It is advised to test for latent TB and if the results are positive treatment should be given for latent TB before initiating tofacitinib.[30] Since both isoniazid and tofacitinib can cause liver parameter derangements, a close look should be maintained during the treatment. Even if the patient's initial latent tuberculosis infection (LTBI) tests are negative, it is imperative that the signs of active tuberculosis should be looked for during the course of treatment.

Hepatitis B virus (HBV) carriers on tofacitinib may experience reactivation of the virus while on therapy. Rescue nucleotide analog therapy may be administered if this occurs to maintain patients on therapy. However, HBV carriers on tofacitinib who receive pre-emptive nucleotide analog therapy may be able to forestall reactivation altogether. The patients should be tested for hepatitis B and C before initiating treatment.[31]

In case of serious infection, drug should be stopped till the infection is controlled.

- *Malignancies*: Clinical trials have reported the occurrence of various malignancies in patients taking tofacitinib, with a rate of 0.4 events per 100 patient-years for the 5 mg twice daily dosing and 0.6 events per 100 patient-years for the 10 mg twice daily dosing.[30,32] These rates may reflect the normal background rates observed in these patient populations. Among the reported malignancies, nonmelanoma skin cancers were the most prevalent, occurring more frequently in patients also taking other DMARDs.[33] Aside from nonmelanoma skin cancers, the most commonly observed malignancies included lung and breast cancers, colorectal, gastric, renal, prostate, and pancreatic cancers, as well as lymphomas and melanomas. The risk of malignancy is likely to be higher in patients receiving other immunosuppressive medications, including post-transplant patients.[34]
- *Gastrointestinal complications*: Gastrointestinal (GI) perforations, including diverticulitis, gastric ulcer perforation, and perforated appendix, have been reported in RA patients taking tofacitinib in long-term extension studies.[9] However, it is important to consider that RA patients are often concomitantly treated with nonsteroidal anti-inflammatory drugs (NSAIDs), which are known to be associated with an increased risk of GI perforations. The risk of GI perforation in PsA patients treated with tofacitinib has not yet been fully elucidated.[35]

- *Hematologic effects*: Laboratory abnormalities may occur during tofacitinib therapy. While cytopenias are generally uncommon with tofacitinib due to its weak JAK2 inhibition, particularly in patients with healthy bone marrow reserves, studies involving tofacitinib for RA and UC have reported anemia and a decrease in red blood cell, neutrophil, and lymphocyte counts.[36] Elevations in creatine phosphokinase enzyme and liver enzymes (transaminases) exceeding three times the upper limit of normal have also been observed in patients treated with tofacitinib. Stopping concomitant DMARDs, decreasing the dose of tofacitinib, or interrupting tofacitinib usually brings the enzyme levels down. Tofacitinib is known to cause dyslipidemia, characterized by minor elevations in low-density lipoprotein, high-density lipoprotein, total cholesterol, and serum triglyceride levels. Despite an increased risk of hypertension and dyslipidemia, tofacitinib has not been associated with an increased risk of major adverse cardiovascular events.[36] Tofacitinib-induced hyperlipidemia may persist for up to 12 weeks before stabilizing. Persistent hyperlipidemia should be managed according to standard clinical guidelines. The use of lipid-lowering agents such as statins can improve dyslipidemia, but regular monitoring of hepatic enzymes is mandatory in these cases.[11]
- *Hypersensitivity reactions and miscellaneous*: Urticaria, angioedema, headache, hypertension, distal symmetric polyneuropathy, and musculoskeletal complaints such as arthralgia, back pain, and pain in extremities have also been reported in various studies.[11,36]
- *Pulmonary effects*: Caution is recommended in patients with a history of chronic lung disease, or in those who develop interstitial lung disease (ILD), as they may be more prone to infections. Concomitant use of tofacitinib and methotrexate should also be approached with caution due to the potential for an increased risk of ILD, a serious adverse effect that can be associated with each medication individually.[1]
- *Other*: Nasopharyngitis, upper respiratory tract infection, headache, diarrhea, and hypertension have also been reported to be associated with tofacitinib therapy.

MONITORING

The monitoring guidelines are mentioned in **Table 6**.

CONTRAINDICATIONS

There are no absolute contraindications to tofacitinib. However, there is boxed warning for OIs, latent tuberculosis, and EBV-associated post-transplant lymphomas tofacitinib with other immunosuppressive medications. Clinical situation where tofacitinib should not be initiated or interrupted is mentioned in **Boxes 1 and 2**.

TABLE 6: Monitoring guidelines of tofacitinib.

Baseline clinical	Baseline lab	Follow-up clinical
• Discuss risk/benefit/adverse effects • Discuss alternative treatments • Requirement of multiple blood tests • History of malignancy/lymphoproliferative disorder • History of herpes infection, ILD, MTX therapy, diverticulitis, renal dysfunction	• CBC/TLC/DLC • LFT • Lipid profile • Hepatitis B • Anti HCV • RFT/GFR • R/o latent TB • UPT (reproductive age group women)	• Every visit – look for signs of infection • Annual examination with special attention to NMSC/lymphoma/TB *Follow-up lab @ 4–8 weeks then 3 monthly* • CBC • LFT • Lipid profile

(CBC: complete blood count; DLC: differential leucocyte count; GFR: glomerular filtration rate; HCV: hepatitis C virus; ILD: interstitial lung disease; LFT: liver function test; MTX: methotrexate; NMSC: nonmelanoma skin cancer; RFT: renal function test; TB: tuberculosis; TLC: total leucocyte count; UPT: urine pregnancy test)

BOX 1 Hematological parameters that warrant avoiding initiation or interruption.

- Avoid initiation
- Absolute lymphocyte count < 500 cells/mm^3
- Absolute neutrophil count < 1,000 cells/mm^3
- Hemoglobin levels < 9 g/dL
- Dose interruption is recommended for management of lymphopenia, neutropenia, and anemia developing in course of treatment
- *ALC/ANC < 500*: No resumption
- *Persistent ANC 500–1,000*: Interrupt treatment till ANC increases to more than 1,000
- Hb < 8 g/dL or whose hemoglobin level drops > 2 g/dL on treatment

BOX 2 Other conditions that warrant avoiding initiation or interruption.

- Avoid initiation
- *Active infections*: Presence of active tuberculosis (TB), serious localized infections such as cellulitis, sepsis, or opportunistic infections
- *Severe hepatic impairment*: Grade C impairment by Child–Pugh scoring (10–50 points)
- Hypersensitivity to the active substance or to any of the excipients
- *Infectious seropositivity*: Positive serology for hepatitis C, HIV
- *Dosage reduction*: 5 mg once a day in moderate liver/renal impairment
- Moderate and severe renal insufficiency-creatine clearance 30–49 mL/min and < 30 mL/min, respectively
- *Moderate hepatic impairment*: Child–Pugh score grade B (7–9 points)

IMMUNIZATION

- *For live attenuated vaccines*: Must wait least 3 months after therapy complete to immunize.
- *Killed/Recombinant vaccine*: Immunize at least 2 weeks prior starting tofacitinib; not adequate immune response, repeat in 3 months.

CONCLUSION

The emergence of novel small-molecule drugs is expanding the therapeutic landscape for a range of challenging skin conditions. The JAK pathway has been implicated in various dermatological disorders, and its inhibition leads to anti-inflammatory effects that have demonstrated clinical benefits in AD, vitiligo, psoriasis, and potentially many other cutaneous conditions. In general, the safety profiles of JAK inhibitors are favorable. As more clinical trials are conducted, we can anticipate the approval of additional JAK inhibitors as well as existing JAKi as tofacitinib for more indications in the near future, further broadening the armamentarium of medications available to dermatologists for managing a wider spectrum of dermatological diseases.

REFERENCES

1. US Food and Drug Administration. Xeljanz prescribing information. [online] Available from https://www.accessdata.fda.gov/drugsatfda_docs/label/2018/203214s018lbl.pdf. [Last accessed January, 2024]
2. Bachelez H, van de Kerkhof PCM, Strohal R, Kubanov A, Valenzuela F, Lee JH, et al. Tofacitinib versus etanercept or placebo in moderate-to-severe chronic plaque psoriasis: A phase 3 randomised non-inferiority trial. Lancet Lond Engl. 2015;386: 552-61.
3. Valenzuela F, Paul C, Mallbris L, Tan H, Papacharalambous J, Valdez H, et al. Tofacitinib versus etanercept or placebo in patients with moderate to severe chronic plaque psoriasis: Patient-reported outcomes from a Phase 3 study. J Eur Acad Dermatol Venereol. 2016;30:1753-9.
4. Lloyd-Lavery A. Long-term safety data for tofacitinib, an oral Janus kinase inhibitor, for the treatment for psoriasis. Br J Dermatol. 2018;179:815-6.
5. Merola JF, Elewski B, Tatulych S, Lan S, Tallman A, Kaur M. Efficacy of tofacitinib for the treatment of nail psoriasis: two 52-week, randomized, controlled phase 3 studies in patients with moderate-to-severe plaque psoriasis. J Am Acad Dermatol. 2017;77(1): 79-87.e1.
6. Ports WC, Feldman SR, Gupta P, Tan H, Johnson TR, Bissonnette R. Randomized pilot clinical trial of tofacitinib solution for plaque psoriasis: challenges of the intra-subject study design. J Drugs Dermatol. 2015;14:777-84.
7. Ports WC, Khan S, Lan S, Lamba M, Bolduc C, Bissonnette R, et al. A randomized phase 2a efficacy and safety trial of the topical Janus kinase inhibitor tofacitinib in the treatment of chronic plaque psoriasis. Br J Dermatol. 2013;169:137-45.
8. Papp KA, Bissonnette R, Gooderham M, Feldman SR, Iversen L, Soung J, et al. Treatment of plaque psoriasis with an ointment formulation of the Janus kinase inhibitor, tofacitinib: a Phase 2b randomized clinical trial. BMC Dermatol. 2016;16:15.

9. Mease P, Hall S, FitzGerald O, van der Heijde D, Merola JF, AvilaZapata F, et al. Tofacitinib or adalimumab versus placebo for psoriatic arthritis. N Engl J Med. 2017;377:1537-50.
10. Gladman D, Rigby W, Azevedo VF, Behrens F, Blanco R, Kaszuba A, et al. Tofacitinib for psoriatic arthritis in patients with an inadequate response to TNF inhibitors. N Engl J Med. 2017;377:1525-36.
11. Berekmeri A, Mahmood F, Wittmann M, Helliwell P. Tofacitinib for the treatment of psoriasis and psoriatic arthritis. Expert Rev Clin Immunol. 2018;14:719-30.
12. Liu LY, Craiglow BG, Dai F, King BA. Tofacitinib for the treatment of severe alopecia areata and variants: A study of 90 patients. J Am Acad Dermatol. 2017;76:22-8.
13. Jabbari A, Sansaricq F, Cerise J, Chen JC, Bitterman A, Ulerio G, et al. An open-label pilot study to evaluate the efficacy of tofacitinib in moderate to severe patch-type alopecia areata, totalis, and universalis. J Invest Dermatol. 2018;138:1539-45.
14. Shin JW, Huh CH, Kim MW, Lee JS, Kwon O, Cho S, et al. Comparison of the treatment outcome of oral tofacitinib with other conventional therapies in refractory alopecia totalis and universalis: A retrospective study. Acta Derm Venereol. 2019;99:41-6.
15. Liu LY, Craiglow BG, King BA. Tofacitinib 2% ointment, a topical Janus kinase inhibitor, for the treatment of alopecia areata: A pilot study of 10 patients. J Am Acad Dermatol. 2018;78:403-4.e1
16. Hosking AM, Juhasz M, Mesinkovska NA. Topical Janus kinase inhibitors: A review of applications in dermatology. J Am Acad Dermatol. 2018;79:535-44.
17. Craiglow BG. Topical tofacitinib solution for the treatment of alopecia areata affecting eyelashes. JAAD Case Rep. 2018;4:988-9.
18. Craiglow BG, King BA. Tofacitinib citrate for the treatment of vitiligo: A pathogenesis-directed therapy. JAMA Dermatol. 2015;151:1110.
19. Liu LY, Strassner JP, Refat MA, Harris JE, King BA. Repigmentation in vitiligo using the Janus kinase inhibitor tofacitinib may require concomitant light exposure. J Am Acad Dermatol. 2017;77:675-82.
20. Kim SR, Heaton H, Liu LY, King BA. Rapid repigmentation of vitiligo using tofacitinib plus lowdose, narrowband UVB phototherapy. JAMA Dermatol. 2018;154:370.
21. Bissonnette R, Papp KA, Poulin Y, Gooderham M, Raman M, Mallbris L, et al. Topical tofacitinib for atopic dermatitis: a phase IIa randomized trial. Br J Dermatol. 2016;175(5):902-11.
22. Levy LL, Urban J, King BA. Treatment of recalcitrant atopic dermatitis with the oral Janus kinase inhibitor tofacitinib citrate. J Am Acad Dermatol. 2015;73(3):395-9.
23. Vu M, Heyes C, Robertson SJ, Varigos GA, Ross G. Oral tofacitinib: a promising treatment in atopic dermatitis, alopecia areata and vitiligo. Clin Exp Dermatol. 2017;42:942-4.
24. Kurtzman DJB, Wright NA, Lin J, Femia AN, Merola JF, Patel M, et al. Tofacitinib citrate for refractory cutaneous dermatomyositis: an alternative treatment. JAMA Dermatol. 2016;152:944-5.
25. Moghadam-Kia S, Charlton D, Aggarwal R, Oddis CV. Management of refractory cutaneous dermatomyositis: potential role of Janus kinase inhibition with tofacitinib. Rheumatology (Oxford). 2019;58:1011-5.
26. Yang CC, Khanna T, Sallee B, Christiano AM, Bordone LA. Tofacitinib for the treatment of lichen planopilaris: a case series. Dermatol Ther. 2018;31:e12656.
27. Jaller JA, Jaller JJ, Jaller AM, Jaller-Char JJ, Ferreira SB, Ferreira R, et al. Recovery of nail dystrophy potential new therapeutic indication of tofacitinib. Clin Rheumatol. 2017;36:971-3.
28. Dhayalan A, King BA. Tofacitinib citrate for the treatment of nail dystrophy associated with alopecia universalis. JAMA Dermatol. 2016;152:492-3.
29. Kochar B, Herfarth N, Mamie C, Navarini AA, Scharl M, Herfarth HH. Tofacitinib for the treatment of pyoderma gangrenosum. Clin Gastroenterol Hepatol. 2019;17:991-3.

30. Cohen SB, Tanaka Y, Mariette X, Curtis JR, Lee EB, Nash P, et al. Long-term safety of tofacitinib for the treatment of rheumatoid arthritis up to 8.5 years: integrated analysis of data from the global clinical trials. Ann Rheum Dis. 2017;76:1253-62.
31. Chen YM, Huang WN, Wu YD, Lin CT, Chen YH, Chen DY, et al. Reactivation of hepatitis B virus infection in patients with rheumatoid arthritis receiving tofacitinib: a real-world study. Ann Rheum Dis. 2018;77:780-2.
32. Cohen S, Curtis JR, DeMasi R, Chen Y, Fan H, Soonasra A, et al. Worldwide, 3-year, postmarketing surveillance experience with tofacitinib in rheumatoid arthritis. Rheumatol Ther. 2018;5:283-91.
33. Fleischmann R, Wollenhaupt J, Takiya L, Maniccia A, Kwok K, Wang L, et al. Safety and maintenance of response for tofacitinib monotherapy and combination therapy in rheumatoid arthritis: an analysis of pooled data from open-label long-term extension studies. RMD Open. 2017;3:e000491.
34. Vincenti F, Tedesco Silva H, Busque S, O'Connell P, Friedewald J, Cibrik D, et al. Randomized phase 2b trial of tofacitinib (CP-690,550) in de novo kidney transplant patients: efficacy, renal function and safety at 1 year. Am J Transplant. 2012;12:2446-56.
35. Damsky W, King BA. JAK inhibitors in dermatology: The promise of a new drug class. J Am Acad Dermatol. 2017;76:736-44.
36. Valenzuela F, Korman NJ, Bissonnette R, Bakos N, Tsai TF, Harper MK, et al. Tofacitinib in patients with moderate-to-severe chronic plaque psoriasis: Long-term safety and efficacy in an open-label extension study. Br J Dermatol. 2018;179(4):853-62.

Part C: Other JAK Inhibitors: Baricitinib, Abrocitinib, and Upadacitinib

Ruchi Hemdani

INTRODUCTION

Janus kinase–signal transducers and activators of transcription (JAK-STAT) is a common signal transduction pathway involved not only in cell proliferation, migration, differentiation, and apoptosis but also in cellular messaging, which is why JAK inhibitors have broader immune-suppressing effects than monoclonal antibodies.[1-4] Targeting this pathway has become the cornerstone of management for many inflammatory disorders with therapy having evolved manifold over recent years. JAK inhibitors stop the intracellular signaling pathway by inhibiting JAK protein phosphorylation catalyzed by the kinase component of JAK.[1,2] Newer JAK-STAT inhibitors are being studied and getting approved increasingly. In this chapter, abrocitinib, baricitinib, and upadacitinib are discussed. All three are newer JAK-STAT inhibitors with various approved dermatological indications as shown in **Table 1**.

TABLE 1: FDA approvals for JAK-STAT inhibitors for dermatological disorders.[1,2]				
JAK inhibitor	**Generation**	**Approved indications**	**Approving authority**	**Year**
Abrocitinib: Selective JAK 1 inhibitor	Second	Atopic dermatitis (moderate to severe)	FDA	September 2023
Baricitinib: JAK 1,2 inhibitor	*First*: Low specificity, relatively higher risk of side effects, block multiple JAKi	Alopecia areata	FDA	June 2022
Upadacitinib: JAK1 inhibitor	Second	Moderate to severe atopic dermatitis in >12 years age	FDA	Jan 2022
Deucravacitinib: Another second-generation selective JAK inhibitor which targets TYK2 and is also FDA (September 2022) approved for moderate to severe psoriasis. It is not discussed in this chapter				

(JAK-STAT: Janus kinase–signal transducers and activators of transcription; FDA: Food and Drug Administration)

PHARMACOLOGY

Abrocitinib is a selective JAK1 inhibitor. It is associated with reduction in platelets (returns to normal after 4 weeks) and inflammatory markers but with increase in the level of low-density lipoprotein (LDL), high-density lipoprotein (HDL), and total cholesterol in a dose-dependent manner. By sparing JAK2, it does not cause anemia and leukopenia. It reaches maximum plasma concentration within an hour.[5,6]

Baricitinib acts on JAK1,2,3 and causes a dose-dependent inhibition of interleukin-6 (IL-6) induced STAT3 phosphorylation (maximum at 1 hour post drug intake), which returns to near baseline by 24 hours. The mean values of serum IgG, IgM, and IgA decrease by 12 weeks on treatment with baricitinib, and then remain stable till 52 weeks. It also causes sustained reduction in serum C-reactive protein (CRP) while on treatment.[7]

Upadacitinib is a reversible inhibitor with greater inhibitory potency for JAK1 than JAK2,3 or TYK2 which causes a dose-dependent inhibition of IL-6 (JAK1/JAK2)-induced STAT3 and IL-7 (JAK1/JAK3)-induced STAT5 phosphorylation (maximum at 1 hour after dosing) which returns to near baseline by the end of 24 hours. Body weight, age, gender, race, and ethnicity did not have a clinically meaningful effect on upadacitinib exposure. It can be used in patients with mild and moderate renal impairment and mild hepatic impairment. However, caution is to be exercised with moderate hepatic impairment and no data is currently available on use in severely impaired cases.[8]

Pharmacological characteristics have been highlighted in **Table 2** and the dose modification with drug interactions and renal impairment in **Tables 3 and 4**, respectively.

USES

Uses of JAK inhibitor are given in **Table 5**.

All three drugs have been strongly recommended in treatment of moderate-to-severe atopic dermatitis (AD) in guidelines of care for treatment of adults with AD.[17]

Abrocitinib for Atopic Dermatitis[5,6,18-21]

Abrocitinib received its first approval on 9 September 2021 for the treatment of moderate-to-severe AD in adults and adolescents 12 years and older who are candidates for systemic therapy in the UK. Abrocitinib was also approved in Japan for the same indication on 27 September 2021. Abrocitinib received a positive CHMP opinion in the EU on 14 October 2021 for the treatment of moderate-to-severe AD in adults who are candidates for systemic therapy. Abrocitinib was approved for management of refractory, moderate-to-severe AD in adolescents (12–18 years) by Food and Drug Administration

TABLE 2: Pharmacological characteristics.[5-8]

JAK inhibitor	Bioavailability and absorption post oral intake	Peak plasma and steady state concentration	Half-life (hours)	Distribution	Metabolism	Elimination
Abrocitinib	91%, rapid and unaffected by meals	Achieves peak plasma concentration within an hour	Half-lives of abrocitinib and its two active metabolites range from 3 to 5 hours	Distribution of abrocitinib and its two active metabolites (3-hydroxypropyl and 2-hydroxypropyl) is equal between red blood cells and plasma	Metabolic clearance by CYP450 enzymes (CYP2C19 and CYP2C9) into three major and one minor metabolite	<1% drug excreted unchanged in urine. Its active metabolites are primarily excreted in urine
Baricitinib	80%	Achieved in approximately 1 hour and 2–3 days respectively; minimal accumulation after once daily administration	10–12	Approximately 50% bound to plasma proteins and 45% bound to serum proteins	CYP3A4 enzymes	Renal
Upadacitinib	Rapid within 2–4 hours of intake, unaffected by meals	Achieved and in 4 days respectively; minimal accumulation after once daily administration	8–14	52% bound to plasma proteins, partitions similarly between plasma and blood cellular components	Metabolized primarily by CYP3A4 and minimally by CYP2D6 enzymes; no active metabolites	Predominantly excreted as unchanged drug in urine (24%) and feces (38%)

(JAK: Janus kinase)

TABLE 3: Drug interactions.[5-8]

	Inducers/Substrate interaction	Inhibitors
Abrocitinib	P-gp substrate where small concentration changes may lead to serious or life-threatening toxicities—monitor or titrate dosage of P-gp substrate	• Strong inhibitors of CYP2C19: dose modification to 50 mg daily • Moderate to strong inhibitors of both CYP2C19 and CYP2C9, or strong CYP2C19 or CYP2C9 inducers—avoid concomitant use
Baricitinib	Baricitinib is OAT3 substrate hence dose to be reduced to half when coadministered with strong OAT3 inhibitors (probenecid)	Nil. No significant inhibition of cytochrome P450 enzymes
Upadacitinib	Coadministration with strong CYP3A4 inducers is not recommended	When indicated for AD, coadministration with strong CYP3A4 inhibitors not recommended

TABLE 4: Dose modifications as per renal impairment.[5-8]

Renal impairment stage	Estimated glomerular filtration rate (eGFR: mL/min/1.73 m²)	Recommended dose as per renal impairment		
		Abrocitinib	Baricitinib	Upadacitinib
Mild	60–90	100 mg od	2 mg od	No dose modification
Moderate	30–60	50 mg od	1 mg od	No dose modification
Severe	15–30	Not recommended	Not recommended	15 mg od
ESRD	<15	Not recommended	Not recommended	Not recommended

(ESRD: end-stage renal disease)

(FDA) in September 2023.[18-20] Signaling cytokines mediated by JAK1 (IL-4,6,12,13,31) are all involved in AD pathogenesis and thus targeted effectively by abrocitinib resulting in rapid relief from pruritus and better sleep thereby improving quality of life in AD patients especially those unresponsive to IL-4 receptor, IL-13, and IL-31 receptor inhibitors.[21] Flexible dosing regimen was assessed in the JADE REGIMEN clinical trial[5,6,18] and considered a valid option. Induction with 200 mg followed by maintenance with 100 mg seems practical as most patients did not flare for at least 40 weeks in JADE regimen trial. This way the adverse effects (AEs) associated with higher dose can be avoided.

Intermittent therapy is not recommended as it was associated with a high relapse rate. Discontinuation of treatment should be considered in patients with no evidence of therapeutic benefit after 24 weeks.

TABLE 5: US FDA approved and off-label indications of JAK inhibitors.

JAK inhibitor	Approved indications	Off-label indications[1,2,9-16]
Abrocitinib	Atopic dermatitis	Alopecia areata, contact dermatitis
Baricitinib	• Alopecia areata • Rheumatoid arthritis • COVID-19	Atopic dermatitis, autoinflammatory disorders, recalcitrant lichen planopilaris, dermatomyositis, systemic sclerosis, familial chilblain lupus, subacute cutaneous lupus erythematosus, chronic nodular prurigo, immunobullous disorders, chronic graft-versus-host disease, chronic hand eczema, eosinophilic fasciitis, generalized morphea, granuloma annulare, hypereosinophilic syndrome, livedoid vasculopathy, psoriasis, lichen planus, vitiligo, sweet syndrome, pyoderma gangrenosum
Upadacitinib	Atopic dermatitis, psoriatic arthritis, rheumatoid arthritis, ulcerative colitis, Crohn's disease, ankylosing spondylitis, nonradiographic axial spondyloarthropathy	Alopecia areata, erosive oral lichen planus, granuloma annulare, hidradenitis suppurativa, persistent erythema multiforme, cutaneous lupus erythematosus, amyopathic dermatomyositis, vitiligo, Hailey–Hailey disease

(JAK: Janus kinase; US FDA: United States Food and Drug Administration)

Monotherapy

Abrocitinib has shown efficacy in patients with moderate-to-severe AD with monotherapy (MONO-1 and 2 clinical trials). 200 mg monotherapy was found to be most effective in maintaining disease control.[20]

Combination Therapy with Topicals

Effective in combination with topical therapies as well in comparison with placebo (COMPARE clinical trial);[5,6] furthermore, efficacy has also been demonstrated in adolescents in combination with topical therapies (JADE TEEN clinical TRIAL).[5,6,18,19]

Baricitinib for Alopecia Areata[7]

Alopecia areata is the only FDA approved dermatological indication for use of baricitinib based on the results of TRIAL AA1, TRIAL AA2, and TRIAL AA3. Baricitinib was shown to be effective in alopecia areata at doses 2 mg and 4 mg in these trials by targeting JAK1, 2, and 3. 4 mg doses were associated with a better response although lesser side effects were reported in the 2 mg group.

Baricitinib for Atopic Dermatitis[22,23]

It is approved in Europe for the treatment of moderate-to-severe AD, and is approved and available in the US for other immune-mediated conditions, but is not approved by the FDA to treat AD. Network meta-analysis suggests baricitinib is less efficacious than upadacitinib and abrocitinib for treating AD.

Upadacitinib for Atopic Dermatitis[8,23]

Being a selective JAK1 inhibitor, it finds many uses in dermatology, but is FDA approved in dermatology currently for AD. The efficacy of upadacitinib was assessed in three phase III randomized, double-blind, multicenter trials (AD-1, AD-2, AD-3, respectively) in a total of 2,584 patients (age > 12 years) with moderate-to-severe AD not adequately controlled by topical medication. Two other phase III clinical trials: MEASURE UP 1 and 2 were done. The results from these studies have suggested good efficacy with safety in moderate-to-severe cases of recalcitrant AD. It is indicated for the treatment of adults and pediatric patients 12 years of age and older with refractory, moderate-to-severe AD whose disease is not adequately controlled with other systemic drug products, including biologics, or when use of those therapies is inadvisable.

DOSE AND ADMINISTRATION[1,2,5-8]

Dose and administration of different drugs are given in **Table 6**.

TESTS/EVALUATION TO BE DONE PRIOR TO ADMINISTRATION (COMMON TO ALL THREE)[1,2]

- Complete medical history and baseline examination for skin cancer
- *Complete blood count (CBC)*: To rule out active infections and preexisting cytopenias
- *Liver function test (LFT)*: Doses may need modification with hepatic impairment
- *Blood urea, serum creatinine*: Doses may need modification with renal impairment
- Fasting lipid profile
- *Viral hepatitis screening as per clinical guidelines*: Hepatitis B surface antigen, anti-hepatitis C virus immunoglobulin M
- Pregnancy test in females of reproductive age group
- Check vaccination status
- *Rule out active and latent tuberculosis*:
  - History of past tuberculosis, history of contact with active case of tuberculosis
  - History of fever, weight loss, night sweats
  - Chest X-ray PA view
  - Purified protein derivative (PPD) or interferon-gamma release assays (IGRA)

TABLE 6: Dose and administration of different drugs.

Drug (brand)	Dosage form	Strength	Dose and frequency of administration
Abrocitinib (Pfizer:CIBINQO)	Film coated tablet oval (50, 200 mg) to round (100 mg) with abr 50/100/200 embossed as per strength	Three strengths each pink in color: 50, 100, 200 mg	• 100 mg once a day (od), can be increased to 200 mg od if inadequate response • 100 mg od for patient > 65 years • *Moderate renal impairment:* 50 mg od, can be increased to 100 mg od
Baricitinib (Eli Lilly: Olumiant)	Debossed, film-coated, immediate-release round (1, 4 mg) to oblong (2 mg) tablets with recessed area on each face of the tablet surface	Three strengths each different shade of pink in color: 1, 2, 4 mg	• AA: 2 mg od as monotherapy or in combination, can be increased to 4 mg od if no response • Age > 75 years: 2 mg od
Upadacitinib (AbbVie: Rinvoq)	Biconvex oblong extended-release tablets (dimensions of 14 × 8 mm) debossed with 'a15'/'a30'/'a45' on one side as per the strength	Three strengths each of different color: 15 mg (purple), 30 mg (red), 45 mg (yellow to mottled yellow)	• AD patients aged 12–65 years and weighing at least 40 kg: 15 mg orally od. If inadequate response, increase to 30 mg od • AD patients > 65 years of age or with severe renal impairment: 15 mg od

Patient must not chew, crush, or split tablets
Patients must avoid food or drink containing grapefruit with upadacitinib
Medicine residue in stool has been noticed with upadacitinib

Any patient with latent TB needs to be treated for same prior to use of JAK inhibitor

Prescription information: Additionally for abrocitinib, those with a negative latent TB test at screening but at high risk for TB, must be started on preventive therapy for latent TB prior to initiation.

MONITORING DURING THERAPY (COMMON TO ALL THREE)[1,2]

Patients who are on JAK-STAT inhibitors should be closely monitored for development of any infection, especially tuberculosis, hepatic, renal function status, dyslipidemia and venous thrombosis or pulmonary embolism. Patients at high risk of developing extrapulmonary or disseminated tuberculosis should be asked for history of weight loss, fever, and night sweats during each visit. Tests to be done:
- Regular skin examination
- Blood tests (4 weeks and 12 weeks on therapy, then periodically such as every 3 months)
  - CBC: additionally at 4 weeks after dose increase and thereafter according to routine patient management
  - Fasting lipid profile: Dose-dependent increases in blood lipid parameters, specifically LDL cholesterol, have been reported in AD patients treated with abrocitinib. Lipid parameters should also be assessed approximately 4 weeks after initiation of therapy and thereafter according to the cardiovascular disease risk of each patient.
  - LFT and RFT: To monitor patients for changes from baseline as dose modification may be required based on hepatic and renal impairment.
- Chest X-ray PA view, IGRA—preferably annually

ADVERSE EFFECTS[5-8]

JAK inhibitors-associated AEs seem to be dose-dependent with higher doses associated with more side effects specifically for abrocitinib. AEs to each drug are delineated in **Table 7** other than black box warning which is common to all three drugs and mentioned below:
- *Serious infections*: Increased risk of serious bacterial, fungal, viral, and opportunistic infections leading to hospitalization or death exists with these drugs especially increased risk of reactivation of latent tuberculosis, extrapulmonary and disseminated tuberculosis, invasive cryptococcosis and pneumocystosis. Herpes simplex, herpes zoster, and pneumonia have been reported with increased risk during therapy with abrocitinib and upadacitinib. If a patient develops a serious or opportunistic infection, discontinue therapy. Initiate complete diagnostic testing and appropriate antimicrobial therapy.

TABLE 7: Adverse effects.	
JAK inhibitor	Adverse effects
Abrocitinib	Nausea, vomiting, dizziness, upper abdominal pain, abdominal discomfort, influenza, gastroenteritis, fatigue, headache, oropharyngeal pain, nasopharyngitis, impetigo, herpes simplex, herpes zoster, urinary tract infection, acne, hypertension, contact dermatitis, increased blood creatinine phosphokinase, thrombocytopenia, lymphopenia, lipid elevation, retinal detachment
Baricitinib	Nausea, upper respiratory infections, herpes simplex, gastrointestinal perforations, lipid elevation, liver enzyme abnormalities, anemia, lymphopenia, neutropenia, increased serum creatine phosphokinase, angioedema, urticaria, and rash
Upadacitinib	Acne is the most frequent adverse event which is usually mild/moderate and managed with topical therapies or no intervention.[24] Other adverse events are: Hypersensitivity/allergic reaction, gastrointestinal perforation, anemia, neutropenia, lymphopenia, upper respiratory tract infections, herpes simplex, headache, blood creatine phosphokinase increased, cough, hypersensitivity, folliculitis, nausea, abdominal pain, pyrexia, increased weight, herpes zoster, influenza, fatigue, neutropenia, myalgia, and influenza-like illness, eczema herpeticum

(JAK: Janus kinase)

- *Malignancy*: Nonmelanoma skin cancers have been reported in patients on therapy with either of these drugs. Periodic skin examination is recommended for patients who are at increased risk for skin cancer. Exposure to sunlight and UV light should be limited by wearing protective clothing and using a broad-spectrum sunscreen. Increased risk of malignancies, including lymphomas, exists which has been reported previously in patients receiving JAK inhibitors used to treat inflammatory conditions.
- *Major adverse cardiac effect (MACE)*: Possibility of MACE exists with all three drugs. Higher rate of MACE [defined as cardiovascular death, myocardial infarction (MI), and stroke] with JAK inhibitor as compared to tumor necrosis factor (TNF) blockers in rheumatoid arthritis (RA) patients. Patients who smoke currently or in past are at increased risk. Discontinue drug if MI or stroke occurs.
- *Mortality*: Higher rate of all-cause mortality, including sudden cardiovascular death, with another JAK inhibitor versus TNF blockers in RA patients.
- *Thrombosis*: Thrombosis including pulmonary embolism and deep venous thrombosis has been observed at increased incidence with above three drugs. Patients with symptoms of thrombosis must discontinue drug.

TABLE 8: Contraindications.

JAK inhibitor	Absolute contraindications[5-8]	Relative contraindications[1,2]
Abrocitinib	• Severe hepatic impairment (drug not evaluated in this population), severe renal impairment and end-stage renal disease on dialysis • Antiplatelet therapies except for low-dose aspirin (≤81 mg daily), during the first 3 months of treatment	*Use with caution in patients at risk of thrombosis*: older age, obesity, a medical history of DVT/PE, prothrombotic disorder, combined hormonal contraceptives or hormone replacement therapy, and major surgery or prolonged immobilization
Baricitinib	• Severe hepatic impairment • Severe renal impairment	
Upadacitinib	Anaphylaxis, severe hepatic impairment	

(DVT: deep vein thrombosis; JAK: Janus kinase; PE: pulmonary embolism)

CONTRAINDICATIONS

Common contraindications to all three drugs[5-8] are mentioned below and specific to each are given in **Table 8**:
- Active serious infection including localized infection
- Hypersensitivity to the active substance or any of the excipients
- *Hematological*: Abrocitinib, baricitinib, and upadacitinib are not recommended in patients with absolute lymphocyte (ALC) <500/mm^3, absolute neutrophil count (ANC) <1000/mm^3, or hemoglobin (Hb) < 8 g/dL. Additionally, abrocitinib is not recommended in patients with a platelet count <1.5 lakh/mm^3, and baricitinib is not recommended in patients with COVID-19 with ALC <200/mm^3, ANC < 500/mm^3
- Pregnancy

SPECIAL SITUATIONS[5-8]

Special situations are described in **Table 9**.

LIMITATIONS

Not to be used in conjunction with other JAK–STAT inhibitors, potent systemic immunomodulators, and biologics.

ADVANTAGES OVER BIOLOGICS

- *Oral formulation*: Ease of administration
- Less frequent monitoring
- Relatively inexpensive
- Wider spectrum

TABLE 9: Special situations.

Special situation	Abrocitinib	Baricitinib	Upadacitinib
Pregnancy and lactation	Avoid use in pregnancy. Data regarding excretion in human milk not available. Breastfeeding not recommended during therapy and for one day after the last dose	• Avoid use in pregnancy • Data regarding excretion in human milk not available. Breastfeeding not recommended during therapy	Avoid use in pregnancy. Advise female patients of reproductive potential to use effective contraception during treatment and for 4 weeks after the final dose. Breastfeeding is not recommended during treatment and for 6 days (approximately 10 half-lives) after the last dose
Pediatric	Use established in >12 years old with atopic dermatitis	Safety and efficacy not established	Use established in atopic patients >12 years old weighing at least 40 kg
Latent tuberculosis	Not to be used in patients with latent TB unless treated. Screen for latent TB before and during therapy; treat latent TB prior to use. Monitor all patients for active TB during treatment, even patients with initial negative, latent TB test		
Viral hepatitis: Hepatitis B and Hepatitis C	JAK inhibitors can lead to flare of hepatitis in patients with chronic hepatitis B carrier state. These drugs are not recommended for use in patients with active hepatitis B or hepatitis C. Therefore, patients need to be screened prior to therapy and monitored for reactivation during therapy as per clinical guidelines. Viral hepatitis patients to be managed by hepatologist before therapy and use in chronic carrier state/inactive HBV expression, is to be done in consultation with hepatologist. Regular monitoring of aminotransferases and prophylactic antiviral therapy should be used if indicated		
Immunization	Avoid live, attenuated vaccines while patient is on therapy. Prior to therapy, it is recommended that patients be immunized adequately including prophylactic herpes zoster vaccinations in adults 50 years or older, in accordance with official recommendations		
DVT/PTE	Lower risk associated with selective JAK inhibitors, such as upadacitinib and abrocitinib, in younger and healthier populations of AD. EMA Pharmacovigilance Risk Assessment Committee (PRAC) has recommended that JAK inhibitors should be used only if no suitable treatment alternatives are available in patients >65 years, patients with increased risk of MACE, smokers (current/old), and patients with increased risk of cancer. These recommendations apply to all approved uses of JAK inhibitors in chronic inflammatory disorders		

(DVT: deep vein thrombosis; EMA: European Medicines Agency; JAK: Janus kinase; MACE: major adverse cardiac effect; PTE: pulmonary thromboembolism; TB: tuberculosis)

CONCLUSION

With upcoming JAK inhibitors, the need for injectable biologics is gradually subsiding. These drugs also serve as effective replacement for existing immunosuppressives. Being small molecules that can be administered orally, these drugs are more suitable for patients willing to avoid injections. Adequate monitoring and consideration of use in patients with cardiovascular disease, a history of thrombotic events, and a history of herpes infection will be necessary to minimize safety concerns. Long-term follow-up studies will better define the safety profile of these JAK inhibitors.

REFERENCES

1. Rygula I, Pikiewicz W, Kaminiów K. Novel Janus Kinase Inhibitors in the Treatment of Dermatologic Conditions. Molecules. 2023;28:8064.
2. Corbella-Bagot L, Riquelme-McLoughlina C, D Morgado-Carrasco. Long-Term Safety Profile and Off-Label Use of JAK Inhibitors in Dermatological Disorders. ACTAS Dermo-Sifiliográficas. 2023;114;784-801.
3. Chapman S, Kwa M, Gold LS, Lim HW. Janus kinase inhibitors in dermatology: Part I. A comprehensive review. J Am Acad Dermatol. 2022;86:406-13.
4. Chapman S, Kwa M, Gold LS, Lim HW. Janus kinase inhibitors in dermatology: Part II. A comprehensive review. J Am Acad Dermatol. 2022;86:414-22.
5. Deeks ED, Duggan S. Abrocitinib: First Approval. Drugs. 2021;81:2149-57.
6. Perche PO, Cook MK, Feldman SR. Abrocitinib: a new FDA approved drug for moderate-to-severe atopic dermatitis. Ann Pharmacother. 2023;57(1):86-98.
7. King B, Ohyama M, Kwon O, Zlotogorski A, Ko J, Mesinkovska NA, et al. Two phase 3 trials of baricitinib for alopecia areata. N Engl J Med. 2022;386(18):1687-99.
8. Guttman Yassky E, Texeira HD, Simpson EL, Papp KA, Pangman AL, Blauvelt A, et al. once daily Upadacitinib versus placebo in adolescents and adults with moderate to severe atopic dermatitis: results from two replicate double blind, randomized controlled phase 3 trials. Lancet. 2021;397(10290):2151-68.
9. Cotter DG, Schairer D, Eichenfield L. Emerging therapies for atopic dermatitis: JAK inhibitors. J Am Acad Dermatol. 2018;78:S53-62.
10. Gilhar A, Keren A, Paus R. JAK inhibitors and alopecia areata. The Lancet. 2019;393(10169):318-9.
11. Sanchez GAM, Reinhardt A, Ramsey S, Wittkowski H, Hashkes PJ, Berkun Y, et al. JAK1/2 inhibition with baricitinib in the treatment of autoinflammatory interferonopathies. J Clin Invest. 2018;128(7):3041-52.
12. Peterson D, Powell M, King B. Less is more? Failure of one JAK inhibitor does not predict failure of another one in a patient with alopecia areata. Dermatol Ther. 2021;34(5):e15062.
13. Boyadzhiev M, Marinov L, Boyadzhiev V, Iotova V, Aksentijevich I, Hambleton S. Disease course and treatment effects of a JAK inhibitor in a patient with CANDLE syndrome. Pediatr Rheumatol Online J. 2019;17(1):19.
14. Ramanan AV, Quartier P, Okamoto N, Foeldvari I, Spindler A, Fingerhutová S, et al. Baricitinib in juvenile idiopathic arthritis: an international, phase 3, randomised, double-blind, placebo-controlled, withdrawal, efficacy, and safety trial. Lancet. 2023;402:555-70.
15. Chong BF, Werth V. Cutaneous lupus erythematosus and dermatomyositis: utilizing assessment tools for treatment efficacy. J Invest Dermatol. 2022;142(3 Pt B):936-43.

16. Fetter T, Smith P, Guel T, Braegelmann C, Bieber T, Wenzel J. Selective Janus kinase 1 inhibition is a promising therapeutic approach for lupus erythematosus skin lesions. Front Immunol. 2020;11:344.
17. Davis DMR, Drucker AM, Alikhan A, Bercovitch L, Cohen DE, Darr JM, et al. Guidelines of care for the management of atopic dermatitis in adults with phototherapy and systemic therapies. J Am Acad Dermatol. 2024;90(2):e43-e56.
18. Iznardo H, Roe E, Serra-Baldrich E, Puig L. Efficacy and safety of JAK1 inhibitor Abrocitinib in atopic dermatitis. Pharmaceutics. 2023;15:385.
19. Silverberg JI, Simpson EL, Thyssen JP, Gooderham M, Chan G, Feeney C, et al. Efficacy and safety of Abrocitinib in patients with moderate-to-severe atopic dermatitis. JAMA Dermatol. 2020;156(8):1-11.
20. Simpson EL, Sinclair R, Forman S, Wollenberg A, Aschoff R, Cork M, et al. Efficacy and safety of abrocitinib in adults and adolescents with moderate-to-severe atopic dermatitis (JADE MONO-1): a multicentre, double-blind, randomised, placebo-controlled, phase 3 trial. Lancet. 2020;396:255-66.
21. Beiber T, Simpson EL, Silverberg JI, Thaci D, Paul C, Pink AE, et al. Abrocitinib versus Placebo or Dupilumab for Atopic Dermatitis. N Engl J Med. 2021;384:1101-12.
22. Simpson EL, Forman S, Silverberg JI, Zirwas M, Maverakis E, Han G, et al. Baricitinib in patients with moderate-to-severe atopic dermatitis: Results from a randomized monotherapy phase 3 trial in the United States and Canada (BREEZE-AD5). J Am Acad Dermatol. 2023;85:62-70.
23. Nogueira M, Torres T. Janus kinase inhibitors for the treatment of atopic dermatitis: focus on abrocitinib, baricitinib, and upadacitinib. Dermatol Pract Concept. 2021;11(4):e2021145.
24. Mendes-Bastos P, Ladizinski B, Guttman-Yassky E, Jiang P, Liu J, Prajapati VH, et al. Characterization of acne associated with upadacitinib treatment in patients with moderate-to-severe atopic dermatitis: A post hoc integrated analysis of 3 phase 3 randomized, double-blind, placebo-controlled trial. J Am Acad Dermatol. 2022;87:784-91.

Part D: Newer Janus Kinase Inhibitors

Padmapriya Srinivasan

INTRODUCTION

Janus kinase (JAK) proteins were historically named after the Greek god of gateways due to their intracellular association with membrane receptors. Small-molecule therapies that inhibit JAK proteins have emerged as efficacious treatment options in rheumatic and dermatologic diseases. JAK inhibitors (JAKis) exhibit anti-inflammatory effects through suppressing cytokine production involved in T helper 1 (Th1), Th2, Th17, and Th22 immune pathways. Broadly, they have been classified into first-generation JAKi that include tofacitinib, ruxolitinib, baricitinib, and oclacitinib; and second-generation JAKi that comprise decernotinib, peficitinib, filgotinib, fedratinib, momelotinib, and lestaurtinib.

In addition to the JAK STAT (signal transducer and activator of transcription) inhibitors mentioned in the previous parts of this chapter, there are many others that are not yet approved or under study for various dermatological indications. The main ones will be discussed further in this chapter.

NEWER JAK INHIBITORS

The list of newer JAKi along with their approved indications are mentioned in **Table 1**.

Table 2 shows new JAKi with dermatological indications approved by United States Food and Drug Administration (US FDA).

TABLE 1: The list of newer Janus kinase (JAK) inhibitors along with their approved indications.

Name	Subspecificity	Approved indications	Application
Ruxolitinib	JAK1/2	• Nonsegmental vitiligo (topical 1.5%) • Myelofibrosis • Post-polycythemia vera myelofibrosis • Postessential thrombocythemia myelofibrosis	Oral, topical
Peficitinib	Pan JAK	None	Oral
Delgocitinib	Pan JAK	None	Topical
Gusacitinib	Pan JAK	None	Oral

Continued

Continued

Name	Subspecificity	Approved indications	Application
Ifidancitinib	JAK1/3	None	Topical
Filgotinib	JAK1/3	RA	Oral
Itacitinib	JAK1/3	None	Oral
Solcitinib		None	Oral
Deucravacitinib (BMS986165)	Tyrosine kinase 2 (TYK2)	Moderate-to-severe plaque psoriasis	Oral
Brepocitinib	TYK2	None	Oral
PF-06826647	TYK2	None	Oral
Ritlecitinib	JAK3	Severe alopecia areata	Oral

TABLE 2: Newer Janus kinase (JAK) inhibitors with United States Food and Drug Administration (US FDA)-approved dermatological indications.

Inhibitor	Drug target	Indications	Dosage	FDA approval
Ruxolitinib	JAK1/2	• Atopic dermatitis • Nonsegmental vitiligo • Acute graft-versus-host disease • Chronic graft-versus-host disease	• Topical ruxolitinib 1.5% cream twice daily • Topical ruxolitinib 1.5% cream twice daily • Oral ruxolitinib 5 mg twice daily • Oral ruxolitinib 10 mg twice daily	• 2021 • 2022 • 2019 • 2021
Deucravacitinib	Tyrosine kinase 2 (TYK2)	Plaque psoriasis	Oral deucravacitinib 6 mg once daily	2022
Ritlecitinib	JAK3	Severe alopecia areata	Oral ritlecitinib 50 mg once daily	2023

PSORIASIS

Oral deucravacitinib, a FDA-approved inhibitor targeting the tyrosine kinase 2 (TYK2) enzyme through selective allosteric modulation, possesses a distinctive mechanism of action. This compound interacts specifically with the regulatory domain of TYK2, which exhibits structural dissimilarity from the regulatory domains found in other JAK family members. This structural specificity enables a more precise and targeted inhibition of TYK2 while minimizing cross-reactivity with JAK1, JAK2, and JAK3.[1,2] In the context of two phase III trials (POETYK PSO-1 and PSO-2), the administration of oral deucravacitinib at a daily dose of 6 mg demonstrated notable efficacy and maintained a tolerable safety profile, as summarized in **Table 3**.[3-5] Notably,

TABLE 3: A summary of trials investigating deucravacitinib for the treatment of psoriasis on ClinicalTrials.gov.

Study number	Study design	Treatment regimen	Results
NCT03624127	Phase III, double-blind, randomized study of 666 patients (POETYK PSO-1)[3]	• Deucravacitinib 6 mg QD • Apremilast 30 mg BID for initial 24 weeks; at week 24, patients who did not achieve PASI-50 were switched to deucravacitinib 6 mg QD, and patients who achieved PASI-50 continued apremilast 30 mg BID • Placebo for initial 16 weeks, followed by deucravacitinib 6 mg QD • All were treated for 52 weeks	• At week 16, PASI-75 and sPGA (0 or 1) response rates were significantly higher in patients on deucravacitinib versus placebo or apremilast (58.4% vs. 12.7% vs. 35.1%; $p < 0.0001$) and (53.6% vs. 7.2% vs. 32.1%; $p < 0.0001$) • Efficacy of deucravacitinib improved beyond week 16 and was maintained through week 52
NCT03611751	Phase III, double-blind, randomized study of 1,020 patients (POETYK PSO-2)[4]	• Deucravacitinib 6 mg QD for initial 24 weeks. At week 24, patients who achieved PASI-75 were re-randomized 1:1 to placebo or deucravacitinib 6 mg QD, and those who did not achieve PASI-75 continued deucravacitinib 6 mg QD; apremilast 30 mg BID for initial 24 weeks; at week 24, patients who did not achieve PASI-75 were switched in a blinded fashion to deucravacitinib 6 mg QD, and patients who achieved PASI-75 were continued on placebo • Placebo for initial 16 weeks, followed by deucravacitinib 6 mg QD • All were treated for 52 weeks	• At week 16, PASI-75 and sPGA (0 or 1) response rates were significantly higher in patients on deucravacitinib versus placebo or apremilast (53.0% vs. 9.4% vs. 39.8%; $p < 0.0001$) and (49.5% vs. 8.6% vs. 33.9%; $p < 0.0001$) • Among deucravacitinib-treated patients who achieved PASI-75 at week 24 and were randomized to continue deucravacitinib, PASI-75 responses were maintained through week 52 [80.4% (119/148); sPGA 0 or 1, 70.3% 83/118)]
NCT03881059	Phase II, double-blind, randomized study of 203 patients[5]	• Deucravacitinib 6 mg QD • Deucravacitinib 12 mg QD • Placebo QD • All were treated for 16 weeks.	• At week 16, ACR-20 response was significantly higher in deucravacitinib 6 mg (52.9%, $p = 0.0134$) and 12 mg (62.7%, $p = 0.0004$) compared to placebo (31.8%)

[ACR-20: American College of Rheumatology-20; BID: twice daily; HAQ-DI: Health Assessment Questionnaire-Disability Index; PASI-50: ≥50% improvement from baseline in Psoriasis Area and Severity Index (PASI) scores; PASI-75: ≥75% improvement from baseline in PASI scores; QD: once daily; QOD: every other day; SF-36 PCS: Short Form-36 (SF-36) Physical Component Summary (PCS) score; sPGA (0 or 1): static Physician's Global Assessment score of clear or almost clear; TYK2: tyrosine kinase 2] in the PSO-1 trial, a significant proportion of patients (58.4% and 53.6%) achieved a ≥75% improvement in the Psoriasis Area and Severity Index (PASI) and static Physician's Global Assessment (PGA) (clear or almost clear) scores when compared to the placebo (12.7% and 7.2%, respectively) or apremilast (35.1% and 32.1%). This therapeutic efficacy persisted throughout the 52-week treatment period. While infrequent occurrences of herpes zoster- and acne-related side effects were noted, the majority of cases did not necessitate discontinuation of treatment. Additionally, ongoing investigations involve allosteric TYK2 inhibitors such as VTX-958 and NDI-034858, showcasing their potential in addressing psoriasis (PsO) and/or psoriatic arthritis (PsA).[6-8]

Apart from deucravacitinib, brepocitinib and ropsacitinib, which are orthosteric inhibitors of TYK2, are also being tried for this indication **(Fig. 1)**.

Ropsacitinib has been tried in individuals with moderate-to-severe PsO through both a phase I trial and a phase IIb trial. In the phase I trial, a double-blind, placebo-controlled study, 40 patients exhibiting moderate-to-severe PsO were randomly assigned to receive either ropsacitinib (at doses of 100 or 400 mg) or a placebo once daily for 28 days (ClinicalTrials.gov Identifier: NCT03210961). Results indicated that ropsacitinib was well-tolerated and effective in reducing disease activity at 28 days, as evidenced by improvements in PASI-75, target plaque severity score, and body surface area.[9]

In the subsequent phase IIb trial, also a double-blind, placebo-controlled study, 179 patients were allocated in a 1:1:2:2:2 ratio to receive ropsacitinib (at doses of 50, 100, 200, or 400 mg) or a placebo once daily for 16 weeks.[10]

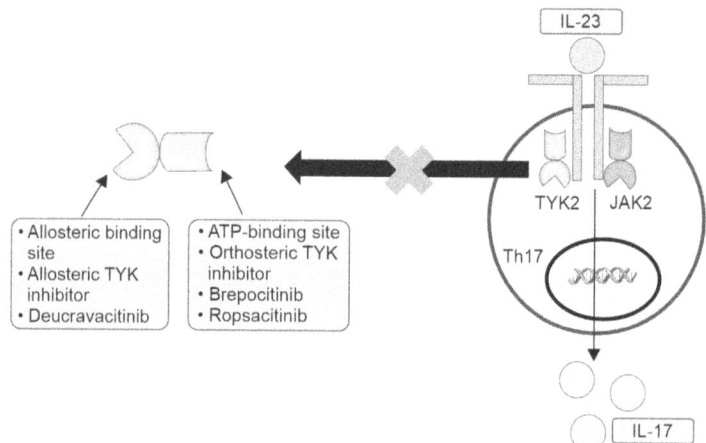

FIG. 1: Site of binding and mechanism of action of deucravacitinib, brepocitinib, and Ropsacitinib.
(ATP: adenosine triphosphate; IL-23: interleukin 23; JAK: Janus kinase; TYK2: tyrosine kinase 2)

Following this initial period, patients on the 200 or 400 mg dose continued with the same dosage, while those initially assigned to other doses were re-randomized to receive 200 or 400 mg once daily (ClinicalTrials.gov Identifier: NCT03895372). By week 16, a significantly greater percentage of patients achieved the primary endpoint of PASI-90 with ropsacitinib at the 200 mg (33.0%, $p = 0.0004$) and 400 mg (46.5%, $p < 0.0001$) doses compared to the placebo. Similarly, significant improvements were observed for PASI-75 at week 16 for ropsacitinib at 200 and 400 mg versus placebo. Moreover, a PGA response, defined as a PGA score of 0/1 (clear/almost clear) with a decrease from baseline ≥2 points, was achieved by a numerically greater proportion of patients across all treatment groups compared to placebo from weeks 6 to 16.

Brepocitinib, has successfully completed phase I and II trials in individuals with moderate-to-severe PsO. While the oral form of brepocitinib is not being pursued further for PsO, ongoing phase II trials are set to assess the efficacy of the topical formulation in cases of mild-to-moderate PsO (ClinicalTrials.gov Identifier: NCT03850483).

In a phase I trial involving healthy subjects and patients with moderate-to-severe PsO (ClinicalTrials.gov Identifier: NCT02310750), brepocitinib demonstrated a generally safe and well-tolerated profile. Subsequently, a phase IIa trial in patients with moderate-to-severe PsO enrolled 212 participants who were randomized to receive brepocitinib (at doses of 30 or 60 mg) or a placebo once daily for a 4-week induction period, followed by maintenance doses of 10 mg once daily, 30 mg once daily, 100 mg once weekly, or a placebo for an additional 8 weeks (ClinicalTrials.gov Identifier: NCT02969018).[11] At week 12, brepocitinib-treated patients exhibited significantly greater changes in PASI compared to the placebo group (least square mean change of –17.3 with 30 mg once daily continuous treatment; $p < 0.05$).[12]

Furthermore, at week 12, all brepocitinib treatment groups showed a higher proportion of patients achieving PASI-75 and PASI-90 compared to the placebo, with the most notable achievements observed in the 30 mg once daily continuous treatment group (PASI-75: 25 out of 29, 86.2%; PASI-90: 15 out of 29, 51.7%).

Biomarker analyses indicated that brepocitinib treatment led to a reduction in inflammatory gene expression in PsO lesions, reaching levels observed in nonlesional skin. These reductions in inflammatory gene expression correlated with improvements in histologic and clinical outcomes.[13]

VITILIGO

The 1.5% cream formulation of ruxolitinib serves as an inhibitor of JAK1/2 and has received FDA approval for the treatment of depigmentation in non-segmental vitiligo (NSV) patients.[10] This approval is substantiated by the outcomes of two phase III trials, namely TRuE-V1 and TRuE-V2. In these studies, 30.7% of individuals utilizing ruxolitinib 1.5% cream twice daily (BID) achieved a ≥75% improvement in the facial Vitiligo Area Scoring Index at week 24, as opposed to 9.9% of patients using the vehicle cream BID.[14] Noteworthy adverse events (AEs) primarily included reactions at the application site.

Significantly, sun-exposed regions, particularly the face, exhibited preferential repigmentation, as evidenced in multiple case studies.[15-17] A meta-analysis involving 45 patients revealed that 88.9% of those subjected to both JAKi and phototherapy experienced superior repigmentation outcomes compared to the 11.1% patients solely undergoing JAKi monotherapy.[18] Consequently, the concurrent administration of JAKi (to suppress immune responses) and light therapy (to stimulate melanocyte regeneration) may be imperative for achieving optimal repigmentation results. This paradigm is supported by the evaluation of the efficacy of other JAKi in numerous case studies.

Summary of clinical trials, case reports, and cohort studies investigating JAKi for the treatment of vitiligo is shown in **Table 4**.

Apart from abovementioned small molecules ritlecitinib, an irreversible inhibitor targeting JAK3 and TYK, designed for treating moderate-to-severe rheumatoid arthritis (RA) and brepocitinib, an inhibitor of TYK2/JAK1, are presently under scrutiny to assess their effectiveness and safety in managing active NSV when combined with phototherapy. Cerdulatinib, an SYK/JAK dual kinase inhibitor, has also been assessed (NCT04103060) for its safety and tolerability for vitiligo treatment in topical formation (0.37% cerdulatinib gel BID).[19]

SYSTEMIC LUPUS ERYTHEMATOSUS

The various mechanisms via which JAK STAT pathway is involved in systemic lupus erythematosus (SLE) is shown in **Figure 2**.

The efficacy of baricitinib was evaluated in two parallel phase III studies, SLE-BRAVE-I and SLE-BRAVE-II.[20,21] Given that type 1 interferons (IFNs) transmit signals through TYK2, inhibitors targeting TYK2, such as deucravacitinib, emerge as promising therapeutic agents. In a phase II study, notable proportions of patients administered oral deucravacitinib at doses of 3 mg BID and 6 mg BID demonstrated significant SRI-4 (Systemic Lupus Erythematosus Responder Index-4) responses in comparison to those on a placebo, as detailed in **Table 5**.[22,23] Furthermore, ongoing investigations involve brepocitinib, characterized as a TYK2/JAK1 inhibitor, and elsubrutinib, an inhibitor of Bruton's TYK.[24,25] These compounds are currently subjects of exploration and evaluation within the scientific community.

TABLE 4: Summary of clinical trials, case reports, and cohort studies investigating Janus kinase (JAK) inhibitors for the treatment of vitiligo.

Inhibitor	Drug target	Study number	Study design	Treatment regimen	Results
Topical ruxolitinib	JAK1/2	• NCT04052425 • NCT04057573	Two phase III, double-blind, randomized, parallel studies of 330 and 334 patients (TRuE-V1 and TRuE-V2)[15]	• Ruxolitinib 1.5% cream BID • Placebo BID • All were treated for 24 weeks (primary), 52 weeks (secondary)	• At week 24, significantly greater proportions of patients applying ruxolitinib cream BID achieved F-VASI75 compared to those on vehicle BID (30.7% vs. 9.9%; $p < 0.0001$) • At week 52, approximately 50% of patients showed ≥75% improvement in F-VASI compared to 30% of patients at week 24 • At week 52, approximately 75% of patients showed ≥50% improvement in F-VASI compared to 51% of patients at week 24 • At week 52, approximately 30% of patients showed ≥90% improvement in F-VASI compared to 15% of patients at week 24
Topical ruxolitinib	JAK1/2	NCT03099304	Phase II, double-blind, randomized study of 157 patients	• Ruxolitinib 1.5% cream BID • Ruxolitinib 1.5% cream QD • Ruxolitinib 0.5% cream QD • Ruxolitinib 0.15% cream QD • Matched placebo • All were treated for 24 weeks.	At week 24, patients on ruxolitinib cream 1.5% BID and 1.5% QD demonstrated a ≥50% improvement from baseline F-VASI (1.5% cream BID, OR 24.7; 95% CI 3.3–1121.4; $p = 0.0001$) and (1.5% cream QD, OR 28.5; 95% CI 3.7–1305.2; $p = 0.0001$) compared to patients on placebo.
Topical ifidancitinib (ATI-50002)	JAK1/3	NCT03468855	Phase II, open-label, nonrandomized, single-group study of 34 patients	Ifidancitinib 0.46% solution BID for 24 weeks	At week 24, there was an improvement in mean F-VASI: −0.067 (SD: 0.2411). The VNS scale change was 2.2 (SD 0.66)
Topical delgocitinib	JAK1/2/3; TYK2	–	Case report of two patients	• *Patient 1*: Delgocitinib cream BID for 8 weeks • *Patient 2*: Delgocitinib cream BID for 12 weeks	At week 8, patient 1 showed significant repigmentation of the neck. At week 12, patient 2 did not show repigmentation of left elbow

(BID: twice daily; CI: confidence interval; F-VASI: facial Vitiligo Area Scoring Index; F-VASI75: ≥75% improvement in the F-VASI; JAK: Janus kinase; NB-UVB: narrow-band ultraviolet; OR: odds ratio; PUVA: psoralen-ultraviolet A; QD: once daily; SD: standard deviation; TCI: topical calcineurin inhibitor; TCS: topical corticosteroid; TYK2: tyrosine kinase 2; VNS: Vitiligo Noticeability Scale)

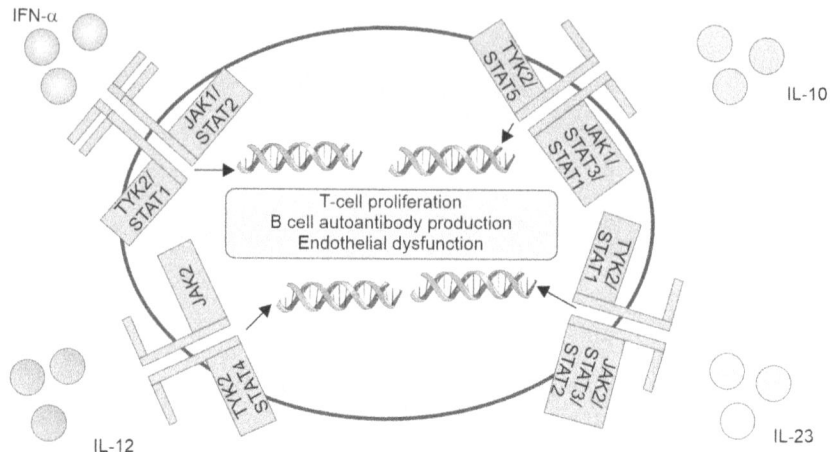

FIG. 2: Pathogenesis of systemic lupus erythematosus (SLE).
(IFN-α: interferon-alpha; IL-10: interleukin 10; STAT1: signal transducer and activator of transcription 1; TYK2: tyrosine kinase 2)

HIDRADENITIS SUPPURATIVA

In a phase II, randomized, double-blind, dose-ranging, placebo-controlled study out of 209 patients who were randomly assigned to different doses (15 mg, n = 52; 45 mg, n = 52; 75 mg, n = 53; placebo, n = 52), 83.3% successfully completed the 16-week treatment.[24] By week 16, povorcitinib demonstrated a significant reduction in abscess and inflammatory nodule count compared to baseline [least squares mean standard error change: 15 mg, –5.2 (0.9), p = 0.0277; 45 mg, –6.9 (0.9), p = 0.0006; 75 mg, –6.3 (0.9), p = 0.0021] in contrast to the placebo group [2.5 (0.9)]. More patients treated with povorcitinib achieved a hidradenitis suppurativa (HS) clinical response at week 16 (15 mg, 48.1%, p = 0.0445; 45 mg, 44.2%, p = 0.0998; 75 mg, 45.3%, p = 0.0829) compared to the placebo group (28.8%).[24] AEs were reported in 60.0% and 65.4% of povorcitinib- and placebo-treated patients, respectively. INCB054707, a JAK1 inhibitor, underwent evaluation in two phase II trials (NCT03569371 and NCT03607487) involving patients with moderate-to-severe HS.[25,26] In the NCT03607487 study, participants were randomly assigned to receive INCB054707 orally once daily in three different doses (30, 60, 90 mg) or a placebo.[25] 80% of patients treated with 30 and 60 mg of INCB054707 experienced grade 1–2 AEs (nonlethal events that are not life-threatening and do not necessitate inpatient hospitalization). For those treated with 90 mg, 50% had grade 1–2 AEs, and 37% experienced grade 3 AEs (events resulting in death, being life-threatening, or requiring inpatient hospitalization). Another ongoing phase II trial (NCT04476043) aims to assess the effectiveness and safety of INCB054707 in patients with HS.[27]

TABLE 5: A summary of trials investigating Janus kinase (JAK) inhibitors for the treatment of systemic lupus erythematosus as found on ClinicalTrials.gov.

Inhibitor	Drug target	Study number	Study design	Treatment regimen	Results
Oral Deucravacitinib (BMS-986165)	TYK2	NCT03252587	Phase II, double-blind, randomized study of 314 patients (PAISLEY)	• Deucravacitinib 3 mg BID • Deucravacitinib 6 mg BID • Deucravacitinib 12 mg QD • Placebo BID • All were treated for 32 weeks	• At week 32, significantly greater proportions of patients in the 3-mg and 6-mg group achieved SRI-4 compared to placebo (deucravacitinib 3 mg BID: 58.2%, $p = 0.0006$; deucravacitinib 6 mg BID: 49.5%, $p = 0.0210$; placebo: 34.4%). The 12-mg group had numerically higher SRI-4 response rates than placebo, but differences were nonsignificant • The efficacy of deucravacitinib was maintained through 48 weeks

(BID: twice daily; CI: confidence interval; OR: odds ratios; QD: once daily; SRI-4: Systemic Lupus Erythematosus Responder Index-4; TYK2: tyrosine kinase 2)

Signals from cytokines IL-23, IL-12, and type I IFNs activate TYK2. Ropsacitinib (PF-06826647) TYK2 inhibitor and brepocitinib (PF-06700841) TYK2/JAK1 inhibitor are part of phase II study with three kinase inhibitors (NCT04092452).[23]

DERMATOMYOSITIS

Effective interventions for refractory dermatomyositis have been demonstrated through the administration of oral tofacitinib and oral ruxolitinib.[28] Furthermore, investigations into potential treatments are ongoing, with oral baricitinib and oral brepocitinib currently under scrutiny in phase II and III trials.[28-32]

LICHEN PLANUS AND LICHEN PLANOPILARIS

Recent investigations have unveiled elevated expression of IFN-γ in lichen planus (LP) skin samples, indicating potential therapeutic applications for JAKi.[33] In a phase II pilot study, noteworthy outcomes were observed in 12 patients who underwent an 8-week treatment regimen with topical ruxolitinib 1.5% cream administered BID.[34] These patients demonstrated substantial improvements in both lesion severity and count, suggesting the therapeutic promise of JAK inhibition in addressing the manifestations of LP.

GRAFT-VERSUS-HOST DISEASE

Oral ruxolitinib, functioning as a JAK1/2 inhibitor, has obtained approval for the treatment of acute graft-versus-host disease (aGvHD) and chronic graft-versus-host disease (cGvHD). A pivotal phase III trial, known as REACH-2, demonstrated that patients with aGvHD receiving oral ruxolitinib at a dose of 10 mg BID achieved a significantly higher overall response rate (ORR) and prolonged median survival when compared to the control group, which received the best available therapy. The overall response was notably superior in the ruxolitinib-treated cohort, with 62% (96 patients) exhibiting a positive response, as opposed to 39% (61 patients) in the control group [odds ratio (OR) 2.64; 95% confidence interval (CI) 1.65–4.22; $p < 0.001$].[35]

In a separate phase III trial, REACH-3, involving patients with steroid-refractory cGvHD, those treated with ruxolitinib at a dosage of 10 mg BID demonstrated a higher ORR compared to the control group.[36] Noteworthy AEs observed in both studies included thrombocytopenia and anemia. These findings underscore the efficacy of oral ruxolitinib in addressing aGvHD and cGvHD, with a favorable overall response profile, albeit with the recognition of common AEs associated with its use.

In a multicenter, phase II trial (NCT03846479), itacitinib, a selective JAK1 inhibitor, was used to treat low risk aGvHD and it was compared with systemic corticosteroids. More patients responded to itacitinib within 7 days (81% vs. 66%, $p = 0.02$), and response rates at day 28 were very high for both groups (89% vs. 86%, $p = 0.67$).[37]

ATOPIC DERMATITIS

Multiple JAKi have been used for atopic dermatitis (AD), as mentioned in the previous sections. In addition, studies (presently in phase III trials) revealed that following topical application for a duration of 24 weeks, both delgocitinib (a pan JAKi) and ruxolitinib (a JAK1/2 inhibitor or JAK1/2i) exhibited significant improvements in pruritus and the Eczema Area and Severity Index (EASI) among individuals with moderate-to-severe AD.[38] These findings suggest that both JAKi have a positive impact on itchiness and overall disease severity in patients with this skin condition.

Gusacitinib (ASN002) is a potent oral dual JAK/spleen tyrosine kinase (SYK) inhibitor that has primarily been studied in malignancies and lymphoproliferative disorders due to its antiproliferative effects.[39,40] In a phase Ib dose escalation study involving patients with moderate-to-severe AD, where patients were administered either 20, 40, or 80 mg of gusacitinib or a placebo once daily, gusacitinib was found to be well-tolerated and effective, especially at higher dosages. Significant and rapid improvements in clinical measures (EASI-50) were observed in the 40 and 80 mg groups after 4 weeks of treatment, and pruritus measures [baseline itch-NRS (Numeric Rating Scale)] in the 80 mg group showed early improvement as early as day 8. Specifically, 100% and 83% of patients receiving 40 and 80 mg gusacitinib, respectively, achieved EASI-50 after 4 weeks. EASI-75 results did not reach significance. Results from a larger 12-week phase IIb extension study in moderate-to-severe AD (RADIANT) further support the efficacy of gusacitinib, as patients receiving gusacitinib demonstrated a significant reduction in EASI, particularly at 60 and 80 mg doses, and rapid and significant decreases in pruritus compared with the placebo at week 12.

ALOPECIA AREATA

Increasing evidence indicates toward efficacy of JAKi in the treatment of alopecia areata (AA). A notable limitation of the promising approach in treating AA with oral JAKi is the preliminary observation that the efficacy of JAK inhibition appears to be temporally restricted. In a significant number of patients, hair loss has been reported to recur upon discontinuation of pharmacological JAK inhibition.[41] The newer drugs are summarized in **Table 6** along with the studies.

TABLE 6: Summary of Janus kinase (JAK) inhibitors that have been reported in the literature for the treatment of alopecia areata.

Drug	Mechanism of action	Dosing regimens
Ruxolitinib[41-44]	JAK1/JAK2 Inhibitor	*Oral*: • 20 mg twice daily • 5–15 mg twice daily • 10–25 mg twice daily *Topical*: • 0.6% twice daily • 1% twice daily • 1.5% twice daily
Ritlecitinib[45]	JAK3/TEC inhibitor	*Oral*: • 200 mg once daily for 4 weeks, then 50 mg once daily for 20 weeks • 50 mg, 30 mg, or 10 mg once daily
Brepocitinib[45]	TYK2/JAK1 inhibitor	*Oral*: 60 mg once daily for 4 weeks, then 30 mg once daily for 20 weeks
Ifidancitinib[46]	JAK1/JAK3 inhibitor	*Topical*: 0.5% or 0.1% twice daily
Delgocitinib[47]	JAK1/JAK2/JAK3/TYK2 inhibitor	*Topical*: 30 mg/g twice daily

(TEC: tyrosine kinase expressed in hepatocellular carcinoma; TYK2: tyrosine kinase 2)

CONCLUSION

Janus kinase inhibitors are the most promising treatment options for the management of dermatological diseases. Newer JAKi and newer indications for JAKi are being developed very rapidly. Treating physicians should understand the risk and opportunities that these molecules bring for their patients.

REFERENCES

1. Shang L, Cao J, Zhao S, Zhang J, He Y. TYK2 in immune responses and treatment of psoriasis. J Inflamm Res. 2022;15:5373-85.
2. Nogueira M, Puig L, Torres T. JAK inhibitors for treatment of psoriasis: Focus on selective TYK2 inhibitors. Drugs. 2020;80:341-52.
3. Armstrong AW, Gooderham M, Warren RB, Papp KA, Strober B, Thaçi D, et al. Deucravacitinib versus placebo and apremilast in moderate to severe plaque psoriasis: efficacy and safety results from the 52-week, randomized, double-blinded, placebo-controlled phase 3 POETYK PSO-1 trial. J Am Acad Dermatol. 2023;88(1):29-39.
4. Strober B, Thaçi D, Sofen H, Kircik L, Gordon KB, Foley P, et al. Deucravacitinib versus placebo and apremilast in moderate to severe plaque psoriasis: efficacy and safety results from the 52-week, randomized, double-blinded, phase 3 Program fOr Evaluation of TYK2 inhibitor psoriasis second trial. J Am Acad Dermatol. 2023;88(1):40-51.
5. Mease PJ, Deodhar AA, van der Heijde D, Behrens F, Kivitz AJ, Neal J, et al. Efficacy and safety of selective TYK2 inhibitor, deucravacitinib, in a phase II trial in psoriatic arthritis. Ann Rheum Dis. 2022;81:815-22.

6. Ventyx Biosciences. (2022). Ventyx biosciences announces positive topline phase 1 data for its selective allosteric TYK2 inhibitor VTX958. [online] Available from https://ir.ventyxbio.com/news-releases/news-release-details/ventyx-biosciences-announces-positive-topline-phase-1-data-its-0 [Last accessed February, 2024].
7. Nimbus Therapeutics. (2022). Nimbus therapeutics announces expansion of oral allosteric TYK2 inhibitor program and provides additional business updates. Nimbus therapeutics. [online] Available from https://www.nimbustx.com/2022/01/06/nimbus-therapeutics-announces-expansion-of-oral-allosteric-tyk2-inhibitor-program-and-provides-additional-business-updates/ [Last accessed February, 2024].
8. Takeda. (2023). Study of NDI-034858 in participants with moderate to severe plaque psoriasis. Identifier NCT04999839. [online] Available from https://classic.clinicaltrials.gov/ct2/show/NCT04999839?cond=NCT04999839&draw=2&rank=1 [Last accessed February, 2024].
9. Tehlirian C, Peeva E, Kieras E, Scaramozza M, Roberts ES, Singh RSP, et al. Safety, tolerability, efficacy, pharmacokinetics, and pharmacodynamics of the oral TYK2 inhibitor PF-06826647 in participants with plaque psoriasis: a phase 1, randomised, double-blind, placebo-controlled, parallel-group study. Lancet Rheumatol. 2021;3(3):e204-13.
10. Tehlirian C, Singh RSP, Pradhan V, Roberts ES, Tarabar S, Peeva E, et al. Oral tyrosine kinase 2 inhibitor PF-06826647 demonstrates efficacy and an acceptable safety profile in participants with moderate-to-severe plaque psoriasis in a phase 2b, randomized, double-blind, placebo-controlled study. J Am Acad Dermatol. 2022;87(2):333-42.
11. Banfield C, Scaramozza M, Zhang W, Kieras E, Page KM, Fensome A, et al. The safety, tolerability, pharmacokinetics, and pharmacodynamics of a TYK2/JAK1 inhibitor (PF-06700841) in healthy subjects and patients with plaque psoriasis. J Clin Pharmacol. 2018;58(4):434-47.
12. Forman SB, Pariser DM, Poulin Y, Vincent MS, Gilbert SA, Kieras EM, et al. TYK2/JAK1 inhibitor PF-06700841 in patients with plaque psoriasis: phase IIa, randomized, double-blind, placebo-controlled trial. J Invest Dermatol. 2020;140(12):2359-70.e5.
13. Page KM, Suarez-Farinas M, Suprun M, Zhang W, Garcet S, Fuentes-Duculan J, et al. Molecular and cellular responses to the TYK2/JAK1 inhibitor PF-06700841 reveal reduction of skin inflammation in plaque psoriasis. J Invest Dermatol. 2020;140:1546-55.
14. Sheikh A, Rafique W, Owais R, Malik F, Ali E. FDA approves Ruxolitinib (Opzelura) for Vitiligo Therapy: A breakthrough in the field of dermatology. Ann Med Surg (Lond). 2022;81:104499.
15. Incyte Corporation. (2022). Topical ruxolitinib evaluation in vitiligo study 2 (TRuE-V2). [online] Available from https://www.clinicaltrials.gov/study/NCT04057573 [Last accessed February, 2024].
16. Liu LY, Strassner JP, Refat MA, Harris JE, King BA. Repigmentation in vitiligo using the Janus kinase inhibitor tofacitinib may require concomitant light exposure. J Am Acad Dermatol. 2017;77:675-82.e1.
17. Kim SR, Heaton H, Liu LY, King BA. Rapid repigmentation of vitiligo using tofacitinib plus low-dose, narrowband UV-B phototherapy. JAMA Dermatol. 2018;154:370-1.
18. Rosmarin D, Pandya AG, Lebwohl M, Grimes P, Hamzavi I, Gottlieb AB, et al. Ruxolitinib cream for treatment of vitiligo: a randomised, controlled, phase 2 trial. Lancet. 2020;396:110-20.
19. Pfizer. (2022). A phase 2b study to evaluate the efficacy and safety profile of PF-06651600 and PF-06700841 in active non-segmental vitiligo subjects. [online] Available from https://clinicaltrials.gov/ct2/show/NCT03715829 [Last accessed February, 2024].
20. Aarts P, Dudink K, Vossen ARJV, van Straalen KR, Ardon CB, Prens EP, et al. Clinical implementation of biologics and small molecules in the treatment of hidradenitis suppurativa. Drugs. 2021;81:1397-410.

21. Milton S. Hershey Medical Center. (2023). Topical Ruxolitinib 1.5% for hidradenitis suppurativa treatment. [online] Available from https://clinicaltrials.gov/study/NCT04414514 [Last accessed February, 2024].
22. AbbVie. (2023). A study of oral upadacitinib tablet compared to placebo in adult participants with moderate to severe hidradenitis suppurativa to assess change in disease symptoms. [online] Available from https://clinicaltrials.gov/study/NCT04430855 [Last accessed February, 2024].
23. Pfizer. (2023). A Phase 2A, Multicenter, Randomized, Double-Blind, Placebo-Controlled, 16-Week Study Evaluating the Safety and Efficacy of PF-06650833, PF-06700841, and PF-06826647 in Adults with Moderate to Severe Hidradenitis Suppurativa. [online] Available from https://clinicaltrials.gov/ct2/show/NCT04092452 [Last accessed February, 2024].
24. Kirby JS, Okun MM, Alavi A, Bechara FG, Zouboulis CC, Brown K, et al. Efficacy and safety of the oral Janus kinase 1 inhibitor povorcitinib (INCB054707) in patients with hidradenitis suppurativa in a phase 2, randomized, double-blind, dose-ranging, placebo-controlled study. J Am Acad Dermatol. 2023;21:S0190-9622(23)03037-2.
25. Incyte Corporation. (2022). A Phase 2, Open-Label, Single-Arm Study of the Safety of INCB054707 in Participants With Hidradenitis Suppurativa. [online] Available from https://clinicaltrials.gov/show/NCT03569371 [Last accessed February, 2024].
26. Incyte Corporation. (2022). A Phase 2, Dose-Escalation, Placebo-Controlled Study of the Safety of INCB054707 in Participants With Hidradenitis [online] Available from https://clinicaltrials.gov/ct2/show/NCT03607487 [Last accessed February, 2024].
27. Incyte Corporation. (2023). A Phase 2, Randomized, Double-Blind, Placebo-Controlled, Dose-Ranging Study of the Efficacy and Safety of INCB054707 in Participants with Hidradenitis Suppurativa. [online] Available from https://clinicaltrials.gov/ct2/show/NCT04476043 [Last accessed February, 2024].
28. Hornung T, Janzen V, Heidgen FJ, Wolf D, Bieber T, Wenzel J. Remission of recalcitrant dermatomyositis treated with ruxolitinib. N Engl J Med. 2014;371:2537-8.
29. First Affiliated Hospital Xi'an Jiaotong University. (2021). The efficacy and safety of JAK inhibitor in the treatment of anti-MDA5 antibody-positive dermatomyositis patients. [online] Available from https://classic.clinicaltrials.gov/ct2/show/NCT04966884 [Last accessed February, 2024].
30. University of Washington. (2023). Baricitinib for cutaneous dermatomyositis. [online] Available from https://clinicaltrials.gov/study/NCT05361109 [Last accessed February, 2024].
31. Assistance Publique - Hôpitaux de Paris. (2022). Baricitinib in patients with relapsing or naïve dermatomyositis (BIRD). [online] Available from https://clinicaltrials.gov/study/NCT04972760 [Last accessed February, 2024].
32. Priovant Therapeutics, Inc. (2024). A study to investigate the efficacy and safety of brepocitinib in adults with dermatomyositis (VALOR). [online] Available from https://clinicaltrials.gov/study/NCT05437263 [Last accessed February, 2024].
33. Damsky W, Wang A, Olamiju B, Peterson D, Galan A, King B. Treatment of severe lichen planus with the JAK inhibitor tofacitinib. J Allergy Clin Immunol. 2020;145:1708-1710.e2.
34. Brumfiel CM, Patel MH, Severson KJ, Zhang N, Li X, Quillen JK, et al. Ruxolitinib cream in the treatment of cutaneous lichen planus: a prospective, open-label study. J Invest Dermatol. 2022;142:2109-16.e4.
35. Zeiser R, von Bubnoff N, Butler J, Mohty M, Niederwieser D, Or R, et al; REACH2 Trial Group. Ruxolitinib for glucocorticoid-refractory acute graft-versus-host disease. N Engl J Med. 2020;382:1800-10.
36. Le RQ, Wang X, Zhang H, Li H, Przepiorka D, Vallejo J, et al. FDA approval summary: ruxolitinib for treatment of chronic graft-versus-host disease after failure of one or two lines of systemic therapy. Oncologist. 2022;27:493-500.

37. Etra A, Capellini A, Alousi A, Al Malki MM, Choe H, DeFilipp Z, et al. Effective treatment of low-risk acute GVHD with itacitinib monotherapy. Blood. 2023;141:481-9.
38. Nakagawa H, Nemoto O, Igarashi A, Saeki H, Kaino H, Nagata T. Delgocitinib ointment, a topical Janus kinase inhibitor, in adult patients with moderate to severe atopic dermatitis: A phase 3, randomized, double-blind, vehicle-controlled study and an open-label, long-term extension study. J Am Acad Dermatol. 2020;82:823-31.
39. Bissonnette R, Maari C, Forman S, Bhatia N, Lee M, Fowler J, et al. The oral Janus kinase/spleen tyrosine kinase inhibitor ASN002 demonstrates efficacy and improves associated systemic inflammation in patients with moderate-to-severe atopic dermatitis: results from a randomized double-blind placebo-controlled study. Br J Dermatol. 2019;181(4):733-42.
40. Asana BioSciences. (2023). Phase 2B study to evaluate ASN002 in subjects with moderate to severe atopic dermatitis (RADIANT). [online] Available from https://clinicaltrials.gov/ct2/show/NCT03531957?cond=NCT03531957 [Last accessed February, 2024].
41. Gilhar A, Keren A, Paus R. JAK inhibitors and alopecia areata. Lancet. 2019;393:318-9.
42. Mackay-Wiggan J, Jabbari A, Nguyen N, Cerise JE, Clark C, Ulerio G, et al. Oral ruxolitinib induces hair regrowth in patients with moderate-to-severe alopecia areata. JCI Insight. 2016;1:e89790.
43. Vandiver A, Girardi N, Alhariri J, Garza LA. Two cases of alopecia areata treated with ruxolitinib: A discussion of ideal dosing and laboratory monitoring. Int J Dermatol. 2017;56:833-5.
44. Liu LY, King BA. Ruxolitinib for the treatment of severe alopecia areata. J Am Acad Dermatol. 2019;80:566-8.
45. Guttman-Yassky E, Pavel AB, Diaz A, Zhang N, Del Duca E, Estrada Y, et al. Ritlecitinib and brepocitinib demonstrate significant improvement in scalp alopecia areata biomarkers. J Allergy Clin Immunol. 2022;149:1318-28.
46. Aclaris Therapeutics, Inc. (2020). A study of ATI-50002 topical solution for the treatment of alopecia areata. [online] Available from https://clinicaltrials.gov/study/NCT03354637 [Last accessed February, 2024].
47. Leo Pharma. LEO 124249 Ointment in the treatment of alopecia areata. [online] Available from https://classic.clinicaltrials.gov/ct2/show/NCT02561585 [Last accessed February, 2024].

CHAPTER 32

Phosphodiesterase-4 Inhibitors

Anupam Das, Kingshuk Chatterjee

INTRODUCTION

Apremilast is an oral phosphodiesterase-4 (PDE4) enzyme inhibitor. It reduces the proinflammatory cytokine production by increasing the anti-inflammatory cytokines and the intracellular levels of cyclic adenosine monophosphate (cAMP). It was synthesized by Celgene Corporation (Summit, NJ, USA). Apremilast was approved by the Food and Drug Administration in 2014 for the treatment of active psoriatic arthritis (PsA) and moderate-to-severe plaque psoriasis.

PHARMACOLOGY

Apremilast is chemically identified as N-[2-[(1S)-1-(3-ethoxy-4-methoxyphenyl)-2-(methylsulfonyl) ethyl]-2, 3-dihydro-1, 3-dioxo-1H-isoindol-4-yl] acetamide. The empirical formula is $C_{22}H_{24}N_2O_7S$, with a molecular weight of approximately 460.5 g/mole **(Fig. 1)**.

The absolute bioavailability of apremilast is ~73%. The peak plasma concentration (C_{max}) is achieved in a median time (t_{max}) of ~2.5 hours.

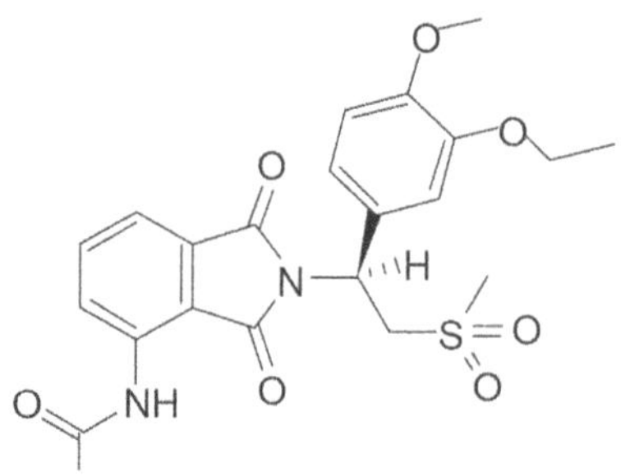

FIG. 1: Chemical structure of apremilast.[1]

Absorption is not altered by coadministration with food. Human plasma protein binding of apremilast is approximately 68%. Following oral administration, apremilast is metabolized by cytochrome (CYP) oxidative metabolism with subsequent glucuronidation as well as non-CYP-mediated hydrolysis. In vitro, the CYP metabolism is primarily mediated by CYP3A4, with minor contributions from CYP1A2 and CYP2A6. It is eliminated through urine and feces.

MECHANISM OF ACTION

Apremilast regulates immune response that causes inflammation and skin disease associated with psoriasis and PsA, by selective inhibition of PDE4. By inhibition of PDE4, a key regulator of inflammatory processes, apremilast prevents the degradation of cAMP. Elevated cAMP level, in turn, stimulates anti-inflammatory mediators and antagonizes the production of proinflammatory cytokines, such as tumor necrosis factor alpha (TNF-α), interleukin 23 (IL-23), IL-17, interferon gamma (IFN-γ), various chemokines from peripheral blood mononuclear cells (PBMCs), and polymorphonuclear leukocytes, including neutrophils, monocytes, natural killer cells, and plasmacytoid dendritic cells. Chemokines and cytokines produced by toll-like receptors (TLR-2 and TLR-4) stimulated PBMC are also susceptible to PDE4 inhibition. TNF-α produced by rheumatoid synovial membrane as well as keratinocyte in vitro is also inhibited by apremilast due to the expression of PDE4 in cell types resident in the joints and skin. An increase in anti-inflammatory cytokines, for example IL-10 is also caused by apremilast. Thus, apremilast leads to intracellular interruption of inflammatory cascade at an early point, in contrast to biologic agents that act as target-specific (e.g., TNF-α) inhibitors.[2-4]

Currently, research is being conducted on PDE4 inhibitors and their immune-modulating effects in a variety of inflammatory conditions, such as chronic obstructive pulmonary disease (COPD), atopic dermatitis, asthma, psoriasis, and PsA.[2,5]

USES

Food and drug administration-approved indications:
- Active PsA in adults
- Patients with moderate-to-severe plaque psoriasis who are suitable for phototherapy or systemic therapy
- Adult with Behçet's disease associated with oral ulcers[6]

Other uses:
- Atopic dermatitis[7]
- Lichen planus[8]

TABLE 1: Apremilast dosage.									
Day 1	Day 2		Day 3		Day 4		Day 5		Day 6 and thereafter
AM	AM	PM	AM	PM	AM	PM	AM	PM	AM	PM
10 mg	10 mg	10 mg	10 mg	20 mg	20 mg	20 mg	20 mg	30 mg	30 mg	30 mg

- Discoid lupus erythematosus[9]
- Sarcoidosis[10]
- Chronic recalcitrant erythema nodosum leprosum[11]
- Hidradenitis suppurativa[12]
- Rosacea[13]
- Epidermolysis bullosa simplex[14]
- Hailey–Hailey disease[15]
- Frontal fibrosing alopecia[16]
- Recurrent erythema multiforme[17]
- Pityriasis rubra pilaris[18]
- Pyoderma gangrenosum[18]
- Synovitis, acne, pustulosis, hyperostosis, and osteitis (SAPHO) syndrome[19]
- Vitiligo[20]
- Pityriasis lichenoides chronica

ADMINISTRATION

- *Availability*: It is available as 10, 20, and 30 mg tablets.
- *Storage and handling*: It is stored below 30°C (86°F).
- *Dosage (Table 1)*: The tablet should not be chewed or crushed and should be swallowed without regard to meals.

CURRENT EVIDENCE

Plaque Psoriasis

A study was conducted by Paul et al. (ESTEEM 2) in which the safety and efficacy of apremilast were evaluated over 52 weeks. Subgroup analysis of this study revealed that Psoriasis Area and Severity Index (PASI)-75 score with apremilast 30 mg BD was achieved in 33.3% patients when they did not have any exposure to conventional therapy, 31.9% when patients did not have any previous biologic exposure, and 22.8% in patients with previous biologic exposure. In a real-word data of Japanese patients, 33.3% patients achieved PASI-75/90. However, 32% patients had to stop the drug. There were no reports of serious adverse events, most common ones being gastrointestinal side effects like diarrhea and nausea.[21-25]

Psoriatic Arthritis

Psoriatic arthritis long-term assessment of clinical efficacy (PALACE) studies were conducted to assess the efficacy of apremilast in the treatment of PsA. In PALACE 1 study, an American College of Rheumatology 20% (ACR20) response rate was found to be 31.8% and 39.8% for 20 and 30 mg BD group, respectively. This efficacy was maintained till 52 weeks across these studies. Therefore, apremilast promises to be a very effective molecule in the management of PsA.[26,27]

Palmoplantar Psoriasis and Pustulosis

Seventeen original studies including five placebo-controlled randomized clinical trials (RCTs), one phase II clinical trial, two randomized methotrexate comparative trials, six cohort studies, and three case series have been analyzed in a meta-analysis. Apremilast has been found to be better than placebo, and similar to methotrexate in achieving clinically satisfactory improvement.[28]

Other indications: Apremilast has been used in numerous dermatological conditions as isolated cases. However, the real effectiveness can be adjudged only after conducting well-designed RCTs

Apremilast in Pediatric Age Group

The molecule has been successfully tried in multiple conditions in the pediatric age group, including plaque psoriasis, atopic dermatitis, alopecia areata, vitiligo, and active oral ulcers associated with Behçet's disease.[29]

ADVERSE REACTIONS

Apremilast was generally well tolerated up to 52 weeks in plaque psoriasis patients and possesses an acceptable safety profile. The majority of the adverse reactions encountered were mild-to-moderate in severity and no significant changes in laboratory values were observed in any of the trials.

- *Gastrointestinal*: It includes diarrhea (most common adverse reaction requiring dose titration as mentioned before), upper abdominal pain, nausea, vomiting, frequent bowel movement, dyspepsia, and gastroesophageal reflux disease. Nausea and diarrhea occur in the first week of treatment and generally resolve by 1 month of treatment. Loperamide can be used in patients who developed diarrhea due to apremilast.
- *Respiratory*: Upper respiratory tract infection, nasopharyngitis, cough, and bronchitis
- *Nervous system*: Headache, depression, or depressed mood has been reported in almost 1% of patients taking apremilast
- *Immunological*: Hypersensitivity and skin rash
- *Others*: Loss of weight (weight loss > 10% is an indication to stop the drug), decreased appetite, fatigue, back pain, tooth abscess, and insomnia[30]

CONTRAINDICATIONS

- Known hypersensitivity to apremilast or the formulation excipients
- Renal impairment
- History of depression or suicidal ideation

DOSE ADJUSTMENT[1]

Renal Impairment
- *Mild or moderate renal impairment*: No dose adjustment is required.
- *Severe renal impairment [creatinine clearance (CrCl) <30 mL/min]*: Reduce dose to 30 mg OD.

Hepatic Impairment
No dose adjustment is required. In multiple, large-scale RCTs of apremilast in psoriasis and PsA, the likelihood of elevations of liver enzymes was not higher than the placebo group. Therefore, as per recent literature, apremilast is safe in liver disease.

DRUG INTERACTIONS[1]

Coadministration of CYP450 enzyme inducers (e.g., phenobarbital, carbamazepine, phenytoin, and rifampicin) with apremilast resulted in reduced levels of the drug with loss of its efficacy.

INVESTIGATIONS

Investigations include:
- Weight of the patient
- Liver function test
- Renal function test

SPECIAL SITUATIONS

Pregnancy Category C
The safety and efficacy of apremilast in pregnancy and lactation are not known. Hence, it should not be prescribed to women who are planning to conceive, pregnant, or lactating mother.

CONCLUSION

Apremilast is an oral PDE4 inhibitor and belongs to a new class of drugs. Its novel mechanism of action, oral formulation, and safety make it an interesting drug for the management of psoriasis and many other indications.

Apremilast is a well-tolerated, effective, and safe drug for moderate psoriasis due to less requirement of stringent monitoring (unlike methotrexate, cyclosporine, and acitretin) and no end-organ damage. It is also used as an add-on therapy in psoriasis.

REFERENCES

1. Celgene Corporation. (2014). Otezla® (apremilast)—Highlights of full prescribing information. [online] Available from http://www.otezla.com/otezla-prescribing-information.pdf. [Last accessed February, 2024].
2. Schafer P. Apremilast mechanism of action and application to psoriasis and psoriatic arthritis. Biochem Pharmacol. 2012;83(12):1583-90.
3. Kavanaugh A, Adebajo AO, Gladman DD, Gomez-Reino JJ, Hall S, Lespessailles E, et al. Long-Term (156-Week) efficacy and safety profile of apremilast, an oral phosphodiesterase 4 inhibitor, in patients with psoriatic arthritis: Results from a phase III, randomized, controlled trial and open-label extension (PALACE 1). Arthritis Rheumatol. 2015;67(suppl 10).
4. Schafer PH, Parton A, Gandhi AK, Capone L, Adams M, Wu L, et al. Apremilast, a cAMP phosphodiesterase-4 inhibitor, demonstrates anti-inflammatory activity in vitro and in a model of psoriasis. Brit J Pharm. 2010;159:842-55.
5. Bäumer W, Hoppmann J, Rundfeldt C, Kietzmann M. Highly selective phosphodiesterase 4 inhibitors for the treatment of allergic skin diseases and psoriasis. Inflamm Allergy Drug Targets. 2007;6(1):17-26.
6. Hatemi G, Melikoglu M, Tunc R, Korkmaz C, Turgut Ozturk B, Mat C. Apremilast for the treatment of Behcet's syndrome: A phase II randomized, placebo-controlled, double blind study. Arthritis Rheum. 2013;65(10 Suppl):S322.
7. Samrao A, Berry TM, Goreshi R, Simpson EL. A pilot study of an oral phosphodiesterase inhibitor (apremilast) for atopic dermatitis in adults. Arch Dermatol. 2012;148(8):890-7.
8. Paul J, Foss CE, Hirano SA, Cunningham TD, Pariser DM. An open-label pilot study of apremilast for the treatment of moderate to severe lichen planus: A case series. J Am Acad Dermatol. 2013;68(2):255-61.
9. De Souza A, Strober BE, Merola JF, Oliver S, Franks AG Jr. Apremilast for discoid lupus erythematosus: Results of a phase 2, open-label, single-arm, pilot study. J Drugs Dermatol. 2012;11(10):1224-6.
10. Baughman RP, Judson MA, Ingledue R, Craft NL, Lower EE. Efficacy and safety of apremilast in chronic cutaneous sarcoidosis. Arch Dermatol. 2012;148(2):262-4.
11. Narang T, Kaushik A, Dogra S. Apremilast in chronic recalcitrant erythema nodosum leprosum: A report of two cases. Br J Dermatol. 2020;182(4):1034-7.
12. Vossen ARJV, van Doorn MBA, van der Zee HH, Prens EP. Apremilast for moderate hidradenitis suppurativa: Results of a randomized controlled trial. J Am Acad Dermatol. 2019;80(1):80-8.
13. Thompson BJ, Furniss M, Zhao W, Chakraborty B, Mackay-Wiggan J. An oral phosphodiesterase inhibitor (apremilast) for inflammatory rosacea in adults: A pilot study. JAMA Dermatol. 2014;150(9):1013-4.
14. Castela E, Tulic MK, Rozieres A, Rozières A, Bourrat E, Nicolas JF, et al. Epidermolysis bullosa simplex generalized severe induces a T helper 17 response and is improved by Apremilast treatment. Br J Dermatol. 2019;180(2):357-64.
15. Kieffer J, Le Duff F, Montaudié H, Chiaverini C, Lacour JP, Passeron T. Treatment of severe hailey-hailey disease with apremilast. JAMA Dermatology. 2018;154(12):1453-6.
16. Hadi A, Lebwohl M. Apremilast for lichen planopilaris and frontal fibrosing alopecia: A case series. Ski J Cutan Med. 2017;1:32-6.

17. Chen T, Levitt J, Geller L. Apremilast for treatment of recurrent erythema multiforme. Dermatol Online J. 2017;23(1):13030.
18. Molina-Figuera E, Gonzalez-Cantero A, Martinez-Lorenzo E, Sánchez-Moya AI, García-Olmedo O, Gómez-Dorado B, et al. Successful treatment of refractory type 1 pityriasis rubra pilaris with apremilast. J Cutan Med Surg. 2018;22(1):104-5.
19. Adamo S, Nilsson J, Krebs A, Steiner U, Cozzio A, French LE, et al. Successful treatment of SAPHO syndrome with apremilast. Br J Dermatol. 2018;179(4):959-62.
20. Huff SB, Gottwald LD. Repigmentation of tenacious vitiligo on apremilast. Case Rep Dermatol Med. 2017;2017:2386234.
21. Papp K, Reich K, Leonardi CL, Kircik L, Chimenti S, Langley RG, et al. Apremilast, an oral phosphodiesterase 4 (PDE4) inhibitor, in patients with moderate to severe plaque psoriasis: Results of a phase III, randomized, controlled trial (Efficacy and Safety Trial Evaluating the Effects of Apremilast in Psoriasis [ESTEEM] 1). J Am Acad Dermatol. 2015;73(1):37-49.
22. Edwards CJ, Blanco FJ, Crowley J, Birbara CA, Jaworski J, Aelion J, et al. Apremilast, an oral phosphodiesterase 4 inhibitor, in patients with psoriatic arthritis and current skin involvement: A phase III, randomised, controlled trial (PALACE 3). Ann Rheum Dis. 2016;75(6):1065-73.
23. Paul C, Cather J, Gooderham M, Poulin Y, Mrowietz U, Ferrandiz C, et al. Efficacy and safety of apremilast, an oral phosphodiesterase 4 inhibitor, in patients with moderate-to-severe plaque psoriasis over 52 weeks: A phase III, randomized controlled trial (ESTEEM 2). Br J Dermatol. 2015;173(6):1387-99.
24. Ohata C, Ohyama B, Kuwahara F, Katayama E, Nakama T. Real-world data on the efficacy and safety of apremilast in Japanese patients with plaque psoriasis. J Dermatolog Treat. 2019;30(4):383-6.
25. Kishimoto M, Komine M, Hioki T, Kamiya K, Sugai J, Ohtsuki M. Real-world use of apremilast for patients with psoriasis in Japan. J Dermatol. 2018;45(11):1345-8.
26. Cutolo M, Myerson GE, Fleischmann RM, Lioté F, Díaz-González F, Van den Bosch F, et al. A Phase III, Randomized, Controlled Trial of Apremilast in Patients with Psoriatic Arthritis: Results of the PALACE 2 Trial. J Rheumatol. 2016;43(9):1724-34.
27. Sandhu VK, Eder L, Yeung J. Apremilast and its role in psoriatic arthritis. G Ital Dermatol Venereol. 2020;155(4):386-99.
28. Spencer RK, Elhage KG, Jin JQ, Davis MS, Hakimi M, Bhutani T, et al. Apremilast in Palmoplantar Psoriasis and Palmoplantar Pustulosis: A Systematic Review and Meta-analysis. Dermatol Ther (Heidelb). 2023;13(2):437-51.
29. Patro N, Panda M, Dash M, Das A. Apremilast in Paediatric Dermatoses-A Comprehensive Review. Indian J Dermatol. 2022;67(2):206.
30. Crowley J, Thac D, Joly P, Peris K, Papp KA, Goncalves J, et al. Long-term safety and tolerability of apremilast in patients with psoriasis: Pooled safety analysis for ≥156 weeks from 2 phase 3, randomized, controlled trials (ESTEEM 1 and 2). J Am Acad Dermatol. 2017;77(2):310-7.

CHAPTER 33

Mammalian Target of Rapamycin Inhibitors: Sirolimus

Riti Bhatia, Vishal Gupta

INTRODUCTION

Sirolimus is a pleiotropic molecule having immunosuppressive, antiproliferative, and antifungal properties. It was named rapamycin after the native name of Easter Island, Rapa Nui, where *Streptomyces hygroscopicus* (a soil fungus) was discovered to produce this antibiotic. Its antifungal properties were also discovered here.[1] After receiving United States Food and Drug Administration (US FDA) approval for renal transplant in 1999, it has been used for preventing graft rejection in heart and liver transplant recipients as well.[1] It is also used in drug-eluting stents after cardiac procedures to prevent restenosis. Structurally, sirolimus is a crystalline lipophilic macrolide lactone. Its molecular weight is 290 kDa (914.2 g/mol) and the chemical formula is $C_{51}H_{79}NO_{13}$.[1]

MECHANISM OF ACTION

Sirolimus shares structural similarity with tacrolimus and cyclosporine. Like these molecules, it also acts by binding to immunophilins, which are intracellular binding proteins [FK506 binding proteins (FKBPs)], specifically FKBP-12. However, the further mode of its action is different. While cyclosporine–immunophilin complex acts via calcineurin, rapamycin–immunophilin complex acts via another protein called the mammalian target of rapamycin (mTOR). mTOR is a 289-kDa multifunctional serine/threonine kinase involved in the transduction of cytokines like interleukin-2 (IL-2) and cell growth. Thus, inhibition of mTOR leads to inhibition of cytokine-mediated immune response. Inhibition of mTOR also blocks its downstream pathways, resulting in the arrest of cell cycle progression between G1 and S phase.[2] Newer mTOR inhibitors, like temsirolimus and everolimus, have been developed with broader applications in oncology and transplant medicine. **Flowchart 1** illustrates the various mechanisms of action of sirolimus.

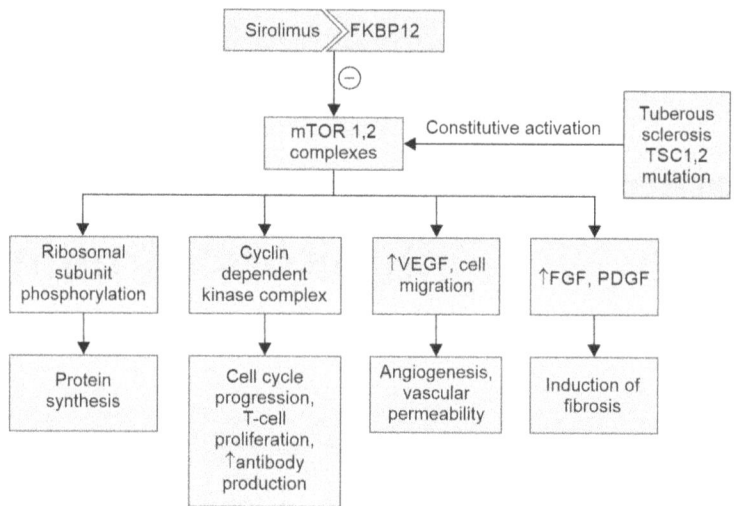

FLOWCHART 1: Various mechanisms of action of sirolimus.
(FGF: fibroblast growth factor; mTOR: mammalian target of rapamycin; PDGF: platelet-derived growth factor; VEGF: vascular endothelial growth factor)

PHARMACOKINETICS

Sirolimus is rapidly absorbed orally, reaching its peak serum concentration in 1 hour in healthy individuals and 2–3 hours in renal transplant recipients.[3] After oral absorption, 95% of the drug is bound to serum proteins, primarily albumin (97%). It is metabolized by the hepatic cytochrome P450 3A4 enzyme and p-glycoprotein intestinal pump.[4] Oral bioavailability is poor (~14%), owing to extensive intestinal and hepatic first-pass metabolism. It is primarily excreted by the fecal route (90%) and has a half-life of 57–62 hours.[5,6] Sirolimus is commercially available as oral tablets (1, 2, and 5 mg) and solution (1 mg/mL).

CLINICAL USES

Till recently, there was no FDA-approved dermatological indication of sirolimus. In 2022, topical sirolimus (0.2% gel) was approved for the treatment of facial angiofibromas with tuberous sclerosis complex in patients aged 6 years or more. Some of its better-known uses in dermatology include treating facial angiofibromas [level of evidence (LOE) I] and vascular anomalies (large case series). Apart from these, it has shown encouraging results in treating various other skin disorders (case reports and small case series), which is a subject of further investigation. The list of various indications for sirolimus in dermatology is summarized in **Table 1**.

CHAPTER 33: Mammalian Target of Rapamycin Inhibitors: Sirolimus

TABLE 1: Sirolimus: Indications in dermatology.

Food and Drug Administration (FDA) approved uses	Off-label uses
Dermatology: 0.2% topical sirolimus for facial angiofibromas of tuberous sclerosis complex *Nondermatology:* • Prevention of transplant rejection • Lymphangioleiomyomatosis • Albumin-bound sirolimus particles for intravenous injection for unresectable or metastatic perivascular epithelioid cell tumor (PEComa)	• Kaposiform hemangioendothelioma • Kasabach–Merritt phenomenon • Lymphatic malformations • Venous malformations • Kaposi's sarcoma • Graft-versus-host disease • Chemoprevention of cutaneous malignancies in transplant recipients
Investigational role: • Antiaging • Genodermatoses such as Birt–Hogg–Dube syndrome, multiple trichoepitheliomas, pachyonychia congenita, Cowden syndrome, and neurofibromatosis • Keloids and hypertrophic scars • Lichen planus • Chronic urticaria • Connective tissue disorders such as systemic lupus erythematosus, scleroderma, and dermatomyositis • Pemphigus vulgaris • Cutaneous T-cell lymphoma • Melanoma	

TUBEROUS SCLEROSIS

In a serendipitous discovery, immunosuppressive treatment with sirolimus in a renal transplant recipient with tuberous sclerosis led to improvement in facial angiofibromas.[7] Defects in the products of *TSC1* or *TSC2* (mutations in these genes are implicated in tuberous sclerosis) lead to unregulated activation of the downstream mTOR signaling pathway. Thus, sirolimus by virtue of its inhibitory effect on mTOR pathway can have a beneficial effect on different manifestations of tuberous sclerosis. Multiple studies have demonstrated the efficacy of topical sirolimus ointment in treating angiofibromas (LOE I).[8,9] As it is not available commercially, the topical formulation of sirolimus has to be compounded by mixing the crushed tablet in petrolatum. A split-face trial comparing the efficacy of topical sirolimus (gel and ointment) with emollient for 12 weeks on 11 patients with tuberous sclerosis showed significantly better improvement in the sirolimus-treated side. The gel form was found to be more effective and less irritating than the ointment. Higher percutaneous absorption of sirolimus in gel form than ointment was also demonstrated on a human skin model.[10] A prospective single-blinded crossover split-face study on 12 patients comparing 0.1% sirolimus ointment with petrolatum for 12 weeks also found significantly better results with sirolimus. There was statistically significant reduction in the redness and size of the lesions. Notably, the facial angiofibromas started to increase in size after stopping the treatment for 6 months, suggesting only a temporary effect of sirolimus. Retreatment with topical sirolimus again led to improvement.[11] The response may be better in early lesions and may be apparent as early as few (4-8) weeks.[12,13] A wide variety of topical formulations, namely ointment, gel, solution, and cream, in varying concentrations (0.003-1%) have been tried. In a review, Balestri et al. concluded that ointment and gel formulations should be preferred, but the optimum concentration is not clear.[8] A randomized controlled trial (RCT) involving 179 patients comparing topical sirolimus 1% versus 0.1% versus vehicle reported better results with 1% formulation as compared to 0.1% and vehicle. The clinical photographs at the end of 6 months were rated better than at baseline by 82% in 1% sirolimus group (17 points mean reduction in angiofibroma grading scale), 66% in 0.1% group (11 points mean reduction), and 26% (2 points mean reduction) in vehicle group ($p < 0.001$; all three pairwise comparisons). Both 1% and 0.1% topical sirolimus were well tolerated with no measurable systemic levels.[14] A recent systematic review and meta-analysis (including 3 RCTs and 23 observational studies) suggest its beneficial effect on facial angiofibromas with topical sirolimus in about 95% patients [patient reported improvement risk ratio (RR) 2.52; 95% confidence interval (CI) 1.27-5]. The median sirolimus concentration was 0.1%, with a median of two applications per day for a median period of 16 weeks. Recurrence was reported in 18 out of 20 patients, for whom the follow-up data was available, 2-12 weeks after discontinuing treatment.[9] Side effects are minimal and include redness and irritation at the site of application, which can be managed with mild topical corticosteroid and Vaseline, acne, and allergic contact dermatitis. Serum sirolimus levels with topical use have been detected in up to 10% patients, with none reaching the threshold for immunosuppression (≥ 4 ng/mL).[9] Good improvement with topical application of commercially available oral solution (1 mg/mL) once daily has also been reported in two patients.[15] Using commercially available oral solution may be more cost-effective than the compounded ointments; however, it causes more irritation.

There are reports of topical sirolimus improving hypomelanotic macules and subungual fibromas related to tuberous sclerosis complex.[16,17]

Apart from topical formulation, oral sirolimus has also been found to be effective in treating angiofibromas, renal angiomyolipomas, pulmonary lymphangiomyomatosis, and brain astrocytomas and may even have a disease-modifying effect in patients with tuberous sclerosis.[18-20]

OTHER GENODERMATOSES

Apart from tuberous sclerosis complex, anecdotal reports of topical or oral sirolimus improving benign cutaneous tumors and hamartomas associated with other genodermatoses as well, such as Birt–Hogg–Dube syndrome, familial trichoepitheliomas, multiple familial discoid fibromas, Cowden syndrome, and other PTEN (phosphatase and tensin homolog) hamartoma syndromes, have emerged in the literature.[21] Painful palmoplantar keratoderma of pachyonychia congenita improves with both oral and topical sirolimus.[22,23] Oral sirolimus has also been shown to slow down the progression of neurofibromatosis type 1 (NF-1)-associated plexiform neurofibromas by half in 30% patients ($n = 7/23$).[24] A pilot double-blind, placebo-controlled randomized trial ($n = 18$) reported a statistically significant difference in the size of cutaneous neurofibromas with sirolimus gel as compared to placebo.[16]

VASCULAR ANOMALIES

Based on the role of mTOR pathway in the proliferation and growth of endothelial cells, sirolimus can have antiangiogenic effects. Successful use of sirolimus in the treatment of refractory kaposiform hemangioendothelioma and Kasabach–Merritt phenomenon (KMP) was first reported by Blatt et al. in 2010.[25] Since then, reports of good results with sirolimus in the treatment of different vascular anomalies, mainly kaposiform hemangioendothelioma and lymphatic malformations, have emerged in the literature.[26,27] In a retrospective review of six children with different vascular anomalies [(kaposiform hemangioendothelioma ($n = 2$), lymphatic–venous malformation ($n = 2$), pulmonary lymphangiectasias ($n = 1$), and orbital lymphatic malformation ($n = 1$)], oral sirolimus (0.05 mg/kg twice daily, and subsequently dose adjusted to achieve serum levels between 5 and 15 ng/mL) produced complete and partial remission in three patients each (median duration: 10 months, range 3–53 months). The coagulation profile and platelet counts in three patients with KMP normalized within 1 month. Mild-reversible leukopenia was seen in all the patients. In a phase II trial involving patients with complicated vascular anomalies (like lymphatic malformations, lymphangiomatosis, kaposiform hemangioendotheliomas), oral sirolimus (0.8 mg/m^2 twice daily) administered for 12 courses, each course lasting 28 days, was found to be effective. Of the 61 patients enrolled, 57 could be evaluated. Partial improvement was seen in 47 (of 57, 83%) patients after 6 courses and 45 (of 53, 85%) patients after 12 courses. Stability was achieved in three (5%) patients at 6 months, while lesions remained progressive in seven (12%) and eight (15%) patients at 6 and 12 months, respectively. None of the patients had a complete clinical response. Bone marrow toxicity was seen in 27% of patients, gastrointestinal toxicity in 3%, and metabolic/

laboratory toxicity in 3%. Dose reduction was needed in two patients due to toxicity and two patients were taken off the study for the same reason. No toxicity-related deaths occurred.[28] As many patients achieved only partial improvement at the end of study period, the optimum duration for complete remission needs further investigation. The initial results suggest that the improvement may be sustained after cessation of treatment.[29] Topical sirolimus has also been used in the treatment of microcystic lymphatic malformations. Topical sirolimus 0.8% ointment in petrolatum used on microcystic lymphatic malformation on scrotum once daily led to complete resolution in 3 months. No recurrence was noted in the next 2 months of follow-up.[30]

Overall, sirolimus causes a reduction in the size of vascular anomalies and improvement in symptoms, particularly in lymphatic malformations as well as venous malformations. Though complete response is rare, partial size reduction is seen in about 75–80% patients with lymphatic malformations, both microcystic and macrocystic. Venous malformations also respond to sirolimus, but the response is not as consistent as in lymphatic malformations; 67% patients with common venous malformations and 93% patients with blue rubber bleb syndrome experienced size reduction. The efficacy of sirolimus in capillary malformations is unclear, and there is conflicting data suggesting better response with a combination of pulsed dye laser (PDL) and sirolimus versus either as monotherapy alone. Arteriovenous malformations do not show favorable response to sirolimus.[31]

Oral sirolimus has been reported to be effective in treating KMP, refractory to previous treatment (including steroids and vincristine) as well, in the dose of 0.8 mg/m^2 twice daily with subsequent dose adjustments to maintain trough levels of 10–15 ng/mL.[27,32] In a series of six patients with refractory kaposiform hemangioendothelioma with life-threatening KMP, the average time to respond was only 5.3 days (range 4–7 days) and platelet counts stabilized on an average of 15 days (range 5–28 days),[18] though it may take as long as 3–4 months.[32] The optimum duration of use of sirolimus, and whether it should be used alone or in combination with steroids, is currently not clear. A recent randomized trial including 73 patients with kaposiform hemangioendothelioma with KMP reported better efficacy of the combination of oral sirolimus with a short course of prednisolone (4–6 weeks) versus sirolimus alone (LOE I). A higher proportion of patients in the combination arm had a durable platelet response at 4 weeks than the sirolimus monotherapy arm (95% vs. 67%). The combination group fared better in terms of overall lesion response (92% vs. 81%) and KMP rebound rates (5% vs. 17%) at 12 months. Adverse events between the two groups were comparable, and common ones included upper respiratory infections, mucositis, and nausea/vomiting. This study used sirolimus for at least 12 months, and if no further improvement was noted, it was tapered and discontinued.[33]

CHEMOPREVENTION OF CUTANEOUS MALIGNANCIES IN TRANSPLANT RECIPIENTS

Organ transplant recipients are at a higher risk of developing cutaneous malignancies, the risk being highest for squamous cell carcinoma. Immunosuppression with sirolimus, as opposed to cyclosporine, to prevent graft rejection reduces the risk of nonmelanoma skin cancers (LOE I). In a recent meta-analysis involving 20 RCTs and two observational studies, including 39,039 kidney recipients overall, sirolimus was associated with a 51% lower incidence of nonmelanoma skin cancer [incidence rate ratio (IRR) 0.49; 95% CI 0.32–0.76]. This protective effect of sirolimus on nonmelanoma skin cancer risk was most notable in studies comparing sirolimus against cyclosporine (IRR 0.19; 95% CI 0.04–0.84).[34,35]

KAPOSI'S SARCOMA

Because of its antiangiogenic properties, sirolimus has been used in the treatment of Kaposi's sarcoma (KS) (LOE III). In addition, sirolimus has been demonstrated to suppress human herpesvirus-8 (HHV-8) lytic master switch protein, thereby impairing virion production.[36] In a series of 15 renal transplant recipients with KS treated with sirolimus (0.15 mg/kg, followed by a dose of 0.04–0.06 mg/kg to maintain drug trough levels of 6–10 ng/mL), complete clinical and histological remission was seen in all the patients after 3 and 6 months, respectively.[37] It has also been used in human immunodeficiency virus (HIV) patients with KS, and three out of seven patients had partial improvement. All these three patients were on protease inhibitor-based regimens, which led to higher serum sirolimus levels, due to drug interactions. No change was observed in HIV load, but CD4 count decreased transiently in five (out of six) patients.[38] In a patient of pemphigus vulgaris with iatrogenic KS, clinical and histological remission was maintained at 24 months with low-dose prednisone, dapsone, and sirolimus.[39]

PSORIASIS

An RCT compared oral sirolimus (0.5, 1.5, and 3 mg/m^2), cyclosporine (5 mg/kg), and a combination of the two agents (sirolimus 3 mg/m^2 and subtherapeutic dose of cyclosporine 1.25 mg/kg) for 8 weeks in the treatment of severe plaque psoriasis [psoriasis area severity index (PASI) ≥ 12] for duration of at least 6 months in 150 patients. While the combination treatment was comparable to cyclosporine monotherapy (63.7% and 70.5% reduction in PASI, respectively), sirolimus monotherapy led to <30% reduction in PASI for any dose. These results suggest that sirolimus monotherapy is ineffective, but adding sirolimus to cyclosporine may reduce its dose (LOE I).[40] Another randomized double-blind, left-right comparative clinical trial tested the efficacy of topical sirolimus versus its vehicle in the treatment of stable chronic plaque psoriasis. In vitro studies showed topical sirolimus to penetrate the skin and decrease the number of CD4+ T cells in the epidermis. 24 patients were treated first with a lower concentration of 2.2% for 6 weeks, followed by a higher concentration of 8% for an additional 6 weeks. The area treated with sirolimus showed significant reduction in a composite clinical score based on erythema, induration, and scaling, but there was no significant change in plaque thickness (measured by ultrasound) and redness (reflectance erythema meter).[41]

GRAFT-VERSUS-HOST DISEASE

Sirolimus has been found to be a safe and effective alternative to glucocorticoids in graft-versus-host disease (GVHD). A similar response rate to glucocorticoids (of 50%) was found in a series of 32 cases with acute GVHD. These patients were also on tacrolimus and methotrexate/mycophenolate mofetil in addition, for prophylaxis of acute GVHD.[42] It was also found to be effective in steroid-refractory acute GVHD with a response rate of 44% for a minimum of 1 month, without additional immunosuppressants.[43] In a retrospective review of 22 cases with steroid-refractory acute GVHD, sirolimus treatment produced a sustained remission rate of 72%.[44]

OTHER DERMATOLOGICAL INDICATIONS

Apart from the abovementioned indications, the utility of sirolimus is being studied in a variety of other conditions as well. With the evidence for involvement of mTOR pathway in aging, there is a growing interest in sirolimus and its analogs as antiaging agents. Sirolimus has been found to enhance the life span of genetically engineered mice.[45] Post-transplant immunosuppression with cyclosporine or tacrolimus but not with sirolimus, in patients with Muir–Torre syndrome, was seen to exacerbate sebaceous adenomas.[46] Sirolimus appears to have the advantage of reducing the risk of malignancies over cyclosporine in transplant recipients. It is being investigated for its role in keloids and hypertrophic scars, lichen planus, chronic urticaria, systemic lupus erythematosus, dermatomyositis, scleroderma, eosinophilic fasciitis, nephrogenic systemic fibrosis, pemphigus vulgaris, cutaneous T-cell lymphoma, and melanoma.[21,47]

ADVERSE EFFECTS AND MONITORING

Common side effects seen in >30% cases, include anemia, thrombocytopenia, fever, arthralgia, hypertension, hypertriglyceridemia, hypercholesterolemia, headache, gastrointestinal effects, (such as anorexia, abdominal pain, and diarrhea) impaired wound healing, lymphedema, infections like urinary tract infections, and reactivation of latent viral infections.[37] Serious adverse

> **BOX 1** **Monitoring guidelines for oral sirolimus.**
>
> *Investigations prior to starting sirolimus treatment:*
> - Complete blood count, liver and renal function tests, and fasting lipid profile
> - Blood pressure measurement
> - *Consider screening for infections in high-risk patients:* Tuberculosis, hepatitis B, hepatitis C, and human immunodeficiency virus (HIV)
>
> *Investigations while on sirolimus treatment:*
> - Complete blood count, liver and renal function tests, and fasting lipid profile
> - Blood pressure measurement
> - Serum or whole blood sirolimus trough levels. Dose adjustment can be done to maintain trough levels 5–15 ng/mL (every week in the 1st month, every 2 weeks in the 2nd month; thereafter, it can be continued only in patients who undergo dose changes or may have drug interactions)

events include upper respiratory infections and noninfective pneumonitis. Common cutaneous side effects include acneiform eruption, oral ulcers, and nail changes. In a study involving 80 renal transplant patients receiving sirolimus, 79 (99%) patients experienced cutaneous side effects, including pilosebaceous apparatus disorders like acneiform lesions (46%), scalp folliculitis (26%), and hidradenitis suppurativa (12%); edematous complaints including chronic edema (55%) and angioedemas (15%); mucosal involvement like aphthous ulcers (60%), epistaxis (60%), chronic gingivitis (20%), and chronic fissuring of lips (11%); and nail involvement like chronic dystrophic nails (74%) and periungual infections (16%). Serious events were seen in 20 (25%) patients, while 6 (7%) patients stopped sirolimus primarily due to cutaneous adverse effects.[48] Most of this information comes from the experience of using sirolimus in renal transplant patients.

Being an immunosuppressive drug, sirolimus puts patients at risk of infectious complications. Some authors recommend antibiotic prophylaxis against *Pneumocystis* pneumonia, but it is not a universal practice. A multicentric retrospective chart review of 113 patients treated with sirolimus for vascular anomalies reported 17 serious adverse events in 14 (12.4%) patients. Respiratory infections were the most common (47%), most commonly viral, followed by foreign body infections, pneumococcal meningitis, and sepsis.[49]

The recommended monitoring guidelines for sirolimus are summarized in **Box 1**.

CONCLUSION

Sirolimus, an mTOR inhibitor, appears to be a promising new agent for the treatment of many often difficult-to-treat skin diseases, particularly vascular malformations and tumors (lymphatic and venous malformations, kaposiform hemangioendothelioma, and KMP), and genodermatoses (tuberous sclerosis complex). Its role in the management of inflammatory dermatoses needs further studies. Topical application, which can bypass the side effects of oral treatment, may be preferred for superficial cutaneous lesions. The optimum formulation and concentration of topical sirolimus are not clear and warrant further investigation. Prospective clinical trials evaluating the efficacy and safety of oral as well as topical sirolimus in various dermatological conditions are currently being conducted. Good-quality, randomized, placebo-controlled studies are required to validate its status in dermatology pharmacotherapeutics.

REFERENCES

1. Vézina C, Kudelski A, Sehgal SN. Rapamycin (AY-22,989), a new antifungal antibiotic. I. Taxonomy of the producing streptomycete and isolation of the active principle. J Antibiot (Tokyo). 1975;28(10):721-6.
2. Sehgal SN. Sirolimus: Its discovery, biological properties, and mechanism of action. Transplant Proc. 2003;35(3):S7-14.
3. Wyeth TM. (2014). Rapamune® (Sirolimus) oral solution and tablets. [online] Available from www.pfizer.ca/sites/g/files/g10017036/f/201410/Rapamune_0.pdf [Last accessed January, 2024].
4. Zimmerman JJ, Kahan BD. Pharmacokinetics of sirolimus in stable renal transplant patients after multiple oral dose administration. J Clin Pharmacol. 1997;37(5):405-15.
5. Paghdal KV, Schwartz RA. Sirolimus (rapamycin): From the soil of Easter Island to a bright future. J Am Acad Dermatol. 2007;57(6):1046-50.
6. MacDonald A, Scarola J, Burke JT, Zimmerman JJ. Clinical pharmacokinetics and therapeutic drug monitoring of sirolimus. Clin Ther. 2000;22(Suppl B):B101-21.
7. Hofbauer GFL, Marcollo-Pini A, Corsenca A, Kistler AD, French LE, Wüthrich RP, et al. The mTOR inhibitor rapamycin significantly improves facial angiofibroma lesions in a patient with tuberous sclerosis. Br J Dermatol. 2008;159(2):473-5.
8. Balestri R, Neri I, Patrizi A, Angileri L, Ricci L, Magnano M. Analysis of current data on the use of topical rapamycin in the treatment of facial angiofibromas in tuberous sclerosis complex. J Eur Acad Dermatol Venereol. 2015;29(1):14-20.
9. Leducq S, Giraudeau B, Tavernier E, Maruani A. Topical use of mammalian target of rapamycin inhibitors in dermatology: A systematic review with meta-analysis. J Am Acad Dermatol. 2019;80(3):735-42.
10. Tanaka M, Wataya-Kaneda M, Nakamura A, Matsumoto S, Katayama I. First left-right comparative study of topical rapamycin vs. vehicle for facial angiofibromas in patients with tuberous sclerosis complex. Br J Dermatol. 2013;169(6):1314-8.
11. Cinar SL, Kartal D, Bayram AK, Canpolat M, Borlu M, Ferahbas A, et al. Topical sirolimus for the treatment of angiofibromas in tuberous sclerosis. Indian J Dermatol Venereol Leprol. 2017;83(1):27-32.
12. Samanta D. Topical mTOR (mechanistic target of rapamycin) inhibitor therapy in facial angiofibroma. Indian J Dermatol Venereol Leprol. 2015;81(5):540-1.
13. Salido R, Garnacho-Saucedo G, Cuevas-Asencio I, Ruano J, Galán-Gutierrez M, Vélez A, et al. Sustained clinical effectiveness and favorable safety profile of topical sirolimus for tuberous sclerosis—associated facial angiofibroma. J Eur Acad Dermatol Venereol. 2012;26(10):1315-8.
14. Koenig MK, Bell CS, Hebert AA, Roberson J, Samuels JA, Slopis JM, et al.; TREATMENT Trial Collaborators. Efficacy and safety of topical rapamycin in patients with facial

angiofibromas secondary to tuberous sclerosis complex: The TREATMENT randomized clinical trial. JAMA Dermatology. 2018;154(7):773-80.
15. Mutizwa MM, Berk DR, Anadkat MJ. Treatment of facial angiofibromas with topical application of oral rapamycin solution (1 mgmL(-1)) in two patients with tuberous sclerosis. Br J Dermatol. 2011;165(4):922-3.
16. Wataya-Kaneda M, Tanaka M, Yang L, Yang F, Tsuruta D, Nakamura A, et al. Clinical and histologic analysis of the efficacy of topical rapamycin therapy against hypomelanotic macules in tuberous sclerosis complex. JAMA Dermatol. 2015;151(7):722-30.
17. Muzic JG, Kindle SA, Tollefson MM. Successful treatment of subungual fibromas of tuberous sclerosis with topical rapamycin. JAMA Dermatol. 2014;150(9):1024-5.
18. Micozkadioglu H, Koc Z, Ozelsancak R, Yildiz I. Rapamycin therapy for renal, brain, and skin lesions in a tuberous sclerosis patient. Ren Fail. 2010;32(10):1233-6.
19. Bissler JJ, McCormack FX, Young LR, Elwing JM, Chuck G, Leonard JM, et al. Sirolimus for angiomyolipoma in tuberous sclerosis complex or lymphangioleiomyomatosis. N Engl J Med. 2008;358(2):140-51.
20. Sadowski K, Kotulska K, Schwartz RA, Jóźwiak S. Systemic effects of treatment with mTOR inhibitors in tuberous sclerosis complex: A comprehensive review. J Eur Acad Dermatol Venereol. 2016;30(4):586-94.
21. Swarbrick AW, Frederiks AJ, Foster RS. Systematic review of sirolimus in dermatological conditions. Australasian J Dermatol. 2021;62(4):461-9.
22. Teng JM, Bartholomew FB, Patel V, Sun G. Novel treatment of painful plantar keratoderma in pachyonychia congenita using topical sirolimus. Clin Exp Dermatol. 2018;43(8):968-71.
23. Daroach M, Dogra S, Bhattacharjee R, Tp A, Smith F, Mahajan R. Pachyonychia congenita responding favorably to a combination of surgical and medical therapies. Dermatol Ther. 2019;32(5):e13045.
24. Weiss B, Widemann BC, Wolters P, Dombi E, Vinks A, Cantor A, et al. Sirolimus for progressive neurofibromatosis type 1–associated plexiform neurofibromas: A neurofibromatosis clinical trials consortium phase ii study. Neuro Oncol. 2015;17(4):596-603.
25. Blatt J, Stavas J, Moats-Staats B, Woosley J, Morrell DS. Treatment of childhood kaposiform hemangioendothelioma with sirolimus. Pediatr Blood Cancer. 2010;55(7):1396-8.
26. Lackner H, Karastaneva A, Schwinger W, Benesch M, Sovinz P, Seidel M, et al. Sirolimus for the treatment of children with various complicated vascular anomalies. Eur J Pediatr. 2015;174(12):1579-84.
27. Kai L, Wang Z, Yao W, Dong K, Xiao X. Sirolimus, a promising treatment for refractory kaposiform hemangioendothelioma. J Cancer Res Clin Oncol. 2014;140(3):471-6.
28. Adams DM, Trenor CC 3rd, Hammill AM, Vinks AA, Patel MN, et al. Efficacy and safety of sirolimus in the treatment of complicated vascular anomalies. Pediatrics. 2016;137(2):e20153257.
29. Yesil S, Bozkurt C, Tanyildiz HG, Tekgunduz SA, Candir MO, Toprak S, et al. Successful treatment of macroglossia due to lymphatic malformation with sirolimus. Ann Otol Rhinol Laryngol. 2015;124(10):820-3.
30. Ivars M, Redondo P. Efficacy of topical sirolimus (rapamycin) for the treatment of microcystic lymphatic malformations. JAMA Dermatol. 2017;153(1):103-5.
31. Geeurickx M, Labarque V. A narrative review of the role of sirolimus in the treatment of congenital vascular malformations. J Vasc Surg Venous Lymphat Disord. 2021;9(5):1321-33.
32. Wang Z, Li K, Dong K, Xiao X, Zheng S. Refractory Kasabach-Merritt phenomenon successfully treated with sirolimus and a mini-review of the published work. J Dermatol. 2015;42(4):401-4.

33. Ji Y, Chen S, Zhou J, Yang K, Zhang X, Xiang B, et al. Sirolimus plus prednisolone vs sirolimus monotherapy for kaposiform hemangioendothelioma: A randomized clinical trial. Blood. 2022;139(11):1619-30.
34. Mathew T, Kreis H, Friend P. Two-year incidence of malignancy in sirolimus-treated renal transplant recipients: Results from five multicenter studies. Clin Transplant. 2004;18(4):446-9.
35. Yanik EL, Siddiqui K, Engels EA. Sirolimus effects on cancer incidence after kidney transplantation: A meta-analysis. Cancer Med. 2015;4(9):1448-59.
36. Nichols LA, Adang LA, Kedes DH. Rapamycin blocks production of KSHV/HHV8: Insights into the anti-tumor activity of an immunosuppressant drug. PLoS One. 2011;6(1):e14535.
37. Stallone G, Schena A, Infante B, Di Paolo S, Loverre A, Maggio G, et al. Sirolimus for Kaposi's sarcoma in renal-transplant recipients. N Engl J Med. 2005;352(13):1317-23.
38. Krown SE, Roy D, Lee JY, Dezube BJ, Reid EG, Venkataramanan R, et al. Rapamycin with antiretroviral therapy in AIDS-associated Kaposi sarcoma: An AIDS Malignancy Consortium study. J Acquir Immune Defic Syndr. 2012;59(5):447-54.
39. Saggar S, Zeichner JA, Brown TT, Phelps RG, Cohen SR. Kaposi's sarcoma resolves after sirolimus therapy in a patient with pemphigus vulgaris. Arch Dermatol. 2008;144(5):654-57.
40. Reitamo S, Spuls P, Sassolas B, Lahfa M, Claudy A, Griffiths CE; Sirolimus European Psoriasis Study Group. Efficacy of sirolimus (rapamycin) administered concomitantly with a subtherapeutic dose of cyclosporin in the treatment of severe psoriasis: A randomized controlled trial. Br J Dermatol. 2001;145(3):438-45.
41. Ormerod AD, Shah SA, Copeland P, Omar G, Winfield A. Treatment of psoriasis with topical sirolimus: Preclinical development and a randomized, double-blind trial. Br J Dermatol. 2005;152(4):758-64.
42. Pidala J, Tomblyn M, Nishihori T, Field T, Ayala E, Perkins J, et al. Sirolimus demonstrates activity in the primary therapy of acute graft-versus-host disease without systemic glucocorticoids. Haematologica. 2011;96(9):1351-6.
43. Benito AI, Furlong T, Martin PJ, Anasetti C, Appelbaum FR, Doney K, et al. Sirolimus (rapamycin) for the treatment of steroid-refractory acute graft-versus-host disease. Transplantation. 2001;72(12):1924-9.
44. Ghez D, Rubio MT, Maillard N, Suarez F, Chandesris MO, Delarue R, et al. Rapamycin for refractory acute graft-versus-host disease. Transplantation. 2009;88(9):1081-7.
45. Harrison DE, Strong R, Sharp ZD, Nelson JF, Astle CM, Flurkey K, et al. Rapamycin fed late in life extends lifespan in genetically heterogeneous mice. Nature. 2009;460(7253):392-5.
46. Levi Z, Hazazi R, Kedar-Barnes I, Hodak E, Gal E, Mor E, et al. Switching from tacrolimus to sirolimus halts the appearance of new sebaceous neoplasms in Muir-Torre syndrome. Am J Transplant. 2007;7(2):476-9.
47. Fogel AL, Hill S, Teng JM. Advances in the therapeutic use of mammalian target of rapamycin (mTOR) inhibitors in dermatology. J Am Acad Dermatol. 2015;72(5):879-89.
48. Mahé E, Morelon E, Lechaton S, Sang KH, Mansouri R, Ducasse MF, et al. Cutaneous adverse events in renal transplant recipients receiving sirolimus-based therapy. Transplantation. 2005;79(4):476-82.
49. Rössler J, Baselga E, Davila V, Celis V, Diociaiuti A, El Hachem M, et al. Severe adverse events during sirolimus "off-label" therapy for vascular anomalies. Pediatr Blood Cancer. 2021;68(8):e28936.

CHAPTER 34

Newer Small Molecules in Pipeline

Bhavni Oberoi

INTRODUCTION

Small molecules are low molecular weight compounds that can easily diffuse into cells and modulate specific cellular pathways. In dermatology, small molecules are being increasingly used for the treatment of various skin conditions. The most important small molecules that are clubbed with biologics include Janus Kinase–signal transducer and activator of transcription (JAK-STAT), phosphodiesterase-4 (PDE-4), and mTOR (mammalian target of rapamycin) inhibitors, which have already been discussed in detail in individual chapters.

Some other newer molecules that are being used or studied in dermatology include novel drugs for psoriasis, atopic dermatitis, pruritus, melanoma, T-cell lymphoma, etc. These can be broadly divided into small molecules in dermatological oncology, small molecules in inflammatory dermatosis, and small molecules in chronic pruritus. We shall be discussing them one by one.

SMALL MOLECULES IN DERMATOLOGICAL ONCOLOGY

The mitogen activated protein kinase (MAPK) pathway is responsible for normal cell growth and multiplication. Any mutations in this pathway can cause uncontrolled cell growth and have been implicated in a large number of metastatic melanomas **(Fig. 1)**.[1]

The MAPK signaling is initiated via cell surface tyrosine kinase (TYK) receptor and subsequent activation of RAS, a membrane-bound GTPase. A sequential cascade of phosphorylation reactions lead to the activation of specific kinases, out of which the most important ones are RAF (rapidly accelerated fibrosarcoma). The three RAFs (ARAF/BRAF/CRAF) lead to further phosphorylation of mitogen activated protein kinase (MEK) and extracellular signal regulated kinase (ERK), which are responsible for cell

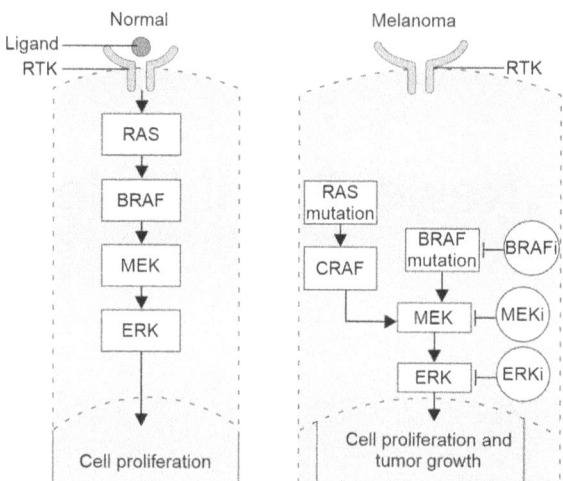

FIG. 1: Signaling pathway implicated in the development of melanoma.
(BRAF and CRAF: rapidly activated fibrosarcoma kinase family isoforms B and C; BRAFi: BRAF inhibitor; ERK: extracellular signal regulated kinase; ERKi: ERK inhibitor; MEK: mitogen activated protein kinase; MEKi: MEK inhibitor; RAS: rat sarcoma virus-associated proto-oncogene protein; RTK: receptor tyrosine kinase)

growth, proliferation, differentiation, and death. Out of these, overactivation of BRAF (V600E) is the most common mutation in melanoma.

The MAPK pathway mutation also plays a role in making the melanoma immunologically cold via various immune escape mechanism.

This knowledge led to the development of a number of targeted therapies using molecules that inhibit this pathway at various levels.

BRAF Inhibitors

- *Molecules available*: Vemurafenib and dabrafenib
- *Mechanism of action*: More than 50% of the metastatic melanomas have a BRAF (proto-oncogene encoding for BRAF protein[2]) mutation, which encodes for a serine threonine kinase within the MAPK pathway[3] and the BRAF inhibitors target this. These mutations lead to constitutive activation of the pathway and cause uncontrollable cell proliferation and tumor growth. This growth can be halted by molecules targeting this gene or formation of its protein.

Vemurafenib

- *Approval*: It was approved by the United States Food and Drug Administration (USFDA) in 2011 and by the European Medicines Agency (EMA) in 2012 for the treatment of patients with unresectable or metastatic melanoma with BRAF V600 mutations (only V600E mutation in the case of FDA).[4]
- *Recommended dose*: 960 mg BID.

- *Clinical response*: In phase 1 ($n = 87$), 69% response on dose escalation and 81% in extension phase was noted. Progression-free survival was >7 months.

  In phase 2 ($n = 132$), 53% response rate was noted. Progression-free survival was 6.8 months and overall survival was 15.9 months.
- *Adverse effects*: Arthralgia (53%), photosensitivity (49%), rash (45%), fatigue (40%), alopecia (36%), diarrhea (21%), dizziness (21%), muscular weakness (21%), paresthesia (21%), solar dermatitis (21%), vomiting (21%), and cutaneous squamous cell carcinomas or keratoacanthomas (26%)[4]

Dabrafenib

Dabrafenib is a reversible, small molecule, which is ATP-competitive and selectively inhibits BRAF V600E.[5]

- *Approval*: The US FDA approved its use in 2013. It also received accelerated approval for combination with trametinib. (Even though BRAF inhibitors have shown excellent promise, there have been gradual reports of early development of resistance due to multiple mechanisms, including BRAF amplification or downstream activating mutations in the MAPK pathway. Addition of MEK inhibitors such as trametinib and cobimetinib to BRAF inhibitors has shown to improve survival rates in multiple phase II and III randomized controlled trials, and has now become the standard of care.)
- *Dose*: 150 mg twice daily (1 hour before or 2 hours after meals)[6]
- *Clinical response*: Similar to vemurafenib of 55–60% with progression-free survival of 6–7 months.
- *Adverse effects*: The adverse effects of BRAF inhibitors are mentioned in **Table 1**.

Toxicity is the main reported difference between dabrafenib and vemurafenib. Cutaneous toxicities, such as rash, hyperkeratosis, squamous cell carcinoma (SCC), and cutaneous keratoacanthoma, occur with both drugs, but less frequently with dabrafenib. Other toxicities such as arthralgia, fatigue, photosensitivity, and hepatitis were also reported to be higher with vemurafenib. Pyrexia is one adverse effect that has been reported to be higher with dabrafenib than vemurafenib.[8]

The need for dose reduction or interruption in view of toxicity is approximately 30–40% for both drugs, but very few patients need to permanently discontinue therapy due to toxicity.

Mitogen Activated Protein Kinase Inhibitors

- *Molecules available*: Trametinib and cobimetinib
- *Mechanism of action*: Inhibition of MEK in MAPK pathway. MEK1 and MEK2 are dual-specificity kinases that catalyze activating phosphorylation at the tyrosine and threonine residues in ERK1 and ERK2. These activated ERK1/2 further catalyze the phosphorylation of cytoplasmic and nuclear

TABLE 1: Adverse effects of BRAF inhibitors.	
Cutaneous	• Photosensitivity • Photodermatosis • Rash (erythema, maculopapular rash, folliculitis, acneiform eruption, nipple hyperkeratosis, not otherwise specified) • Palmoplantar hyperkeratosis • Palmoplantar dysesthesia • Alopecia • Abnormalities in hair texture • Actinic keratosis • Keratosis pilaris • Pruritus • Verruca • Xerosis • Panniculitis • Seborrheic keratosis • Milia • Eruptive nevi • Mucosal, vulvar, and gingival hyperkeratosis • Cutaneous SCC • Keratoacanthoma • BCC
Ophthalmic	• Uveitis • Keratoconjunctivitis sicca • Central serous retinopathy (rare)
Paradoxical oncogenesis	• Cutaneous malignancies[7] • RAS mutant leukemia • Metastatic recurrence of RAS mutant colorectal cancer • Gastric polyp
Renal	• Acute tubular necrosis • Fanconi syndrome • Hypophosphatemia • Hyponatremia • Hypokalemia • Subnephrotic-range proteinuria • Acute/subacute decrease in GFR by 20–40%
Others	• Arthralgia and arthritis • Vomiting • Diarrhea • Muscle weakness • Fatigue • Paresthesia

(BCC: basal cell carcinoma; GFR: glomerular filtration rate; RAS: rat sarcoma virus; SCC: squamous cell carcinoma)

substrates leading to cellular response important in tumorigenesis. MEK1 and MEK2 are 86% identical in structure, thus currently available MEK inhibitors are not selective for either isoform.[9]

Trametinib
- *Approval*: FDA approved in 2013[10]
- *Dose*: 2 mg once a day[10]
- *Clinical response*: 65% tumor reduction with a progression-free survival of 4.8 months[10]
- *Adverse effects*: Common adverse effects in phase I and II trials were rash (57%), diarrhea (43%), peripheral edema (26%), fatigue (26%), and acneiform eruptions (19%). Overall, 14 (7%) patients had decreased ejection fraction or ventricular dysfunction, and two patients had serious grade 3 cardiac-related events leading to discontinuation of drug. Ocular events occurred in 9% of patients, mainly grade 1 and 2. Adverse events led to dose reduction in 27% of patients and dose interruption in 35% of the patients.[9]

Cobemetinib
- *Approval*: The US FDA approved in November 2015 for use in combination with vemurafenib for unresectable/metastatic melanoma.[11]
- *Dose*: 60 mg once a day used in combination with vemurafenib (Vemurafenib 960 mg twice a day and cobimetinib 60 mg daily, 21 days on/7 days off)
- *Clinical response*: There was 68% response rate in the combination group with vemurafenib and median progression-free survival for 9.9 months with combination.
- *Adverse effects*: Adverse effects in patients who had progressed on vemurafenib and those who were naïve to BRAF inhibitors were nonacneiform rash (33% and 87%), diarrhea (47% and 83%), fatigue (27% and 70%), photosensitivity (15% and 67%), and liver enzyme abnormalities (33% and 67%), respectively.[12]
  BRAF inhibitor–naïve patients had a higher incidence of typical MEK inhibitor toxicities, including eye disorders [retinal detachment (2%), chorioretinopathy (5%), retinopathy (3%), and macular edema (2%)]. Elevated creatine phosphokinase (CPK) level is another known class effect of MEK inhibitors.[11]
  Recently,[13] in phase III COLUMBUS trial encorafenib and binimetinib, a new BRAF–MEK inhibitor combination has demonstrated survival benefit as compared with single agent BRAF inhibitors.

Cyclin-dependent Kinase 4/6 Inhibitors
- *Mechanism of action*: Cyclin-dependent kinase (CDK)4/6 are a class of serine/threonine kinases expressed in most cell types and control the first

TABLE 2: Src and Syk family drugs under trial.

Drug	Trade name	Clinical indication/trial	Clinical trial number
Fostamatinib		Hidradenitis suppurativa	NCT05040698
		Rheumatoid Arthritis	NCT02092961
			NCT01725230
Lapatinib	Tykerb	Malignant melanoma	NCT01264081
Dasatinib	Sprycel	Systemic mastocytosis	NCT00979160

gap phase (G1 to S) of the cell cycle, thus establishing their importance in both tumorigenesis as well as normal cellular processes. Approximately 90% of melanoma patients have some mutations affecting various parts of CDK4/6 pathway. Also, high frequency mutations in the CDK4 pathway have been identified in rare variants of melanoma such as acral and mucosal melanoma. Thus, inhibitors of this pathway form promising anticancer therapies.[14]

- *Molecules available*: Most common is abemaciclib. Others under investigation include palbociclib and ribociclib.[15]

Src Family and Syk Tyrosine Kinase

- *Mechanism*: Src gene encodes the nonreceptor TYK proteins, which have a role to play in cell cycle progression, motility, proliferation, differentiation, and survival, among other cellular processes.

The *Syk* gene family is responsible for neutrophil/macrophage integrin signaling and responses to immune complexes.

They are implicated not only in malignancies such as melanoma but also in disorders such as pemphigus vulgaris, hidradenitis suppurativa, systemic mastocytosis, and neutrophilic dermatosis.

The drugs currently under trial are mentioned in **Table 2**.

SMALL MOLECULES IN INFLAMMATORY DERMATOSIS

Aryl Hydrocarbon Receptor Agonists

- *Molecules available*: Tapinarof
- *Approval*: 1% tapinarof cream approved by the USFDA in May 2022 for psoriasis.[16]

Mechanism of Action

Tapiranof is an aryl hydrocarbon receptor (AHR) agonist. Its molecular action points and pathways are depicted in **Fig. 2**. AHR can get activated by various oxidative and antioxidative ligands. On activation, the cytoplasmic AHR translocates to the nucleus where it heterodimerizes with an AHR-nuclear

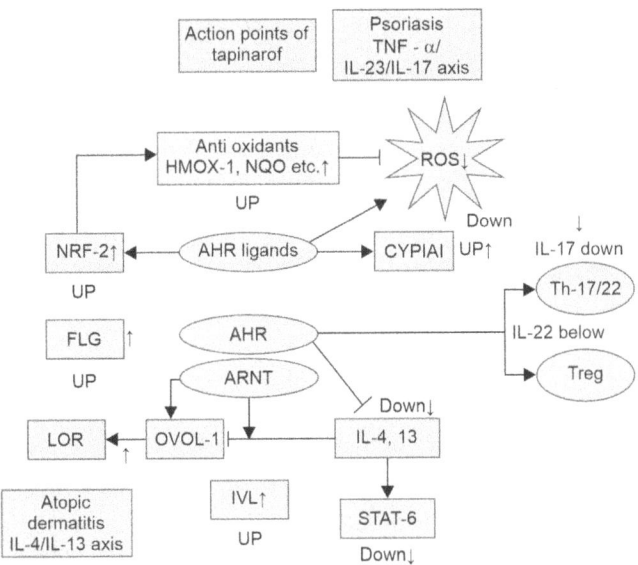

FIG. 2: Mechanism of action of AHR agonists.[17]
(AHR: aryl hydrocarbon receptor; ARNT: AHR nuclear translocator; FLG: filaggrin; HMOX-1: heme oxygenase 1; IVL: involucrin; LOR: loricrin; NQO: NAD(P)H:quinone acceptor oxidoreductase; NRF-2: nuclear factor E2-related factor 2; OVOL-1: OVO like 1 transcription factor; ROS: reactive oxygen species)

translocator (ARNT). This induces the transcription of AHR-responsive genes such as cytochrome P450 1A1 (CYP1A1), which degrades AHR ligands. This produces long-lived ligands such as dioxins, which generate reactive oxygen species (ROS) and some antioxidative AHR ligands, which activate nuclear factor-erythroid 2-related factor-2 (NRF2) transcription factor. This leads to upregulation of genetic expression of various antioxidative enzymes, such as heme oxygenase-1 (HMOX-1), NAD(P)H dehydrogenase, and quinone 1 (NQO-1), and these neutralize ROS.

The AHR/ARNT signaling also activates transcription factors such as OVO-like-1 (OVOL-1) and upregulates the expression of filaggrin (FLG), loricrin (LOR), and involucrin (IVL) in an OVOL1-independent manner. Interleukin (IL)-4 and IL-13 are activators of STAT6 and inhibitors of the OVOL1/FLG, OVOL1/LOR, and AHR/IVL axes. Activation of AHR can inhibit IL-4/IL-13-mediated pathways, thereby restoring the expression of FLG, LOR, and IVL. AHR signaling also affects T-helper (Th17) and Treg cell differentiation and is required for IL-22 production. This explains their role in psoriasis and atopic dermatitis.

Thus, to summarize, AHR pathway activation is responsible for upregulation of various antioxidant enzymes. It has an important role in suppression of inflammatory cytokines such as IL4/13, suppression of Th17 pathway, and modulation of skin barrier protein (upregulation of filaggrin, loricrin, and involucrin), thereby making it efficacious in psoriasis and atopic dermatitis.[17]

Clinical Response
Good efficacy, fast onset of action, and clinical response maintained for an average of 130 days beyond treatment discontinuation in patients with psoriasis in phase 3 studies.[18]

Adverse Effects
The adverse effects include folliculitis, nasopharyngitis, contact dermatitis, headache, and pruritus.[19]

Tyrosine Kinase-2 Inhibitors
Molecules Available
Three TYK2 inhibitors that have advanced in clinical trials are deucravacitinib (BMS-986165), brepocitinib/PF-06700841(both oral and topical), and ropsacitinib/PF-06826647 (oral), and others such as NDI-034858 and ESK-001 are being investigated.[20,21]

Mechanism of Action
Tyrosine kinase-2 forms a part of the JAK-STAT pathway (**Fig. 3**). It pairs with JAK2 and mediates signal transduction pathways downstream of IL-12 and IL-23. Out of these, IL-12 is essential for Th1 cells, which in turn release the proinflammatory cytokines [tumor necrosis factor and interferon gamma (IFN-γ)]. IL-23 controls the expansion and survival of Th17 cells. Cytokines derived in turn from Th1 and Th17 cells combine to amplify keratinocyte proliferation and activation. TYK2 also pairs with JAK1 to mediate signal transduction pathways downstream of type I IFN receptors. This explains their role in psoriasis similar to JAK-2 inhibitors.[22]
- *Deucravacitinib*: Selective TYK2 inhibitor; binds to the pseudokinase regulatory domain (allosteric inhibition)[22]
- *Brepocitinib*: It is a dual TYK2/JAK1 inhibitor with partial selectivity over JAK2, and binds to the active sites in the catalytic domains of TYK2, JAK1, and JAK2.[22]
- *Ropsacitinib*: Dual TYK2/JAK2 inhibitor; binds to the active site in the catalytic domain[22]

Clinical Uses
Psoriasis and psoriatic arthritis, also being evaluated for inflammatory bowel disease (IBD) and systemic lupus erythematosus (SLE).

With deucravacitinib, psoriasis area and severity index (PASI) 75 at 12 weeks with 3 mg twice daily was 69%, 6 mg twice daily was 67%, and 12 mg once daily was 75%. Other two drugs also showed significant reduction in PASI 75 at 12 weeks.[22]

CHAPTER 34: Newer Small Molecules in Pipeline

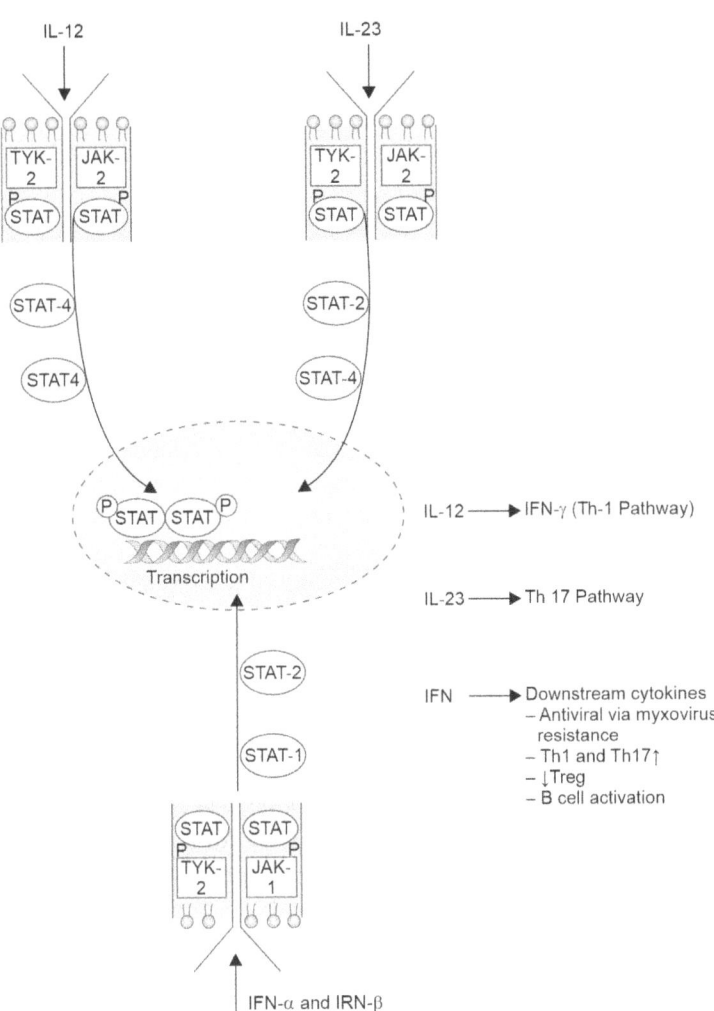

FIG. 3: Mechanism of action of JAK STAT/TYK-2 pathway.
(IFN: interferon; IL: interleukin; JAK: Janus Kinase; STAT: signal transducers and activators of transcription; TYK: tyrosine kinase)

Adverse Effects and Monitoring

- *Brepocitinib*: Platelet and reticulocyte counts were reduced due to concomitant JAK2 inhibition[22]
- *Deucravacitinib*: Side effects observed were nasopharyngitis, headache, diarrhea, nausea, and upper respiratory tract infection. No significant adverse effects were seen on the hematological parameters.[22]
- *Ropsacitinib*: Side effects seen were increased blood creatinine levels, increased alanine aminotransferase levels, and headache.[22]

SMALL MOLECULES IN CHRONIC PRURITUS

Neurokinin 1 Receptor Antagonist
- *Molecules available*: serlopitant and aprepitant
- *Mechanism of action*: The tachykinin substance P (SP) and its receptor, neurokinin 1 receptor (NK1R), are well established as a pivotal pathway in histamine-independent pruritus. Activation of this receptor (NK-1R) on mast cells can lead to degranulation and secretion of histamine, leukotriene B4, prostaglandin D2, tumor necrosis factor A, and vascular endothelial growth factor (VEGF), while on vessels it can induce vasodilatation and neurogenic inflammation with clinical symptoms including erythema, edema, and pruritus.[23]
- *Doses*: Aprepitant (oral: 125 mg on day 1, 80 mg on day 2-3 twice/week, topical: 5% gel); serlopitant (0.25, 1, or 5 mg oral)
- *Clinical uses*: Serlopitant can result in a dose-dependent decrease in pruritus. The mean percentage decreases were significantly larger with the 1 and 5 mg doses of serlopitant ($p = 0.022$ and $p = 0.013$, respectively) than with placebo at week 6.[24]
- *Adverse effects and monitoring*: Nasopharyngitis, diarrhea, somnolence, and fatigue

CONCLUSION

Thus, we a can see that a large number of small molecules that are considered with biologics but not clubbed with them are finding a multitude of use in various streams of dermatology and dermatological oncology. Many more molecules are under investigation and will soon surface to slowly side track conventional drugs if they can surpass the side effects of the conventional drugs.

REFERENCES

1. Fernandez A. Dermatology update: The dawn of targeted treatment. Cleve Clin J Med. 2015;82(5):309-20.
2. Liu Q, Zhu H, Tiruthani K, Shen L, Chen F, Gao K, et al. Nanoparticle-mediated trapping of Wnt family member 5A in tumor microenvironments enhances immunotherapy for B-Raf proto-oncogene mutant melanoma. ACS Nano. 2018;12(2):1250-61.
3. Davies H, Bignell GR, Cox C, Stephens P, Edkins S, Clegg S, et al. Mutations of the BRAF gene in human cancer. Nature. 2002;417(6892):949-54.
4. Martin-Liberal J, Larkin J. Vemurafenib for the treatment of BRAF mutant metastatic melanoma. Future Oncol. 2015;11(4):579-89.
5. King AJ, Arnone MR, Bleam MR, Moss KG, Yang J, Fedorowicz KE, et al. Dabrafenib; preclinical characterization, increased efficacy when combined with trametinib, while BRAF/MEK tool combination reduced skin lesions. PLoS One. 2013;8(7):e67583.
6. Dhillon S. Dabrafenib plus trametinib: A review in advanced melanoma with a BRAF (V600) mutation. Target Oncol. 2016;11(3):417-28.

7. Gibney GT, Messina JL, Fedorenko IV, Sondak VK, Smalley KS. Paradoxical oncogenesis—the long-term effects of BRAF inhibition in melanoma. Nat Rev Clin Oncol. 2013;10(7):390-9.
8. Menzies AM, Long GV. Dabrafenib and trametinib, alone and in combination for BRAF-mutant metastatic melanoma. Clin Cancer Res. 2014;20(8):2035-43.
9. McCain J. The MAPK (ERK) pathway, investigational combinations for the treatment of BRAF-mutated metastatic melanoma. P T. 2013;38(2):96-108.
10. Chopra N, Nathan PD. Trametinib in metastatic melanoma. Expert Rev Anticancer Ther. 2015;15(7):749-60.
11. Signorelli J, Gandhi AS. Cobimetinib. Ann Pharmacother. 2017;51(2):146-53.
12. Ribas A, Gonzalez R, Pavlick A, Hamid O, Gajewski TF, Daud A, et al. Combination of vemurafenib and cobimetinib in patients with advanced BRAF(V600)-mutated melanoma: a phase 1b study. Lancet Oncol. 2014;15(9):954-65.
13. Dummer R, Ascierto PA, Gogas HJ, Arance A, Mandala M, Liszkay G, et al. Encorafenib plus binimetinib versus vemurafenib or encorafenib in patients with BRAF-mutant melanoma (COLUMBUS): a multicentre, open-label, randomised phase 3 trial. Lancet Oncol. 2018;19(5):603-15.
14. Guo L, Qi J, Wang H, Jiang X, Liu Y. Getting under the skin: The role of CDK4/6 in melanomas. Eur J Med Chem. 2020;204:112531.
15. Julve M, Clark JJ, Lythgoe MP. Advances in cyclin-dependent kinase inhibitors for the treatment of melanoma. Expert Opin Pharmacother. 2021;22(3):351-61.
16. Keam SJ. Tapinarof cream 1%: First approval. Drugs. 2022;82(11):1221-8.
17. Furue M, Hashimoto-Hachiya A, Tsuji G. Aryl hydrocarbon receptor in atopic dermatitis and psoriasis. Int J Mol Sci. 2019;20(21):5424.
18. Bissonnette R, Saint-Cyr Proulx E, Jack C, Maari C. Tapinarof for psoriasis and atopic dermatitis: 15 years of clinical research. J Eur Acad Dermatol Venereol. 2023;37(6):1168-74.
19. Nogueira S, Rodrigues MA, Vender R, Torres T. Tapinarof for the treatment of psoriasis. Dermatol Ther. 2022;35(12):e15931.
20. Jo CE, Gooderham M, Beecker J. TYK 2 inhibitors for the treatment of dermatologic conditions: the evolution of JAK inhibitors. Int J Dermatol. 2022;61(2):139-47.
21. Loo WJ, Turchin I, Prajapati VH, Gooderham MJ, Grewal P, Hong CH, et al. Clinical implications of targeting the JAK-STAT pathway in psoriatic disease: Emphasis on the TYK2 pathway. J Cutan Med Surg. 2023;27(1_suppl):3S-24S.
22. Krueger JG, McInnes IB, Blauvelt A. Tyrosine kinase 2 and Janus kinase–signal transducer and activator of transcription signaling and inhibition in plaque psoriasis. J Am Acad Dermatol. 2022;86(1):148-57.
23. Pojawa-Gołąb M, Jaworecka K, Reich A. NK-1 Receptor Antagonists and Pruritus: Review of Current Literature. Dermatol Ther (Heidelb). 2019;9(3):391-405.
24. Yosipovitch G, Ständer S, Kerby MB, Larrick JW, Perlman AJ, Schnipper EF, et al. Serlopitant for the treatment of chronic pruritus: Results of a randomized, multicenter, placebo-controlled phase 2 clinical trial. J Am Acad Dermatol. 2018;78(5):882-91.e10.

CHAPTER 35

Intravenous Immunoglobulins

Rohit Kothari, Rajesh Verma

INTRODUCTION

Intravenous immunoglobulin (IVIg) was originally used for antibody replacement therapies in primary immune deficiencies and treatment of viral infections. A multitude of dermatologic disorders have shown potential for treatment with this unique treatment modality. The dermatoses where IVIg has been used with success include autoimmune bullous diseases, connective tissue diseases, vasculitis, Stevens–Johnson syndrome (SJS), toxic epidermal necrolysis (TEN), and infectious disorders such as streptococcal toxic shock syndrome.[1,2] High cost and thereby a lack of randomized controlled trials, except for pemphigus vulgaris and dermatomyositis, is a hindrance to the regular use of IVIg. Nevertheless, there is a significant body of evidence demonstrating the efficacy of IVIg in patients with skin diseases that are resistant to treatment with standard agents.

STRUCTURE OF IMMUNOGLOBULIN

Immunoglobulins are produced by plasma cells in response to an immunogen and are glycoprotein molecules. The structure and the components of an immunoglobulin are depicted in **Figures 1A and B**.[3]

METHODS OF PREPARATION OF INTRAVENOUS IMMUNOGLOBULIN

Intravenous immunoglobulin contains supraphysiologic levels of IgG and is derived from fractionated human plasma. It is obtained from purified human plasma of 3,000 to approximately 10,000 individual donors per batch. Pooling is performed to provide repertoire representing all antibodies and natural autoantibodies.[4] The donors are screened for bloodborne viruses and parvovirus and there is a "look back" screening period of 60 days for donors.

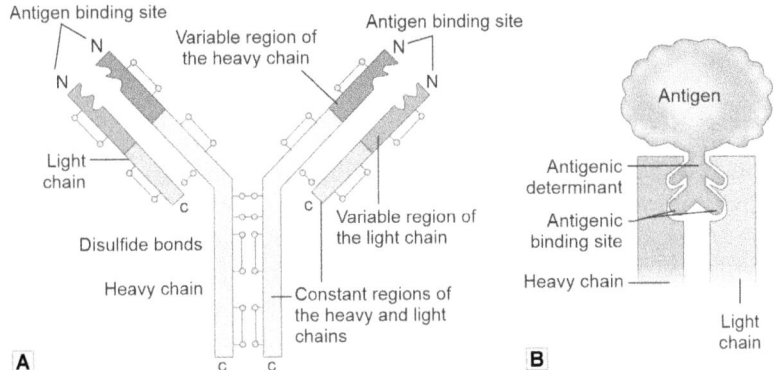

FIGS. 1A AND B: Structure of immunoglobulin.[3] (A) Structure; (B) Antigen binding site.[3]

Any seroconversion of a donor during this period would result in quarantine and destruction of the plasma obtained.[5,6]

COMPOSITION OF INTRAVENOUS IMMUNOGLOBULIN

Intravenous immunoglobulin is a highly purified IgG preparation which typically contains >95% of unmodified IgG with functionally intact Fc-dependent effector functions and only trace amounts of IgA, IgE, and IgM.[2] Subclass distribution may vary between preparations, with some products having less than physiological levels of IgG3 and/or IgG4.[5] It may also contain small amounts of albumin, sugars, salts, solvents, detergents, and buffers.[5] Variability of the manufacturing processes may lead to differences in the marketed IVIg products. Factors affecting the biological activity and integrity of the IgG molecule, tolerability, and yield depends on production steps such as stabilization and purification. Sodium-containing IVIg preparation reduces the proportion of coronary artery abnormalities and IVIg resistance in Kawasaki disease when compared with sodium-trace preparation.[7]

PHARMACOKINETICS

Peak serum concentrations occur immediately after intravenous (IV) injection and are dose related. Up to 30% of the dose may be removed by catabolism and distribution within 24 hours. IVIg distributes in the intravascular (60%) and extravascular (40%) compartments and can cross placenta and is excreted in milk. The serum half-life is 3–5 weeks.[8,9] The higher the concentration of the IVIg product, the less volume is required for infusion. For example, a 70 kg individual receiving 1 g/kg would require either 700 mL of a 10% solution or 1,400 mL of a 5% solution. In high-risk patients, such as those with cardiac or renal failure, these factors must be taken into consideration. In selecting the most appropriate IVIg for the patient, convenience, efficacy, safety, and tolerability of different products must be considered.

MECHANISM OF ACTION

The mechanism by which high-dose IVIg mediates anti-inflammatory activity is not well-understood. The effects are mediated via the Fc portion of IgG or the antigen-binding site and the variable regions of the antibody molecule.[2]

The proposed mechanism of action of IVIg is discussed in **Table 1**. The complex interplay of these effects is diagrammatically represented in **Figure 2**.

TABLE 1: Mechanism of action of high-dose IVIg.[5,10,11]

Mechanism	Remarks	Example
Reduced antibody production	By IgG binding via its Fc fragment (crystallizable) to corresponding cellular surface receptors on B lymphocytes	Autoantibodies directed against factor VIII, DNA, intrinsic factor, thyroglobulin and ANCA
	Downregulation of pathogenic autoantibody production	
Increased catabolism of antibodies	Reduced half-life of circulating immunoglobulins, probably by saturating the protective neonatal Fc receptor (FcRn)	
Effect on complement system	Bind to complement components C3b and C4b	Dermatomyositis
	Block complement activation at an early stage and inhibits complement deposition	
	Interfere with the formation of the terminal MAC	
Effect on granulocytes	Induce apoptosis and decrease neutrophil count within 24 hours of infusion	Kawasaki disease
Functional blockade of Fc receptors	Fc receptors are saturated by "anti-idiotypic" antibodies in IVIg	Idiopathic thrombocytopenic purpura
	Decreased cellular destruction as a consequence of Fc-mediated phagocytosis of antibody-coated cells in auto-antibody mediated diseases	
Effect on T-cell activation	IVIg preparations contain amounts of soluble CD4, CD8, MHC-I and MHC-II molecules which may have the ability to inhibit autoreactive T lymphocytes	–

Continued

Continued

Mechanism	Remarks	Example
	Modulates the production of IL-1, -2, -3, -4, -5, -10, TNF-α, GM-CSF, and IL-1 receptor antagonist by monocytes, macrophages, and lymphocytes	
	Restoration of a Th1/Th2 cytokine balance by supplying neutralizing antibodies	
	Induction of T-regulatory cells	
Activation or functional blockade of the death receptor Fas (CD95)	IVIg can either inhibit or activate cell death by binding to the death receptor Fas	SJS/TEN
	Mediated by agonistic anti-Fas IgG and antagonistic anti-Fas IgG	
	Inhibitory Fc receptor, FcγRIIB, is shown to be required for protection	
Synergistic effect with corticosteroids	Adjunctive use of IVIg has led to reduced dose requirements for systemic corticosteroids	–
	Because of increased glucocorticoid receptor sensitivity	
	IVIg and corticosteroids can synergistically suppress the lymphocyte activation	

(ANCA: antineutrophil cytoplasmic antibodies; CD: Cluster of differentiation; FcγRIIB: Fcγ receptor IIB; GM-CSF: granulocyte-macrophage colony-stimulating factor; IL: interleukin; IVIg: intravenous immunoglobulin; MAC: membrane attack complex; MHC: major histocompatibility complex; IL: TNF-α: tumor necrosis factor-alpha; SJS: Stevens–Johnson syndrome; TEN: toxic epidermal necrolysis)

INDICATIONS IN DERMATOLOGY

The only Food and Drug Administration (FDA) approved indication for use of IVIg from a dermatology point of view is Kawasaki disease. The other indications and contraindications for use of IVIg in dermatology are listed in **Box 1 and Table 2**. Indications for high-dose IVIg in autoimmune bullous diseases are given in **Box 2 and Table 3**.

DOSAGE REGIMEN

The most used dosage regimen in dermatology to produce desired or expected results is 2 g/kg/cycle, divided into three equal doses, given on each of 3 consecutive days. Some studies have advocated the use of 400 mg/kg daily given over a course of 5 days to constitute a cycle. The infusion is given slowly over 4–4.5 hours and vital signs are monitored frequently.[10]

As the half-life of IVIg ranges from 3 to 5 weeks, the infusions are generally spaced at monthly intervals. But in very aggressive diseases, it

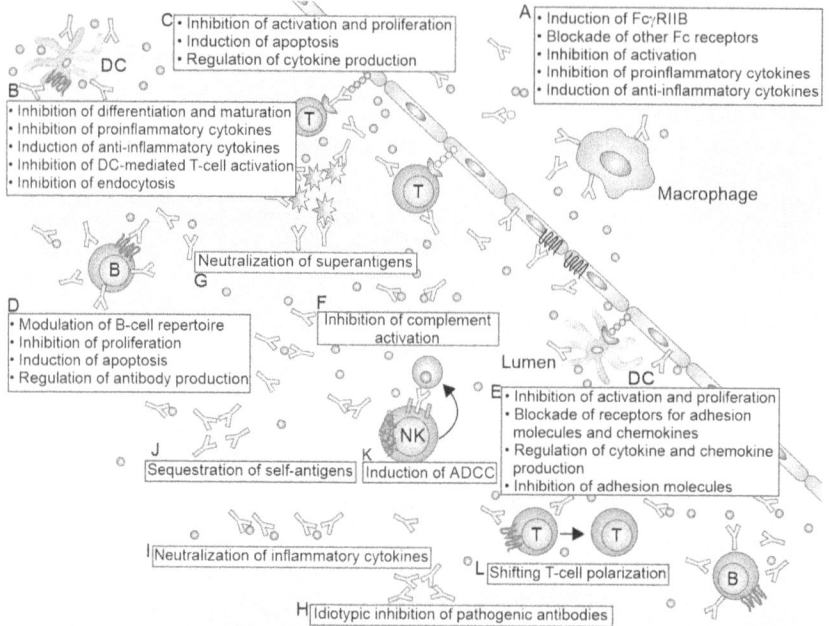

FIG. 2: The complex interplay of various effects of high-dose intravenous immunoglobulin (IVIg).[12]

The mechanisms that underlie the beneficial effects of IVIg involve its direct interaction with various cellular and soluble components of the immune system. IVIg stimulates the expression of FcγRIIB on a subset of macrophages while blocking the expression of FcγRIIA (A) IVIg also modulates cytokine secretion, blocks the expression of Fc receptors, and inhibits the activation of macrophages (A) and dendritic cells (B). (C) In addition to inhibition of the activation and production of proinflammatory cytokines by T cells, IVIg downregulates DC-mediated T-cell proliferation. (D) At the B-cell level, IVIg modulates antibody synthesis and the B-cell repertoire, inhibits B-cell proliferation, and induces B-cell apoptosis. (E) In endothelial cells, IVIg blocks the expression of proinflammatory cytokines, chemokines, and adhesion molecules. Several other mechanisms of action of IVIg exist: (F) interference with complement activation; (G) neutralization of superantigens; (H) pathogenic autoantibodies; and (I) cytokines; (J) sequestration of self-antigens; (K) induction of ADCC; and (L) shifting the balance between T-helper cell subsets. The area encompassed by endothelial cells represents the vascular lumen. Adhesion molecules on endothelial cells are depicted. IVIg is depicted in the form of antibody structures with different colors to highlight the fact that it is a polyclonal IgG obtained from pooled plasma from a large number of healthy blood donors. Soluble factors such as complement proteins and cytokines are indicated by colored circles.

(ADCC: antibody-dependent cell-mediated cytotoxicity; B: B-cell; DC: dendritic cell; EC: endothelial cell; Fc: crystallizable fragment; FcγR: Fcγ receptors; IVIg: intravenous immunoglobulin; NK: Natural killer cell; T: T-cell)

may be shortened up to once in every 2 weeks. A maintenance schedule which has been proposed is to increase the interval between two infusions in the increment of 2 weeks keeping the dose of the infusion the same, till a maximum interval of 16 weeks is achieved.[10,12,37,38] Low-dose IVIg at 1 g/kg/cycle has also been postulated for several dermatoses.

> **BOX 1** **Indications for use of high-dose intravenous immunoglobulin (IVIg).**[13-18]
>
> - Food and Drug Administration (FDA) approved indication:
>   - Kawasaki disease
>   - Prevention of graft versus host disease
>
> **Off-label indications**
> - Autoimmune connective tissue disorders:
>   - Systemic lupus erythematosus
>   - Scleroderma
>   - Generalized morphea
>   - Dermatomyositis/polymyositis
> - Autoimmune bullous dermatoses:
>   - Pemphigus vulgaris and foliaceous
>   - Bullous pemphigoid
>   - Pemphigoid gestationis
>   - Cicatricial pemphigoid
>   - Linear IgA bullous dermatoses
>   - Epidermolysis bullosa acquisita
>   - Stevens–Johnson syndrome/toxic epidermal necrolysis
> - Other inflammatory dermatoses:
>   - Chronic autoimmune urticaria
>   - Atopic dermatitis
>   - Psoriasis
>   - Pyoderma gangrenosum
>   - Graft versus host disease
> - Other dermatoses:
>   - Scleromyxedema
>   - Scleroderma
>   - Pretibial myxedema
>   - Livedoid vasculopathy
>   - Necrobiotic xanthogranuloma
>   - Netherton syndrome
>   - Drug reaction with eosinophilia and systemic symptoms

Intravenous Immunoglobulin with Rituximab

Intravenous immunoglobulin has been successfully combined with rituximab (Rtx) for the management of various bullous dermatoses. Ahmed et al. suggested a protocol (Ahmed protocol) for the management of autoimmune bullous dermatosis with this combination. This has been shown to benefit in pemphigus vulgaris, bullous pemphigoid, mucous membrane pemphigoid, and epidermolysis bullosa acquisita. The protocol is divided into the following three phases:
1. *B-cell depletion phase*: A cycle of IVIg is given first followed by eight infusions of Rtx at a weekly interval. Four additional Rtx infusions are

TABLE 2: Contraindications for use of high-dose intravenous immunoglobulin (IVIg).[10]

Absolute	Relative
Anaphylaxis secondary to previous infections Hypersensitivity to IVIg products	• Renal failure (risk of fluid overload) • IgA deficiency (risk of anaphylaxis) • Congestive cardiac failure • Rheumatoid arthritis (risk of renal failure) • Cryoglobulinemia (risk of renal failure) • Hypercoagulability (risk of thrombosis)
Pregnancy category C (New rating: Compatible)	
Clinical experience does not suggest harmful effect on pregnancy or fetus and it should be used if benefit outweighs the risk.	

BOX 2: Indications for high-dose intravenous immunoglobulin (IVIg) in autoimmune bullous diseases.[37]

- Disease is progressive in spite of administering appropriate maximum yet safe conventional systemic therapy
- Significant adverse effects of conventional therapy
- Conventional therapy has failed
- Absolute and relative contraindications to the use of high-dose long-term systemic steroids or immunosuppressive agents

given at monthly (preferably 3 monthly) interval. IVIg is continued at monthly interval. Previous treatment with corticosteroids (CS) and immunosuppressive agents is tapered in this phase.

2. *B-cell reconstitution phase*: IVIg was continued on a monthly basis till the time B-cell repopulated. This usually lasted till 24 months.
3. *Immune restoration phase*: Each patient received a total of six cycles of IVIg at 6-, 8-, 10-, 12-, and 14-week interval. The last cycle was at 16-week interval, thus making the total duration of this phase to 16.5 months.

Intravenous Immunoglobulin with Corticosteroids

The combination has been used in a wide range of dermatologic diseases. The adjunctive use of IVIg has led to a reduced dose requirement of systemic CS due to the increased glucocorticoid receptor sensitivity, and both IVIg and CS synergistically suppressing the lymphocyte activation.

ADVERSE EFFECTS

High-dose IVIg infusion is a complex therapy and can lead to various adverse effects. Fortunately, most IVIg infusion reactions are mild and cause back or abdominal aching or pain, nausea, rhinitis, asthma, chills, low-grade

TABLE 3: Summary of evidence and recommended dosing schedule of high-dose intravenous immunoglobulin (IVIg) in various dermatological indications.[4,18-31]

Indications	Summary of evidence	Dosing	Response time	Remarks
Dermatomyositis	Level of evidence I-b, grade of recommendation grade A	2 g/kg (over 2 days) Initially given every month for 6–10 cycles	1–2 months to response; maximal response at 3 months	Resistant or intolerant to prednisolone or immunosuppressives; watch for thromboembolism
Kawasaki disease	Level of evidence Ia, recommendation grade A	2 g/kg (over 6–12 hours) for a period of 3–6 months 1 g/kg may also be tried with good results	Clinical response in 4.5 months	In addition, acetylsalicylic acid with an initial dose of 50 mg/kg body weight per day is administered
Toxic epidermal necrolysis	Case series, evidence level II a, recommendation grade B	2–3 g/kg over 3–5 days	Mean time to response: 2.3 days Mean time for skin healing: 15 days Objective response rate: 90% Survival rate: 88%	Administered at the earliest on confirmation of the diagnosis. The onset of re-epithelialization is the best clinical parameter for evaluating treatment efficacy. No significant survival benefit demonstrated[31]
Pemphigus variants	Case series, anecdotal evidence	2 g/kg (over 2–3 days) Initially given every month, maintenance schedule individualized	Clinical response in 4.5 months	Adjunctive or second-line therapy
Bullous pemphigoid	Case series, anecdotal evidence	2 g/kg (over 2–3 days) Initially given every month, maintenance schedule individualized	Mean effective clinical response: 2.9 months	Adjunctive or second-line therapy Good response in steroid-resistant cases[24]

Continued

Continued

Indications	Summary of evidence	Dosing	Response time	Remarks
Mucous membrane pemphigoid	Case series, anecdotal evidence	2–3 g/kg (over 3 days) Initially given every 2–6 weeks, maintenance schedule individualized	Maximum response between 4 cycles and 12 cycles	Adjunctive or second-line therapy
Epidermolysis bullosa acquisita	Case series, anecdotal evidence	2 g/kg over 3–5 days May require up to 16–22 cycles	-	Adjunctive or second-line therapy
Granulomatosis with polyangiitis and microscopic polyangiitis	Level of evidence I a, recommendation grade B	2 g/kg (over 2–3 days). Initially given every month, for a period of 3–6 months, maintenance schedule individualized	-	IVIg prevents massive tissue destruction and thus reduce the extent of defects in Wegener granulomatosis

Other off-label indications:[32-36]

Vascular diseases: Antineutrophil cytoplasmic antibody associated vasculitis, livedoid vasculopathy

Autoimmune connective tissue disorders: Scleroderma, scleromyxedema, systemic lupus erythematosus

Other inflammatory dermatoses: MIS-c (multisystem inflammatory syndrome in children) post COVID, chronic autoimmune urticaria, atopic dermatitis, graft versus host disease, pyoderma gangrenosum, DRESS (Drug reaction with eosinophilia and systemic symptoms) syndrome, necrobiotic xanthogranuloma, pretibial myxedema, febrile ulcerative Mucha Habermann disease

(IVIg: Intravenous immunoglobulin)

CHAPTER 35: Intravenous Immunoglobulins

TABLE 4: Common adverse reactions and precautions to high-dose intravenous immunoglobulin (IVIg).[10]

Adverse reaction	Remarks
Infusion-related general effects	Generally mild, 30–60 minutes after initiation of infusion
	Easily managed by slowing down the infusion rate or temporarily discontinuing the infusion
Anaphylaxis and other hypersensitivity reactions	Increased risk in patients with IgA deficiency with anti-IgA antibodies and those with previous infections
	Erythema multiforme, purpura, and alopecia have also been reported
Risk of fluid overload	Acute renal failure due to "osmotic nephrosis", noncardiogenic pulmonary edema
Hematological side effects	Neutropenia and hemolysis in patients with autoantibodies against blood group antigens of the ABO and Rhesus (Rh) system. Caution for patients with thrombocytopenia and bleeding disorders
Neurologic side effects	Aseptic meningitis (11% of neurological patients)
Thromboembolic events	Because of high osmolality and viscosity of the preparation, cerebral and myocardial infarctions reported
	Risk may be reduced by slowing down the rate of infusion
Miscellaneous	Pompholyx, beau's line, eczematous reactions, hyperviscosity, hyponatremia, hyperproteinemia, tubulointerstitial nephritis, central retinal artery occlusion

fever, myalgia, and/or headache. Mild reactions can be reversed by slowing or stopping the infusion for 15–30 minutes.[10] Recalcitrant reactions can be managed by 50–100 mg of injection hydrocortisone and oral nonsteroidal anti-inflammatory drugs (NSAIDs). Adverse reactions are particularly likely in patients who have not received IVIg previously and who have or recently have had a bacterial infection. Irrespective of an individual patient's personal experience with IVIg, vigilance needs to be maintained for detecting and managing reactions. The common adverse reactions and precautions to use high-dose IVIg are listed in **Table 4**.

MONITORING GUIDELINES

The monitoring guidelines have been illustrated in **Box 3**.

CONCLUSION

As more and more studies are collated, the understanding of the role of IVIg is increasing. Our knowledge of the properties, clinical management, and potential benefits of IVIg has increased greatly over the past several years. Newer processing techniques have improved the quality of the IVIg.

BOX 3	Monitoring guidelines for use of high-dose intravenous immunoglobulin (IVIg).[10]

Baseline

History and physical examination
- Complete history and physical with emphasis on cardiopulmonary and renal status
- Weigh patient prior to treatment for comparison if at risk of fluid overload

Laboratory
- Complete blood count (CBC)
- Assess liver function and renal function—liver function test (LFT) and renal function test (RFT)
- Immunoglobulin levels—particularly IgA (if defective, anti-IgA titers of the IVIg preparation need to be assessed)
- Screen for rheumatoid factor (RA factor) and cryoglobulins
- Screening for hepatitis B and C and human immunodeficiency virus (HIV)

Follow-up

During infusion
- Monitor blood pressure and heart rate frequently
- *Assess for fluid overload*: weight of the patient, auscultate lungs and heart

Laboratory

No specific follow-up laboratory testing required

Although evidence-based data supporting the use of high dose IVIg is lacking in many indications, one has to bear in mind the fact that its use is beneficial in many dermatological conditions if risk–benefit ratio is considered. Careful matching of the most appropriate IVIg preparation with each patient and the risk factors and consideration of the actual cost–benefit ratio of treatment with IVIg compared with alternative therapeutic options are a must before undertaking treatment.

REFERENCES

1. Orange JS, Hossny EM, Weiler CR, Ballow M, Berger M, Bonilla FA, et al. Use of intravenous immunoglobulin in human disease: a review of evidence by members of the Primary Immunodeficiency Committee of the American Academy of Allergy, Asthma and Immunology. J Allergy Clin Immunol. 2006;117(4 Suppl):S525-53.
2. Sandipan Dhar. IVIG in dermatology. Indian J Dermatol. 2009;54(1):77-9.
3. Poljak RJ, Amzel LM, Avey HP, Chen BL, Phizackerley RP, Saul F. Three-dimensional structure of the Fab' fragment of a human immunoglobulin at 2.8-Å resolution. Proc Natl Acad Sci U S A. 1973;70(12):3305-10.
4. Enk A. Guideline on the use of high-dose intravenous immunoglobulin in dermatology: developed by the Guideline Subcommittee of the European Dermatology Forum. Eur J Dermatol. 2009;19(1):90-8.
5. Norris PAA, Kaur G, Lazarus AH. New insights into IVIg mechanisms and alternatives in autoimmune and inflammatory diseases. Curr Opin Hematol. 2020;27(6):392-8.
6. Martin TD. IVIG: contents, properties, and methods of industrial production—evolving closer to a more physiologic product. Int Immunopharmacol. 2006;6(4):517-22.

7. Suzuki T, Michihata N, Aso S, Yoshikawa T, Saito K, Matsui H, et al. Sodium-containing versus sodium-trace preparations of IVIG for children with Kawasaki disease in the acute phase. Eur J Pediatr. 2021;180(11):3279-86.
8. Morell A, Schürch B, Ryser D, Hofer F, Skvaril F, Barandun S. In vivo behaviour of gamma globulin preparations. Vox Sang. 1980;38(5):272-83.
9. Morell A, Riesen W, Nydegger UE. Structure, Function and Catabolism of Immunoglobulins in Immunotherapy. London: Academic Press; 1981.
10. Sulk M, Goerge T, Luger TA. Intravenous immunoglobulin therapy. In: Wolverton SE, Wu JJ (Eds). Comprehensive Dermatologic Drug Therapy, 4th Edition. US: Elsevier; 2021. p. 399.
11. Graeter S, Simon HU, von Gunten S. Granulocyte death mediated by specific antibodies in intravenous immunoglobulin (IVIG). Pharmacol Res. 2020;154:104168.
12. Bayry J, Lacroix-Desmazes S, Kazatchkine MD, Kaveri SV. Monoclonal antibody and intravenous immunoglobulin therapy for rheumatic diseases: rationale and mechanisms of action. Nat Clin Pract Rheumatol. 2007;3(5):262-72.
13. Mydlarski PR, Mittmann N, Shear NH. Intravenous immunoglobulin: use in dermatology. Skin Therapy Lett. 2004;9(5):1-6.
14. Jolles S, Hughes J, Whittaker S. Dermatological uses of high-dose intravenous immunoglobulin. Arch Dermatol. 1998;134(1):80-6.
15. Rutter A, Luger TA. Intravenous immunoglobulin: an emerging treatment for immune-mediated skin diseases. Curr Opin Investig Drugs. 2002;3(5):713-9.
16. Bussel JB, Eldor A, Kelton JG, Varon D, Brenner B, Gillis S, et al. IGIV-C, a novel intravenous immunoglobulin: evaluation of safety, efficacy, mechanisms of action, and impact on quality of life. Thromb Haemost. 2004;91(4):771-8.
17. Ibanez C, Montoro-Ronsano JB. Intravenous immunoglobulin preparations and autoimmune disorders: mechanisms of action. Curr Pharm Biotechnol. 2003;4(4):239-47.
18. Kromer C, Mitterlechner L, Langer N, Schön MP, Mössner R. Response of recalcitrant generalized morphea to intravenous immunoglobulins (IVIg): three cases and a review of the literature. Eur J Dermatol. 2021;31(6):822-9.
19. Winston DJ, Antin JH, Wolff SN, Bierer BE, Small T, Miller KB, et al. A multicenter, randomized, double-blind comparison of different doses of intravenous immuno-globulin for prevention of graft-versus host disease and infection after allogeneic bone marrow transplantation. Bone Marrow Transplant. 2001;28(2):187-96.
20. Oates-Whitehead R, Baumer J, Haines L, Love S, Maconochie IK, Gupta A, et al. Intravenous immunoglobulin for the treatment of Kawasaki disease in children. Cochrane Database Syst Rev. 2003;2003(4):CD004000.
21. Aggarwal R, Charles-Schoeman C, Schessl J, Bata-Csörgő Z, Dimachkie MM, Griger Z, et al. Trial of intravenous immune globulin in dermatomyositis. N Engl J Med. 2022;387(14):1264-78.
22. Ahmed AR. Intravenous immunoglobulin therapy in the treatment of patients with pemphigus vulgaris unresponsive to conventional immunosuppressive treatment. J Am Acad Dermatol. 2001;45(5):679-90.
23. Svecova D. IVIG therapy in pemphigus vulgaris has corticosteroid-sparing and immunomodulatory effects. Australas J Dermatol. 2016;57(2):141-4.
24. Ujiie H, Arakawa M, Aoyama Y. Intravenous immunoglobulin in patients with bullous pemphigoid insufficient response to corticosteroids: Nationwide post-marketing surveillance in Japan. J Dermatol Sci. 2023;109(1):22-29.
25. Lytvyn Y, Rahat S, Mufti A, Witol A, Bagit A, Sachdeva M, et al. Biologic treatment outcomes in mucous membrane pemphigoid: A systematic review. J Am Acad Dermatol. 2022;87(1):110-20.

26. Trent JT, Kirsner RS, Romanelli P, Kerdel FA. Analysis of intravenous immunoglobulin for the treatment of toxic epidermal necrolysis using SCORTEN: The University of Miami Experience. Arch Dermatol. 2003;139(1):39-43.
27. Prins C, Kerdel FA, Padilla RS, Hunziker T, Chimenti S, Viard I, et al. Treatment of toxic epidermal necrolysis with high-dose intravenous immunoglobulins: multicenter retrospective analysis of 48 consecutive cases. Arch Dermatol. 2003;139(1):26-32.
28. Bachot N, Revuz J, Roujeau JC. Intravenous immunoglobulin treatment for Stevens-Johnson syndrome and toxic epidermal necrolysis: a prospective noncomparative study showing no benefit on mortality or progression. Arch Dermatol. 2003;139(1):33-6.
29. He L, Liu F, Yan W, Huang M, Huang M, Xie L, et al. Randomized trial of different initial intravenous immunoglobulin regimens in Kawasaki disease. Pediatr Int. 2021;63(7):757-63.
30. Miyamoto D, Gordilho JO, Santi CG, Porro AM. Epidermolysis bullosa acquisita. An Bras Dermatol. 2022;97(4):409-23.
31. Chang HC, Wang TJ, Lin MH, Chen TJ. A Review of the systemic treatment of Stevens-Johnson syndrome and toxic epidermal necrolysis. Biomedicines. 2022;10(9):2105.
32. Gardette E, Moguelet P, Bouaziz JD, Lipsker D, Dereure O, Le Pelletier F, et al. Livedoid vasculopathy: a French observational study including therapeutic options. Acta Derm Venereol. 2018;98(9):842-7.
33. Sanges S, Riviere S, Mekinian A, Martin T, Le Quellec A, Chatelus E, et al. Intravenous immunoglobulins in systemic sclerosis: Data from a French nationwide cohort of 46 patients and review of the literature. Autoimmun Rev. 2017;16(4):377-84.
34. Guarneri A, Cioni M, Rongioletti F. High-dose intravenous immunoglobulin therapy for scleromyxoedema: a prospective open-label clinical trial using an objective score of clinical evaluation system. J Eur Acad Dermatol Venereol. 2017;31(7):1157-60.
35. Mitzel-Kaoukhov H, Staubach P, Muller-Brenne T. Effect of high-dose intravenous immunoglobulin treatment in therapy resistant chronic spontaneous urticaria. Ann Allergy Asthma Immunol. 2010;104(3):253-8.
36. Singer EM, Wanat KA, Rosenbach MA. A case of recalcitrant DRESS syndrome with multiple autoimmune sequelae treated with intravenous immunoglobulins. JAMA Dermatol. 2013;149(4):494-5.
37. Ahmed AR, Dahl MV. Consensus statement in the use of intravenous immunoglobulin therapy in the treatment of autoimmune mucocutaneous blistering disease. Arch Dermatol. 2003;139(8):1051-9.
38. Goodfield M, Davison K, Bowden K. Intravenous immunoglobulin (IVIg) for therapy-resistant cutaneous lupus erythematosus (LE). J Dermatolog Treat. 2004;15(1):46-50.

CHAPTER 36

Ready Reckoner for Biologics and Small Molecules

Bhavni Oberoi, Shekhar Neema

AVAILABLE BIOLOGICS FOR PSORIASIS

Baseline investigations:
- CBC
- Blood urea, serum creatinine
- LFT with enzymes
- *Hepatitis serology*: HBsAg, anti HCV-IgM, anti-HBC
- ELISA for HIV
- Chest radiograph, IGRA/Mantoux test

Drug	Pregnancy category/ permissible age	Availability and preparation	Adult dose
Etanercept	Category B/>4 years	PFS: 25 mg/50 mg	50 mg SC twice a week for 3 months and once a week thereafter
Adalimumab	Category B/>4 years	PFS: 40 mg	*Psoriasis*: • Day 0: 80 mg SC stat • Day 8 and every other week: 40 mg SC *Hidradenitis suppurativa*: • Day 0: 160 mg; day 15: 80 mg • Day 29 and every other week: 80 mg SC
Infliximab	Category B	• Lyophilized powder 100 mg/vial • Reconstitute 100 mg in 10 mL sterile water for injection • Solution to be mixed with 250 mL 0.9% normal saline	• 5 mg/kg IV infusion • 0, 2, 6 weeks and 8 weekly thereafter • Start within 3 hours of reconstitution • Infuse slowly at least over 2 hours

Continued

Continued

Drug	Pregnancy category/ permissible age	Availability and preparation	Adult dose
Secukinumab	Category B/>6 years	Lyophilized powder 150 mg/vial; to be diluted with 1 mL water for injection	300 mg SC; 0, 1, 2, 3, and 4 weeks and 4 weekly thereafter
Ixekizumab	Category B/>6 years	Autoinjector pen 80 mg	• 160 mg at week 0; 80 mg at week 2, 4, 6, 8, 10, 12 • 80 mg every 4 weeks

Monitoring
- Infliximab requires monitoring during and till 2 hours after infusion
- Rest biologics patient should be monitored for at least 2 hours after first injection; later 30 minutes monitoring after injection is enough
- CBC, LFT every 3 month
- Annual chest radiograph, IGRA, and hepatitis serology

(anti-HBc: anti-hepatitis B core antibody; CBC: complete blood count; ELISA: enzyme-linked immunosorbent assay; HBsAg: hepatitis B surface antigen; HCV: hepatitis C virus; HIV: human immunodeficiency virus; IGRA: interferon gamma release assay; IV: intravenous; LFT: liver function test; PFS: progression-free survival; SC: subcutaneous)

RITUXIMAB

Baseline investigations:
- CBC
- Blood urea, serum creatinine
- LFT with enzymes
- *Hepatitis serology*: HBsAg, anti HCV-IgM, anti-HBc
- ELISA for HIV
- Chest radiograph, IGRA/Mantoux test
- ECG, echocardiography
- CD19+ flowcytometry, desmoglein levels in pemphigus patients

Pregnancy category: C

Availability and preparation: • *Vial*: 500 mg/50 mL (10 mg/mL) *Premedication*: • Baseline temperature, pulse, RR, BP, and SpO$_2$ • Prehydration: 2 × 500 mL of NS • Injection hydrocortisone 200 mg IV stat • Tablet paracetamol 1 g stat • Start test dose after 30 minutes	*Dosage*: • *RA protocol*: 1 g at 0 and 15 day • *Lymphoma protocol*: 375 mg/m^2 every week for 4 weeks • RA protocol—most commonly used • Maintenance—500 mg at 6 and 12 months

Continued

CHAPTER 36: Ready Reckoner for Biologics and Small Molecules

Continued

Test dose: • Mix 100 mg (10 mL) in 90 mL of NS (discard 410 mL from 500 mL) • *Resulting concentration*: 1 mg/mL • Start @13–14 drops/min and increase to 26–28 drops/min after 30 minutes • *Approximate time for completion*: 90 minutes *Main dose:* • 900 mg (90 mL) in 360 mL of NS (discard 140 mL from 500 mL) • *Resulting concentration*: 2 mg/mL • Start @ 20 drops/min and keep increasing by 7 drops every 30 minutes till a maximum rate of 50 drops/min is reached	*Infusion reaction:* • Mild—very common, fever, chills; reduce the speed of infusion • Severe—anaphylaxis, hypotension, bronchospasm, acute respiratory distress syndrome; stop infusion immediately and resuscitate *Monitoring:* • CBC, LFT—every month for 6 months • Annual—hepatitis serology, HIV, and chest radiograph

(anti-HBc: anti-hepatitis B core antibody; BP: blood pressure; CBC: complete blood count; ECG: electrocardiography; ELISA: enzyme-linked immunosorbent assay; HBsAg: hepatitis B surface antigen; HCV: hepatitis C virus; HIV: human immunodeficiency virus; IGRA: interferon gamma release assay; IV: intravenous; LFT: liver function test; NS: normal saline; PFS: progression-free survival; RA: rheumatoid arthritis; RR: respiratory rate)

INTRAVENOUS IMMUNOGLOBULIN

Baseline investigations: • CBC • Blood urea, serum creatinine • Blood sugar fasting and postprandial • LFT with enzymes • Hepatitis serology—HBsAg, anti HCV-IgM, ELISA for HIV • ECG, echocardiography • Serum IgA level *Pregnancy category*: C	
Availability and preparation: • *Vial*: 5 g/100 mL; 10 g/100 mL *Infusion*: • Baseline temperature, pulse, RR, BP, SpO$_2$, and weight • Start @15 mg/kg/h • After 30 minutes—increase to 30 mg/kg/h • After 30 minutes—increase to 60 mg/kg/h • Do not increase >75 mL/h	*Dosage*: • 400 mg/kg/day for 5 days • Monthly cycle *Infusion reaction*: • Mild—fever, chills; reduce the speed of infusion • Severe—anaphylaxis, hypotension, bronchospasm, acute respiratory distress syndrome; stop infusion immediately and resuscitate *Monitoring*: • CBC and LFT—every month for 6 months • Annual—hepatitis serology, HIV, and chest radiograph

(BP: blood pressure; CBC: complete blood count; ECG: electrocardiography; ELISA: enzyme-linked immunosorbent assay; HBsAg: hepatitis B surface antigen; HCV: hepatitis C virus; HIV: human immunodeficiency virus; LFT: liver function test; RR: respiratory rate)

OMALIZUMAB

Baseline investigations:
- No baseline investigations required
- Serum IgE levels (not mandatory)

Pregnancy category: B
Age approval: For >12 years

Availability and preparation: • *Vial*: 150 mg lyophilized powder and solvent water (1.2 mL) • *Reconstituted*: 125 mg/mL (150 mg in 1.2 mL) *Administration*: • Reconstitute with solvent (1.4 mL of water transferred into the vial) • Vial swirled in upright position for 5–10 seconds every 5 minutes to dissolve contents (do not shake) • Dissolves in 15–20 minutes to form a viscous solution • Withdraw with 18 gauge needle and replace with 25 gauge • Excess solution expelled to get 1.2 mL dose • Injected subcutaneously over 5–10 seconds	*Dosage*: 300 mg every 4 weeks *Infusion reaction*: • High risk of anaphylaxis (0.2%); always keep anaphylactic tray ready *Monitoring*: • Observe for 2 hours after first 3 injections and for 30 minutes after subsequent injections • Monitor platelet count (known to cause thrombocytopenia)

JANUS KINASE INHIBITORS

Baseline investigations:
- CBC
- Blood urea, serum creatinine
- LFT with enzymes
- Hepatitis serology—HBsAg, anti HCV-IgM, anti-HBc
- ELISA for HIV
- Fasting lipid profile
- Urine routine and microscopic examination
- Chest radiograph, IGRA/Mantoux test

Drug	Pregnancy category/permissible age	Availability and preparation	Adult dose
Tofacitinib (JAK1/3)	Category C/ >2 years	• *Tablet*: 5 mg, 11 mg (ER) • *Ointment*: 2%	• *Alopecia areata*: 5 mg BD/11 mg OD • *Atopic dermatitis*: 5 mg BD • *Psoriasis*: 10 mg BD • *Vitiligo*: 5 mg BD • Application twice daily

Continued

CHAPTER 36: Ready Reckoner for Biologics and Small Molecules

Continued

Drug	Pregnancy category/ permissible age	Availability and preparation	Adult dose
Baricitinib (JAK1/2)	Not assigned/ >9 years	*Tablet*: 1 mg, 2 mg, and 4 mg	2 mg OD
Ruxolitinib (JAK1/2)	Category C/ >12 years	• *Tablet*: 5 mg, 10 mg, 15 mg, 20 mg, and 25 mg • *Cream*: 1.5%	• *Acute and chronic GVHD*: Start from 5 mg BD • Application twice daily
Upadacitinib (JAK1)	Category D/ >12 years	*Tablet*: 15 mg, 30 mg, and 45 mg	• *Atopic dermatitis and psoriatic arthritis*: 15 mg OD • Can increase to 30 mg OD
Abrocitinib (JAK1)	Not assigned/ >12 years	*Tablet*: 50 mg, 100 mg, and 200 mg	• *Atopic dermatitis*: 100 mg OD • Can increase to BD if inadequate response
Deucravacitinib (Tyk2)	Not assigned/not established	*Tablet*: 3 mg and 6 mg	*Psoriasis*: 6 mg OD
Monitoring			
CBC, LFT, RFT, and fasting lipid profile after 1 month and then every 3 months; annual chest radiograph and IGRA			

(anti-HBc: anti-hepatitis B core antibody; CBC: complete blood count; ECG: electrocardiography; ELISA: enzyme-linked immunosorbent assay; HBsAg: hepatitis B surface antigen; HCV: hepatitis C virus; HIV: human immunodeficiency virus; IGRA: interferon gamma release assay; JAK: Janus Kinase; LFT: liver function test; RFT: renal function test; RR: respiratory rate; TyK: tyrosine kinase)

Index

Page numbers followed by *b* refer to box, *f* refer to figure, *fc* refer to flowchart, and *t* refer to table.

A

Abatacept 14, 209
Abbott's adalimumab 5
Abrocitinib 439, 454-458, 460, 462-464, 529
Absolute neutrophil count 463
Acetazolamide 35
Acid-fast bacillus 239
Acitretin 54, 233, 241, 242, 411, 416, 417
Acne 53, 66, 462, 484
    conglobata 362
Acneiform eruption 379, 504
Acquired immunodeficiency syndrome 401
Actinic keratosis 504
Activated lymphocyte cell adhesion molecule 108, 109
Adalimumab 25, 75, 77, 79-82, 87, 233, 235, 236, 241, 247, 248, 266, 303, 314, 317, 318, 323, 324, 345, 358, 371, 372, 381, 414, 416, 417, 419, 424, 426, 525
    efficacy of 76*t*, 78*t*
    therapy 82
Adenosine triphosphate 470
Adverse drug reactions 110
    classification of 370
Alanine aminotransferase 301
Alcohol 35
    consumption 35
Alefacept 14
Allergenic products 9
Allergic contact dermatitis 203
Allergic reaction 80, 462
Alopecia 504
    areata 203, 333, 358, 379, 398, 439, 440, 443, 445, 446*t*, 458
    extensive 313

refractory 313
    severe 468
    treatment of 478*t*
    totalis 445
    universalis 445
Ampicillin 35
Anakinra 80, 271
Analgesia 253
Anaphylaxis 387, 463
Androsterone 4
Anemia 462
Angioedema 90, 462
Angiofibroma 491
Angiogenesis 40
Angiotensin-converting enzyme inhibitors 35
Ankylosing spondylitis 24, 52, 65, 76, 84, 85, 209, 440, 442, 443, 458
Antibodies 10
    antidrug 70, 100, 380
    dependent cell-mediated
        cytolysis 145
        cytotoxicity 516
Anti-CD20 monoclonal antibody 145, 308, 372
Anti-CD6 monoclonal antibody 106, 108
Anti-desmoglein 153
Antigen 108
    presenting cell 33, 34, 38-40, 45, 108, 109
    migration of 38
Antiglomerular basement membrane 348
Anti-hepatitis
    B core antibody 526, 527, 529
    C
        antibody 153
        virus 82, 89, 99, 234

Antihistamines 429
  oral 199
Anti-interleukin 358
Antimalarial inhibit enzyme
  transglutaminase 35
Antineutrophil cytoplasmic antibodies
  348, 515
Anti-nuclear
  antibody 56, 239, 254, 378
  matrix protein 2 150
Antiphospholipid antibody syndrome
  334
Antiplatelet therapy 463
Antiretroviral therapy 61
Antirheumatic drugs, disease-modifying
  99, 351, 381, 402, 445
Anti-secukinumab antibodies 89
Anti-sialic acid-binding agent 192
Antitoxin 9
Anti-tumor necrosis factor alpha 192,
  342, 346
Antiviral therapy 304
Antiviral treatment, oral 159
Aphthous stomatitis 52
Apoptosis 145
Appetite 485
Apremilast 412, 416, 417, 482, 484t, 487
Armamentarium 231
Arrhythmia 154
Arterial thromboembolic events, risk
  of 183
Arthralgia 208, 503, 504
Arthritis 504
  bacterial 375
  polyarticular 375
  psoriatic 17, 36, 37, 51, 52, 55, 56, 67,
    76-78, 84, 87, 323, 440, 443, 445,
    458, 482, 485
Arthropathy 57
  psoriatic 238
Aryl hydrocarbon receptor 506, 507
  agonists 506
    action of 507f
Ascorbic acid 4
Aspartate aminotransferase 303
Asthma 203, 483
  moderate-to-severe 218
Atacicept 168, 360

Atopic dermatitis 116, 151, 180, 181,
  197, 199, 203, 204t, 205, 209, 212,
  213, 214f, 218, 223, 313, 315, 328,
  334, 372, 439, 440, 443, 446, 454, 455,
  458, 459, 468, 477, 483, 517
  management of 212
  moderate-to-severe 223, 454
  scoring of 446
  therapy for 223
Atopic eczema 199
Autoantibodies 380
Autoimmune
  adverse events 375
  blistering diseases 155, 349
  bullous
    dermatoses 168t, 359, 360t, 372,
      517
    diseases 147, 149, 331, 512, 518b
    disorders 167, 171, 313
  connective tissue
    diseases 149
    disorders 517
  diseases 84, 238, 397, 399, 404
  disorders 157, 334
  hemolytic anemia 147
  inflammatory syndrome 405
  neuropathies 147
  rheumatic diseases 275
  thrombocytopenia 147
  vesiculobullous disorders 398
Autoimmunity 71, 80
Autoinflammatory
  circuit 115f
  disorders 458
Autoinjector injection 99
Avdoralimab 173
Azathioprine 70, 252, 419, 420, 422
  low-dose 398

B

Bacillus Calmette-Guérin 292, 399, 400
  vaccine 343
Back pain 485
Bacterial infection, secondary 160
Baricitinib 439, 454, 456-458, 460, 462-
  464, 529
Barzolvolimab 192

Basal cell carcinoma 504
Baseline epidermal hyperplasia 223
Basophil 171
   degranulation 186
B-cell 170, 516
   activating factor 170, 360, 361
   depletion 157, 517
   lymphomas, cutaneous 147
   molecules targeting 167, 170
   reconstitution phase 518
Behçet's disease 52, 57, 68, 76, 364
Belimumab 168, 170, 315, 325, 334, 360
   intravenous 334
Benralizumab 190
Bermekimab 363
Bertilimumab 168, 172, 360
Beta-blockers 35
Beta-cell lymphoma, primary cutaneous 151
Bevacizumab 5
Bifidobacterium
   lactis 46
   longum 46
Bilirubin, serum 301
Bimekizumab 123, 132, 247, 363, 372
Biologics
   classification of 9, 9fc
   drugs 370
   infections 285
   therapy 224, 240, 409
      initiation of 397
Biologische arzneimittel 3
Biomimics 20
Biopharmaceuticals 23
Birt-Hogg-Dube syndrome 491
Bisphosphonate therapy 253
Blinatumomab 168, 169, 360
Blood
   basophils 181
   creatine phosphokinase 462
   pressure 527
   sugar
      fasting 100, 234, 527
      postprandial 100
   urea 234, 459, 527, 528
B-lymphocytes, cell membranes of 145
Body
   surface area 103, 316
   weight 207

Bone protection 253
BRAF inhibitors, adverse effects of 504t
Brazikumab 123, 130
Breast milk 81
Breastfeeding 91, 119
Brepocitinib 468, 470, 478, 508, 509
Briakinumab 123, 127
Brodalumab 123, 131, 247, 314, 321, 322, 363, 372
   efficacy of 132t
Bronchial asthma 180
Bronchitis 485
Bruton's tyrosine kinases 170
   inhibitors 168, 170
Bullous dermatoses 52
Bullous pemphigoid 52, 149, 171, 180, 182, 203, 252, 258, 334, 379, 517, 519
   management of 258

C

Calcineurin inhibitor, topical 473
Calcium 253
   channel blockers 35
Canakinumab 192
Cancer 239, 350
Candida infections 384
Carbamazepine 35
Carcinoma
   colorectal 209
   hepatocellular 305, 478
Cardiac disease 56, 350
Cardiac failure 59
   congestive 234
Cardiomyopathy 154
Cardiovascular disease 35, 59, 382, 380
Cell
   surface receptors 167
   types 44, 45
Central serous retinopathy 504
Cerebrospinal fluids 42
Certolizumab 123
   pegol 247, 322, 323, 372
Cetirizine 429
Cetuximab 5, 209, 371
Chemokine 42, 108, 109
   activation-regulated 216
   inhibitors of 172

Chest radiograph 528
Chimeric
  antibodies 10
  autoantibody receptor 360
  murine 145
Chinese hamster ovary cells 51, 84, 114
Chronic obstructive pulmonary disease 483
Chronic plaque psoriasis 35, 52, 65, 66t, 76, 232-234
  management of 76t
Cicatricial pemphigoid 52, 517
Cirrhosis
  development of 302
  high risk of development of 302
Clindamycin 426
  combination therapy 425
Clonidine 35
Cobemetinib 505
Complement system inhibitors 172
Complete blood count 234, 317, 450, 459, 522, 526, 527, 529
Conjunctivitis 387
Connective tissue
  diseases 53, 68, 359, 512
  disorders 334, 372, 491
Contact dermatitis 443, 458, 462
Continuous therapy 55, 66
Conventional immunosuppressive therapies 313
Conventional systemic therapy 232
  toxicity of 231
Conventional therapy, ineffectiveness of 213
Corbevax 406t
Coronary artery disease 238
Coronavirus disease 2019 (COVID-19) 399, 406, 458
  elevated risk of 155
  vaccination 404
  vaccines 404
    therapeutic effect of 161
Corticosteroids 148, 518
  low-dose 398
  oral 448
  topical 205, 213, 217, 473
Cough 462, 485
Covaxin 406t
Covishield 406t
Covovax 406t

Cowden syndrome 491
C-reactive protein 136, 455
Crohn's disease 76, 91, 101, 116, 318, 458
  treatment of 65
Cryoglobulinemia, mixed 147
Cryopyrin-associated periodic syndromes 402
Cryptococcosis 379, 447
Crystallizable fragment 516f
Cyclic adenosine monophosphate 35, 122, 482
Cyclin dependent kinase inhibitors 505
Cyclo-oxygenase pathway 35
Cyclophosphamide 160, 252, 419, 420, 422
Cyclosporine 54, 70, 187, 202, 233, 241, 242, 306, 411, 412, 416, 417
Cytochrome 483
Cytokines 15, 44t, 45, 439f
  binding of 438f
  inflammatory 438f
  inhibitors of 172
  levels of 102
  production 44
  release reactions 373
Cytotoxic T-lymphocyte antigen 4-immunoglobulin 40

D

Dabrafenib 503
Damage-associated molecular patterns 38
Dapsone 252
Dasatinib 506
Deep vein thrombosis 463, 464
Delgocitinib 439, 467, 478
  topical 473
Demodex 388
Demyelinating diseases 59, 71, 380
Dendritic cell 516
Denileukin diftitox 14
Deoxyribonucleic acid 301, 305
  recombinant 51, 114
Depression 485
Dermatitis herpetiformis 252
Dermatological disorders 334, 454t
Dermatology life quality index 136, 188, 327, 418, 444

Dermatomyositis 53, 58, 147, 150, 359, 361, 379, 398, 443, 458, 476, 491, 517, 519
 amyopathic 458
 juvenile 334
Dermoepidermal junction 167
Desmogleins 256
Deucravacitinib 454, 468, 469t, 470, 508, 509, 529
 oral 468, 475
Dexamethasone-cyclophosphamide pulse 421, 422
Diarrhea 449, 485, 504, 510
Differential leucocyte count 450
Digoxin 35
Dimethyl fumarate 173
Diphtheria 399
 vaccines 403
Discoid lupus erythematosus 484
Dizziness 462
Doxorubicin 160
Doxycycline 425, 426
Dupilumab 168, 172, 191, 199-201, 201, 207, 208, 259, 315, 325, 329, 331, 360, 372, 387
 clinical trials of 206t
 contraindications of 208
 development of 200, 201fc
 device 207f
 dosage of 207t
 facial redness 208
 indication of 203t
 injection 206
 pharmacodynamic action 202
Dysrhythmia 375

E

Ebdarokimab 123, 128
Eczema 209, 217
 area and severity index scores 216, 446
 herpeticum 462
 nummular 203
 tralokinumab trial 217
Efalizumab 10
Efgartigimod 168, 171
Electrocardiography 100, 153, 527, 529
Elevated creatine phosphokinase 505
Emollients, topical 199

Emzumab 25
Enbrel 416, 417
Endocytosis 179
Endothelial cell 516
 stimulating angiogenesis factor 41
Enthesopathy 67
Enzyme 527
 inhibitors 15
Enzyme-linked immunosorbent assay 256, 526, 527, 529
 method 153
Eosinophilia 208, 517
Epidermal innate immune system 38
Epidermal keratinocyte-derived cytokine 222
Epidermolysis bullosa
 acquisita 149, 252, 334, 517, 520
 simplex 484
Epratuzumab 168, 169, 360
Erosive oral lichen planus 458
Ertapenem rescue therapy 425, 426
Eruptive nevi 504
Erythema 208, 504
 multiforme, recurrent 484
 nodosum leprosum 53
Erythrocyte sedimentation rate 317
Erythrodermic psoriasis 35, 55, 66, 67, 98, 246
Erythropoietin 439
Escherichia coli 5
Esophageal candidiasis 447
Esophagitis, eosinophilic 203
Estimated glomerular filtration rate 457
Estrone 4
Etacept 413
Etanercept 14, 25, 33, 51, 52, 54, 60, 61, 97, 131, 233, 235, 236, 248, 269, 314, 316-348, 323, 324, 334, 345, 372, 382, 413, 418, 525
 biosimilar of 58
 efficacy of 53t
 subcutaneous 52
 therapy 59
Evolocumab 209
Exacerbate psoriatic skin disease 35
Exacerbations 9, 101
Excretion 145
Exemptia 25, 414, 424
Extracellular signal regulated kinase 501

F

Facial vitiligo area scoring index 473
Familial chilblain lupus 458*t*
Fanconi syndrome 504
Fasciitis, eosinophilic 458
Fasting lipid profile 459, 528
Fatigue 462, 485, 504, 510
Fedratinib 440
Fertility 91, 119
  status 388
Fever 153
Fezakinumab 224, 372
Fibroblast growth factor 490
Filgotinib 440, 468
Fingerprint match 25
Fluid overload, risk of 521
Folic acid 411
Follicular occlusion, disorders of 361
Folliculitis 462, 504
Food allergy 180
Fostamatinib 168, 174, 506
Free omalizumab 179
Frontal fibrosing alopecia 484
Fusion protein, type of 14

G

Gain effector phenotypes 43
Gastric polyp 504
Gastritis diarrhea 208
Gastroenteritis 462
Gastrointestinal
  intolerance 233
  perforation 462
  side effects 376
Gene therapy 9
Genodermatoses 491, 493
Gingival hyperkeratosis 504
Gliptins 258
Glomerular filtration rate 450, 504
Glucocorticoid 315
  replacement therapy 398
Golimumab 123, 124, 372
Graft-versus-host disease 53, 57, 147, 151, 476, 491, 496, 517
  acute 440, 468, 476
  chronic 440, 458, 468, 476
  prevention of 517

Granulocyte-macrophage colony stimulating factor 9, 15, 39, 265, 361, 363, 515
Granuloma annulare 53, 57, 358, 379, 443, 458
Granulomatosis 146, 315, 332, 520
Granulomatous dermatoses 53, 68, 76, 357
Growth hormone 439
Guillain-Barré syndrome 405, 406
Gusacitinib 467, 477
Guselkumab 123, 128, 168, 247, 322, 363, 372
Gut microbiota 46
Guttate psoriasis 37

H

Haemophilus influenzae infection 384
Hailey–Hailey disease 458, 484
Hair texture, abnormalities in 504
Hand eczema, chronic 203, 458
Headache 100, 208, 388, 449, 462, 485
Heart failure, congestive 70, 80, 238, 350
Helicobacter pylori 35
Helminthic infections 208, 387
Helper T cell 214
Hematologic reactions 80
Hematological side effects 376, 521
Hepadnaviridae 301
Hepatic impairment 183, 486
  severe 463
Hepatitis
  A 399
  B 92, 237, 399, 405, 448, 464
    core antibody 234, 301, 305
    reactivation 79
    vaccine 403
  B envelope
    antibody 300, 301, 305
    antigen 300, 301, 305
  B infection 61, 70, 72, 158, 300, 302
    chronic 349
    reactivation of 302
  B surface
    antibody 301, 305
    antigen 82, 89, 99, 153, 234, 300, 301, 305, 317, 403, 526, 527, 529

B virus 59, 300, 301, 305, 349, 397, 448
  infection 300, 301t, 302
  reactivation 158, 202
  surface antigen 239, 301
C 92, 237, 448, 464
  chronic 305
  infection 61, 72, 92, 159, 300, 308
C virus 300, 305, 307, 317, 349, 450, 526, 527, 529
  infection 306, 307fc
  panel 59
  reactivation 159
  infection, rule out 153
  serology 527, 528
  viral 464
Hepatotoxicity 71, 233, 381
Herpes simplex 462
Herpes zoster 399, 400, 405, 462
  vaccine 402
Hidradenitis suppurativa 53, 57, 68, 76, 77, 98, 116, 236, 262, 265, 266, 334, 361, 363t, 372, 398, 423, 424t, 426t, 458, 474, 484, 506
  clinical response 78, 423
  management of 78t, 264, 423
  moderate-to-severe 314
  pediatric 272
  treatment of 267b
High-dose intravenous immunoglobulin 516f, 522b
Histamine release 186
Histoplasma infection 384
Histoplasmosis 379, 447
Human antichimeric antibodies 156
Human herpesvirus 379
Human immunodeficiency virus 35, 59, 72, 82, 89, 99, 160, 239, 276, 292, 317, 376, 526, 527, 529
  coinfection 92
  infection 61, 72, 153, 237
Human immunoglobulin
  E 179
  G 170
Human leukocyte antigen 37
Human papillomavirus 397, 399, 406
  infection 404
  vaccine 404
Human tumor necrosis factor-alpha 51
Hurley's staging system 263, 263f
Hypercholesterolemia, primary familial 209

Hypereosinophilic syndrome 443, 458
Hyperimmunoglobulin E syndrome 180, 182
Hyperkeratosis 503
Hyperostosis 53, 66, 484
Hypersensitivity 79, 90, 101, 215, 462
  reactions 100, 334, 372, 385, 388, 449
  severe 90
Hypertension 449, 462
Hypertrophic scars 491
Hypogammaglobulinemia 375
Hypokalemia 504t
Hyponatremia 504t
Hypophosphatemia 504t

I

Ibrutinib 168
Idiopathic arthritis, juvenile 52, 75, 318, 440, 443
Idiopathic chronic eczematous eruption 203
Ifidancitinib 468, 478
  topical 473
Immune
  adaptive 44
  cells, recruitment of 34
  humoral 160
  inhibitors 332
  innate 44, 45
  mediated diseases 102
  modulatory neurotransmitters 36
  restoration phase 518
  system 44t, 199
    dysfunction 212
    juvenile 157
Immunization 61, 72, 451
  adult 397
Immunobullous diseases 259
Immunobullous disorders 17, 143, 252, 458
  management of 167
  pathogenesis of 167
  treatment of 174
Immunogenicity 22, 23, 115, 344, 382
  E 156, 168, 214, 372, 373
  G 65, 106, 214, 301, 342
  M 155, 234, 301
  structure of 512, 513f
Immunological synapse 38, 39t

Immunosuppressants 187, 257
  systemic 199
Immunosuppression, low-dose 255
Impetigo 462
In vitro studies 21
Inebilizumab 168, 169, 360
Infections 33, 34, 70, 79, 90, 100, 111, 120, 155, 237, 381, 324, 325, 382, 383, 385, 386, 447
  asymptomatic nature of 300
  early detection of 157
  herpetic 253
  opportunistic 447
  parasitic 215
  severe 160
  tuberculous 288
Infimab 414, 416, 417, 424, 426
Inflammation 43
Inflammatory
  arthritis 359
  bowel disease 56, 91, 100, 234, 236, 238, 378, 384, 508
  cells 171
  dermatoses 357, 506
  pathways 212
    levels of 122
  response 44, 212
  stimuli 43
Infliximab 10, 24, 25, 33, 65, 67, 71, 72, 192, 233, 235, 247, 266, 269, 303, 314, 317, 323, 321, 324, 334, 345, 358, 361, 371, 372, 374t, 377, 379, 413, 424, 426, 525
  efficacy of 66t
  infusion 357, 380
  multinational psoriatic arthritis controlled trial 67
  therapy 69, 71
Influenza 399, 405, 462
  vaccine 402
Infusion
  reactions 70, 153, 372, 377, 385
    acute 111
  speed of 257
Inhibitor 457, 468, 473, 475
Injection site reactions 90, 100, 183, 381, 382
Insomnia 485
Intacept 413, 416, 417
Intercellular adhesion molecule 39, 40, 108

Interferon 15, 122, 276, 361, 371, 509
Interferon-alpha 9
Interferon-gamma 39, 45, 294, 373, 483, 508
  release assays 59, 69, 89, 234, 239, 293, 317, 411, 526, 527, 529, 459
Interleukin 9, 15, 39, 42, 85, 114, 122, 123, 168, 187, 202, 214, 221, 276, 315, 360, 361, 363, 371, 372, 474, 509, 515
  blocker 220
  receptor 39, 40
Intermittent therapy 55, 66, 457
International hidradenitis suppurativa severity scoring system 423
Interstitial granulomatous dermatitis 379
Interstitial lung disease 449, 450
Intravenous immunoglobulin 15, 253, 375, 400, 512, 513, 515-517, 517b, 518, 518b, 518t, 519t, 520, 521t, 527
  composition of 513
  methods of preparation of 512
Invasive fungal infections 70
Investigator's global assessment 209, 217
  score 216
Ipilimumab 315, 333
Isoniazid 71, 239
Itacitinib 468
Itching 208
Itolizumab 106, 108, 109t, 111, 112, 233, 372, 415-417
  adverse effects of 111t
  dosage of 112
  mechanism of action of 108f
Ixekizumab 96-98, 100-102, 103t, 104, 123, 130, 131, 168, 233, 235, 236, 246, 247, 303, 304, 308, 314, 320, 322, 325, 344, 345, 358, 360, 372, 385, 415-417, 526
  contraindications of 100
  efficacy of 96, 131
  injections of 173

J

Janus kinase 363, 437-440, 454, 456, 458, 462-464, 470, 509, 529
  inhibitors 437, 442, 454, 456, 458, 462, 463, 467, 467t, 468t, 473t, 478, 478t, 528

classification of 438
first-generation 438
irreversible 439
second-generation 438
use of 440, 455
proteins 467
signal transducer 43, 454, 501
role of 43
Japanese encephalitis 399
Juvenile collagen vascular diseases 313

K

Kaposi's sarcoma 491, 495
Kaposiform hemangioendothelioma 491
refractory 493
Kappa antibody against 145
Kasabach–Merritt phenomenon 491, 493
Kawasaki disease 53, 334, 515, 517, 519
Keloids 491
Keratinization, abnormal 43
Keratinocyte 41, 45
derived factors 107
proliferation 34
release cytokines 40
role of 40
Keratoacanthoma 504t
cutaneous 503
Keratoconjunctivitis sicca 504t
Keratosis pilaris 504
Kimura disease 180
Koebner's phenomenon 36, 37

L

Lactation 60, 71, 81, 91, 102, 112, 157, 184, 464
Lactobacillus rhamnosus 46
Langerhans cells 45
Lapatinib 506
Latent tuberculosis 71, 89, 92, 100, 118, 158, 237, 459
infection 289, 290, 448
management of 287
screening for 290
treatment of 296
reactivation of 92
Latex allergy 180

Lebrikizumab 214, 218-220, 315, 329, 372
efficacy 218
epitopes distinguish 220
groups 219
loading dose 218
pharmacokinetics 218
treatment 219
Lesions
eczematous 199
psoriatic 35
Leukemia, chronic lymphocytic 146
Leukoencephalopathy, progressive multifocal 276, 371, 375
Leukotrienes, accumulation of 35
Lichen
planopilaris 443, 476
planus 379, 443, 458, 476, 483, 491
Lichenoid
dermatosis 156
eruptions 379
Life-threatening hypersensitivity reactions 118
Ligelizumab 168, 171, 187, 188, 224, 328, 372
efficacy of 188
Lipocalin-2 108
Lipoprotein
high-density 455
low-density 455
Lirentelimab 192
Listeria monocytogenes sepsis 375
Live attenuated vaccines 400, 451
Livedoid vasculopathy 281, 458, 517
Liver
cancer 397
damage, acute 300
disease, chronic 348
enzyme
abnormalities 462
derangement 159
function test 59, 81, 99, 234, 239, 305, 307, 308, 317, 411, 450, 459, 486, 522, 526, 527, 529
injury, drug-induced 349
Loop diuretics 258
Loricrin 507
Lupus
erythematosus, cutaneous 150, 458
pernio 57
syndrome 379, 382

Lymph nodes 38
Lymphatic malformations 491
Lymphocyte function antigen 39, 40, 108
Lymphoma 159, 382, 383
  protocol 146
Lymphomatoid granulomatosis 147
Lymphopenia 462

M

Macrophages 45
Maculopapular rash 504
Major histocompatibility complex 39, 40, 45, 108, 276, 515
Malassezia 35
Malignancy 56, 59, 70, 80, 380, 397, 448, 462
  cutaneous 504
Mantoux test 59, 528
Mast cells 45, 192
Mastocytosis 362
  systemic 180, 182, 506
Measles, mumps, and rubella 399, 400
Melanoma 315, 332, 491
  development of 502f
  malignant 332, 506
  metastatic 315
Membrane attack complex 515
Mepolizumab 168, 172, 360, 372
Mercaptopurine, low-dose 398
Metabolic dysfunction 233
Metabolism 111, 456
Methotrexate 54, 67, 70, 76, 87, 99, 232, 233, 241, 242, 258, 411, 416, 417, 419, 450
  low-dose 398
Microbiota dysbiosis 46
Microheterogeneity 18
Milia 504
Mirikizumab 123t, 130, 372
Mitogen activated protein kinase 115, 501, 502
  inhibitors 503
  pathway 501
Molecular weight 65, 145
Mometasone furoate 217
Monoclonal antibody 5, 10, 17, 21, 65, 209, 179, 214, 266, 315, 363
  nomenclature of 10, 10t
  type of 11-13

Monotherapy 53, 458
Morphea 359, 360, 443
  generalized 458, 517
Morphine 35
Mucocutaneous candidiasis 384
Mucocutaneous reactions 156
  severe 377
Mucous membrane pemphigoid 58, 149, 252, 334, 520
Muir-Torre syndrome 496
Murine 10
  antibodies 10
Muromonab 10
Muscle weakness 504
Myalgia 208, 462
Mycobacterium tuberculosis infection 158
Mycophenolate 258
  mofetil 252, 419, 420, 422
Myelofibrosis 440, 467
Myeloid dendritic cells 45
Myocardial
  infarction 462
  ischemia 375
Myocarditis 154
Myositis, inflammatory 280
Myxedema, pretibial 517

N

Nail
  dystrophy 443
  psoriasis 35, 56, 66, 68, 77, 85, 87, 245
  severity index 56, 87, 443
Narrowband ultraviolet B 54, 242
Nasal polyp 180
Nasopharyngitis 208, 223, 388, 449, 462, 485, 510
Natural killer cell 45, 516
  bind 145
  receptors 37
Nausea 462, 485
Necrobiosis lipoidica 358
  diabeticorum 57t
Necrobiotic xanthogranuloma 517
Necrolysis, epidermal 53
Necrosis, cutaneous 334
Nemolizumab 221, 222, 329, 330, 372
Neoplasia 376
Neoplastic disorders 334

Nervous system 111
Netakimab 123, 133
Netherton syndrome 517
Neurofibromatosis 491
Neurokinin receptor 510
  antagonist 510
Neurological disorders 59
Neutropenia 90, 100, 384, 462
  late-onset 156, 376
Neutrophil 45
  accumulation 40
  extracellular trap 115
Neutrophilic dermatoses 52, 66, 68, 76, 359
Nipple hyperkeratosis 504
Nivolumab 315, 333
Nodular prurigo disorder, chronic 458
Nomacopan 173
Non-Hodgkin's lymphoma 146
Nonmelanoma skin cancer 450, 462
Nonradiographic axial spondyloarthropathy 458
Nonreceptor tyrosine kinases 170
Nonsteroidal anti-inflammatory drugs 35, 190, 265, 347, 448
  oral 521
Nuclear factor-kappa 122
Nucleotide-binding oligomerization domain 38
Numeric rating scale 217, 477
Nutrition disorders 111

O

Obesity 239
Obinutuzumab 161, 169, 360
Ofatumumab 161, 169, 360, 371
Omalirel 25t
Omalizumab 25, 151, 168, 171, 179-182, 184, 187, 224, 259, 314, 325, 327, 327t, 330, 334, 344, 347, 360, 386, 389, 427, 428, 428t, 429, 528
  administration of 182
Oncogenesis, paradoxical 504
Optic neuritis 375
Organ failure assessment score 160
Oropharyngeal discomfort 208
Orthoclone 5
Osteitis syndrome 484

P

Pachyonychia congenita 491t
Pacritinib 440
Pain visual analog scale 136
Pain
  abdominal 462
  muscle 153
  oropharyngeal 462
Palmoplantar
  dysesthesia 504
  hyperkeratosis 504
  psoriasis 35, 77, 85, 88, 245, 485
  pustulosis 36, 116
Panniculitis 504t
Papules 208
Paracetamol 257
Paradoxical reactions 378, 381, 382, 386
Paraneoplastic pemphigus 149, 170, 257
Paresthesia 504
Pathogen-associated molecular patterns interact 38
Peak plasma 456
Peficitinib 440, 467
Pegylated certolizumab 124
Pembrolizumab 315, 333
Pemphigoid
  gestationis 517
  group 167
Pemphigus 160, 252, 255, 256, 331, 419, 420t
  disease activity index 419
  foliaceus 147, 203, 252, 334
  management of 145, 252, 254
  moderate 253
  moderate-to-severe 256
  severe 253
  treatment options for 256
  variants 519
  vulgaris 52, 147, 203, 252, 334, 491, 517
  management of 419
Penicillin 4, 35
Peptides 38
Perianal streptococcal infection 35
Periodic fever syndromes 313
Peripheral blood mononuclear cells 483
Persistent erythema multiforme 458
Pharmacokinetics 21

Pheniramine 257
Phosphodiesterase 501
  enzyme inhibitor, oral 482
  inhibitors 233, 482
Photodermatosis 504
Photosensitivity 503, 504
Phototherapy 242, 416, 417
Pityriasis
  lichenoides chronica 484
  rubra pilaris 53, 57, 98, 334, 358, 484
Plaque psoriasis 78, 123, 322*t*, 468, 484
  chronic 35, 52, 65, 66*t*, 76, 232-234
  management of 233
  moderate-to-severe 85, 468
  skin of 85
  treatment of 112
Plasma cells 170
Plasmacytoid dendritic cells 41, 45
Plasmapheresis 256
Platelet derived growth factor 9, 15, 41, 490
Pleuritis 375
Pneumococcal
  conjugate vaccine 401
  polysaccharide vaccine 401
  vaccine 401
Pneumococcus 160
Pneumocystis
  carinii pneumonia 155
  jirovecii pneumonia 375
  pneumonia 379
Pneumocystosis 447
Poliovirus vaccine, oral 343
Polyangiitis 146, 315, 332, 520
  microscopic 146, 315, 332, 520
  nodosa, cutaneous 334
Polychondritis, relapsing 53
Polycythemia vera 440
Polymerase chain reaction 301
Polymyositis 147, 517
Postessential thrombocythemia myelofibrosis 467
Post-polycythemia vera myelofibrosis 467
Potassium iodide 35
Pregnancy 60, 71, 81, 91, 101, 112, 119, 157, 184, 341, 342, 463, 464
  category 157, 345, 486, 525-527, 529
  outcomes 256
  test 59, 459

Principal monoclonal antibodies 11*t*
Progesterone 4, 35, 526
Proinflammatory cytokines 42
  secretion of 106
Proteins, antimicrobial 38, 44
Proteinuria, subnephrotic-range 504
Proteolysis 60
Prurigo nodularis 206, 206*t*
Pruritus 219, 504, 510
Psoriasis 25, 31, 33, 35-37, 42, 43, 46, 53, 53*t*, 56, 66, 76, 84, 85, 109*f*, 110, 122, 136, 231, 232, 236, 289, 314, 316, 347, 348, 350, 372, 398, 410, 443, 444*t*, 458, 468, 470, 483, 495, 517, 525
  area 53, 66, 103, 131, 132, 242
    severity index 26, 66, 77, 107, 232, 316, 410, 443, 470, 484, 495, 508
  aspect of 26
  biologic therapy for 410, 416*t*, 417*t*
  biosimilar of 26
  common forms of 245
  etiology of 34
  induction of 71
  management of 17, 231, 348
  moderate-to-severe 35
  pathogenesis of 33, 34*f*
  pediatric 316, 323
  severe 232
  susceptibility 33, 37
  symptom scale 136
  systemic therapy in 410, 411*t*
  treatment of 469*t*
  understanding of 46
  variants of 245
Psoriatic arthritis 17, 36, 37, 51, 52, 55, 56, 67, 76-78, 84, 87, 323, 440, 443, 445, 458, 482, 485
  management of 78*t*
Psychiatric disorder 111
Purified protein derivative 69, 89, 459
Pustular psoriasis 35, 38, 88, 114, 372
  generalized 67, 98, 116, 136, 233, 247, 318
Pustulosis 53, 66, 484, 485
Pyoderma gangrenosum 52, 57, 66, 76, 116, 236, 334, 359, 379, 443, 458, 484, 517
Pyrexia 462

Q

Quality-of-life score 232
Quilizumab 189
Quinone acceptor oxidoreductase 507

R

Randomized controlled trial 358, 363, 443, 444, 492
Rapamycin inhibitors, mammalian target of 489, 490
Rash 462
Rasmussen's encephalitis 147
Rat sarcoma virus 502, 504
Reactive oxygen species 507
Recalcitrant
  erythema nodosum leprosum, chronic 484
  lichen planopilaris 458
Receptor tyrosine kinase 502
Reditux 25
Reiter's syndrome 69
Remicade 413, 416, 417, 424
Renal disease, end-stage 348, 457
Renal failure, chronic 239, 347
Renal function test 59, 239, 317, 450, 486, 529
Renal impairment 102, 183, 486
  mild 486
  moderate 486
  severe 463, 486
  stage 457
Reslizumab 190
Respiratory disorders 111
Respiratory rate 527, 529
Reticulohistiocytosis, multicentric 53
Retinoid failure, systemic 362
Reversible posterior leukoencephalopathy syndrome 386
Rheumatoid arthritis 24, 52, 65, 75, 81, 85, 146, 209, 255, 343, 439, 440, 442, 443, 458, 462, 506, 527
  protocol 146
Rhinosinusitis, chronic 180
Ribonucleic acid 307
  virus, single-stranded 305
Rifampicin 71, 425, 426

Risankizumab 123, 129, 247, 322, 363, 372
Ritlecitinib 440, 468, 478
  oral 468
Rituximab 5, 25, 145, 148fc, 150, 151, 155-157, 159-161, 191, 252, 253, 255-257, 290, 304, 308, 315, 331, 334, 344, 345, 347, 360, 372, 373, 374t, 376, 388, 398, 420, 422, 517, 526
  biosimilar drugs of 423
  cardioprotective effects of 154
  dermatological uses of 147
  infusion of 254, 257
  therapy 153, 156
  use of 256
Ropsacitinib 470f, 508, 509
Rosacea 484
Rotational therapy 240
Rotavirus vaccine 343
Rozanolixizumab 168, 171
Ruxolitinib 440, 467, 468, 478, 529
  topical 468, 473

S

Sarcoidosis 53, 357, 379, 484
  psychological 57
Sartorius staging system, modified 263, 263t
Scalp psoriasis 35, 88, 245
Scleroderma 53, 58, 359, 398, 491, 517
Scleromyxedema 517
Sclerosis
  multiple 56, 234, 238
  systemic 150, 279, 458
Seborrheic keratosis 504
Secukinumab 84, 87, 91, 92, 192, 209, 233, 235, 236, 246-248, 270, 303, 308, 314, 317, 319, 322, 324, 344, 345, 358, 364, 372, 383, 389, 416, 417, 425, 426, 526
  effect of 91
  efficacy of 86t
  mechanism of action of 85f
  originator molecule 415
  selectively binds 85
  superiority of 86
  therapy 89
Selective interleukin inhibitors 214

Sepsis 160
Sequential switch therapy 151
Serum creatinine 234, 459, 527, 528
Serum glutamic
   oxaloacetic transaminase 305, 307
   pyruvic transaminase 305, 307
Severe refractory eosinophilic asthma, treatment of 190
Short-chain fatty acids 46
Sickness, serum 71, 156, 375
Sinus tachycardia 375
Sinusitis 381
Sirolimus 489, 490, 491*t*
   mechanisms of action of 490*fc*
   oral 497*b*
Sjögren's syndrome 147
Skin
   barrier
      maintenance of 213
      role of 43
   clearance 219
   disease
      chronic 409
      rapid control of 235
   inflammatory 199
   persistent 199
   psoriatic 40
Sleeplessness 208
Sleep-loss scale score 219
Small molecule 501, 506, 510
   drugs 369
Social engagement, facilitation of 210
Sodium chloride injection 118
Solcitinib 468
Soluble receptor fusion proteins 17
Somatic cells 9
Somnolence 510
Sonelokimab 123, 134
Spesolimab 114, 115, 116*t*, 118, 119, 119*t*, 120, 134, 233, 372
   indication of 233
   metabolic pathway of 115
Spleen tyrosine kinase 477
   inhibitors 173
Sputnik V 406
Squamous cell carcinoma 397, 503, 504
   cutaneous 504
Staphylococcus aureus 35
Steatotic liver disease 233
Sterile pustules, development of 247

Steroid
   side effects, risk of 213
   sparing agent 254
   sparing agents, role of 252
   systemic 253
   tapering of 258
   topical 213, 398
Stevens-Johnson syndrome 53, 57, 156, 374, 512, 515, 517
Streptomyces hygroscopicus 489
Stress 33
   psychological 36
Subacute cutaneous lupus erythematosus disorder 458
Sun exposure 36
Sutimlimab 168, 172, 360
Sweet's syndrome 57, 359, 458
Synovitis 53, 66, 484
Systemic lupus erythematosus 56, 147, 170, 275, 332, 334, 359, 397, 472, 491, 508, 517
   pathogenesis of 474*f*
   systemic manifestations of 170
   treatment of 475*t*
Systemic therapy 232, 240, 419
   cost analysis for 420*t*

T

T helper cell 122, 108
Target plaque severity score 443
T-cell 41, 516
   activation, inhibition of 40*f*
   disorder 212
   lymphoma, cutaneous 491
   maturation of 39
   receptor 39, 40, 45, 108, 276
   regulatory 42
Tendon rheumatic symptoms 55
Tetanus 403
   and diphtheria 406
   toxoid vaccinations 160
Tezepelumab 192, 222, 223, 372
Thiopurine methyltransferase enzyme level 254
Thrombocytopenia 100
Thromboembolism, psychological 464
Thrombosis 462
Thymic stromal lymphopoietin 192, 214
Thymidine phosphorylase 41

Thymus 388
Tick-borne encephalitis 399
Tildrakizumab 123, 128, 168, 322, 372
T-lymphocyte activation 106
Tofacitinib 440, 442, 445, 446t, 450t, 528
  indication of 443t
  pharmacological properties of 442t
  studies of 443
  use of 444t, 447t
  XR 442
Tooth abscess 485
Toothache 208
Tositumomab 169, 360
Total leucocyte count 450
Toxic epidermal necrolysis 57, 156, 362, 374, 512, 515, 517, 519
Toxic shock syndrome 512
Toxin 9
Tralokinumab 214, 218, 330, 372
  competitively inhibits 214
Trametinib 505
Transcription pathway, activator of 43
Transforming growth factor
  alpha 41
  beta 45
Trastuzumab 5
Treg cells retain 43
Trichoepitheliomas, multiple 491
Trimethylamine-N-oxide 46
T-spot 294
Tuberculin skin test 291, 292
  reaction, classification of 292b
Tuberculosis 70, 79, 92, 120, 234, 237, 254, 276, 292, 379, 448, 450, 464
  active 237
  latent 71, 89, 92, 100, 118, 158, 237, 459
  reactivation of 71, 82
Tuberous sclerosis 491
  complex 493, 498
Tubular necrosis, acute 504
Tumor 92
  lysis syndrome 154
  malignant 92
Tumor necrosis factor 116, 122, 170, 266, 371, 462
  alpha 33, 39, 45, 65, 75, 106, 109, 115, 123, 187, 192, 239, 292, 315, 358, 363, 372, 373, 398, 515

blockers, concentration of 81
  inhibitors 124, 303, 306, 316, 377, 445
  use of 236
  inhibitors 343
Tyrosine kinase 43, 439, 468, 470, 473, 474, 478, 501, 509, 529
  inhibitors 508

U

Ulcerative colitis 65, 76, 101, 116, 318, 440, 442, 443, 458
Ultraviolet therapy 25, 36
Upadacitinib 440, 454-460, 462-464, 529
Upper abdominal pain 462
Upper respiratory tract infection 375, 381, 388, 449, 462, 485
Urinary tract infection 381, 462
Urine
  pregnancy test 100, 153, 450
  routine 528
Urticaria 90, 177, 180, 186, 372, 377, 462
  activity score 188
  cholinergic 203
  chronic 184, 186, 187f, 398, 427, 491
    autoimmune 517
    spontaneous 180, 186, 203, 313, 314, 327, 427, 428t, 429t, 430t
Urticarial vasculitis 180
Ustekinumab 10, 123, 125, 168, 269, 314, 317, 319, 322, 325, 333, 334, 358, 372, 385
Uveitis 76, 375, 504

V

Vaccination, timing for 255
Vaccine 9, 399, 404-406
  efficacy of 401
  safety of 404
Valproic acid 35
Vascular anomalies 493
Vascular endothelial growth factor 40, 41, 490, 510

Vasculitis 57, 150, 375, 412
  cutaneous 76, 280, 378
  disorders 334
  flare 377
  renal 348
  systemic 66, 68, 375
Veltuzumab 169, 360
Vemurafenib 502
Verruca 504t
Vesiculobullous dermatitis 156
Vincristine 160
Viral hepatitis 464
  screening 459
Vitamin 4, 253
Vitiligo 398, 440, 443, 445, 458, 471-473, 484
  area scoring index 447
  nonsegmental 467, 468, 471
  treatment of 473t
Vomiting 462, 504

W

Warfarin 202
Wegener's granulomatosis 146, 315

X

Xerosis 504

Y

Yellow fever 399

Z

Zoster vaccine 402
  live 402, 406
  recombinant 406

EU GSPR Authorised Reprsentative
Logos Europe, 9 rue Nicolas Poussin
1700, La Rochelle, France
Phone: +33 (0) 6 67 93 73 78
E-mail: contact@logoseurope.eu

www.ingramcontent.com/pod-product-compliance
Ingram Content Group UK Ltd.
Pitfield, Milton Keynes, MK11 3LW, UK
UKHW050455150426
5217IPUK00025B/1698